Manual of
Clinical Oncology

Manual of Clinical Oncology

Third Edition

Edited by

Dennis A. Casciato, M.D.

Clinical Professor of Medicine,
University of California, Los Angeles,
UCLA School of Medicine, Los Angeles;
Chief of Medicine, Encino-Tarzana
Regional Medical Center, and Director,
Shared Medical Research Foundation,
Tarzana, California

Barry B. Lowitz, M.D.

Emeritus Associate Clinical Professor of
Medicine, University of California, Los
Angeles, UCLA School of Medicine,
Los Angeles

Little, Brown and Company
Boston New York Toronto London

Library of Congress Cataloging-in-Publication Data

Manual of clinical oncology / edited by Dennis A. Casciato, Barry
    B. Lowitz. — 3rd ed.
        p.   cm.
    Includes bibliographical references and index.
    ISBN 0-316-13279-9
    1. Oncology—Handbooks, manuals, etc.   I. Casciato, Dennis
    Albert.   II. Lowitz, Barry Bennett.
    [DNLM: 1. Medical Oncology—handbooks.   2. Neoplasms—handbooks.
    QZ 39 M2943 1995]
    RC263.M263 1995
    616.99′4—dc20
    DNLM/DLC
    for Library of Congress   95-9993
                                                              CIP

Printed in the United States of America

10 9 8 7 6 5 4 3

Editorial: Nancy Megley, Richard L. Wilcox
Copyeditor: Martha Cushman
Indexer: AlphaByte
Production Supervisor: Michael A. Granger
Cover Designer: Linda Willis and Patrick Newbery

Foremost, we consider ourselves fathers, husbands, physicians, and teachers. Recognizing that we are what we are because of our past, we dedicate this edition of the *Manual of Clinical Oncology* to those teachers who most influenced what we have become.

To **Frank and Ida Casciato,** who were role models for industriousness, organization, and the virtues of family bonds; to **Ms. Grace Harper,** who introduced me to creative writing and the thrills of bylines in junior high school; to **Ms. Elizabeth Coffelt,** who, like Auntie Mame, exposed me to the worlds of photography, fonts, and publishing; to **Dr. Carl Shepherd,** Professor of Art History, whose course was the most applied that I ever had; to **Dr. Melkowitz,** Professor of Physics, who imparted the power of the basic laws of physics with more drama than the Nobel laureates who followed; to **Dr. Seymour Dayton,** an internist who taught that one gathers strength not only by one's own achievements but also through carefully selected associates; to **Dr. Ben Fishkin and Dr. James Scott,** who taught the power and beauty of a simple tool—the microscope; to **Dr. Sydney Finegold and Dr. Lucien Guze,** both specialists in infectious disease, who glorified the rewards, excitement, and influence of teaching and research; to **Dr. William Valentine and Dr. Charles Craddock,** inspirational teachers of classical hematology; and finally to **Dr. Barry Lowitz,** the most *compleat* oncologist, who taught me that treating patients with solid tumors could be as gratifying as treating those with hematologic disorders.

D.A.C.

To **Joseph and Frieda Lowitz,** my role models for lifelong scholarship and community responsibility; to **Mrs. Lucille Murphy and Mr. Eugene Salisbury,** grammar school and high school English teachers, who taught me how to communicate; to **Mr. Alfred Lustgarten and Mr. Sheldon Steinberg,** who helped me discover human spirituality through music and art; to **Chaplain Charles Pickens,** a teacher of support and comfort of each person in his own terms; to **Mr. Jerry Coash,** who taught spirituality through mental clarity, personal insight, and caring for others without prejudice or judgment; to **Dr. Raymond Redheffer,** Professor of Mathematics and teacher of the fun and excitement of disciplined study and development of ideas; to **Dr. Lucien Guze and Dr. Vasant Udhoji,** quintessential teachers, caregivers, and role models for medical practice; to **Mr. Thomas Jefferson and Mr. Alexander Hamilton,** teachers of the unique value of every human being; to **Mr. William Shakespeare,** everyone's teacher about what we human beings are; and to **Mr. Sherlock Holmes,** instructor of observation and deduction.

B.B.L.

Contents

Contributing Authors

Jonathan S. Berek, M.D.	Professor of Obstetrics and Gynecology, University of California, Los Angeles, UCLA School of Medicine; Vice Chair, Department of Obstetrics and Gynecology, UCLA Medical Center, Los Angeles
James R. Berenson, M.D.	Associate Professor of Medicine, University of California, Los Angeles, UCLA School of Medicine, Los Angeles; Chief, Hematology-Oncology Section, Wadsworth VA Medical Center, West Los Angeles
Harold E. Carlson, M.D.	Professor of Medicine, State University of New York at Stony Brook, Health Sciences Center School of Medicine, Stony Brook; Chief, Endocrinology Section, Veterans Administration Medical Center, Northport, New York
Dennis A. Casciato, M.D.	Clinical Professor of Medicine, University of California, Los Angeles, UCLA School of Medicine, Los Angeles; Chief of Medicine, Encino-Tarzana Regional Medical Center, and Director, Shared Medical Research Foundation, Tarzana, California
Jean B. deKernion, M.D.	The Fran and Ray Stark Professor of Urology, University of California, Los Angeles, UCLA School of Medicine; Chief, Division of Urology, UCLA Medical Center, Los Angeles
Lawrence H. Einhorn, M.D.	Distinguished Professor of Medicine, Indiana University School of Medicine; Attending Physician, Indiana University Hospital, Indianapolis
Robin P. Farias-Eisner, M.D.	Assistant Professor of Obstetrics and Gynecology, University of California, Los Angeles, UCLA School of Medicine; Attending Physician, Division of Gynecologic Oncology, UCLA Medical Center, Los Angeles

Robert A. Figlin, M.D.   Associate Professor of Medicine, University of California, Los Angeles, UCLA School of Medicine; Director, Clinical Research Unit, UCLA Jonsson Comprehensive Cancer Center, Los Angeles

Kenneth A. Foon, M.D.   Professor of Medicine, University of Kentucky College of Medicine; Chief, Division of Hematology and Oncology, University of Kentucky A.B. Chandler Medical Center, and Director, Lucille P. Markey Cancer Center, Lexington, Kentucky

Jeffrey E. Galpin, M.D.   Clinical Associate Professor of Medicine, University of Southern California School of Medicine, Los Angeles; Attending Physician, Encino-Tarzana Regional Medical Center, and President, Shared Medical Research Foundation, Tarzana, California

Charles M. Haskell, M.D.   Professor of Medicine, University of California, Los Angeles, UCLA School of Medicine, Los Angeles; Director, Wadsworth Cancer Center and VA Medical Center, West Los Angeles

Carole G. H. Hurvitz, M.D.   Professor of Pediatrics, University of California, Los Angeles, UCLA School of Medicine; Director, Department of Pediatric Hematology/Oncology, Cedars-Sinai Medical Center, Los Angeles

David W. Knutson, M.D.   Professor of Medicine, Pennsylvania State University College of Medicine, Hershey; Chief, Medical Service, Lebanon Veterans Medical Center, Lebanon, Pennsylvania

Steven M. Larson, M.D.   Professor of Radiology, Cornell University Medical College; Chief, Nuclear Medicine Service, Department of Radiology, Memorial Sloan Kettering Cancer Center, New York

Alexandra M. Levine, M.D.   Professor of Medicine, University of Southern California School of Medicine; Chief, Division of Hematology, Kenneth Norris, Jr. Cancer Hospital and Research Institute, Los Angeles

Robert B. Livingston, M.D.   Professor of Medicine, University of Washington School of Medicine; Head, Division of Oncology, University of Washington Medical Center, Seattle

Barry B. Lowitz, M.D.

Emeritus Associate Clinical Professor of Medicine, University of California, Los Angeles, UCLA School of Medicine, Los Angeles

Ellen E. Mack, M.D., M.P.H.

Assistant Clinical Professor of Neurology, University of California, San Francisco, School of Medicine; Attending Surgeon, Department of Neurosurgery, Mount Zion Medical Center of UC-San Francisco, San Francisco

Mimi Mott-Smith, M.S.N., F.N.P.

Clinical Instructor of Internal Medicine, University of California, San Francisco, School of Medicine, San Francisco; Attending Physician, Department of Internal Medicine, Valley Medical Center, Fresno, California

Robert G. Parker, M.D.

Professor of Radiation Oncology, University of California, Los Angeles, UCLA School of Medicine; Chairman, Department of Radiation Oncology, UCLA Medical Center, Los Angeles

Dale H. Rice, M.D.

Tiber/Alpert Professor, University of Southern California School of Medicine; Chair, Department of Otolaryngology-Head and Neck Surgery, Los Angeles County USC Medical Center, Los Angeles

Peter J. Rosen, M.D.

Professor of Clinical Medicine, University of California, Los Angeles, School of Medicine; Director, Solid Oncology Program, UCLA Medical Center, Los Angeles

Lawrence Stolberg, M.D.

Associate Clinical Professor of Medicine, University of California, San Francisco, School of Medicine, San Francisco; Attending Physician, Department of Internal Medicine, Valley Medical Center, Fresno, California

Hassan J. Tabbarah, M.D.

Professor of Medicine, University of California, Los Angeles, UCLA School of Medicine, Los Angeles; Assistant Chairman, Department of Medicine, Harbor-UCLA Medical Center, Torrance, California

Richard F. Wagner, Jr., M.D.

Professor of Dermatology, University of Texas Medical Branch, Galveston, Texas

Donna L. Walker, M.D.   Clinical Researcher, Division of
Gynecologic Oncology, UCLA Medical
Center, Los Angeles

Preface

The *Manual of Clinical Oncology,* which has attained popularity as a major reference source for medical students, residents, and fellows in oncology, is completely revised for its third edition to reflect advances in clinical and molecular oncology. The focus of the new edition, like its predecessors, is on information useful for participating in rounds and for making diagnostic and therapeutic decisions at the bedside of patients with malignancies. Our goal is for the Manual to remain comprehensive, concise, and current without being susceptible to rapid obsolescence. Evanescent aspects of oncology, such as combination chemotherapy "regimens of the month," have been assiduously avoided.

The chapters remain grouped into four parts. Part I presents the principles of diagnosis and treatment of cancer. Part IV presents complications of cancer according to end-organ involvement, whether by local invasion, metastasis, paraneoplasia, or therapy.

Parts II and III address the specific malignancies in the following uniform format:

I. **Epidemiology and etiology** emphasizes predisposing factors.

II. **Pathology and natural history** emphasizes the breadth of histopathologies, the usual modes of tumor spread, and common complications.

III. **Diagnosis** emphasizes the selection and limitations of special studies.

IV. **Staging systems and prognostic factors** use the most familiar or most informative systems and present survival data.

V. **Prevention and early detection** are discussed when applicable.

VI. **Management** discusses the roles of surgery, radiotherapy, and chemotherapy for early and late disease.

Several chapters were completely rewritten: Chapter 1, Principles of Cancer Biology and Management (including expansion of interpretation of clinical trials and statistics); Chapter 4, Cancer Chemotherapeutic Agents; Chapter 9, Gastrointestinal Tract Cancers; Chapter 14, Neurologic Tumors; Chapter 20, Metastases of Unknown Origin; Chapter 32, Neuromuscular Complications; Chapter 35, Infectious Complications; and Chapter 36, Acquired Immunodeficiency Syndrome (AIDS). Two new chapters—Chapter 2, Nuclear Medicine and Chapter 37, AIDS-Related Malignancies—have been added to reflect important advances in these fields. The remaining chapters have been significantly updated and revised.

The first edition was written primarily by the two editors. A few contributors were added in the second edition. New authors contributed Chapters 2, 8, 11, 13, 14, 18, 26, 31, 32, and 37 in this edition and significantly expanded the geographic and institutional distribution of the faculty. Every line of the entire book, however, was punctiliously reviewed by a single editor to ensure consistency in both style and philosophy.

The appendixes were entirely reconstructed to present the most useful combination chemotherapeutic regimens in a condensed format (Appendix A); the complications of such treatment and toxicity criteria for evaluating both individual patients and those in clinical trials (Appendix B); tumor identifiers, such as leukocyte differentiation antigens and cytogenetic nomenclature (Appendix C); and a unique "primer" on carcinogenic viruses and oncogenes (Appendix D).

Approaches to clinical problems in oncology are frequently controversial; none of the alternatives may be ideal or scientifically validated. The authors of this text avoid equivocation in the face of uncertainty; they provide grounds for understanding diagnostic and therapeutic interventions and guidelines for managing difficult problems, even if standard approaches are nonexistent.

The physician must go beyond the axiom of doing no harm and has the additional responsibility of actively keeping cancer patients out of harm's way—physically, psychologically, and financially. Despite the technical nature of the material discussed, the editors have maintained an underlying approach in caring for cancer patients that may be summarized by the following:

The decision of one is more useful than the opinions of many.

Life is most valuable when there is little of it left.

D.A.C.
B.B.L.

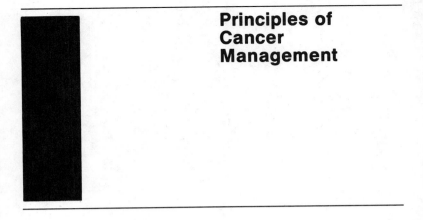

Principles of
Cancer
Management

Principles of Cancer Biology and Management

Barry B. Lowitz and
Dennis A. Casciato

*In medical practice, as in most of life, a lot
can be done, a little should be done, and a
vanishingly small amount must be done.*

I. Epidemiology and etiology

A. Epidemiology. Epidemiology is the study of the relationship of cancer incidence and mortality to a variety of factors to determine possible causes or risk factors for cancers. Risk factors include behavioral patterns, socioeconomic status, geographic and demographic data, and changing patterns of cancer incidence either with emigration or over time.

1. Incidence and mortality rates

a. Incidence is the overall number of persons developing cancer in a particular time frame, usually one year.

b. Incidence rate is the number of persons developing cancer per 100,000 persons per year.

c. Mortality rate is the number of persons dying of cancer per 100,000 persons in a year.

d. Case fatality rate is the percentage of persons with a particular cancer who die of that cancer.

2. Overall incidence of cancer in the United States in 1992 was approximately 1,200,000, and the number of persons dying of cancer was about 500,000. The overall incidence rate of cancer is increasing slowly, possibly as a result of better methods of detection.

3. Survival. Palliative treatment is essential to cancer care, but treatment in an epidemiologic context is important only as it relates to survival.

a. Lethality. More than 50 percent of cancer deaths are caused by lung, colorectal, breast, and prostate malignancies.

b. The overall five-year survival rate for all cancers has improved by about 10% in the past 20 years (Table 1-1). Most of the treatment-related improvement in survival has occurred as the result of early detection and treatment for uncommon cancers, such as childhood leukemia and testicular cancer. With the exception of small cell lung cancer and breast cancer, improvement in five-year survival has been negligible in the advanced stages of most of the common lethal malignancies.

(1) Early detection and diagnosis of cancers that appear histologically identical but are biologically less lethal can yield misleading survival figures.

(2) Lead time bias. Patients appear to live longer from the time of diagnosis only because the cancer was detected earlier rather than because of treatment.

B. Etiology. At least 80 percent of cancers in Americans are caused by living habits (smoking, alcohol consumption, and diet) and environmental carcinogens.

*Of the natural catastrophes that can befall us,
the most distressing are those caused by our
own behavior.*

Table 1-1. Five-year survival expectancy in Caucasian Americans with cancer

Malignancy	Prevalence	1970 survival	1988 survival	Change in five-year survival
Lung cancer	15%	10%	14%	+ 4%
Colon cancer	14%	49%	58%	+ 9%
Breast cancer	16%	68%	78%	+10%
Prostate cancer	12%	63%	76%	+13%
Endometrial cancer	4%	81%	84%	+ 3%
Pancreatic cancer	2%	3%	5%	+ 2%
Bladder cancer	5%	61%	79%	+28%
Ovarian cancer	2%	36%	38%	+ 2%
Testicular cancer	0.5%	72%	93%	+21%
Hodgkin's disease	0.04%	67%	77%	+10%

1. **Tobacco.** Smoking and other tobacco use unequivocally cause about 30 percent of all cancer deaths in the United States.
   a. At least 90 percent of lung cancer deaths are due to smoking. Smoking is also clearly causative for cancers of the upper respiratory tract, genitourinary tract, gastrointestinal tract, and pancreas. Chewing tobacco and snuff cause cancers in the upper respiratory passages.
   b. Passive smoke (smoke produced by smokers and inhaled by nonsmokers) accounts for approximately 6000 cancer deaths in the United States annually. Most of these deaths result from lung cancers, with some deaths due to leukemia, urinary tract, and other cancers. Passive smoke may also cause as many as 50,000 deaths annually from nonmalignant causes, particularly cardiovascular disease.
2. **Alcohol,** although not a carcinogen, can cause cancers in the upper respiratory passages and esophagus, apparently by increasing the permeability of the mucosa to active carcinogens, especially in smokers. Alcoholic cirrhosis predisposes individuals to hepatocellular cancer. Beer drinking, some homemade brandies, and possibly Eau de Vie are associated with esophageal cancer in France.
3. **Ionizing radiation exposure** causes about 5 percent of cancer deaths. Its etiologic role was well-established with the development of leukemias in populations exposed to the atomic bomb, in patients who were treated with radiotherapy for ankylosing spondylitis, and in radiologists prior to the advent of safety measures. The cancer risk appears to be higher if the same radiation dose is accumulated over a short period of time rather than over long periods.
   a. The risk of leukemia, particularly in children, is higher for those living near nuclear plants or exposed to diagnostic and therapeutic radiation.
   b. Premenopausal Japanese women exposed to radiation from the atomic bomb blast have had an increased risk of breast cancer.
   c. Ambient radon gas is produced as the result of naturally occurring nuclear fission deep within the earth. The gas finds its way to the surface in various geographic locations, where the risk of lung cancer and other malignancies is increased. In areas where radon is detectable, persons living closest to the ground floor appear to be at a higher risk for cancer. Radon is chemically inert, but it has reportedly been found in tobacco.
   d. A report of an increased risk of lung cancer (especially the small cell

variety) in nonsmoking uranium miners in Colorado suggests that some of the 10 percent of lung cancer patients who never smoked may have acquired the disease from radiation, possibly arising from ambient radon gas.

   4. Solar ultraviolet radiation (UV-B) is clearly related to an increased risk of skin cancers, namely melanomas and squamous or basal cell carcinomas.

   5. Electromagnetic fields have an unclear relationship to malignancy. Workers on high-voltage electric lines may be at increased risk for gliomas. Clusters of leukemia have been reported in children living or going to school under high-power lines. To date, no excess cancer risk has been reported for magnetic resonance imaging.

   6. Dietary habits, body habitus, and cancer risk.

   a. Dietary substances are associated with cancers in the following sites:

   (1) Fat: breast and colon

   (2) High total caloric intake: breast, endometrium, prostate, colon, and gallbladder

   (3) Animal protein, particularly as red meats: breast, endometrium, and colon

   (4) Alcohol, particularly in smokers: mouth, pharynx, larynx, esophagus, and liver

   (5) Salt-cured, smoked, or charred foods: esophagus and stomach

   (6) Nitrate and nitrite additives: intestine

   b. Dietary elements that appear to reduce the risk of cancer

   (1) High-fiber foods

   (2) High content of vegetables, fruits, and whole grain cereal

   (3) Indole-containing vegetables (e.g., cabbage, cauliflower, broccoli), so-called cruciferous vegetables named for the cross-shaped arrangement of leaves under the edible part of the plant. These decrease the risk of large bowel cancer but may increase the risk of stomach cancer.

   (4) Beans (especially soybeans and lima beans)

   c. Body habitus and exercise. Obesity is associated with an increased risk of breast cancer in women over 40 years. Thin habitus (10% or more below average body weight) is possibly associated with an increased risk of breast cancer in young women. Regular exercise may decrease the risk of colon cancer.

   7. Chemical and microbial agents are discussed with the specific cancers.

   8. Oncogenes and viruses. See Appendix D. *Carcinogenic Viruses and Oncogenes: A Primer.*

II. Natural history, survival, and response to treatment

> *An art of medicine is the ability to make decisions in the face of insufficient information. Obtaining sufficient information would usually alter the host to the point that a different diagnosis and therapy are required.*

A. Importance of natural history. The natural history of a malignancy is the course that a particular tumor usually takes without treatment and the effect of that course on the function of the host. Cognizance of the natural history facilitates making patient management decisions, as follows:

   1. Knowing the first detectable changes associated with early cancer provides a basis for screening programs and permits early removal of certain malignancies.

   2. Knowing which organs are typically involved by metastases permits cost-effective monitoring of those sites (see Table 1-2).

   3. Knowing how specific treatment modalities alter the course of untreated cancer prevents the selection of therapy that provides no advantage over nontreatment.

   4. Knowing how often the cancer in question produces the observed clinical

Table 1-2. Metastases from carcinomas

Primary site	Metastatic site (%)			
	Bone	Lung	Liver	Brain
Lung	30–50	35	30–50	15–30
Breast	50–85	60	45–60	15–25
Thyroid	40	65	60	1
Pancreas	5–10	25–40	50–70	1–5
Liver	10	20		0
Colon and rectum	5–10	25–40	70	1
Stomach	5–10	20–30	35–50	1–5
Kidney	30–50	50–75	35–40	5–10
Ovary	2–5	10	10–15	1
Prostate	50–75	15–50	15	2

Source: Adapted from H. A. Gilbert and A. R. Kagan, Metastases: Incidence, Detection, and Evaluation Without Histologic Confirmation. In L. Weiss (ed.), *Fundamental Aspects of Metastases*. New York: American Elsevier, 1976. Pp. 385–405.

pattern permits the recognition of atypical patterns that may herald an unrelated, treatable benign condition.

5. Knowing how the tumor produces symptoms and death enables the physician to provide optimal palliative care.

B. Evaluation of the clinical course of cancer

1. **Cure** is a statistical term that applies to groups of cancer patients rather than to individuals; it describes those patients who are rendered clinically free of detectable cancer and who have the same survival expectancy as a healthy age-matched control group. A "cure" does not guarantee that the particular patient meeting these criteria will not eventually die from the original cancer.

2. **Survival rates.** Improvement in survival may be attributable more to the method of calculation of the survival rate than to the method of treatment.

   a. **Actuarial survival** (or life table survival) compares patient depletion by death or by loss to follow-up during a specified period of study to patient loss in a matched healthy population that is under continued follow-up. This method projects the chance that an individual will survive for some determined time.

   b. **Observed survival rate** indicates the percentage of patients alive at the end of a specified interval of observation after the time of diagnosis.

   c. **Relative survival rate** corrects the survival rate for the "normal mortality expectation" in a matched population.

   d. **Adjusted survival rate** corrects the survival rate for deaths due to other causes for patients free of cancer at the time of death.

   e. **Median survival** is the time when 50 percent of patients are dead and 50 percent are still alive. Average or mean survival rates are meaningless, since survival of patients with similar tumors may range from a few weeks to years. Median survival may be a useful index for comparison of clinical trials, but can be misleading. In "mature studies," a significant group of patients may survive for many months or years after the time that 50 percent of the patients are dead.

   f. **Disease-free interval.** The time from when the patient is rendered free of clinically detectable cancer until recurrent cancer is diagnosed.

3. **Responses to treatment**

   a. **Complete remission (CR).** No clinically detectable cancer is found following treatment.

   b. **Partial remission (PR).** Measurable tumor (usually the sum of the products of two diameters from all measurable lesions) is decreased by 50 percent following treatment, no new areas of cancer can be found, and no area of tumor shows progression.
   c. **Minimal remission (MR).** Same as partial remission, but not meeting the criteria of 50 percent reduction.
   d. **Progression.** The increase of a tumor mass by more than 25 percent (sum of products of diameters), appearance of new lesions, or tumor-induced death.
   e. **Stable disease.** Measurable tumor does not meet the criteria for CR, PR, MR, or progression.

III. Diagnosis

Use technology to confirm your diagnostic impression, not to rule it out.

A. **Biopsy.** Histologic proof of malignancy is the cornerstone of diagnosis and treatment. Neoplasms can masquerade as benign or inflammatory conditions, and vice versa. The site that is least risky and most likely to provide the necessary information is biopsied. Specimens should not be routinely placed in formalin; suspect lymphomas or metastases of unknown primary site should be placed in a fixative, such as B5, that permits immunohistochemical analysis.

B. **Shortcomings of pathologic diagnosis.** Establishing the type of tumor and whether it is malignant or benign is not an exact science. Errors may occur in selecting, sampling, processing, and interpreting specimens. Some tumors can change with time or appear to be benign histologically but act malignant biologically (and vice versa). Intraepithelial dysplasia and malignancy form a continuous spectrum. Pathologic classifications are being developed that grade neoplastic changes rather than unrealistically committing to a positive or negative diagnosis of cancer. Histopathologic data, therefore, should be regarded as laboratory tests that must be interpreted as only part of the information about the evolving clinical syndrome. **Recommendations:**
   1. Never confuse the ability to name a tumor with the ability to understand its behavior.
   2. Never accept a histopathologic diagnosis as unequivocal.
   3. Never act on verbal reports from anyone.
   4. Review biopsy specimens with the pathologist and communicate important clinical data regarding the patient.
   5. Be sure that the pathologist has reviewed sufficient samples.
   6. When the histologic diagnosis and the biologic course are not in concert
      a. Make certain the tissue came from your patient.
      b. Re-review the slides with the pathologist.
      c. If still equivocal, obtain an opinion from another institution or obtain another biopsy specimen.

C. **Microscopic clues of tumor origin** are presented in Appendix **C-1.**

D. **Tumor markers** are cellular products that are abnormally elaborated by malignancies. These markers can be detected in various body fluids and on the surface of cancer cells. Blood level determinations can be useful in diagnosis and prognosis of cancer and in monitoring of cancer treatment.
   1. **The utility of a tumor marker** depends on its sensitivity, specificity, variability in assays, and probably most importantly, the existence (or absence) of effective tumor treatment. Properties of potentially helpful serum tumor markers are shown in Table 1-3. Most tumor markers are present at low or even moderately high levels in healthy persons, and normal levels, which are somewhat arbitrary, are found in patients with malignancy. Measurements that help define the usefulness of a tumor marker are:
      a. **Sensitivity** is the percentage of patients with cancer who have an abnormal test. **Specificity** is the percentage of people without cancer whose test is negative.
      b. **Positive predictive value** is the probability that patients with an

Table 1-3. Helpful serum tumor markers

Marker	Upper limit	Serum half-life	Application in cancer
α-FP	25 μ/l	3–6 days	Testis, hepatoma
β-HCG	<1 ng/ml	18–24 hours	Testis, trophoblastic neoplasia
β$_2$-microglobulin	2 μg/ml	?	Myeloma, lymphoma
Calcitonin	0.1 ng/ml[a]	12 minutes	Thyroid (medullary carcinoma)
CA 15-3	25 U/ml	<2 weeks	Breast
CA 19-9	37 U/ml	?	Pancreas
CA 72-4[b] (TAG-72)	6 U/ml	?	Breast, ovary
CA 125	35 U/l	4–5 days	Ovary
CEA	5 ng/ml	Weeks	Colorectal, breast, lung (small cell)
NSE[b]	12 μg/l	14 days	Neuroendocrine (oat cell)
PSA	2.5–4.0 ng/ml	2–3 days	Prostate
Thyroglobulin	10 ng/ml	Weeks	Thyroid

[a] Without calcium infusion, 0.10 ng/ml; with calcium infusion, 0.55 ng/ml.
[b] Possibly helpful.
Abbreviations are defined in text.

abnormal test actually have cancer. **Negative predictive value** is the probability that a negative test will predict that a person will not have cancer.

   c. **Prevalence.** The probability that a positive test is truly the result of cancer can be greatly improved if the test is performed in a population where the prevalence of the cancer is high. High prevalence can be achieved by performing the test only in patients with known cancer, with risk factors for cancer, or with imaging studies that suggest the presence of cancer.

2. **Oncofetal proteins** are substances found normally in larger amounts during fetal development. Cancers derived from the fetal counterpart of adult tissues often elaborate these proteins in increased quantities.

   a. **α-fetoprotein (α-FP)** in fetuses is biochemically related to albumin in adults. It is found in fetal liver, yolk sac, and gastrointestinal tract. Consequently, α-FP is correspondingly increased in about 80 percent of patients with hepatomas, 60 percent of patients with nonseminoma germ cell cancers and occasionally in other cancers. α-FP is further discussed in Chap. 12, sec. III.C.2.

   b. **Carcinoma embryonic antigen (CEA)** is a fetal glycoprotein found on cell surfaces. It is chemically related to immunoglobulins. CEA is produced in the fetal gastrointestinal tract, pancreas, and liver. It is present in small quantities in the blood and on cells of many normal adult tissues.

      (1) CEA is a useful marker for monitoring breast, ovary, colon, and small cell lung cancers. CEA is increased in patients with a variety of other endothelial malignancies, where its usefulness is generally limited.

      (2) Elevations of CEA blood levels (usually <10 ng/ml) are found in smokers and in patients with chronic obstructive lung disease, inflammatory or peptic bowel disease, liver inflammation or cirrhosis of any cause, renal failure, and fibrocystic breast disease.

3. **Hormones**

   a. **Human chorionic gonadotropin (β-HCG)** is a glycoprotein produced by placental syncytiotrophoblasts that is found as a normal blood product in women during pregnancy, and *is never found in normal males.* See Chap. 12, sec. **III.C.1.**

b. **Thyrocalcitonin** is produced by thyroid C-cells and medullary thyroid cancer. It is an effective way of screening patients with first-degree relatives affected by this dominantly inherited disease and related forms of multiple endocrine neoplasia (MEN). Elevated levels may also occur in:

   (1) Other cancers: breast, lung, gastrointestinal, carcinoid, gastrinoma

   (2) Benign disorders: diseases of the lung or pancreas, pregnancy, hyperparathyroidism, boney Paget's disease, pernicious anemia

c. **Hormone markers** are often produced by cancers of endocrine organs and in various paraneoplastic syndromes as well. These are discussed with the individual tumors.

4. Enzymes

a. **Prostatic acid phosphatase** is elevated in about 85 percent of men with metastatic prostate cancer, and levels correlate with response to therapy. See Chap. 13, *Prostate Cancer,* sec. **III.C.2.a.**

b. **Prostate-specific antigen (PSA)** is a serine protease which is produced by prostatic alveolar and ductal epithelial cells and correlates closely with tumor bulk and response to therapy for men with prostate cancer. See Chap. 13, *Prostate Cancer,* sec. **III.C.2.b.**

c. **Lactic dehydrogenase (LDH)** blood level is elevated in association with many types of malignancy, including leukemia and melanoma. However, blood levels correlate most closely with disease activity and response to therapy in nonseminomatous germ cell tumors and high-grade lymphomas.

d. **Placental alkaline phosphatase** (Regan isoenzyme) is elevated in seminomas. See Chap. 12, sec. **III.C.3.**

e. **Neuron-specific enolase (NSE)** is a glycolytic enzyme with α, β, and γ forms. The γ form is neuronal in origin and may be useful in following neuroendocrine tumors, small cell lung cancer, and neuroblastoma. NSE levels are also increased in melanoma, islet cell carcinoma, hypernephroma, non–small cell lung cancer, as well as in benign conditions.

5. Cancer antigens (CAs) are glycoproteins with undefined normal counterparts and are elaborated by malignancies. Of the many that have been described, a few are clinically useful in monitoring the course of certain cancers. None of these are useful in general screening for cancer. Some of the more commonly described cancer antigens include:

a. **CA 15-3,** which is a mucinous glycoprotein detected by monoclonal antibodies against breast cancer extracts. It has both low sensitivity and specificity, but does reflect the extent of metastases in breast cancer.

   (1) CA 15-3 levels are also variably elevated in lung (25%), liver (30%), and ovarian (45%) cancers.

   (2) Elevated CA 15-3 levels in patients without cancer are observed in chronic hepatitis (40%), cirrhosis (15%), sarcoidosis, tuberculosis, and systemic lupus erythematosus.

b. **CA 19-9,** which is a mucinous glycoprotein detected by antibodies raised in mice against colon cancer. Although it is not useful in evaluating colon cancer, it is the most accurate marker for monitoring pancreatic cancer.

   (1) CA 19-9 is also increased in biliary, hepatic, gastric, and colon cancers.

   (2) CA 19-9 is elevated in nonmalignant diseases of the liver, in pancreatitis, and in several other nonmalignant conditions.

c. **CA 72-4 (TAG-72),** is commonly associated with elevated blood levels in gastric and colon cancers. Increased blood levels are also found in some patients with lung, breast, ovarian, or prostate cancer. CA 72 is increased in nonmalignant conditions in less than 10 percent of cases.

   d. CA 125, which is a mucinous glycoprotein that is detected by monoclonal antibodies against cystadenocarcinoma cell lines. It is useful for monitoring patients with known ovarian cancer. For ovarian cancer, CA 125 blood levels correlate closely with extent of disease, response to therapy, and recurrence.

   (1) Patients with breast, lung, liver, pancreas, or uterine cancers have a significant prevalence of elevated blood levels of CA 125.

   (2) CA 125 levels are elevated in patients with liver cirrhosis (65%), other liver diseases, pancreatitis, and inflammatory diseases of the gastrointestinal tract. Elevations also occur in pregnancy and in benign diseases of the uterus and adnexa such as fibroids, endometriosis, and pelvic inflammatory disease.

   (3) Less than 1 percent of healthy women have blood levels over 35 U/ml. A cutoff level above 65 U/ml confers a high specificity of 98 percent in excluding normal patients and those with benign disease, but the sensitivity is reduced to 70 percent and the positive predictive value to only 2 percent when a general population is screened.

   (4) Thus, CA 125 is useless as a general screening test for ovarian cancer. When elevated it does not exclude women with diseases other than ovarian cancer.

6. Miscellaneous markers

   a. β_2-microglobulin correlates with tumor burden, prognosis, and response to therapy in myeloma and with disease activity and prognosis in lymphomas. β_2-microglobulin levels are greatly affected by renal function.

   b. Paraproteins, determined by serum protein electrophoresis and immunoelectrophoresis, were the first diagnostically and therapeutically useful tumor markers (for myeloma and lymphomas).

   c. Serum ferritin levels correlate with extent of disease in hepatoma.

   d. Thyroglobulin is a glycoprotein produced by thyroid follicular cells and is increased in all thyroid disorders, including thyroid carcinoma. Thyroglobulin can also be increased in patients with breast or lung cancer. In addition, thyroglobulin levels are useful for following patients with well-differentiated thyroid cancer if residual thyroid tissue is ablated and antithyroid antibodies are determined simultaneously. Antithyroid antibodies, thyroxine, and triiodothyronine can interfere with the test for thyroglobulin. Thyroglobulin is also useful in following nonfunctioning metastases in combination with ^{131}I scanning.

IV. Staging

A. Principles of cancer staging

1. Determining the extent of disease and the organs involved is essential to the proper management of patients with cancer. Staging is necessary for comparing results of cancer research trials and facilitating the exchange of information. Many staging procedures are expensive and must be ordered in a cost-effective manner. The value of performing expensive tests outside of a research context for "prognostic purposes" is generally of questionable value.

2. Staging should describe both the tumor and the host, including

   a. Organ of tumor origin

   b. Histologic type and grade of tumor

   c. Extent of primary tumor (size, invasion of adjacent tissues, involvement of nerves, blood vessels, or lymphatic system)

   d. Sites of metastases

   e. Functional status of the patient (see inside back cover)

B. Staging procedures.
There is no routine set of evaluations to be obtained on all patients. Studies are individually selected with the knowledge of the natural history of the specific tumor type, the impact of results on management decisions, and the needs of the patient.

V. Prevention and early detection

A. Prevention

1. **Cigarette smoking** causes the same yearly morbidity that would occur if one nuclear reactor underwent a complete meltdown in a major city every four months. The death rate from lung cancer alone approximates all the lives lost in Bosnia in the same time.

2. **Diet** is most closely associated with the development of cancers of the gastro-intestinal tract and of cancers that are affected by hormones (breast, endo-metrium, ovary, and prostate). The National Cancer Institute has advocated a well-rounded ("prudent") diet, similar to that recommended for the pre-vention of cardiovascular disease, to possibly reduce the incidence of certain cancers.

3. **Recommendations** that could have a significant impact on the incidence of cancer generally involve attempts to change long-standing patterns of behavior. Recommendations include cessation of smoking, restraint of alco-hol consumption (in moderation if at all), avoidance of sun damage, and change in dietary habits beginning early in life. The risks of occupational and environmental hazards can probably only be reduced by government agencies, because the behavior patterns of business and industry do not appear to be more likely to respond to reason than those of individuals.

B. Early detection

1. **Self-examination**

   a. All women over 20 years old should examine their breasts five days after each menstrual period. Postmenopausal women should examine their breasts on the same day each month.

   b. **Patients exposed to sunlight,** especially light-complexioned individu-als, should search for new moles, changes in old moles, and scaly patches on the skin.

2. **Screening.** Unless the patient reports a specific symptom, screening proce-dures are generally fruitless. Certain procedures have been found adequate to detect potentially curable cancers in asymptomatic individuals in a cost-effective manner.

   a. Annual breast examination in women over 40 years of age and every three years in women between 20 and 40 years of age. Mammography is performed as a single baseline for those from 35 to 39 years of age, every 1 to 2 years for those from 40 to 49 years of age, and yearly for those who are age 50 and older.

   b. Papanicolaou smear of the uterine cervix annually (see Chap. 11, *General Aspects*, sec. **II.A**).

   c. Annual test for occult blood in stool (and, perhaps, biannual proctosig-moidoscopy) for patients more than 45 years old.

   d. Yearly CBC to search for tumor-related iron deficiency anemia and other hematologic problems in older patients.

   e. Periodic chest x-ray film for smokers more than 45 years old (a practice of questionable validity).

VI. Management

> *The withholding of technology requires as much skill and judgment as its employment. Do not use chemicals when time and words are indicated.*

A. Guidelines

1. **Provide comprehensive medical care.** Treat the whole patient, not just the tumor.

2. **Make decisions without subjecting the patient to every available test;** know the relative risks and benefits of diagnostic modalities.

3. **Optimize the patient's functional status** with medical technology and psy-chosocial support.

4. **Prolong life at a functional level tolerable to the patient and individualize**

the goals of therapy. A young patient may be psychologically and socially rehabilitated following hemipelvectomy for sarcoma. The same potentially curable procedure in an elderly patient with residual deficits from a stroke may not be salutary, even if survival were prolonged.

5. **Never threaten or desert a patient** because the patient requests another opinion or refuses to receive the recommended therapy. The physician, however, must set limits on ill-conceived or dangerous treatments desired by the patient.

6. **There is always a positive role for the physician** in the treatment of cancer patients, whether this role involves aggressive therapy, palliative therapy, or psychosocial support.

B. **Oncologic emergencies** may occur as presenting or complicating features in the course of malignancy.

   1. Emergencies that may evolve in a period of hours include
      a. Seizures, cerebral edema (Chap. 14, secs. **III.C.I, IX.A.,** and **IX.E.**)
      b. Spinal cord compression (Chap. 32, sec. **III**)
      c. Pericardial effusion with tamponade (Chap. 29, sec. **V**)
      d. Hyperviscosity states (Chap. 22, sec. **VII.A.1**)
      e. Hypercalcemia (Chap. 27, sec. **I**)
      f. Hyponatremia (Chap. 27, sec. **VI**)
      g. Hypoglycemia (Chap. 27, sec. **XII**)
      h. Infection, especially in leukopenic patients (Chap. 35)

   2. Emergencies that usually evolve over days to weeks but require early therapy to minimize morbidity include
      a. Superior vena cava obstruction (Chap. 29, sec. **I**)
      b. Lymphangitic pulmonary metastases (Chap. 29, sec. **II**)
      c. Brain metastases (Chap. 32, sec. **I**)
      d. Pain (Chap. 5, sec. **I**)
      e. Psychosocial problems (Chap. 6)

C. **Interpretation of results of clinical research trials.** An understanding of statistical design and terminology is important for interpreting research literature in the process of making clinical decisions.

   1. **Sample space** is the number of patients, tests, treatments, or other data points used in an experiment to represent all (the entire "universe") similar patients, tests, treatments, or data points.

   2. **Stratification** is a determination made prior to an experiment of elements that are known or suspected to affect the outcome of the study (e.g., age, sex, extent and sites of disease, functional status).

   3. **Randomization** is the assignment by random chance of a stratified patient to a treatment plan in a study comparing different kinds ("arms") of treatment.

   4. **Blinded study** is a study in which the patient does not know what arm of a study he or she is on. In "double-blinded studies" neither the investigator nor the patient knows what arm the patient is on.

   5. **Placebo trial** is a randomized study in which a group of treated patients is compared to a group of patients who are untreated.

   6. **Drug development trials**
      a. **Phase I trials** determine the optimal dose, frequency of administration, and side effects of a treatment.
      b. **Phase II trials** determine what kinds of cancer, if any, respond to a particular treatment.
      c. **Phase III trials** compare a treatment shown to be effective in phase II studies with either no treatment or another kind of treatment.

   7. *P* **value** is the probability that a difference between two arms of a study is the same when the results appear to be different. When the P value is less than .05, the probability that the difference between two groups occurred by chance alone is less than 5 percent; a high level of confidence that one treatment is better than the other, however, is not necessarily justified. The necessary sample size must be determined before the investigation is

started, and the full complement of patients must be entered into the study to justify statistical comparison. "Interval P values" reported before the planned number of patients are entered are typically misleading false-positives, and should be ignored.

8. **β error** is the probability that two treatment groups that appear to have identical results would be different if more patients were included.

9. **One- and two-tailed (sided) tests.** A one-sided analysis only gives the P value for the hypothesis that one treatment is better than another. A two-tailed test also evaluates the hypothesis that the worse treatment would remain that way if the entire sample space could be tested. Thus, a two-tailed test has much more discriminating power than a one-tailed test but requires twice as many patients to obtain the result.

10. **Power of a statistical test.** Studies done with small numbers of patients are more likely to have P values of less than .05 and may appear positive. The P-value is more likely to increase as the number of patients included in the study is increased. The "power" of a statistical test takes into account the number of patients enrolled, and higher powers give increasing confidence that the difference would be seen no matter how many more patients are treated.

11. **Meta-analysis** is a retrospective study in which data from *multiple randomized clinical trials* are pooled and analyzed. All patients, including those who were considered for study, must be accounted for. Meta-analysis can be helpful (1) in evaluating many similar small or highly stratified trials to look for a treatment effect that is not apparent in an individual study or (2) in identifying a subset of patients who benefit from the treatment.

12. **Critical evaluation of research reports** is essential for clinicians who are deciding whether to use a new treatment for a patient. Just because something is printed in a journal does not necessarily make it valid or useful. Evaluation requires answers to the following questions:

    a. Are patients who benefited from the treatment substantially like your patient with regard to age, sex, stage, performance status, and other prognostic factors?

    b. Does the study exclude certain patients? If so, what were the reasons for exclusion?

    c. Did the study produce toxicity or treatment-related deaths that are unacceptable in view of the potential benefits? On the other hand, was improvement in survival so superior that the risks of toxicity and drug-related death are warranted?

    d. Did the study stratify and randomize patients in such a way that the data can be interpreted? Did the report and conclusions seem to "backtrack" to try to explain why the results were not what the investigator retrospectively thought they should be?

    e. Was the study large enough to provide sufficient confidence that observed differences were not just random chance? Physicians should look for two-sided analysis with P values less than .05 and a power of 80 or greater.

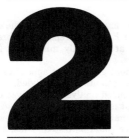

Nuclear Medicine

Steven M. Larson

I. Definitions

A. **Nuclear medicine** is the use of radioactive tracers in the form of unsealed sources for the diagnosis, therapy, and laboratory testing of human diseases. The common radiopharmaceuticals comprise 27 forms for diagnostic imaging applications and five forms for therapy (Table 2-1).

B. **Radioactivity.** Radioactive elements occur when subatomic particles in the nucleus are inherently unstable. The "half-life" ($T_{1/2}$) is the time required for half of the atoms to undergo radioactive decay.

  1. **Forms of radioactive emissions**
     a. **X-rays,** which result from rearrangement of electrons in orbitals around the nucleus.
     b. **Auger electrons,** which are very low energy electrons that are emitted from the orbitals around the nucleus and are capable of traveling only a few microns in tissue.
     c. **Gamma rays,** which are photoelectric energy that is capable of penetrating a meter or more through human tissue.
     d. **Neutrons,** which are proton-sized particles that have no charge.
     e. **Beta rays,** which are particulate emissions with the mass of an electron and a negative charge that are capable of penetrating from a few millimeters to about a centimeter in tissue.
     f. **Positron particles,** which are particulate emissions with the mass of an electron and a positive charge that travel for a few millimeters in tissue and then interact with an electron, forming annihilation radiation.
     g. **Annihilation radiation,** which is two gamma photons traveling at 180 degrees from each other that develops when a beta ray and a positron combine (see **e** and **f**).
     h. **Alpha particles,** which are two neutrons and two protons (a helium nucleus), that are capable of traveling for about 10 to 20 cell diameters in tissues.
     i. **Applications.** Gamma rays and annihilation radiation in particular are useful for various diagnostic imaging applications. The shorter range particles, such as beta rays and even the auger electrons, are used for therapeutic applications.

  2. **Quantity of radioactivity**
     a. **Becquerels (Bq).** One disintegration per second (dps) is defined as one becquerel of radioactivity, in honor of the discoverer of radioactivity. Typical doses used for imaging are often 37 megabecquerels (MBq).
     b. **Curies (Ci).** The curie unit was based on the amount of radioactivity in one gram of radium or 3.7×10^{10} dps. Typical diagnostic doses range from one millicurie (mCi or 37 MBq) to 30 mCi (1110 MBq).
     c. **Rads.** When radioactive emissions interact with matter, a fraction of the total energy is absorbed. The rad is equivalent to one erg of energy absorbed per gram of tissue.
     d. **Grays (Gy)** is the newer unit replacing the "rad." One Gy is 100 rad; one centigray (cGy) is one rad.
     e. **Rem (R)** (roentgen equivalent man) was introduced as a unit because

C	Carbon (^{11}C)	O	Oxygen (^{15}O)
F	Fluorine (^{18}F)	**P**	Phosphorus (^{32}P)
Ga	Gallium (^{67}Ga)	**S**	Sulfur (^{35}S)
I	Iodine (^{123}I, ^{125}I, ^{131}I)	**Sr**	Strontium (^{89}Sr)
In	Indium (^{111}In)	**Tc**	Technetium (^{99m}Tc); "m" = "metastable"
Kr	Krypton (^{81}Kr)	**Tl**	Thallium (^{201}Tl)
Mo	Molybdenum (^{99}Mo)	**U**	Uranium (^{235}U, ^{238}U)
N	Nitrogen (^{13}N)	**Xe**	Xenon (^{127}Xe, ^{133}Xe)

all radiation emitted does not exert equivalent biologic effects for a given amount of radiation dose absorbed. For gamma photons and x-rays, the rad dose and the rem dose are the same; for larger particles (e.g., alpha particles), a quality factor is applied and a very much larger rem is calculated.

   f. Sieverts (Sv). 100 rem is one Sv.
3. **Radiation protection and safety.** How much radiation exposure is safe? The answer is the "ALARA" concept, which means "as low as reasonably achievable." For the occupational worker, 5000 millirem (mR) per year are permitted as a maximum; 25% (1250 mR) is targeted as a goal. The general public in the United States receives an average of 290 mR per year from naturally occurring radiation. Up to 10 times this exposure occurs at high altitudes with no discernible adverse effects.

   The current mandated level for the general public is now set at 100 mR per year. Therapeutic radioisotopes commonly require admission to the hospital with isolation procedures until the radiation levels fall to 5 mR/hr at 1 meter from the treated subject. After that point, the patient is not subjected to any special precautions.

C. **Instrumentation**
1. **Well counters.** A radiation sensitive crystal (usually sodium iodide) is fashioned so that a small test tube containing a body fluid can be placed in a well within the radiation sensitive volume of the crystal. By reference to standards of known radioactivity, the absolute amount of tracer can be determined.
2. **Gamma camera devices** are the most commonly used imaging devices. The gamma camera is designed as a circular sheet of sodium iodide crystal with a collimator device to focus the radiation. A computer calculates the origin of each photon and produces pictures of the distribution of radioactivity within the body. Resolution is about 10 mm for most planar gamma cameras.
3. **Single photon emission computerized tomography (SPECT).** In this form of imaging, radioactivity within the patient is collected at 360 degrees around the patient and the data reconstructed into a three-dimensional representation. SPECT is commonly used for the imaging of ^{67}Ga citrate in the mediastinum of patients with lymphoma, ^{201}Tl in myocardial perfusion studies, hemangiomas within the liver, and radiolabeled antitumor antibodies. The typical in-depth resolution is 16 mm, somewhat more coarse than for planar imaging. The advantage of SPECT over planar gamma camera imaging is that SPECT has much better contrast resolution, so that small deep lesions are much better seen with SPECT imaging.
4. **Positron emission tomography (PET)** has the highest resolution and is the most sensitive imaging device available for nuclear medicine. For reasons related to the physics of positron emission decay, the image can be converted into an accurate, quantitative three-dimensional distribution of radioactiv-

Table 2-1. Diagnostic and therapeutic radiopharmaceuticals

Nuclide	Pharmaceutical	Pharmacology	Dosage	Patient Preparation	Use
Diagnostics					
^{18}F	FDG	Glycolysis	10 mCi	Fasting	Tumor viability
^{67}Ga	Citrate	Transferrin receptor	10 mCi	Laxatives	Lymphoma, inflammation
^{131}I	MIBG	Catecholamine uptake	0.5 mCi	Off α-, β-blockers	Neuroendocrine tumor
^{131}I	Norcholesterol	Steroid biosynthesis	1 mCi	Dexamethasone suppression	Adrenocortical hyperplasia or adenoma
^{123}I	Sodium iodide	Thyroid hormone	50 μCi	Off thyroid hormone, iodides	Thyroid dysfunction
^{111}In	DTPA	CSF circulation	5 mCi	None	CSF clearance
^{111}In	Leukocytes	Target inflammation	5 mCi	None	Abscess
^{111}In	Pentetreotide	Somatostatin receptors	5 mCi	Off steroids and octreotide; laxatives	Endocrine malignancy
^{111}In	Oncoscint	Anti-TAG-72 monoclonal antibody	5 mCi	Laxatives	Colorectal/ovarian cancer
^{99m}Tc	Phosphonates	Bone mineralization	25 mCi	None	Bone disease
^{99m}Tc	Bile acids	Biliary excretion	7 mCi	Fasting	Cholecystitis
^{99m}Tc	Sulfur colloid	Reticuloendothelial clearance	5 mCi	None	Liver/spleen disease
^{99m}Tc	Albumin	Lymphatic clearance	1 mCi	None	Lymphatic drainage

Isotope	Agent	Mechanism	Dose	Preparation	Indication
^{99m}Tc	Aggregated albumin	Capillary blockade	5 mCi	None	Pulmonary emboli
^{99m}Tc	DTPA	Glomerular filtration	5 mCi	Hydration	Renal function
^{99m}Tc	Erythrocytes	Vascular marker	30 mCi	Off β-blockers	Measure LVEF
^{99m}Tc	Pertechnetate	Thyroid iodine trap	10 mCi	Off thyroxine, iodide	Thyroid nodule
^{99m}Tc	MIBI	Lipophilicity and intracellular binding	20 mCi	Fasting; stop xanthines	Tumor viability, cardiac perfusion
^{201}Tl	Chloride	Na$^+$·K$^+$ pump	3 mCi	None	Tumor viability; cardiac perfusion
^{201}Tl	Chloride	Myocardial perfusion	5 mCi	Fasting; stop xanthines	Myocardial ischemia

Therapeutics

Isotope	Agent	Mechanism	Dose	Preparation	Indication
^{131}I	Sodium iodide	Thyroid hormone	7 mCi	Off thyroid medications	Hyperthyroidism
^{131}I	Sodium iodide	Thyroid hormone	25 μCi	Off thyroxine, iodide	Hyper- or hypothyroidism
^{131}I	Sodium iodide	Thyroid hormone	29 mCi	Off thyroid medications	Medical thyroidectomy
^{131}I	Sodium iodide	Thyroid hormone	200 mCi	Low iodide/high TSH levels	Thyroid cancer
^{131}I	MIBG	Catecholamine uptake	50 mCi	Off α-, β-blockers	Neuroblastoma
^{32}P	Chromic phosphate colloid	Sediment on surfaces	20 mCi	Patent catheter	Malignant effusion
^{32}P	Phosphate	Targets proliferating cells	5 mCi	None	Polycythemia vera
^{89}Sr	Chloride	Bone mineralization	40 mCi	None	Bone pain due to malignancy

Key: CSF = cerebrospinal fluid; DTPA = diethylene triamine penta-acetic acid; FDG = fluorodeoxy glucose; LVEF = left ventricular ejection fraction; MIBG = metaiodobenzyl-guandine; MIBI = methoxy isobutyl isonitrile; TSH = thyroid-stimulating hormone.

ity with a resolution of about 3–5 mm for deep-seated lesions within the body. The radiotracers used with PET are ^{18}F, ^{15}O, ^{13}N, and ^{11}C; these elements are readily incorporated into biologic molecules. Most of these radiotracers have half-lives that are too short for shipping. Thus they must be produced in a hospital-based cyclotron.

5. **Cyclotron.** The cyclotron accelerates subatomic particles (e.g., protons, deuterons, helium nuclei, alpha particles) to speeds approaching the speed of light. The particle strikes a "target" atom and artificially produces radioactivity. A large variety of the radiotracers, including ^{11}C, ^{15}O, ^{13}N, ^{67}Ga, ^{111}In, ^{123}I, and even ^{18}F, useful in nuclear medicine are produced by these "accelerator" systems.

6. **Reactors.** The reactor is fueled by heavy elements, such as ^{238}U and ^{235}U, which undergo spontaneous fission; neutrons are emitted from the nucleus and "split" the uranium atoms with the consequent release of large amounts of energy. An entire cascade of radioactive elements are produced in this process which are called "fission products," including ^{99}Mo (from which ^{99m}Tc is derived), ^{131}I, ^{125}I, ^{32}P, and ^{35}S. In some cases, a target element is bombarded with neutrons to produce the radioactive element used in medicine (e.g., ^{89}Sr). In other cases, separation of fission products may produce the radioisotope as a by-product of reactor operation (^{131}I, ^{125}I).

II. Tumor imaging studies

A. Bone scanning

1. **Indication.** To determine the presence and extent of primary and metastatic tumor involving bone.

2. **Radiopharmaceutical agent.** A phosphonate derivative such as pyrophosphate, methylene diphosphonate, or ethylene diphosphonate is labeled with ^{99m}Tc.

3. **Principle.** Primary or metastatic tumor provokes a reaction in the adjacent bone that causes the bone crystal to remodel and in the process take up the ^{99m}Tc bone agent. See Chap. 33, sec. I.D.3.

4. **Procedural notes.** Whole body scans are ordinarily obtained using gamma cameras with large fields of view. SPECT imaging is performed on suspect regions and is particularly helpful in the spine.

5. **Interpretation.** Against a background of bone turnover, a metastatic site stands out as very avid uptake. Bone scans are more sensitive than computerized tomography (CT) or magnetic resonance imaging (MRI) for detection of metastases in cortical bone.

B. ^{67}Gallium imaging

1. **Indications**

   a. To evaluate response to treatment of patients with **Hodgkin's and non-Hodgkin's lymphoma** (intermediate or high-grade). A baseline assessment is performed before therapy and repeated at the time of restaging procedures.

   b. **To evaluate viability selectively** in other tumors (e.g., hepatoma, sarcoma). These patients are studied as far from the completion of treatment as possible.

2. **Radiopharmaceutical agent.** ^{67}Ga citrate.

3. **Principle.** ^{67}Ga is a transition element that shares a variety of properties with iron, including rapid binding to transferrin (TF) following intravenous injection. Thereafter, the ^{67}Ga-TF is taken up by tumor cells through binding to the TF receptor on the membrane of tumor cells. The expression of the TF receptor is proportional to growth; the more rapidly proliferating the tumor, the more avid is the uptake.

4. **Procedural notes.** The patient is imaged 48–72 hours after injection. SPECT is significantly more sensitive than planar imaging for detecting active tumor sites. Anatomic correlation with CT or MRI helps greatly in interpretation. Where available, images from two different imaging modalities can be coregistered ("fused") in the computer. The anatomic image is

used as a template on which the ^{67}Ga image is laid to identify the tumor avid sites.

5. **Interpretation**
    a. ^{67}Ga citrate imaging is not normally used for staging purposes, but a baseline scan in Hodgkin's disease and high-grade lymphomas is helpful for later comparisons to help determine tumor response, particularly in patients with mediastinal involvement. Tumor sites may take up ^{67}Ga with strong avidity, which is greatly reduced when the tumor has responded to treatment. ^{67}Ga scans are almost never positive in low-grade lymphoma and play almost no role in the management of this disease.
    b. ^{67}Ga imaging is quite nonspecific; the isotope is avidly taken up in inflammatory lesions (e.g., diffusely in the lungs with *Pneumocystis carinii* and other pneumonitides). ^{201}Tl has been found to be useful when the cause of uptake on a ^{67}Ga scan is questioned. ^{201}Tl is normally concentrated in viable tumor and is rarely positive in lymphatic inflammation.

C. **^{111}Indium Oncoscint imaging**
    1. **Indication.** To determine the extent and location of extrahepatic abdominal disease in patients with known colorectal and ovarian cancer.
    2. **Radiopharmaceutical agent.** Oncoscint CR/OV (satumomab pendetide) is a conjugate produced from a murine monoclonal antibody (MoAb). The MoAb is an IgG-kappa directed to the nonspecific cancer antigen TAG-72 (or, CA72-4; see Chap. 1, sec. **III.D.5.c**). It contains the site-specific linker chelator that is conjugated to the oxidized oligosaccharide component of the MoAb. ^{111}In is conjugated to this linker chelate.
    3. **Principle.** The injected, radiolabeled MoAb binds to antigen sites (most commonly tumor). Over time sufficient concentration of radioactivity builds up at tumor sites to permit detection by a gamma camera.
    4. **Procedural notes.** The patient is imaged with a planar gamma camera or SPECT camera between 48 and 72 hours after injection. Later imaging and the use of cathartics may help to define a region of abdominal uptake in relationship to bowel or bladder activity.
    5. **Interpretation.** The abnormal focus of uptake in tumor is seen as a hot spot. Comparison to other imaging modalities, such as CT or MRI scans, may be helpful in determining the anatomic location of the uptake.
        a. Compared to CT scanning in patients with colorectal cancer, Oncoscint detected a significantly greater proportion of lesions in the lower abdomen (75% versus 55%) and pelvis (67% versus 28%). CT scanning was better for liver lesions. When the two tests were used in combination, the aggregate sensitivity was 88 percent.
        b. In ovarian cancer, there is improved sensitivity in comparison to CT for detecting peritoneal spread and disease within the pelvis (about 55% versus 35%).

D. **^{111}Indium pentetreotide imaging**
    1. **Indication.** For diagnostic workup of neuroendocrine tumors that bear somatostatin receptors.
    2. **Radiopharmaceutical agent.** Pentetreotide is a diethylene triamine pentaacetic acid conjugate of octreotide, which is a long-acting analog of human somatostatin. ^{111}In is bound to the agent.
    3. **Principle.** ^{111}In pentetreotide binds to somatostatin receptors throughout the body. Neuroendocrine tumors express these receptors and concentrate sufficient amounts of the radioactive agent to be seen by scintigraphy.
    4. **Procedural notes.** The patient undergoes daily planar and SPECT imaging until it is determined whether the agent is helpful. Typical imaging times are 4, 24, and 48 hours after injection. Because the agent is excreted into the bowel, the patient should be given a mild laxative in the evening before the 24- and 48-hour imaging times.
        a. **False-negative results** may occur in patients who are concurrently taking octreotide acetate for control of symptoms related to neuroendocrine

tumors. If possible, patients should stop taking this medication two weeks prior to the scan. Corticosteroids (by prescription or adrenocorticotropic hormone (ACTH)-producing tumors) can reduce the expression of somatostatin receptors and should also be stopped before scanning.

   b. Warnings and adverse reactions. Transient symptoms are occasionally seen, including dizziness, hypotension, and headache. Patients with known or suspected **insulinomas** should have an intravenous line running with 5 percent dextrose in normal saline before and during administration to avoid any possible hypoglycemia.

5. Interpretation. The normal pituitary gland, thyroid gland, and liver are seen. To a lesser extent the gall bladder, kidney, and bladder are also visible. Uptake in tumors bearing somatostatin receptors is apparent beginning at four hours, with the 24- and 48-hour images showing the greatest tissue contrast.

   a. New lesions, which were previously occult, despite extensive workup, were identified in nearly 30 percent of patients. The sensitivity for detecting tumor depends on the frequency of somatostatin receptor. Carcinoid tumors, neuroblastomas, pheochromocytoma, paragangliomas, small cell lung cancer, and meningiomas were detected in about 90 percent of cases. Lymphomas, pituitary tumors, and medullary tumors were detected in high but more variable percentages.

   b. Granulomatous lesions and other types of inflammatory lesions were also strongly positive, including tuberculosis, sarcoidosis, rheumatoid arthritis, and Graves' disease ophthalmopathy.

E. ^{131}**Iodine metaiodobenzylguanidine (MIBG) imaging**

   1. Indication. To identify metastatic and primary tumor sites for pheochromocytoma and neuroblastoma.

   2. Radiopharmaceutical agent. Iobenquane sulfate ^{131}I (metaiodobenzylguanidine sulfate).

   3. Principle. MIBG is normally concentrated by adrenergic tissues in cytoplasmic storage granules that also contain other catecholamines. Anything or any drug that blocks uptake or promotes release of these storage granules can potentially lead to false-negative results (see "Drug interactions").

   4. Procedural notes

   a. The patient is imaged with the whole body camera at 24 and 48 hours, with special attention to the retroperitoneum and adrenal region. Patient preparation consists of administering SSKI beginning 24 hours prior to starting the study and from 1 week after administering the dose.

   b. Warning. Hypertensive crises have occurred after injection of MIBG, especially in patients with pheochromocytoma. Pregnancy is not an absolute contraindication, but the potential risk to the fetus should be carefully assessed.

   5. Interpretation. MIBG is cleared by glomerular filtration from the plasma, and is rapidly taken up in catecholamine storage granules in tissue sites containing sympathetic nerves or adrenergic storage sites. Thus, uptake occurs in the heart, kidneys, liver, and adrenals at most imaging times. Tumors show up as areas of increased uptake.

   6. Drug interactions. The following drugs have the potential to interfere with the uptake of MIBG by neuroblastoma and pheochromocytoma and should be stopped prior to beginning the imaging for a few days to weeks, depending on the pharmacology of the drug.

   a. Antihypertensives: labetalol, reserpine, calcium channel blockers

   b. Amytriptyline, imipramine, and derivatives

   c. Doxepin, lamoxapin, and amoxipen

   d. Sympathetic amines (pseudoephedrine, ephedrine, phenylpropanolamine, phenylephrine)

   e. Cocaine

F. ^{18}**FDG (fluorodeoxyglucose) imaging**

   1. Indications

   a. To distinguish radiation necrosis from recurrent glioblastoma.

  b. To evaluate degeneration of brain tumor from low-grade to high-grade.
  c. To evaluate the potential for recurrence of meningioma.
  d. To assess tumor viability and monitor treatment response.
  e. To differentiate benign from malignant pulmonary nodules.

2. Radiopharmaceutical agent. [^{18}F]-2-fluoro-2-deoxy-D-glucose is an analogue of glucose.

3. Principle. Tumors have a markedly accelerated glycolysis in comparison to the tissues from which they arise. FDG enters the tumor cell via the glucose transporter and is phosphorylated to FDG-6-phosphate (FDG-6P). However, FDG-6P is not a suitable substrate for other glycolytic enzymes, is "metabolically trapped," and accumulates in the tumor tissue in proportion to the rate of phosphorylation. Although FDG-6P can be dephosphorylated by glucose-6-phosphatase, this enzyme is not expressed in actively proliferating tumors. Most normal tissues, with the exception of brain and heart, do have glucose-6-phosphatase and rapidly clear the FDG. Thus a gradient develops between tumor and background over time. A PET scanner can readily detect the tumor deposits.

4. Procedural notes. ^{18}FDG is injected into a fasting patient 45–60 minutes prior to PET scanning.

5. Interpretation. ^{18}FDG PET imaging is likely to be of great use in the scanning of numerous malignancies.

  a. For primary brain tumors, a comparison is made to the "contralateral" white matter; a hyperactive tumor has a ratio of 1.4 times the concentration of FDG. Increased uptake is characteristic of high-grade primary and metastatic neoplasms. The more active the uptake, the more rapid the growth pattern. Areas of decreased uptake are seen with low-grade tumors and radiation necrosis.

  b. Solitary pulmonary nodules are commonly managed with thoracotomy because of uncertainty about the benign or malignant nature of this finding. ^{18}FDG PET uptake can be helpful. If the ratio of uptake between a nodule and a normal control region is 2.5 or greater, the lesion is almost certainly malignant.

G. Tumor viability imaging: ^{201}Tl chloride and ^{99m}Tc "sestaMIBI"

  1. Indications

    a. Differential diagnosis of breast masses
    b. Viability assessment of primary bone tumors after chemotherapy
    c. Monitoring viability of well-differentiated thyroid cancer
    d. Imaging of parathyroid adenomas
    e. Imaging of brain tumors (SPECT)

  2. Radiopharmaceutical agents

    a. ^{201}**Tl (thallous) chloride** is a radioisotope of thallium, which is in the actinide series of elements and behaves in vivo as an analog of potassium.

    b. ^{99m}**Tc methoxy isobutyl isonitrile (MIBI)** is a monovalent cationic form of ^{99m}Tc that is highly lipid soluble. The agent is formed as a central ^{99m}Tc atom surrounded by six isobutyl nitrile. For this reason it is sometimes referred to as "sestaMIBI."

  3. Principle. ^{201}**Tl chloride** is a widely used cardiac perfusion agent that is taken up by most viable cells as a potassium analog and transported by the Na$^+$-K$^+$ pump. ^{99m}**Tc sestaMIBI** is also used to monitor cardiac perfusion. In addition, when taken up into the cell by a different mechanism, it can be used as a marker for cellular viability. After introduction into the blood stream, both of these agents are rapidly cleared from the circulation in proportion to cardiac output.

  4. Procedural notes. For breast imaging, a special breast apparatus permits planar lateral views of the breast in the prone position. This appears to be a technical advance. For brain and other organs SPECT scanning is performed.

  5. Interpretation

    a. Breast masses. Palpable breast masses in patients with mammographically "dense" breasts present a clinical dilemma. [201]Tl scans are reportedly negative in fibrocystic disease and in 96 percent of breast cancer nodules. Although false-positive results do occur, the negative predictive value for breast cancer is 97 percent. This technique is likely to improve the specificity of breast mammography.

   b. Primary bone tumors are frequently treated with chemotherapy before surgery. [201]Tl and ^{99m}Tc sestaMIBI are both taken up with high sensitivity into primary bone tumors and extremity sarcomas. Chondrosarcoma is an exception. MIBI uptake is lost in tumors responding to chemotherapy and has also been shown to correlate well with response to therapy.

   c. Brain tumors. SPECT imaging is accurate for assessing the viability of brain tumors. [201]Tl chloride appears to be the agent of choice for evaluating supratentorial primary brain tumors when FDG-PET is not available. In the author's experience ^{201}Tl is preferred over ^{99m}Tc sestaMIBI because uptake in the choroid plexus is not as marked.

   d. Thyroid cancer imaging. [201]Tl whole body imaging is a good way to monitor the activity of well-differentiated thyroid cancer during the interval when the patient is fully suppressed on thyroid hormone. The total uptake, as a percentage of the total body uptake, monitors the cellular viability of the tumor and can be used to assess the effectiveness of primary cancer treatment.

   e. Parathyroid imaging. With careful comparisons of ^{201}Tl or ^{99m}Tc sestaMIBI imaging it is sometimes possible to detect parathyroid adenomas in the neck or upper mediastinum when other modalities are negative. Still, the sensitivity of these techniques is disappointingly low (about 50%).

III. Other imaging studies

A. Cardiac functional studies. Equilibrium (gated) blood pool imaging is used to evaluate possible cardiac failure and to monitor changes following treatment with cardiotoxic drugs.

   1. Radiopharmaceutical agent. Red blood cells (RBCs) may be labeled in vivo. Stannous pyrophosphate (1 mg) is administered 20 minutes before injecting ^{99m}Tc pertechnetate. The stannous pyrophosphate enters and is trapped in the RBCs. The ^{99m}Tc pertechnetate diffuses into the RBCs, and is bound to the beta chain of hemoglobin. About 75 percent of the dose is labeled to the RBCs. Alternatively, the RBCs are labeled in a test tube attached to the patient (in vitro/in vivo method), wherein more than 95 percent of ^{99m}Tc is bound to RBC. An ECG R-wave signal serves as a physiologic "gate" for collection of timed "frames" (often called "gated blood pool imaging").

   2. Interpretation. Images obtained during rest are interpreted qualitatively to determine areas of abnormal wall motion, size of cardiac chambers, presence of intrinsic or extrinsic compression of the cardiac contour, and size and shape of the outflow tracts. Images are interpreted quantitatively for a physiologic assessment of the quantity of blood ejected from the left ventricle with each beat (the left ventricular ejection fraction [LVEF]). A normal LVEF is usually greater than 50 percent. Ejection fractions (EFs) less than 30 percent are usually but not always associated with clinical congestive heart failure. A decrease of more than 10 percent EF is highly significant. Cardiotoxic chemotherapeutic agents should be stopped when EFs fall to below normal (See Chap. 29, sec. **VI.D**).

B. Cardiac perfusion studies are performed for suspected myocardial ischemia and for evaluation of operative risk. Any tracer that is rapidly cleared from the blood and concentrated into an organ is regionally distributed within that organ according to regional blood flow (the "Saperstein principle"). [201]Tl chloride is rapidly cleared from coronary arteries by the Na^+-K^+-ATPase pump (about 80% in the first pass) and is still the most widely used of these Saperstein tracers. ^{99m}Tc-labeled sestaMIBI and teboroxime also give very high quality images.

C. **Vascular flow and bleeding studies** can be used to detect the patency of venous access in the upper extremities (e.g., postsubclavian catheter-placement swelling, superior vena cava syndrome), to assess for the presence of hemangioma as a space-occupying lesion, or to determine a site for bleeding. ^{99m}Tc pertechnetate or ^{99m}Tc sulfur colloid can be used as transient labels of the vasculature. In vivo labeling of RBCs with ^{99m}Tc may be used as more long-term vascular labels (see sec. **III.A.1**).

D. **Lymphoscintigraphy** can be used to determine the direction of lymph node drainage from truncal skin lesions and to evaluate the status of lymph ducts in regions of lymphedema. Typically, ^{99m}Tc-labeled albumin is injected into the webbing between the fingers or toes to assess the lower limbs or arms, respectively. For a truncal lesion (e.g., of melanoma), injections are made in four divided doses around the lesion. Gamma camera imaging is performed to assess the direction of drainage as a guide to determine which lymph node bearing region should undergo surgical exploration. Careful attention to detail in the early images may show the sites of interruption of draining lymphatic ducts.

E. **^{99m}Tc-macroaggregated albumin for lung perfusion** can be used to evaluate patients suspected of having pulmonary embolism and to determine the lung function capacity prior to pulmonary resection. ^{99m}Tc-labeled to macroaggregates of albumin (30–60 μ in diameter) are injected intravenously and are cleared in the first pass through the pulmonary circulation. The distribution of radioactivity is proportional to blood flow to the lungs.

F. **Studies of pulmonary ventilation** can be used to determine whether a ventilation perfusion "mismatch" exists as an aid in the differential diagnosis of pulmonary embolism and to assess the ventilatory capacity of the human lung. ^{133}Xe gas, ^{127}Xe gas, ^{81m}Kr, and ^{99m}Tc DTPA aerosol are used to label the inspiratory air. As the patient breathes, a gamma camera obtains an image of the distribution of radioactivity. Several minutes of breathing are required to fully achieve equilibrium with bullae and fistulous tracts. Then the washout phase is slowest from the least accessible areas. Particles also closely mimic gas, provided that they are smaller than 2 μ in diameter.

G. **Evaluation of biliary and gall bladder function.** ^{99m}Tc-labeled bile acids (derivatives of iminodiacetic acid), including hydroxyiminodiacetic acid, di-isofenin, and mebrofenin are used. The intravenously injected biliary agents are rapidly extracted by the liver and excreted by the hepatocytes into the biliary ducts. The demonstration of uptake by the gall bladder means that the cystic duct is patent and excludes the diagnosis of acute cholecystitis.

H. **Adrenal imaging** can be used to differentiate hypersecreting adrenocortical adenomas from bilateral hyperplasia, to determine the site of hyperfunctioning adenomas prior to surgery, and to evaluate clinically silent adrenal masses. ^{131}I-6β-iodomethyl-norcholesterol, which is a precursor for hormonal synthesis of gluco- and mineralocorticoids, is taken up in the adrenal gland and hyperfunctioning adenomas. Lesions that have become autonomous are not suppressed by dexamethasone.

I. **Thyroid evaluation** with radionuclides assesses the overall function of the thyroid gland and the functional status of nodules within the thyroid gland (categorized as "hot" or "cold"). Sodium ^{123}I, sodium ^{131}I, and ^{99m}Tc pertechnetate are "trapped" by the first phase of uptake into the thyroid gland within a few minutes. ^{99m}Tc pertechnetate can be displaced from the thyroid with anionic competitors (e.g., perchlorate). The iodide can also be displaced from the gland if there is a defect in organification of iodine, as occurs when patients are treated with organic blocking agents (e.g., methimazole).

The level of hormone production correlates directly with the level of total iodine transport into the gland. Normal uptake values vary according to the food iodine content, which depends on the region of the country. Typical values are now 9–30 percent of the dose taken up into the thyroid gland at 24 hours. In the presence of replacement doses of thyroid hormone, uptakes are suppressed to 1–2 percent at 24 hours; CT contrast dye typically suppresses uptake for up to six weeks.

J. Infection imaging

1. **⁶⁷Ga citrate** appears to be taken up by the cells near the region of the infection. ⁶⁷Ga imaging requires several days to complete and normal physiologic uptake (especially in the abdomen) interferes with interpretation. ⁶⁷Ga citrate imaging is very sensitive for making the diagnosis of *Pneumocystis* pneumonia at a relatively early stage. It is somewhat less sensitive than ¹¹¹In-labeled white blood cells (WBCs) in the postsurgical setting; the normal excretion of ⁶⁷Ga into the bowel is a drawback. Nevertheless, by using imaging methods that increase contrast, such as SPECT, satisfactory imaging can be obtained in the majority of cases.

2. **Radiolabeled (¹¹¹In or ⁹⁹ᵐTc) WBCs** progressively accumulate at the site of infection. The labeled WBC method requires external manipulation and labeling of the patient's blood; this procedure raises the possibility of misadministration, which can be fatal (e.g., if the donor is an acquired immunodeficiency syndrome [AIDS] patient). WBC imaging with ¹¹¹In shows uptake in the liver, spleen, and bone marrow, but not in other sites within the abdomen. Sensitivity for acute infection approaches 90 percent.

3. **New directions for inflammation imaging.** Radiolabeled monoclonal antibodies that label WBC in vivo, a variety of leukotropic peptides (that also label WBC in vivo), and a radiolabeled nonspecific immunoglobulin (accuracy rates: close to 90%) are in various stages of development and approval.

IV. Therapeutic radioisotopes

A. Iodine 131 for well-differentiated thyroid cancer

1. **Radiopharmaceutical agent.** Sodium iodide (¹³¹I), oral solution.

2. **Procedural notes.** (See Chap. 15, sec. III.) There is considerable variation in protocols of study. In most situations some form of testing for the ability of the tumor to concentrate radioactive iodine is performed. At the time of testing, patients are expected to be hypothyroid (thyroid-stimulating hormone [TSH] >30 IU/ml) and to have a low serum iodide (<5 μg/dl). Patients are taken off thyroid hormone (T_4 for six weeks and T_3 for three weeks) and placed on a low-iodide diet for three weeks prior to treatment.

3. **Dose selection.** A thyroid remnant, if present, is ablated with administered doses sufficient to deliver >30,000 rads to the normal thyroid. Several authorities treat with standard doses once uptake in thyroid cancer is demonstrated. Some experts simply treat all high-risk patients after thyroidectomy with more than 100 mCi of ¹³¹I. If lymph nodal metastases are demonstrated in the neck only, a dose of 150 mCi is sometimes used. For pulmonary, bone or CNS metastases, a dose of 200 mCi may be used. At Memorial Sloan Kettering Cancer Center, a protocol has been developed that administers a higher dose and depends on careful dosimetry (the "highest safe dose" approach).

4. **Treatment response.** Patients respond best to treatment when tumor is small (total tumor burden <200 grams) and confined to local or regional areas of the body. The cure rate at MSKCC was more than 95 percent for patients under 40 years of age and 50 percent for those over 40. Even when cure is not achieved, significant palliation can be obtained with ¹³¹I treatment.

5. **Follow-up.** Patients are normally evaluated at yearly intervals. Consideration for retreatment requires taking the patient off thyroid hormone, allowing hypothyroidism to develop, and treating with high-dose ¹³¹I until no appreciable ¹³¹I tissue is present ("clean slate"). Elevation of thyroglobulin levels indicates a high likelihood of recurrence of thyroid cancer at some time in the next five years in patients with well-differentiated thyroid cancer. In patients with unusually aggressive thyroid cancers, retreatment at a shorter interval can be considered (usually at about six months). The author usually requires tumor doses of at least 2000 rads. Ablation of known metastases has occurred with doses as low as 3500 rads, but 10,000 rads is usually required for lymph nodes containing tumor.

6. **Treatment complications.** The most common complication of high-dose ¹³¹I

treatment is sialadenitis, which occurs in about 20 percent of patients at dose above 200 mCi. Treatment with ^{131}I does not significantly increase the risk of leukemia.

B. ^{89}**Strontium chloride for pain from bone metastases**

1. **Radiopharmaceutical agent.** ^{89}Sr chloride [Metastron] (dosage: 4 mCi; 40–60 μCi/kg).

2. **Principle.** Various human tumors produce a strong osteoblastic reaction that results in the deposition of bone-seeking radionuclides in the hydroxyapatite crystal in the region of the tumor. When given in sufficient quantity, the radionuclide radiates the active boney regions near the metastases sufficiently to relieve pain. It is unclear whether the benefits of treatment are due to the irradiation of the bone or of the tumor itself. The usual dose is thought to be about 700–1000 rads.

3. **Procedural notes.** Patients should have platelet counts above 60,000/μL and WBCs above 2400/μL, and an osteoblastic response on bone scan demonstrated within three weeks of the treatment. Patients should not be treated with ^{89}Sr unless their life expectancy is at least three months.

   a. CBCs should be repeated every two weeks for four months. Platelet and WBC counts are typically decreased by about 30 percent and the nadir counts occur 12–16 weeks after injection.

   b. Because the radioactivity is primarily excreted in the urine, the patient should be continent or catheterized to minimize contamination of clothing and the patient's home environment.

   c. Patients may be considered for retreatment, usually after 90 days, if they have responded well to initial therapy, and provided that hematopoietic toxicity has not been excessively severe. Most patients tolerate multiple injections without major side effects.

   d. Pregnancy is an absolute contraindication. Women of childbearing age should have a pregnancy test the day prior to administering ^{89}Sr.

4. **Treatment response.** Patients with cancers of the prostate, breast, and lung have been treated with Metastron, but in principle, any tumor with an osteoblastic component on bone scan could be treated with this agent. The usual onset of pain relief occurs within 7–21 days after administration. Patients should be counseled about the possibility of a "flare response," in which pain is increased for a period of days to weeks following the treatment. A significant proportion of patients (said to be 75–80%) do get significant pain relief, and the typical duration of response is 3–4 months.

C. ^{32}**Phosphorus for polycythemia vera (PV)**

1. **Radiopharmaceutical agent.** The usual form of ^{32}P is a sodium phosphate solution buffered with sodium acetate in isotonic saline.

2. **Dosage.** Intravenous doses of 2.3 mCi/m^2 (dose not to exceed 5.0 mCi) are administered at three-month intervals to induce remission or control excessive cellular proliferation. The dose may be repeated twice if a remission is not achieved and is increased by 25 percent at each dose (not to exceed 7.0 mCi as a single dose).

3. **Treatment response.** About 80 percent of patients with PV achieve remission after one injection of ^{32}P. In comparison to phlebotomy alone, patients treated with ^{32}P survive longer and have fewer thrombotic complications but have an increased incidence of AML.

4. **Contraindications.** Pregnancy is an absolute contraindication because of the possibility of teratogenic effects. In PV, the drug should not be administered when the WBC count is less than 5000/μL or platelets are less than 150,000/μL.

D. Colloidal ^{32}**P for malignant effusions**

1. **Radiopharmaceutical agent.** Chromic phosphate ^{32}P is a colloidal suspension in sterile, pyrogen-free saline.

2. **Dosage.** In a 70-kg patient, 6–12 mCi are used for intrapleural administration and 10–20 mCi for intraperitoneal administration. For interstitial injection, the size of the tumor is used as a guide; doses range from 0.1 to

0.5 mCi/gm. Great care should be taken to ensure that all radioactivity is deposited in the intended body cavity. Large tumor masses or loculation of fluid is a relative contraindication to treatment.

3. **Treatment response.** Most patients receive some benefit from treatment in terms of control of effusions. There is a growing interest in the treatment of low-volume ovarian cancer. Mostly anecdotal reports suggest a longer survival in patients with ovarian cancer who have received ^{32}P.

Selected Reading

Coleman, R. E. (ed.) Nuclear medicine. *Radiol. Clin. North Am.* 31:721, 1993.

Miller, J. H., and Gelfand, M. J. *Pediatric Nuclear Medicine.* Philadelphia: Saunders 1994.

Palmer, E. L., Scott, J. A., and Strauss, H. W. *Practical Nuclear Medicine.* Philadelphia: Saunders 1992.

3

Radiation Therapy

Robert G. Parker

I. Mechanisms of action

A. Induction of damage to cells and tissues. Radiations in the energy range used clinically are absorbed through the physical processes of ionization and excitation of atoms and molecules. This process, which occurs in about 10^{-12} second, is similar for all types of "ionizing" radiations. Differences in observed effects of equal physical doses are related to differences in spatial or temporal distribution. Short-lived free radicals cause molecular damage and biochemical changes.

1. **Radiations** may be electromagnetic (x-rays, gamma rays) or corpuscular (electrons, protons, heavy ions, neutrons, alpha particles). Regardless of their origin (e.g., x-rays from linear accelerators, gamma rays from cobalt 60 or cesium 137, neutrons from a cyclotron), the basic biophysical mechanisms of action of all types of ionizing radiations are similar.

2. **Cell death.** Nearly all radiation-induced cell death results from disruption of the replication process (reproductive death). The direct killing of cells, unrelated to the replication process (interphase death), is infrequent and at clinical dose levels only occurs in highly sensitive cells such as lymphocytes and oocytes. Apoptosis (programmed cell death) following irradiation also appears to be important.

3. **Repair** of nonlethal and potentially lethal cellular damage occurs within a few hours and probably is never complete. While all mammalian cells have a narrow range of radiosensitivity ($D_0 = 110$–240 cGy), the more efficient repair and recovery processes of normal cells, compared to tumor cells, enables clinical exploitation through the application of multiple increments separated by more than 4–6 hours.

B. Radiosensitivity and radiocurability

1. **Radiosensitivity** is a measure of the susceptibility of cells to injury by ionizing (and exciting) radiations. The conventional measurement is the dose required to reduce a population of replicating cells to 37 percent of the initial value on the exponential portion of the cell survival curve. With photons, cellular radiosensitivity varies throughout the replication cycle, with maximal response during the late G_2 and early M phases (see Chap. 4, *Principles*, sec. I). With other radiations, such as neutrons, pions, and heavy ions, which provoke a high intensity of ionization events per unit path (high linear energy transfer), these variations in radiosensitivity throughout the replication cycle are reduced.

2. **Radioresistance** is the reciprocal to radiosensitivity and therefore is relative, not absolute. The terms *radiosensitivity* and *radioresistance* frequently are misused clinically because of the misconception that the rate of gross reduction of a tumor is the measure of effectiveness of treatment. Actually, gross tumor response also relates to other factors such as the rate of clearance of dead cells, tumor cell proliferation, and the proportion of intercellular material.

3. **Molecular oxygen** must be present at the time of irradiation for maximal cell killing. The probable mechanism is "fixation" of free radicals. Hypoxia may reduce cellular radiosensitivity by a factor of up to 3. This is the basis

of investigation of methods that reduce the adverse effects of tumor cell hypoxia, such as irradiation while the patient is in a hyperbaric chamber in 3 atm of oxygen, administration of hypoxic cell sensitizers (e.g., nitroimidazoles), and use of high linear energy transfer radiations.

   4. Cellular responses to ionizing radiations also can be modified by changes of the dose rate, manipulation of the process of repair of damage, synchronization of cells in the replication cycle, and heating cells, especially between 42.5° and 45°C for varying times.

   5. Radiocurability, the issue of importance to patients and their physicians, is more closely related to site and extent of tumor, its inherent biologic behavior, and a range of host-related factors than to radiosensitivity. Actually, the most radiocurable cancers are not those that grossly disappear rapidly, except for a few such as seminoma and dysgerminoma.

C. Dosimetry. For decades, the radiation dose was extrapolated from exposure doses measured in air (i.e., the roentgen). However, the absorbed dose at the anatomic point of interest has clinical relevance. A physical dose is now quantified in units of gray (Gy). One gray (one joule per kilogram of absorber) is equivalent to 100 rad in the old terminology; alternatively, one cGy equals one rad. The biologic effectiveness of a total physical dose is modified by dose rate, dose increment size when the total dose is given as a series of dose fractions, overall time and temporal pattern of application, anatomic part and tissue volume irradiated, and, to some extent, host factors that can influence radiosensitivity.

II. Clinical use. Like surgery and chemotherapy, radiation therapy (RT) has definite indications and contraindications for clinical application. It can be used alone or in combination with other methods, either as the major component of treatment or as an adjuvant. Currently, 50 to 60 percent of all patients with cancer receive RT during the course of their illness. Properly used, the intent of treatment for 50 percent of these patients should be cure. For the other half, incurable by any current method, palliation of specific symptoms and signs can improve the quality of life.

A. Treatment planning

   1. Essential pretreatment evaluation includes establishment of the diagnosis by biopsy, determination of tumor site and extent, and assessment of the host.

   2. After establishing whether the intent of treatment is curative or palliative, treatment planning includes identification of the target volume, which may consist of the primary tumor site and the high-risk sites of spread, selection of the treatment unit, design and verification of the pattern of delivery, and estimation of the dose, time, and pattern of application.

   3. Treatment with curative intent often is complicated, requiring professional skills and facilities that may be distant from the patient's home. Frequently, the doses to the target volume are higher than required for palliation and, consequently, the risks of unfavorable sequelae are higher. Such treatment is likely to be more prolonged and expensive.

   4. In contrast, palliative irradiation should have a specific objective, should minimize cost, inconvenience, discomfort, and risk, and should be completed in the shortest reasonable time.

B. Treatment with curative intent

   1. At this time, RT frequently may be the sole agent used with curative intent for anatomically limited tumors of the retina, optic nerve, brain (craniopharyngioma, medulloblastoma, ependymoma), spinal cord (low-grade glioma), skin, oral cavity, pharynx, larynx, esophagus, uterine cervix, vagina, prostate, and reticuloendothelial system (Hodgkin's disease, stages I, II, and IIIA).

   2. RT is combined with surgery for more extensive cancers of the head and neck, cancers of the lung, uterus, breast, ovary, urinary bladder, testis (seminoma), and rectum, and soft tissue sarcomas and primary bone tumors.

   3. RT is an adjuvant to chemotherapy for some patients with lymphomas, lung cancers, and cancer in children (rhabdomyosarcoma, Wilms' tumor, neuroblastoma).

C. Treatment with palliative intent. Objectives of palliative irradiation include relief of pain, usually from metastases to bone; relief of headache or neurologic dysfunction from intracranial metastases; relief of obstruction, such as from tumors involving the ureter, esophagus, bronchus, lymphatic or blood vessels; promotion of healing of surface wounds by local tumor control; preservation of the weight-bearing skeleton by control of metastases to bone; and preservation of vision by controlling metastasis to or invasion of the eye or of the orbit.

III. Technical modalities

A. Methods of delivery. Ionizing radiations may be delivered clinically in three ways:

1. External beam irradiation from sources at a distance (usually 80–100 cm) from the body. This includes ^{60}Co teletherapy units and x-ray sources, such as linear accelerators.
2. Local irradiation from sources (^{60}Co, ^{137}Cs, ^{192}Ir, ^{125}I) in contact with or near the target volume, such as with interstitial, intracavitary, or surface placement of radioactive isotopes in closed containers and direct x-ray therapy through short-distance cones.
3. Internal or systemic irradiation from radioactive sources (i.e., ^{131}I, ^{32}P, ^{89}Sr) administered enterally, intracavitarily, or intravenously.

B. Beam energy and penetration. Most clinical RT is done with beams of high-energy photons from linear accelerators or ^{60}Co teletherapy units. The radiations are absorbed exponentially in the body, which means that for a single beam, the intensity decreases continually with increasing depth.

1. The **penetration** of the radiations into the body is directly proportional to the generating energy. Penetration is characterized by the thickness of a specific material, such as aluminum, copper, or lead, which reduces the intensity of the radiation beam by 50 percent (half-value layer).
2. Clinically used **energies** range from 85 kV, for the treatment of tumors on the body surface, to 35 million V, for the treatment of tumors within the body. Compared to low-energy photons, high-energy photons are less absorbed in bone and are less side-scattered in the body, resulting in sharper beam margins. Inasmuch as x-rays are generated by high-energy electrons striking a target, removal of the target provides beams of electrons with limited penetration that can be used for tumors on or near the body surface.
3. Radiations such as **pi mesons** or **heavy ions**, currently used experimentally, deliver doses that are greater at the point of interest at a depth in the body than along the path of entry, through exploitation of the Bragg peak. Beams of high-energy **fast neutrons** produce more ionizations per unit path (high linear energy transfer) in an absorber than do high-energy photons. Such fast neutron beams have successfully tested experimentally in several tumors poorly responsive to conventional photon beams. High-energy **protons** have some dosimetric advantages but no clinically detectable radiobiological advantage over high-energy photons and electrons.

C. Brachytherapy (radiation sources in or close to the target volume) can deliver a very high dose to a restricted tissue volume containing tumor with relatively lower doses to adjacent normal tissues because of the proportional reduction of radiation intensity with increasing distance from the source. This method of application requires direct access to the target volume and so is most frequently used for cancers of the oral cavity, oropharynx, uterine cervix, and prostate. The actual placement of the radioactive sources often requires anesthesia of the patient and so generates risks not inherent in external beam irradiation.

IV. Side effects of RT. Every effective therapy may generate undesirable and even dangerous side effects. Although these side effects are inherent in the method, their frequency and severity are influenced by physician competence and philosophy, adequacy of equipment and facilities, operational quality assurance, and attitudes

of the patient and his or her family. Adverse effects of RT are summarized in Table 3-1.

A. Early radiation-induced reactions occur during or immediately following treatment and are self-limiting, although they may last for a few weeks. These sequelae may be local or constitutional and include anorexia, nausea, lassitude, esophagitis, diarrhea, skin reactions (erythema, desquamation), mucosal reactions, epilation, and hematopoietic suppression. The basic mechanism is damage of actively proliferating cells. Treatment is nearly always symptomatic, although the intensity of these temporary reactions usually can be reduced or even avoided by the use of smaller daily radiation doses or treatment of smaller volumes.

B. Late radiation-induced reaction. The clinically important, occasionally severe sequelae of radiation therapy become evident months or years after treatment. They are not proportional to early, acute reactions. Often they are progressive rather than self-limiting. They are local rather than systemic and include myelopathy; necrosis of bone; bowel stenosis; fibrosis of lung; skin devascularization, occasionally with ulceration; renal damage with loss of function; and pericardial and myocardial damage. Such undesirable sequelae should be very infrequent and are minimized by good treatment. Until recently, the primary mechanism was considered to be small vessel endarteritis and connective tissue proliferation. While these may be factors, a major mechanism is the damage of slowly proliferating cells. Since late sequelae often are progressive and treatment is ineffective, they must be anticipated and avoided or minimized whenever possible.

C. Influence of other treatment modalities. The side effects of RT influence other treatment methods and vice versa. For example, acute skin and mucosal radiation reactions are accentuated by concurrent or consecutive administration of dactinomycin, halogenated pyrimidines, or doxorubicin (Adriamycin) and may be reactivated by these drugs months after gross healing. Radiation-induced acute and late bowel damage is accentuated by prior abdominal surgery, presumably because of high doses delivered to segments of the bowel fixed by adhesions. Surgery at any site can be made more difficult by the presence of late radiation-induced small vessel endarteritis and soft tissue fibrosis.

Table 3-1. Adverse effects of radiation therapy

Site	Onset (dose in cGy)	
	Acute or Subacute	Subacute or Late
Head and neck		
Eyes	Corneal ulceration	Cataract (500)[a]
		Xerophthalmia (3000)
		Iridocyclitis, blindness (5000)
Ears, tongue	Otitis media (3000)	Deafness (<6000)
	Loss of taste (3000)	Meniere's syndrome (6000)
Mouth, salivary glands	Decreased saliva (2000)	Xerostomia, permanent (5000)
	Acute sialitis (1000)	
	Painful mucositis (4000)	Mucosal ulcer (6000)
Jaw		Osteonecrosis (6000)[b]
Larynx		Cartilage necrosis (>7000)
Heart	Pancarditis, pericarditis (4000)	Pericardial stricture, myocardiopathy (5000)
Lung	Pneumonitis (2000)	Pulmonary fibrosis (3000)
Gastrointestinal system		
Alimentary canal	Diarrhea (2000)	Strictures, ulcers, perforation, or fistulas (4500–5500)[c]
	Esophagitis (3000)	
	Proctitis (4000)	
		Chronic proctitis (6000)

Table 3-1 (continued)

	Onset (dose in cGy)	
Liver	Hepatitis (2500)	Liver failure (3500)
Biliary tract		Biliary stricture
Pancreas		Exocrine insufficiency
Genitourinary system		
Kidneys	Nephritis (2000)	Chronic nephritis, nephro-sclerosis (>2000)
Ureter		Stricture (7500)
Bladder	Cystitis (4000)	Chronic cystitis, ulcer (6500)
Prostate		Impotence[c]
Vagina		Ulcer, fistula (9000)
Uterus		Necrosis (>10,000)
Endocrine system		
Pituitary gland		Hypopituitarism (4500)[d]
Thyroid gland		Hypothyroidism (4500)
Adrenal gland		Hypoadrenalism (<6000)
Testes	Temporary hypospermia (200)	Sterility (1500)
Ovary	Temporary amenorrhea (300)	Permanent amenorrhea (1200)
Nervous system		
Brain	Somnolence syndrome (4500)	Brain necrosis (5500)
Spinal cord	Lhermitte's syndrome (4500)	Transverse myelitis (5000)[e]
Bone marrow		
Segmental		Marrow aplasia (3000)
Whole body		Marrow aplasia (200–400)
Other tissues		Fibrosis, sarcomas
Skin	Dry desquamation (5000) Moist desquamation (6000)	Atrophy, telangiectasia, induration, ulcer (5500)[f]
Lymphatics		Lymphedema
Breast		Atrophy, induration (5000)
Muscle		Atrophy (>10,000)
Bone, cartilage		Necrosis, fracture (6000)[g]
Fetus	Death (200–450)	
Systemic effect	Fatigue, anorexia, decreased libido	

The tolerance doses listed here (in cGy) are the minimal doses that result in a significant complication within normal tissues in 1–3% of patients within a five-year period after treatment (TD$_{3/5}$). In children, radiation can result in hypoplasia or arrested growth of the breast (1000), cartilage (1000), bone (1500), and muscle (2000).

[a]Incipient cataracts may be accelerated but in the young patient, more than 5000 cGy usually is required to produce a cataract. The development of cataracts is affected by the dose rate, method of irradiation, the patient's age, concomitant medical therapies, and comorbid medical conditions.

[b]The mandible often receives >7000 cGy without osteonecrosis developing; osteonecrosis can follow <6000 cGy with dental extraction or infection.

[c]Our patients receive >7000 cGy with external beam RT for cancer of the prostate; the clinical frequency of permanent rectal problems has been about 1% and most of our patients retain their potency.

[d]Many patients retain their pretreatment reduced pituitary function after 4500 cGy, and this loss is gradual.

[e]Myelopathy is related to dose increment and the segment irradiated. When the cervical cord is irradiated to 6000 cGy, less than 1% of patients develop problems.

[f]Atrophy and telangectasia may develop in the skin after a single increment of 2000 cGy if "superficial" x-rays are used, but the skin may remain pliable and of normal gross appearance after 5000–6000 cGy delivered in 180–200 cGy increments (e.g., the breast).

[g]Bone and cartilage can "tolerate" >6000 cGy until challenged by severe trauma or infection.

Source: Modified with permission from P. Rubin, and C. Poulter. Principles of Radiation Oncology and Cancer Radiotherapy. In P. Rubin (ed.), *Clinical Oncology for Medical Students and Physicians* (5th ed.). New York: American Cancer Society, 1978.

D. Hematosuppression. A major toxicity shared by ionizing radiations and many chemotherapy agents is suppression of bone marrow function. While recovery is usual after chemotherapy, recovery after irradiation is inversely proportional to dose and volume treated and may never be complete. Indeed, after doses in excess of 3000 cGy, the bone marrow may be replaced by fatty and fibrous tissue. The distribution of marrow in the human skeleton is shown in Fig. 34-1. Consequently, radiation therapy and chemotherapy must be carefully integrated so that hematopoietic suppression does not interrupt the therapeutic plan.

A recently recognized concern is the development of leukemia in some patients who receive both radiation therapy and chemotherapy with alkylating agents. For example, although patients curatively irradiated for anatomically limited Hodgkin's disease rarely develop leukemia, five to seven percent of those receiving both alkylating agents and radiation therapy for more extensive disease may develop leukemia.

Selected Reading

Hill, R. P. Cellular basis of radiotherapy. In Tannock, I. F. (ed.), *The Basic Science of Oncology* (2nd ed.), New York: McGraw Hill, 1992. Pp. 259–275.

Perez, C. A., and Brady, L. W. (eds.). *Principles and Practice of Radiation Oncology* (2nd ed.), Philadelphia: Lippincott, 1992.

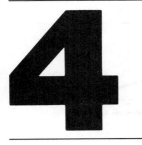

Cancer Chemotherapeutic Agents

Dennis A. Casciato and
Barry B. Lowitz

Principles

I. The cell cycle. The cell cycle is depicted in Fig. 4-1. Cell replication proceeds through a number of phases that are increasingly well-defined biochemically. Many cytotoxic agents act at more than one phase of the cell cycle, including those classified as "phase-specific." Certain oncogenes are activated at specific phases in the cell cycle.

A. In the G_0 phase (gap 0 or resting phase) cells are generally programmed to perform specialized functions. Cells in the G_0 phase are, for the most part, refractory to chemotherapy.

B. In the G_1 phase (gap 1 or interphase) proteins and RNA are synthesized for specialized cell functions. In late G_1 a burst of RNA synthesis occurs and many of the enzymes necessary for DNA synthesis are manufactured. G_1-phase specific drug: L-asparaginase.

C. In the S phase (DNA synthesis) the cellular content of DNA doubles. S-phase specific drugs: procarbazine and antimetabolites.

D. In the G_2 phase (gap 2) DNA synthesis ceases, protein and RNA synthesis continues, and the microtubular precursors of the mitotic spindle are produced. G_2-phase specific drugs: bleomycin and plant alkaloids.

E. In the M phase (mitosis) the rates of protein and RNA synthesis diminish abruptly while the genetic material is segregated into daughter cells. After completion of mitosis, the new cells enter either the G_0 or G_1 phase. M-phase specific drugs: plant alkaloids.

II. Mechanisms of drug activity

A. Categories of drugs. Cytotoxic agents can be *roughly* categorized by their activities relative to the cell generation cycle.

1. Phase nonspecific

a. Cycle-nonspecific drugs kill nondividing cells (e.g., steroid hormones, antitumor antibiotics except bleomycin).

b. Cycle-specific–phase-nonspecific drugs are effective only if the cells proceed through the generation cycle, but they can inflict injury at any point in the cycle (e.g., alkylating agents).

c. Pharmacokinetics. Cycle-nonspecific and cycle-specific–phase-nonspecific drugs generally have a linear dose-response curve: The greater the amount of drug administered, the greater the fraction of cells killed.

2. Phase specific

a. Cycle-specific–phase-specific drugs are effective only if present during a particular phase of the cell cycle.

b. Pharmacokinetics. Cycle-specific–phase-specific drugs reach a limit in cell-killing ability, but their effect is a function of both time and concentration (Fig. 4-2). Above a certain dosage level, further increases in drug dose do not result in more cell killing. If the drug concentration is maintained over a period of time, however, more cells enter the specific lethal phase of the cycle and are killed.

B. Population kinetics. Tumor growth depends on the size of the proliferating pool of cells and the number of cells dying spontaneously. The larger the tumor mass,

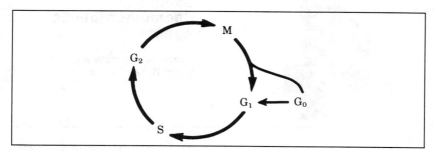

Fig. 4-1. Phases of cell growth.

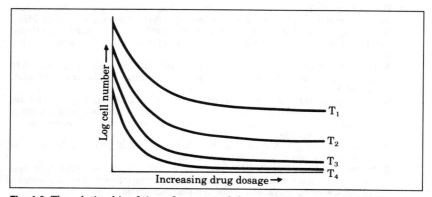

Fig. 4-2. The relationship of time of exposure of phase-specific drugs and cell killing ability. T_1 through T_4 represents progressively increasing lengths of time that cells are exposed to the drug at a particular dosage. These curves contrast with the linear relationship of log cell number and increasing drug dosage seen with phase-nonspecific drugs.

the greater the percentage of nondividing and dying cells and the longer it takes for the average cell to divide. Fig. 4-3 demonstrates the theoretic (Gompertzian) tumor growth curve. Some features of this sigmoid-shaped curve on logarithmic coordinates are:

1. Growth rate (doubling time) is rapid during early and exponential stages of growth. When the tumor is small and growing rapidly, a relatively high proportion of cells are undergoing division; that is, the "growth fraction" (ratio of dividing to total cells) is high.

2. The growth fraction decreases as the tumor gets larger and presumably should increase following therapies that reduce tumor volume. Growth rates eventually plateau because of restrictions of space, nutrient availability, and blood supply.

3. 1×10^9 cells represent one gram of tissue and the smallest number of tumor cells required to be clinically detectable (equivalent to a mass of 1 cm diameter found on chest x-ray film or by breast examination). Tumors with 10^{12} and 10^{13} cells (approximately 2–20 lb of cancer) usually result in damage to vital organs and death of the patient.

4. A 50 percent reduction in tumor mass represents only a one-third log decrease in tumor volume. For example, a tumor mass on x-ray film containing 8×10^{10} cells that is reduced to one-half its volume by chemotherapy still contains 4×10^{10} cells.

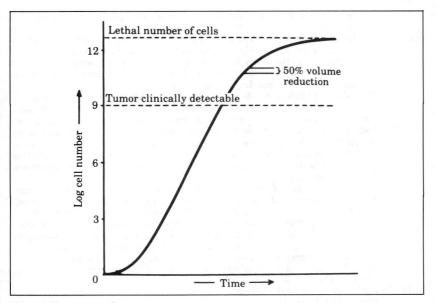

Fig. 4-3. Tumor growth.

III. Mechanisms of drug resistance

A. Tumor cell heterogeneity. Spontaneous genetic mutations occur in subpopulations of cancer cells prior to their exposure to chemotherapy. Some of these subpopulations are drug-resistant and grow to become the predominant cell type after chemotherapy has eliminated the sensitive cell lines. The *Goldie-Coldman hypothesis* indicates that the probability of a tumor population containing resistant cells is a function of the total number of cells present. This hypothesis asserts the high likelihood of the presence of drug-resistant mutants at the time of clinical presentation.

B. Single drug resistance

1. **Catabolic enzymes.** Exposure to a drug can induce the production of catabolic enzymes that result in drug resistance. The drug is catabolized more rapidly inside the cell by gene amplification of DNA for the specific catabolic enzymes. Examples include increased dihydrofolic reductase, which metabolizes methotrexate; deaminase, which deactivates cytarabine; and glutathione, which inactivates alkylating agents.

2. **Glutathione (GSH)** is essential for the synthesis of DNA precursors. Increased levels of GSH enzymes have been found in various cancers and not in their surrounding normal tissues. GSH and its enzymes scavenge free radicals and appear to play some role in inactivation of alkylating agents through direct binding, increased metabolism, detoxification, or repairing DNA damage. Alkylating agents share cross-resistance related to DNA repair in some settings.

3. **DNA topoisomerases.** DNA is attached at regular intervals to the nuclear matrix at sites called "domains," which are wound together with their paired DNA molecules. Topoisomerases participate in the separation and resealing of DNA molecules during cell division. Topoisomerase II is an enzyme believed to promote DNA strand breaks in the presence of amsacrine, anthracyclines, and epipodophyllotoxins.

   Some anticancer drugs (e.g., epipodophyllotoxins) exert their cytotoxic effect by inhibiting topoisomerase enzymes. Resistance to these drugs may develop with decreased drug access to the enzyme, alteration of the enzyme structure or activity, or by other mechanisms.

    4. Transport proteins. Exposure to a drug can induce the production of transport proteins that lead to drug resistance. As a result, smaller amounts of the drug enter the cell or larger amounts are carried out because of adaptive changes in cell membrane transport. Examples include methotrexate transport and the multiple drug resistance gene.

C. Multiple drug resistance. Resistance to many agents, particularly antimetabolites, may result from mutational changes unique to that agent. In other cases, however, a single mutational change following exposure to a single drug may lead to resistance to apparently unrelated chemotherapeutic agents (multidrug resistance [MDR]). The process appears to occur as a result of induction or amplification of the *mdr-1* gene. The gene product is a 170-dalton membrane glycoprotein (P-170), which functions as a pump and rapidly exports hydrophobic chemicals out of the cell.

    P-170 is a normal product of cells with inherent resistance to chemotherapy, including kidney, colon, and adrenal cells. P-170 membrane glycoprotein can be induced by and mediates the efflux of vinca alkaloids, anthracyclines, actinomycin D, epipodophyllotoxins, and colchicine. When exposed to one of these drugs, the cells become resistant to the others but remain sensitive to drugs of other classes (e.g., alkylating agents or antimetabolites). Calcium channel blockers (e.g., verapamil), amiodarone, quinidine, cyclosporine, phenothiazines, and other agents have been studied for their ability to reverse or block the effects of P-170.

IV. Clinical uses of cytotoxic agents

A. Indications. Chemotherapy is used

    1. To cure certain malignancies (see sec. **IV.C.1**)

    2. To palliate symptoms in patients with disseminated cancer when the potential benefits of treatment exceed the side effects of treatment

    3. To treat asymptomatic patients when

        a. The cancer is aggressive and treatable (e.g., acute leukemia, small cell lung cancer), *or*

        b. Treatment has been proved to decrease the rate of relapse and increase the disease-free interval or increase the absolute survival (stage C colon carcinoma, stages I or II breast carcinoma, osteogenic sarcoma)

B. Contraindications. Chemotherapeutic agents are relatively or absolutely contraindicated in the following situations:

    1. Facilities are inadequate to evaluate the patient's response to therapy and to monitor and manage toxic reactions.

    2. The patient is not likely to survive longer even if tumor shrinkage could be accomplished.

    3. The patient is not likely to survive long enough to obtain benefits from the drugs (e.g., severely debilitated patients).

    4. The patient is asymptomatic with slow-growing, incurable tumors, in which case chemotherapy should be postponed until symptoms require palliation.

C. Responsiveness of tumors to chemotherapy

    1. Curable. Tumors that are potentially curable by chemotherapy are

        a. Childhood cancers ($\geq 50\%$): acute lymphocytic leukemia, non-Hodgkin's lymphoma, Wilms' tumor, Ewing's sarcoma, retinoblastoma, rhabdomyosarcoma

        b. Hodgkin's disease, certain aggressive lymphomas ($\geq 50\%$)

        c. Carcinoma of the testis ($\geq 75\%$)

        d. Choriocarcinoma in women ($\geq 90\%$)

        e. Adult acute leukemia, ovarian carcinoma (15–20%)

    2. Improved survival. Tumors for which chemotherapy provides substantial improvement in survival but is rarely curative include

        a. Neuroblastoma (in childhood)

        b. Aggressive non-Hodgkin's lymphomas

        c. Small cell lung cancer

  d. Carcinoma of the breast

  e. Osteogenic sarcoma

3. Palliation. Chemotherapy may substantially palliate symptoms from some tumors even though the effects of treatment on survival are unknown or negligible. Examples include

  a. Non-Hodgkin's lymphoma (low or intermediate grade)

  b. Chronic leukemias

  c. Multiple myeloma

  d. Carcinoma of the prostate

  e. Endocrine gland cancers

4. Occasional responses. Tumors for which chemotherapy occasionally produces responses and, in some cases, modest improvement in survival at the expense of moderate to severe toxicity are

  a. Soft tissue sarcomas

  b. Brain cancers

  c. Non-oat cell lung carcinoma

  d. Carcinoma of the head and neck

  e. Transitional cell carcinomas (of the urinary bladder)

  f. Malignant melanoma (with skin or lymph node involvement)

5. Ineffective. Tumors for which chemotherapy rarely or never produces a meaningful tumor response or improved survival and which are best treated with experimental protocols or symptom management alone are

  a. Malignant melanoma (with visceral involvement)

  b. Pancreatic carcinoma

  c. Hypernephroma

V. Administration of and withholding of chemotherapeutic agents

A. Adjuvant chemotherapy is given to the patient with no evidence of residual disease but who is at high risk for relapse. The justifications for adjuvant chemotherapy are the high recurrence rate after surgery for apparently localized tumors, the inability to identify cured patients at the time of surgery, and the failure of therapy to cure these patients after recurrence of disease. The disadvantages of this therapy are the immediate patient discomfort and the short- and long-term risks of such treatment. To date, the only malignancies for which adjuvant chemotherapy has proven to be beneficial are breast cancer, stage C colon cancer, and osteogenic sarcoma.

B. Dose intensification has received increasing emphasis in recent years as a strategy for overcoming resistance to chemotherapy. This principle has generated the notion that drugs in combination chemotherapy regimens should be given in the highest tolerated dose over the briefest interval, perhaps even with patient rescue maneuvers such as the intensive utilization of hematopoietic growth factors, autologous marrow stem cell infusion, or allogeneic bone marrow transplantation. Although dose intensification is being tested in certain malignancies, such as breast cancer, the concept that more chemotherapy is better than regimens using "standard doses" remains to be proven.

C. Monitoring therapy. Administration of chemotherapeutic agents requires knowledge of the extent of disease, toxicity of the previous treatment courses, and timing of the expected drug toxicity. Flow sheets with dates, doses, responses, side effects, and pertinent laboratory values are mandatory.

D. Administering cytotoxic agents intravenously

1. Vein selection. Large veins in the forearm are preferred. Metacarpal veins on the dorsum of the hand are second choice. If possible, avoid the antecubital fossa and wrist because extravasation in these areas can result in loss of function. Management of patients with insufficient venous access is discussed in Chapter 5, sec. **XI.**

2. Administering irritants and vesicants must be accomplished through a freely flowing intravenous line with extreme caution to avoid extravasation. The management of extravasation is discussed in Chap. 28, sec. **IV.B.**

  a. Irritants may produce burning or inconsequential inflammation during infusion or when extravasated, but usually without necrosis. Irritants include carmustine (BCNU), cisplatin, dacarbazine (DTIC), etoposide, plicamycin, and vinca alkaloids.

b. Vesicants cause pain, edema, induration, ulceration, and eventually necrosis when extravasated. Vesicant drugs are tabulated in Appendix B-1 and particularly include anthracyclines, dactinomycin, mitomycin, and nitrogen mustard.

VI. Adverse effects of chemotherapy

A. General effects. The adverse effects of chemotherapeutic agents are summarized in Appendix B-1. Many patients complain of malaise and fatigue, which may last a week or longer. Fever and chills following certain drugs typically begin six hours after therapy and may last up to 24 hours. Alopecia usually begins two to three weeks after drugs are given.

B. Guidelines for modifying drug dosage

1. **Principles.** Cytotoxic agents should not be prescribed by physicians inexperienced in their use. Cytotoxic drugs must be prescribed in full doses to be effective. Dosages are modified according to the curability of the tumor and to established guidelines for each drug or regimen. Chemotherapy is generally postponed if the patient has an **infection** of any type, persistent **toxicity** from previous treatments, or significant **debility** from cancer (Karnofsky scale performance status less than 50%). Tumors that are highly aggressive but responsive and life-threatening (e.g., acute leukemia, widespread small cell lung cancer) are exceptions to withholding treatment for those problems.

   a. Radiotherapy. Patients previously or simultaneously treated with radiation generally should be started at about 50 percent of the recommended dose of myelosuppressive drugs. Subsequent doses can be escalated if acceptable toxicity results from the initial dose.

   b. In vitro chemosensitivity assays are very expensive, technically problematic, and not yet proven to be clinically useful. Their utility perhaps may lie in identifying which cytotoxic agents should not be used based on extreme resistance of cloned tumor cells. However, that information is frequently useless in patients with malignancies that are substantially responsive only to limited choices of drugs or drug combinations.

2. **Myelosuppression.** The different effects of cytotoxic agents on leukocyte and platelet counts are compared in Appendix B-1. Myelosuppressive drugs generally should not be administered to a patient with a solid tumor who has an absolute neutrophil count (ANC) less than 2000/μL or a platelet count less than 120,000/μL. For such a patient, increasing the interval between doses is preferable to decreasing the dosage. Depending on the goals of treatment, dosage can also be modified based on the severity of the lowest (nadir) counts.

   The length of time it takes after treatment to reach the nadir is different for the various agents. Most myelotoxic agents result in a nadir at 10 days with recovery in 3–4 weeks. For busulfan, melphalan, DTIC and procarbazine the nadir develops in 2–4 weeks with recovery in about six weeks. For nitrosoureas, the nadir (often two separate nadirs) develops in 4–5 weeks with recovery in 6–8 weeks, and the time to recovery usually lengthens with each course of treatment.

3. **Alimentary tract toxicity.** Nausea and vomiting after chemotherapy is discussed in Chap. 5, sec. III.A.2. Drugs that cause mucositis or diarrhea must not be given until the patient has fully recovered from these symptoms. Subsequent dose reduction often is indicated.

4. **Abnormal renal function.** Drugs that cause renal toxicity (particularly methotrexate, cisplatin, and streptozocin) should not be administered unless the creatinine clearance is greater than 55 ml/min; the use of reduced doses with lower clearance rates is not recommended. Other drugs that are excreted in the urine may require dose reduction in the presence of renal dysfunction (see Appendix B-1).

5. **Abnormal liver function.** In the presence of hepatic functional impairment, doses of the vinca alkaloids and anthracyclines (Adriamycin, daunorubicin)

must be reduced. Other drugs that are excreted in the bile require some dose reduction or cautious administration (see Appendix B-1).

Chemotherapeutic Agents

I. Alkylating agents

A. General pharmacology of alkylating agents. Alkylating agents target DNA and are cytotoxic, mutagenic, and carcinogenic. All agents produce alkylation through the formation of intermediates.

1. Alkylating agents impair cell function by transferring alkyl groups to amino, carboxyl, sulfhydryl, or phosphate groups of biologically important molecules. Most importantly, nucleic acids (DNA and RNA) and proteins are alkylated. The number 7 (N-7) position of guanine in DNA and RNA is the most actively alkylated site; the O-6 group of guanine is alkylated by nitrosoureas. Alkylation of guanine results in abnormal nucleotide sequences, miscoding of messenger RNA, cross-linked DNA strands that cannot replicate, breakage of DNA strands, and other damage to the transcription and translation of genetic material.

2. The primary mode of action for most alkylating agents is via cross-linking of DNA strands. Cytotoxicity is probably due to damage to the DNA templates rather than to inactivation of DNA polymerase and other enzymes responsible for DNA synthesis. DNA strand breakage also appears to be a minor determinant of cytotoxicity.

3. Alkylating agents are cell cycle–specific but not phase specific. The drugs kill a fixed percentage of cells at a given dose.

4. Tumor resistance to these drugs appears to be related to the capacity of cells to repair nucleic acid damage and to inactivate the drugs by conjugation with glutathione.

B. Busulfan (Myleran)

1. **Indications.** Chronic myelogenous leukemia, myeloproliferative disorders, bone marrow transplantation (high doses)

2. **Pharmacology**
   a. **Mechanism.** Alkylation (see sec. **A.**)
   b. **Metabolism.** Acts directly; catabolized to inactive products that are excreted in the urine.

3. **Toxicity**
   a. **Dose-limiting.** Reversible and irreversible myelosuppression with slow recovery; blood cell counts fall for about two weeks after discontinuation of drug.
   b. **Common.** Gastrointestinal (GI) upset (mild), sterility
   c. **Occasional.** Skin hyperpigmentation, alopecia, rash; gynecomastia, cataracts, liver function test (LFT) abnormalities
   d. **Rare.** Pulmonary fibrosis ("busulfan lung", see Chap. 29, sec. **IV.A.**), retroperitoneal fibrosis, endocardial fibrosis; Addisonian-like asthenia (without biochemical evidence of adrenal insufficiency); hypotension, impotence, hemorrhagic cystitis, secondary neoplasms

4. **Administration**
   a. **Supplied** as 2-mg tablets
   b. **Dose modification.** Hematologic
   c. **Dose.** Usually 2–8 mg/day PO; *or* 0.05 mg/kg/day

C. Chlorambucil (Leukeran)

1. **Indications.** Chronic lymphocytic leukemia, Waldenström's macroglobulinemia, indolent lymphomas, myeloma, trophoblastic neoplasms, some carcinomas

2. **Pharmacology**
   a. **Mechanism.** Alkylation (see **A**)
   b. **Metabolism.** Acts directly; spontaneously hydrolysed to inactive and active products (e.g., phenylacetic acid mustard); some is also metab-

olized in the liver. Native drug and metabolic products excreted in urine.

3. Toxicity. Least toxic alkylating agent
   a. Dose-limiting. Myelosuppression (usually moderate, gradual, and reversible)
   b. Occasional. GI upset (minimal or absent at usual doses), mild LFT abnormalities, sterility
   c. Rare. Rash, alopecia, fever; cachexia, pulmonary fibrosis, neurologic or ocular toxicity, cystitis; acute leukemia

4. Administration
   a. Supplied as 2-mg tablets
   b. Dose modification. Hematologic
   c. Dose. Various dosage schedules are used. For example, 0.05–0.20 mg/kg/day PO for 3–6 weeks, then decrease dose for maintenance (usually 2 mg/day); *or* 0.4 mg/kg every 2–4 weeks.

D. Cyclophosphamide (Cytoxan, Neosar, Endoxan)
   1. Indications. Used in a wide variety of conditions.
   2. Pharmacology
      a. Mechanism. Alkylation (see **A**); plus it also inhibits DNA synthesis.
      b. Metabolism. Native drug is inactive and requires activation by liver microsomal oxidase system to form an aldehyde that decomposes in plasma and peripheral tissues to yield acrolein and an alkylating metabolite (e.g., phosphoramide mustard). The liver also metabolizes metabolites to inactive compounds. Drugs that induce microsomal enzymes (e.g., barbiturates, griseofulvin) may enhance toxicity; liver disease may decrease toxicity. Native drug is not protein bound, but active products are 50 percent protein bound. Active and inactive metabolites are excreted in urine.
   3. Toxicity
      a. Dose-limiting
         (1) Myelosuppression. Leukopenia develops 8–14 days after administration. Thrombocytopenia occurs but rarely is significant.
         (2) Effects on urinary bladder. Degradative products are responsible for hemorrhagic cystitis, which can be prevented by maintaining a high urine output. Hemorrhagic cystitis is more common and can be severe when massive doses are used (e.g., for bone marrow transplantation); under these circumstances, the use of mesna can be preventative. Bladder fibrosis with telangiectasis of the mucosa can occur (usually after long-term oral therapy) without episodes of cystitis. Bladder carcinoma has occurred.
      b. Side effects
         (1) Common. Alopecia, stomatitis, aspermia, amenorrhea; headache (fast onset, short duration). Nausea and vomiting are common after doses greater than or equal to 700 mg/m^2 beginning 6–10 hours after administration.
         (2) Occasional. Skin or fingernail hyperpigmentation; metallic taste during injection; sneezing or a cold sensation in the nose after injection; abnormal LFTs, dizziness; allergy, fever
         (3) Rare. Transient syndrome of inappropriate secretion of antidiuretic hormone (SAIDH) (especially if given with a large volume of fluid), hypothyroidism, cataracts, jaundice, pulmonary fibrosis; cardiac necrosis and acute myopericarditis (massive doses); secondary neoplasms (acute leukemia, bladder carcinoma)
   4. Administration. The drug should be administered with a large volume of fluid in the morning or early afternoon to avoid cystitis.
      a. Supplied as 25-mg or 50-mg tablets; vials contain 100 to 1000 mg
      b. Dose modification. Hematologic; may be required for hepatic functional impairment
      c. Dose. Cyclophosphamide is frequently employed as part of combination

chemotherapy regimens (see Appendix A). Some common doses are 0.5 to 1.5 g/m^2 IV every 3 weeks or 50–200 mg/m^2 PO for 14 days every 28 days.

    d. Drug interactions. With warfarin to further prolong the prothrombin time; with succinyl choline to increase neuromuscular blockade.

E. Ifosfamide (Isophosphamide, Ifex)

  1. Indications. A wide variety of neoplasms, especially lymphomas, sarcomas, and relapsed testicular carcinoma

  2. Pharmacology

    a. Mechanisms. An alkylating agent (see **A**); DNA cross-linking and chain breakage. Metabolites are alkylating agents that are similar to cyclophosphamide but not cross-resistant.

    b. Metabolism. Inactive until activated by hepatic microsomal enzymes. Like cyclophosphamide, the drug undergoes hepatic activation to an aldehyde form that decomposes in plasma and peripheral tissues to yield acrolein and its alkylating metabolite. Acrolein is highly toxic to urothelial mucosa. The chloroacetaldehyde metabolite may be responsible for much of the neurotoxic effects, particularly in patients with renal dysfunction. Metabolites and unaltered drug (15–55%) are excreted in the urine.

  3. Toxicity

    a. Dose-limiting. Myelosuppression; hemorrhagic cystitis

    b. Common. Alopecia, nausea and vomiting

    c. Neurotoxicity (especially when given in one day rather than five days and when renal dysfunction is present or when sedatives are given); lethargy, dizziness, confusion, ataxia, coma

    d. Occasional. Salivation, stomatitis, diarrhea, constipation; urticaria, hyperpigmentation, nail ridging; abnormal LFTs, phlebitis, fever; hypotension, hypertension, hyponatremia, hypokalemia; renal tubular acidosis (at high doses)

  4. Administration. Aggressive concomitent hydration (2–4 liters per day) and mesna are given to reduce the incidence of hemorrhagic cystitis.

    a. Supplied as 1- and 3-gm vials; mesna is available as 400 mg vials

    b. Dose modification. Hematologic and renal dysfunction

    c. Dose. 1000–1200 mg/m^2 IV over 30 minutes for five days every 3–4 weeks.

    d. Mesna (sodium 2-mercaptoethanesulfonate). The total dose of mesna is 60 percent of the ifosfamide dose. Twenty percent of the ifosfamide dose is given just before, four hours after, and eight hours after ifosfamide. The last dose of mesna can be given PO to allow the patient to leave the hospital sooner. When given as a continuous infusion, mesna and ifosfamide can be mixed in equal dosages, preceded by a mesna loading dose of about 10 percent of the total ifosfamide dose.

F. Melphalan (Alkeran, phenylalanine mustard, L-PAM, L-sarcolysin)

  1. Indications. Multiple myeloma, ovarian carcinoma, other carcinomas. The injection form is used in bone marrow transplantation (BMT) studies and limb perfusion for melanoma.

  2. Pharmacology

    a. Mechanism. Alkylation (see **A**)

    b. Metabolism. Acts directly. Ninety percent of the drug is bound to plasma proteins and undergoes spontaneous hydrolysis in the bloodstream to inert products. Melphalan is excreted in the urine as unchanged drug and metabolites.

  3. Toxicity

    a. Dose-limiting. Myelosuppression may be cumulative and recovery may be prolonged.

    b. Occasional. Anorexia, nausea, vomiting, mucositis, sterility

    c. Rare. Alopecia, pruritus, rash, hypersensitivity; secondary malignancies (acute leukemia); pulmonary fibrosis, vasculitis, cataracts

4. **Administration**
   a. **Supplied** as 2-mg tablets and 50-mg vials
   b. **Dose modification.** Hematologic; administer cautiously in patients with azotemia
   c. **Dose.** If no myelosuppression is observed after oral dosing, poor oral absorption should be suspected.
      (1) **Continuous therapy.** 0.10–0.15 mg/kg PO daily for 2–3 weeks; no therapy for 2–4 weeks, *then* 2–4 mg PO daily *or*
      (2) **Pulse therapy.** 0.25 mg/kg (10 mg/m^2) PO daily for four days every 4–6 weeks (with prednisone for myeloma)

G. **Nitrogen mustard** (mechlorethamine, Mustargen, HN$_2$)
   1. **Indication.** Hodgkin's disease and a variety of other oncologic conditions
   2. **Pharmacology**
      a. **Mechanism.** Rapid alkylation of DNA, RNA, and protein (see **A**)
      b. **Metabolism.** Native drug is highly active and is very rapidly deactivated within the blood by spontaneous hydrolysis; the elimination half-life is 15 minutes. Metabolites are mostly excreted in the urine.
   3. **Toxicity**
      a. **Dose-limiting.** Myelosuppression
      b. **Common.** Severe nausea and vomiting beginning one hour after administration; skin necrosis if extravasated (sodium thiosulfate may be tried); metallic taste; discoloration of the infused vein
      c. **Occasional.** Alopecia, sterility, diarrhea, thrombophlebitis
      d. **Rare.** Neurotoxicity (including hearing loss), angioedema, secondary neoplasms
   4. **Administration.** Patients should always be premedicated with antiemetics. The drug should be administered through the tubing of a running IV line using extravasation precautions.
      a. **Supplied** as 10-mg vials
      b. **Dose modification.** Hematologic; none required for hepatic or renal impairment
      c. **Dose.** 0.2–0.4 mg/kg (10 mg/m^2) as a single or divided dose monthly or 6 mg/m^2 on day one and day eight of the MOPP regimen.

H. **Nitrosoureas.** Carmustine (BCNU, bischlorethyl, nitrosourea); lomustine (CCNU, cyclohexyl chlorethyl nitrosourea, CeeNU); semustine (methyl-CCNU, an investigational agent); streptozocin (streptozotocin), which is a nitrosourea with a different mechanism of action (see sec. **I.I.**)
   1. **Indications.** Brain cancer, Hodgkin's disease, lymphomas, multiple myeloma, melanoma, and some carcinomas
   2. **Pharmacology**
      a. **Mechanism.** Alkylation of DNA and RNA (see **A**); DNA cross-linking; inhibition of DNA polymerase, DNA repair, and RNA synthesis
      b **Metabolism.** Highly lipid-soluble drugs that enter the brain. Rapid spontaneous decomposition to active and inert products; the drugs also undergo metabolic transformation. Most of the intact drug and metabolic products are excreted in urine; some products have an enterohepatic cycle.
   3. **Toxicity**
      a. **Dose-limiting.** Myelosuppression is prolonged, cumulative, and substantially aggravated by concurrent radiation therapy.
      b. **Common.** Nausea and vomiting may last 8–24 hours. BCNU causes local pain during injection or hypotension during a too rapid or concentrated injection.
      c. **Occasional.** Stomatitis, esophagitis, diarrhea, LFT abnormalities; alopecia, facial flushing, brown discoloration of skin; lung fibrosis (with prolonged therapy and higher doses); dizziness, optic neuritis, ataxia, organic brain syndrome; renal insufficiency.
      d. **Rare.** Secondary malignancies.

4. Administration

a. **Supplied** as 100-mg vials of BCNU; 10-, 40-, and 100-mg capsules of CCNU

b. **Dose modification.** Hematologic and renal

c. **Dose**

(1) **BCNU.** 150–200 mg/m^2 IV (as a single dose or divided over two days) every 6–8 weeks. Do not infuse over longer than two hours owing to incompatibility of the drug with IV tubing. If blood and BCNU are mixed in the syringe prior to administration, the painfulness of injection may be decreased.

(2) **CCNU.** 100–130 mg/m^2 PO every 6–8 weeks.

d. **Drug interactions.** With cimetidine to decrease nitrosourea metabolism, resulting in increased hematosuppression

I. Streptozocin (streptozotocin, Zanosar)

1. Indications. Islet cell cancer of the pancreas (in combination with fluorouracil), Hodgkin's disease, carcinoid syndrome

2. Pharmacology

a. **Mechanism.** Alkylating agent (see **A**). Inhibits DNA synthesis and the DNA repair enzyme, guanine-O^6-methyl transferase. Affects pyrimidine nucleotide metabolism and inhibits enzymes involved in gluconeogenesis.

b. **Metabolism.** Drug is a type of nitrosourea that is extensively metabolized and has a short plasma half-life. Crosses the blood-brain barrier. Excreted in urine as metabolites and unchanged drug.

3. Toxicity

a. **Dose-limiting.** Nephrotoxicity initially appears as proteinuria and progresses to glycosuria, aminoaciduria, proximal renal tubular acidosis, and renal failure if the drug is continued.

b. **Common.** Nausea and vomiting (often severe), myelosuppression (mild, but may be cumulative), hypoglycemia following infusion, vein irritation during infusion

c. **Occasional.** Diarrhea, abdominal cramps, LFT abnormalities

d. **Rare.** Central nervous system (CNS) toxicity, fever, secondary malignancies.

4. Administration. Urinalysis and serum creatinine levels are monitored before each dose. Patients are routinely premedicated with antiemetics. The dose is administered slowly over 30–60 minutes to prevent local pain.

a. **Supplied** as 1-gm vials

b. **Dose modification.** Proteinuria or elevated serum creatinine levels contraindicate use of the drug until the abnormalities resolve.

c. **Dose**

(1) 1.0–1.5 gm/m^2 IV weekly, *or*

(2) 0.5–1.0 gm/m^2 IV daily for five days every 3–4 weeks

J. Thiotepa (Thio-TEPA, triethylenethiophosphoramide)

1. Indications. Intracavitary for malignant effusions, intravesicular for urinary bladder, local treatment for skin metastases

2. Pharmacology

a. **Mechanism.** Alkylation (see sec. **A**)

b. **Metabolism.** Rapidly decomposed in plasma and excreted in urine

3. Toxicity

a. **Dose-limiting.** Myelosuppression, which may be cumulative

b. **Common (for intravesicular administration).** Abdominal pain, hematuria, dysuria, frequency, urgency, ureteral obstruction

c. **Occasional.** GI upset, abnormal LFTs, rash, hives

d. **Rare.** Alopecia, fever, angioedema

4. Administration. Thiotepa has been administered IV, IM, intravesicularly, intrathecally, intra-arterially, intrapleurally, intrapericardially, intraperitoneally, intratumorally, and as an ophthalmic instillation.

      a. Supplied as 15-mg vials

      b. Dose modification. Necessary for patients with cytopenias. Apnea can occur in patients receiving succinylcholine.

      c. Dose. Intravenous: 12–16 mg/m^2 every 1–4 weeks; Intravesicular: 15–60 mg every week for four weeks.

II. Other agents with alkylator activity

A. General pharmacology. This group of compounds comprise heavy metal alkylators (platinum complexes) that act predominantly by covalent bonding and "non-classic alkylating agents." The latter usually contain a chloromethyl group and an important N-methyl group. They typically must undergo metabolic transformation to active intermediates that alkylate or covalently bond biologic macromolecules.

B. Amsacrine (m-AMSA, AMSA, acridinylanisidide, 4'-(9-acridinylamino)methanesulfon-m-anisidide)

  1. Indications (experimental). Second-line therapy of acute myelogenous leukemia

  2. Pharmacology

    a. Mechanisms of action. Alkylating agent. Intercalates with DNA and also inhibits topoisomerase II

    b. Metabolism. Metabolized in the liver and excreted in the bile and urine as unchanged drug and metabolites.

  3. Toxicity

    a. Dose-limiting. Leukopenia

    b. Common. Mild thrombocytopenia; tissue damage with infiltration; alopecia, phlebitis, stomatitis, diarrhea; orange urine, yellow skin color

    c. Occasional. Mucositis, vomiting, abnormal LFTs; cardiac arrhythmias, congestive heart failure (cardiac arrests have occurred during infusion of the drug, usually in the presence of hypokalemia)

    d. Rare. Urticaria, rash; headache, dizziness, neuropathy, seizures

  4. Administration. Ensure that serum potassium levels are normal.

    a. Supplied as a 50 mg/ml vial of amsacrine in N,N-dimethylacetamide (DMA) and a vial of diluent. Glass syringes must be used for the concentrated solution because the DMA dissolves plastic.

    b. Dose modification. Use cautiously with hepatic dysfunction.

    c. Dose. 90–150 mg/m^2 IV daily for five days for acute leukemia.

C. Carboplatin (Paraplatin, carboplatinum, CBDCA)

  1. Indications. Ovarian and other carcinomas. Carboplatin is an alternative to cisplatin where renal or neural toxicity are dose-limiting considerations.

  2. Pharmacology

    a. Mechanisms. Heavy metal alkylating-like agent with mechanisms very similar to cisplatin, but with different toxicity profile. Cisplatin and carboplatin exhibit substantial clinical cross-resistance.

    b. Metabolism. Plasma half-life of only 2–3 hours. Excreted in the urine as unchanged drug (60%) and metabolites.

  3. Toxicity

    a. Dose-limiting. Myelosuppression, especially thrombocytopenia, with cumulative suppression of erythropoiesis

    b. Common. Nausea and vomiting (less severe than with cisplatin), pain at injection site

    c. Occasional. Abnormal LFTs, azotemia

    d. Rare. Alopecia, rash, flu-like syndrome, hematuria, hyperamylasemia; peripheral neuropathy (especially in patients >65 years old), hearing loss, optic neuritis

  4. Administration

    a. Supplied as 50-, 150-, 450-mg vials

    b. Dose modification. Reduce dosage for creatinine clearance less than or equal to 60 ml/minute. Be cautious when concomitantly administering other myelosuppressive or nephrotoxic drugs.

    c. Dose. 300–400 mg/m^2 IV over 15–60 minutes every four weeks

D. Cisplatin (cisplatinum, *cis*-diaminedichloroplatinum, CDDP, DDP, Platinol)

1. **Indications.** A wide variety of malignancies

2. **Pharmacology**

   a. **Mechanism.** A heavy metal alkylator of DNA (see sec. **A**). Covalently bonds to proteins, RNA, and especially DNA, forming DNA cross-linking and intrastrand N-7 adducts. The *trans* isomer has virtually no antitumor activity. May augment immune function at therapeutic doses. Acquired resistance to cisplatin involves alterations in transmembrane transport of drugs, intracellular levels of GSH or sulfhydryl-containing proteins, and the capacity to repair cisplatin-DNA lesions.

   b. **Metabolism.** Ninety percent of the drug is protein-bound. Widely distributed in body except the central nervous system. Long half-life in plasma (up to three days); may remain bound in tissues for months. Native drug (30%) and metabolites excreted in urine; biliary excretion accounts for less than 10 percent of the total drug excretion.

3. **Toxicity**

   a. **Dose-limiting**

      (1) **Cumulative renal insufficiency.** The incidence of renal insufficiency is about 5 percent with adequate hydration measures and 25–45 percent without hydration measures. Nephrotoxicity (and perhaps ototoxicity) is increased by concurrent administration of nephrotoxic drugs such as aminoglycoside antibiotics, methotrexate, or amphotericin B.

      (2) **Peripheral sensory neuropathy** develops after the administration of 200 mg/m^2 and can become dose-limiting when the cumulative cisplatin dose exceeds 400 mg/m^2. Symptoms may progress after treatment is discontinued and include loss of proprioception and vibratory senses, hyporeflexia, and Lhermitte's sign. Symptoms may resolve slowly after many months but are aggravated by further dosing.

      (3) **Ototoxicity** with tinnitus and high-frequency hearing loss occurs in 5 percent of patients. Ototoxicity occurs more commonly in patients receiving doses more than 100 mg/m^2 by rapid infusion or high cumulative doses.

   b. **Common.** Severe nausea and vomiting occur in all treated patients and last more than 24 hours without use of effective preventative antiemetic regimens. Hypokalemia, hypomagnesemia (occasionally difficult to correct) and mild myelosuppression

   c. **Occasional.** Alopecia, loss of taste, vein irritation, abnormal LFTs, SIADH, hypophosphatemia, myalgia, fever

   d. **Rare.** Altered color perception and reversible focal encephalopathy that often causes cortical blindness. Raynaud's phenomenon, bradycardia, bundle-branch block, congestive heart failure; anaphylaxis, tetany

4. **Administration**

   a. **Supplied** as 10- and 50-mg vials

   b. **Dose modification.** Renal function must return to normal before cisplatin can be given. Many physicians avoid using cisplatin when the creatinine clearance is less than 40 ml/minute. Cisplatin is relatively contraindicated in patients with documented hearing impairment.

   c. **Dose**

      (1) 40–120 mg/m^2 or more IV every 3–4 weeks *or*

      (2) 20–40 mg/m^2 IV daily for 3–5 days every 3–4 weeks

   d. **Method.** The principles of cisplatin administration are:

      (1) **Monitoring.** Serum creatinine, electrolytes, magnesium, and calcium levels should be measured daily during therapy. Audiometry is usually not necessary.

      (2) **Antiemetics.** Patients should be given antiemetics, such as ondansetron and dexamethasone, before, during, and after cisplatin infusion.

      (3) **Hydration and diuresis** is required when 40 mg/m^2 or more of cis-

platin is given as a short infusion to maintain a urine output of 100–150 ml/hour prior to administration of the drug.
- **(a)** 1.5–2.0 liters 5% dextrose in 0.45% NaCl containing $MgSO_4$ (8 mEq/L) and KCl (20 mEq/L) should be administered prior to cisplatin treatment. The same volume and composition of fluids is also given after cisplatin.
- **(b)** Furosemide, 40 mg IV, should be given if needed, to prevent fluid overload.
- **(c)** Mannitol, 12.5–37.5 grams, should be administered prior to cisplatin if urine output is insufficient.
- **e. Drug interactions.** Cisplatin inhibits renal elimination of bleomycin. Thiosulfates may theoretically inactivate the drug systematically.

E. Dacarbazine (DTIC, DIC, dimethyltriazenoimidazolecarboxamide)
1. **Indications.** Hodgkin's disease, malignant melanoma, sarcomas
2. **Pharmacology**
   - **a. Mechanisms.** Inhibits purine, RNA, and protein synthesis. Has some alkylating activity. Causes DNA methylation and direct DNA damage
   - **b. Metabolism.** Native drug inactive; requires activation by oxidative N-methylation by liver microsomal oxidases. Excreted in urine predominantly; minor hepatobiliary and pulmonary excretion.
3. **Toxicity**
   - **a. Dose-limiting.** Myelosuppression; nadir blood counts occur 2–4 weeks after treatment
   - **b. Common.** Nausea and vomiting (often severe); pain along the injection site, local irritant if injected SQ (not a vesicant)
   - **c. Occasional.** Alopecia, facial flushing, photosensitivity, abnormal LFTs. Flu-like syndrome (malaise, myalgia, chills, and fever developing one week after treatment and lasting 1–3 weeks)
   - **d. Rare.** Diarrhea, stomatitis; cerebral dysfunction; hepatic vein thrombosis, hepatic necrosis; azotemia; anaphylaxis
4. **Administration.** Dacarbazine is often used in combination chemotherapy regimens (see Appendix A). Withdrawing blood into the drug-filled syringe before injecting the mixture reduces the pain of injection.
   - **a. Supplied** as 100-, 200-, and 500-mg vials. Protect from sunlight
   - **b. Dose modification.** Necessary for patients with impaired bone marrow, hepatic, or renal function
   - **c. Dose**
     - (1) 750 mg/m^2 IV as a single injection every 28 days *or*
     - (2) 50–250 mg/m^2 IV daily for five days every 21–28 days *or*
     - (3) 75–125 mg/m^2 IV daily for 10 days every 28 days

F. Hexamethylmelamine (HMM, altretamine, Hexalen)
1. **Indications.** Recurrent ovarian carcinoma
2. **Pharmacology**
   - **a. Mechanism.** Alkylates DNA; also acts as an antimetabolite by inhibiting incorporation of thymidine and uridine into DNA and RNA.
   - **b. Metabolism.** Rapidly demethylated and hydroxylated in the liver by microsomal enzymes. Excreted in urine and hepatobiliary tract as metabolites.
3. **Toxicity**
   - **a. Dose-limiting.** Nausea and vomiting, which may worsen with continued therapy
   - **b. Common.** Myelosuppression (mild) with nadir blood cell counts occurring 3–4 weeks after starting treatment
   - **c. Occasional.** Neurotoxicity, including paresthesias, hypoesthesia, hyperreflexia, motor weakness, agitation, confusion, hallucinations, lethargy, depression, coma
   - **d. Rare.** Alopecia, skin rashes, cystitis, secondary malignancies
4. **Administration**
   - **a. Supplied** as 50-mg capsules.

b. **Dose modification.** Give cautiously to patients with hepatic dysfunction.

c. **Dose.** 150 mg/m^2 PO daily in divided doses for 14 days, then repeated when hematologic recovery permits

d. **Drug interactions.** Cimetidine may inhibit metabolism. Barbiturates may enhance metabolism.

G. **Procarbazine** (Matulane, Natulanar, N-methylhydrazine)

1. **Indications.** Hodgkin's disease, lymphomas, myeloma, brain cancer, small cell lung cancer

2. **Pharmacology**

a. **Mechanism.** DNA alkylation and depolymerization. Methylation of nucleic acids. Inhibition of DNA, RNA, and protein synthesis

b. **Metabolism.** Metabolic activation of the drug is required. Readily enters the cerebrospinal fluid. Degraded in the liver to inactive compounds, which are excreted in urine

3. **Toxicity**

a. **Dose-limiting.** Myelosuppression, which may not begin until several weeks after starting treatment

b. **Common.** Nausea and vomiting, which decrease with continued use; myalgia, arthralgia; sensitizes tissues to radiation

c. **Occasional.** Dermatitis, hyperpigmentation, photosensitivity; stomatitis, dysphagia, diarrhea; hypotension, tachycardia; urinary frequency, hematuria; gynecomastia, sterility

d. **Neurologic.** Procarbazine may result in disorders of consciousness or mild peripheral neuropathies in about 10 percent of cases. These abnormalities are reversible and rarely serious enough to alter drug dosage. Manifestations of toxicity include sedation, depression, agitation, psychosis, decreased deep-tendon reflexes, paresthesias, myalgias, and ataxia.

e. **Rare.** Xerostomia, retinal hemorrhage, photophobia, papilledema; allergic pneumonitis, secondary malignancy

4. **Administration**

a. **Supplied** as 50-mg capsules

b. **Dose modification.** Reduce dose in patients with hepatic, renal, or bone marrow dysfunction.

c. **Dose.** 100 mg/m^2 PO daily for 14 days in combination regimens

d. **Drug interactions.** Procarbazine is a monoamine oxidase inhibitor and interacts with

(1) Alcohol, causing disulfiram (Antabuse)-like reactions

(2) CNS depressants synergistically (antihistamines, phenothiazines, barbiturates)

(3) Tricyclic antidepressants and monamine oxidase inhibitors, causing hyperpyrexia, convulsions

(4) Meperidine and other narcotics, causing hypertension, hypotension, and coma

(5) Hypoglycemic agents, increasing hypoglycemia

(6) Levodopa, causing hypertensive crisis (nullified by carbidopa)

(7) Sympathomimetic amines and tyramine-containing foods, causing hypertensive crises

III. **Antimetabolites**

A. **General pharmacology of antimetabolites**

1. Some antimetabolites are structural analogues of normal molecules that are essential for cell growth and replication. Other antimetabolites inhibit enzymes that are necessary for the synthesis of essential compounds. Their major effect is interfering with the building blocks of DNA synthesis (Fig. 4-4). Their activity, therefore, is greatest in the S phase of the cell cycle. In general, these agents have been most effective where cell proliferation is rapid.

2. The pharmacokinetics of these drugs are characterized by nonlinear dose-

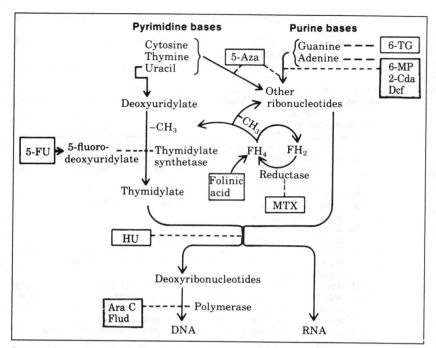

Fig. 4-4. Sites of action of antimetabolites. 2-Cda = 2-chlorodeoxyadenosine, 5-Aza = 5-azacytidine, 5-FU = 5-fluorouracil, 6-MP = 6 mercaptopurine, 6-TG = 6-thioguanine, Ara C = cytosine arabinoside, Dcf = deoxycoformycin, Flud = fludarabine, HU = hydroxyurea, and MTX = methotrexate.

response curves; after a certain dose, no more are killed with increasing doses (fluorouracil is an exception). Because of the entry of new cells into the cycle, the length of the time the cells are exposed to the drug is directly proportional to the killing potential (see Fig. 4-2).

B. Azacitidine (5-azacytidine, ladakamycin)
1. **Indication. AML** (experimental)
2. **Pharmacology**
   a. **Mechanism.** Antimetabolite (cytidine analogue). Rapidly phosphorylated and incorporated into DNA and RNA, thereby inhibiting protein synthesis; also inhibits pyrimidine synthesis and DNA methylation.
   b. **Metabolism.** Activated by phosphorylation and deactivated by deamination; similar to cytarabine. Excreted in urine (20% as unchanged drug).
3. **Toxicity**
   a. **Dose-limiting.** Myelosuppression; nausea and vomiting (severe, but less common with continuous infusion)
   b. **Common.** Hepatic dysfunction, diarrhea, alopecia
   c. **Occasional.** Neurotoxicity (restlessness, confusion), azotemia (transient and reversible), hypophosphatemia with myalgia, stomatitis, phlebitis, fever
   d. **Rare.** Progressive lethargy and coma, renal tubular acidosis, rhabdomyolysis, hypotension, rash
4. **Administration**
   a. **Supplied** as 100-mg vials
   b. **Dose modification.** Necessary for patients with impaired liver function.

Some authorities have warned against the use of azacitidine in patients with serum albumin of less than 3 g/dl. Use with caution in patients with altered mental status.

   c. Dose. 150–300 mg/m^2 IV for five days by continuous infusion

C. Cladribine (2-CdA, CdA, 2-chloro-2-deoxyadenosine, chlordeoxyadenosine, Leustatin)

  1. Indications. Hairy cell leukemia, indolent lymphomas, chronic lymphocytic leukemia, mycosis fungoides

  2. Pharmacology

    a. Mechanism. Antimetabolite. A deoxyadenosine analogue that accumulates in cells, blocks adenosine deaminase, and inhibits RNA synthesis.

    b. Metabolism. Plasma half-life is seven hours. Rapidly distributed and eliminated.

  3. Toxicity

    a. Dose-limiting. Myelosuppression

    b. Common. Nausea, skin reactions at injection site, fever, chills

    c. Occasional. Headache, fatigue

    d. Rare. Neurotoxicity, pancreatitis

  4. Administration

    a. Supplied as 20-mg vials

    b. Dose modification. Hematologic

    c. Dose. Either 0.10 mg/kg/day (4 mg/m^2/day) by continuous IV infusion for seven days, *or* 0.14 mg/kg daily IV over two hours for five days

D. Cytarabine (cytosine arabinoside, arabinosylcytosine, Cytosar, Tarabine, ara-C)

  1. Indications. Acute leukemia, chronic myelogenous leukemia, lymphoma, meningeal involvement with tumor

  2. Pharmacology

    a. Mechanism. Antimetabolite. Phosphorylated derivative of the drug competitively inhibits DNA polymerase, which is involved in the conversion of cytidine to deoxycytidine; some is incorporated into DNA. Blocks DNA repair and terminates DNA chain elongation.

    b. Metabolism. Requires activation to triphosphate by kinase; deactivated by deaminase. Ara-C is rapidly and completely deaminated in liver, plasma, and peripheral tissues. Ara-C antitumor activity depends on relative amounts of kinase and deaminase in cells. In patients with renal insufficiency, one metabolite (uracil arabinoside) has the ability to produce high concentrations of ara-C triphosphate, which may result in CNS toxicity. Excreted in urine as inactive metabolites.

  3. Toxicity

    a. Dose-limiting. Myelosuppression (nadir is expected in 5–7 days and recovery in 2–3 weeks)

    b. Common. Nausea, vomiting, diarrhea (potentiated by the addition of an anthracycline); conjunctivitis (usually within the first three days of high-dose regimens, but reduced with prophylactic glucocorticoid eye drops); hydradenitis, arachnoiditis with intrathecal administration

    c. Cerebellar toxicity begins on the fourth or fifth day of infusion and resolves within seven days. The incidence and severity of toxicity are related to the dose given (especially with total dose >48 gm/m^2), the rate of infusion (least incidence for continuous infusions), age (particularly >60 years), gender (especially males), and the degree of hepatic or renal dysfunction (particularly with creatinine clearance <60 ml/minute). In some cases, it is irreversible or fatal.

    d. Occasional. Alopecia, stomatitis, metallic taste, esophagitis, hepatic dysfunction (mild and reversible), pancreatitis, severe GI ulceration; thrombophlebitis; flu-like syndrome, myalgias, arthralgias, fever, headache; rash, transient skin erythema without exfoliation

    e. Rare. Sudden respiratory distress rapidly progressing to pulmonary edema; pericarditis, cardiomegaly, tamponade; urinary retention

4. Administration
  a. Supplied as 100-mg vials
  b. Dose modification. Use cautiously in patients with liver or renal disease or with risk factors for neurotoxicity.
  c. Dose
    (1) See Chap. 21 for use in lymphomas and Chap. 25 for acute leukemia.
    (2) For intrathecal administration: 50–100 mg in 10 ml saline for 1–3 days weekly.
    (3) Low-dose regimen: 10 mg/m^2 SQ every 12–24 hours for 15–21 days
  d. Drug interactions. Nephrotoxic drugs may reduce the clearance of ara-C. Ara-C enhances activity of alkylating agents.

E. Fludarabine (2-fluoroadenine arabinoside-5-phosphate, Fludara)
  1. Indications. Chronic lymphocytic leukemia and low-grade lymphomas
  2. Pharmacology
    a. Mechanism. Antimetabolite. Its active metabolite, 2-fluoro-ara-A, appears to act by inhibiting DNA primase, DNA polymerase alpha, and ribonucleotide reductase.
    b. Metabolism. The plasma half-life is 9–10 hours. Metabolites are excreted primarily in the urine.
  3. Toxicity
    a. Dose-limiting. Myelosuppression, which may be cumulative
    b. Common. Nausea and vomiting
    c. Occasional. Alopecia (mild), abnormal LFTs, tumor lysis syndrome
    d. Rare. Stomatitis, diarrhea; dermatitis; neurotoxicity (somnolence, transient paresthesias, delayed demyelination); chest pain, hypotension, fever
  4. Administration
    a. Supplied as 50-mg vials
    b. Dose modification. Decrease dosage by 30 percent for patients with creatinine clearance of less than 70 ml/minute.
    c. Dose. 25 mg/m^2 IV over 30 minutes daily for five consecutive days every four weeks

F. Fluorouracil (5-FU, Adrucil, Efudex)
  1. Indications. A wide variety of carcinomas
  2. Pharmacology
    a. Mechanism. Antimetabolite. Interferes with DNA synthesis by blocking thymidylate synthetase, an enzyme involved in the conversion of deoxyuridylic acid to thymidylic acid. It is incorporated into several RNA species, which may thereby interfere with RNA function and protein synthesis. It is cell cycle S-phase specific but acts in other cell cycle phases as well and is unique in having a log linear cell-killing action.
    b. Metabolism. Fluorouracil rapidly enters all tissues, including spinal fluid and malignant effusions. The drug requires intracellular activation by a series of phosphorylating enzymes and phosphoribosyl transferase. Most of the drug degradation occurs in the liver. Responsive tumors appear to lack degradation enzymes. Metabolism eliminates 90 percent of 5-FU. Inactive metabolites are excreted in the urine, bile, and breath (as CO_2).
  3. Toxicity is more common and more severe in patients with dihydropyrimidine dehydrogenase deficiency.
    a. Dose-limiting. Myelosuppression (less common with continuous infusion); mucositis (more common with five-day infusion); diarrhea (may be cholera-like with high doses of leucovorin)
    b. Common. Nasal discharge; eye irritation and excessive lacrimation due to dacrocystitis and lacrimal duct stenosis; vein pigmentation
    c. Reversible cerebellar dysfunction occurs in about 1 percent of patients. Symptoms usually disappear 1–6 weeks after the drug is discontinued,

but they abate after the dose is reduced or even if the same dose is maintained. Manifestations include acute dizziness, dysmetria, slurred speech, ataxia of the trunk or extremities, and coarse nystagmus.

   d. Occasional. Nausea, vomiting, esophagitis; "hand-foot syndrome" with protracted infusion (paresthesia, erythema, and swelling of the palms and soles); myocardial ischemia (particularly in patients with a prior history of myocardial ischemia); thrombophlebitis

   e. Rare. Alopecia, dermatitis, loss of nails, dark bands on nails; photosensitivity, blurred vision, "black hairy tongue" (hypertrophy of filiform papillae), anaphylaxis, fever

4. Administration. The optimal method of administration for fluorouracil is controversial. It is given by IV bolus, IV infusion over 15 minutes, continuous IV infusion, arterial infusion, intracavitarily, topically, or PO mixed with water, juice, or carbonated beverage.

   a. Supplied as
      (1) 500-mg vials
      (2) Topical cream: 5% fluorouracil (Efudex)

   b. Dose modification. Fluorouracil is withheld if the patient has stomatitis, diarrhea, evidence of infection, leukopenia or thrombocytopenia; drug is resumed when these problems have resolved. Dose is permanently reduced 25–50 percent if fluorouracil caused a previous episode of stomatitis, diarrhea, WBC lower than 2000/μL, or platelet count lower than 100,000/μL. Drug should be prescribed cautiously in the presence of hepatic dysfunction.

   c. Dose. Fluorouracil is erratically absorbed orally. Several regimens have been used including the following:
      (1) 300 mg/m^2 IV weekly
      (2) 300–450 mg/m^2 IV daily for five days every 28 days
      (3) 1000 mg/m^2/day by continuous infusion for 4–5 days every 28 days
      (4) 250–300 mg/m^2/day by continuous infusion indefinitely

   d. Drug interactions. Allopurinol inhibits activation of 5-FU and may result in decreased effectiveness. Toxicity is enhanced by leucovorin, methotrexate, and PALA.

G. Hydroxyurea (hydroxycarbamide, Hydrea)

1. Indications. Chronic myelogenous leukemia, myeloproliferative disorders, and as a radiosensitizing agent. Has some activity in solid tumors as well (e.g., melanoma and ovarian carcinoma)

2. Pharmacology

   a. Mechanism. Antimetabolite. Inhibits DNA synthesis by inhibiting nucleotide reductase, the enzyme that converts ribonucleosides to deoxyribonucleosides. Inhibits DNA repair and thymidine incorporation into DNA. Cell cycle S-phase specific, but acts in other phases as well.

   b. Metabolism. Crosses the blood-brain barrier. Half of the drug is rapidly degraded into inactive compounds. Inactive products and unchanged drug (50%) are excreted in urine.

3. Toxicity

   a. Dose-limiting. Myelosuppression, which recovers rapidly when treatment is stopped (prominent megaloblastosis)

   b. Occasional. Nausea, vomiting; skin rash, facial erythema, hyperpigmentation; azotemia, proteinuria; transient LFT abnormalities; radiation recall phenomenon

   c. Rare. Alopecia, mucositis, diarrhea, constipation; neurologic events; pulmonary edema; flu-like syndrome

4. Administration

   a. Supplied as 500-mg capsules.

   b. Dose modification. The drug should be given cautiously in the presence of liver dysfunction or when combined with other antimetabolites. Dosages should be reduced for creatinine clearances less than 50 ml/minute and when given with concomitant radiotherapy.

c. Dose
(1) Chronic myelogenous leukemia: 15–30 mg/kg PO every day *or*
(2) Solid tumors: 80 mg/kg PO every three days

H. Leucovorin (leucovorin calcium, citrovorum factor, folinic acid, 5-formyl tetrahydrofolate)

1. **Indications.** Combined with 5-FU in treatment of colorectal and other adenocarcinomas; the rescue agent for antifol toxicity (e.g., methotrexate)

2. **Pharmacology**
   a. **Mechanism.** Leucovorin is a tetrahydrofolic acid derivative that acts as a cofactor for carbon transfer reactions in the synthesis of purines and pyrimidines. It inhibits the effects of methotrexate and other dihydrofolate reductase antagonists. Leucovorin potentiates the cytotoxic effects of fluorinated pyrimidines (i.e., 5-FU and floxuridine) by increasing the binding of folate cofactor and activated 5-FU to thymidylate synthetase within the cells.
   b. **Metabolism.** Plasma half-life is 2–4 hours. Excreted in the urine as metabolites.

3. **Toxicity.** Potentiates the toxic effects of fluoropyrimidine therapy

4. **Administration**
   a. **Supplied** as 50-, 100-, and 350-mg vials for IV use and as a 60-mg bottle for PO use.
   b. **Dose.** Depends on combination regimen

I. Mercaptopurine (6-MP, Purinethol)

1. **Indication.** Acute lymphoblastic leukemia (maintenance therapy)

2. **Pharmacology**
   a. **Mechanism.** Purine antimetabolite. Undergoes extensive metabolic changes; mechanisms of cytotoxicity are complex. Inhibits de novo purine synthesis and purine interconversion. Competes with ribotides for enzymes responsible for conversion of inosinic acid to adenine and xanthine ribotides. Its incorporation into DNA or RNA are of uncertain significance.
   b. **Metabolism.** Mercaptopurine is slowly degraded in the liver, largely by xanthine oxidase. Allopurinol, a xanthine oxidase inhibitor, causes marked increase in its toxicity. Clearance is primarily hepatic with conventional doses.

3. **Toxicity**
   a. **Dose-limiting.** Myelosuppression
   b. **Common.** Nausea, vomiting, anorexia (25%); usually reversible cholestasis (30%)
   c. **Rare.** Stomatitis, diarrhea, dermatitis, fever, hematuria, Budd-Chiari-like syndrome, hepatic necrosis

4. **Administration**
   a. **Supplied** as 50-mg tablets.
   b. **Dose modification.** Dose is reduced by 50–75 percent for patients with hepatic dysfunction.
   c. **Dose.** 70–100 mg/m^2 PO daily until patient responds or toxic effects are seen; then adjust for maintenance therapy.
   d. **Drug interactions.** If given the allopurinol, the 6-MP dose must be reduced by 75 percent. Dosage may also need to be modified if other hepatotoxic drugs are given. Warfarin dosages may be affected by 6-MP.

J. Methotrexate (amethopterin, MTX)

1. **Indications.** A wide variety of conditions

2. **Pharmacology**
   a. **Mechanism.** Antifol metabolite. MTX blocks the enzyme dihydrofolate reductase, preventing formation of reduced (tetrahydro-) folic acid; tetrahydrofolic acid is critical to the transfer of carbon units in a variety of biochemical reactions (see Fig. 4-4). MTX thus blocks formation of thymidylate from deoxyuridylate and prevents synthesis of DNA. The

drug also inhibits RNA and protein synthesis and prevents cells from entering the S phase of the cell cycle, thus inhibiting its own killing action.

   b. Metabolism. MTX is minimally metabolized by the human species. The drug is distributed to body water; patients with significant effusions eliminate the drug much more slowly. Since 50 to 70 percent of the drug is bound to plasma proteins, displacement by other drugs (e.g., aspirin, sulfonamides) may result in an increase in toxic effects. The intracellular levels of MTX must be high enough to saturate all substances that can bind the drug, otherwise the drug will not be fully cytotoxic. Excreted in urine as unchanged drug (90%). Renal dysfunction results in dangerous blood levels of MTX and possible further renal damage.

3. Toxicity. Leucovorin (also called citrovorum factor, 5-formyltetrahydrofolic acid, folinic acid) can reverse the immediate cytotoxic effects of MTX; generally, 1 mg of leucovorin is given for each 1 mg of MTX.

   a. Dose-limiting. Myelosuppression, stomatitis (may be preventable by sucking ice during the injection), renal dysfunction (especially patients with dehydration or preexisting renal dysfunction)

   b. High-dose regimens. Nausea, vomiting, renal tubular necrosis, cortical blindness

   c. Previously irradiated areas. Skin erythema, pulmonary fibrosis, transverse myelitis, cerebritis

   d. Chronic therapy. Liver cirrhosis (subclinical and reversible hepatic dysfunction occurs with short-term intermittent therapy); osteoporosis (in children)

   e. Neurotoxicity. MTX neurotoxicity depends on dose and route of administration. Within a few hours after intrathecal administration, MTX can produce an acute aseptic meningitis that is usually self-limited. A subacute encephalopathy and myelopathy can also occur after intrathecal administration; this disorder can be reversible but sometimes progresses to a fixed deficit.

   High-dose systemic administration can cause a reversible encephalopathy of rapid onset and resolution that lasts from minutes to hours ("stroke-like" episodes). Chronic intrathecal combined with high-dose systemic administration can produce a more serious and irreversible leukoencephalopathy that develops months after treatment, is more likely to occur after brain irradiation, and causes dementia, seizures, spasticity, and ataxia. Long-term complications in children treated for acute leukemia are discussed in Chap. 25, sec. **V.B.3.b.**

   f. Occasional. Nausea, vomiting, diarrhea (GI ulceration, hemorrhage and perforation can occur if therapy is continued after the onset of diarrhea); dermatitis, photosensitivity, altered pigmentation, furunculosis; allergic conjunctivitis, photophobia, excessive lacrimation, cataracts; fever, reversible oligospermia, flank pain (associated with rapid IV infusion)

   g. Rare. Alopecia, MTX pneumonitis (see Chap. 29, sec. **IV.A.** for further details)

4. Administration

   a. Supplied as 2.5-mg tablets and 20-mg–1000-mg vials.

   b. Dose modification. The drug must not be administered to any patient with a creatinine clearance less than 60 ml/min (serum creatinine >1.5 mg/dl).

   c. Dose. Commonly used schedules are

   (1) Low-to-medium-dose regimens

      (a) 2.5–5.0 mg PO daily, *or*

      (b) 5–25 mg/m^2 PO, IM, or IV twice weekly *or*

      (c) 500 mg/m^2 IV every 2–3 weeks with leucovorin rescue

   (2) High-dose regimens use supralethal doses of MTX followed by administration of the antidote leucovorin. This treatment is complex and requires experience on the part of the clinician and use of special monitoring techniques.

- **(3) Intrathecal administration.** $5–10$ mg/m^2 (maximum 15 mg) in $7–15$ ml of preservative-free saline (3 ml if given via an Ommaya reservoir) every $3–7$ days.

   d. Drug interactions
   - **(1)** Leucovorin rescues normal tissues from high-dose toxicity,
   - **(2)** L-asparaginase blocks MTX toxicity and antitumor action.
   - **(3)** Aspirin, other nonsteroidal anti-inflammatory agents, and probenecid decrease renal clearance of MTX and increase its toxicity.
   - **(4)** Sulfonamides displace MTX from protein binding sites and enhance its toxicity.
   - **(5)** Trimethoprim is also an inhibitor of dihydrofolate reductase and can enhance MTX toxicity.

K. Mitoguazone (Methyl-GAG, methylglyoxal-bis[guanylhydrazone])
   1. **Indications.** Investigational agent for lymphomas, myeloma, and certain carcinomas
   2. **Pharmacology**
      - **a. Mechanism.** An antimetabolite that inhibits 5'-adenosylmethionine decarboxylase, which is important in the production of spermidine, which inhibits DNA and RNA synthesis
      - **b. Metabolism.** Triphasic elimination pattern
   3. **Toxicity**
      - **a. Dose-limiting.** Mucositis (severe); diarrhea (sometimes severe or bloody), nausea and vomiting (rarely severe)
      - **b. Common.** Flushing during infusion, myelosuppression
      - **c. Other.** Polyneuropathy and myopathy (may be dose-limiting at higher doses); vasculitis, hypoglycemia
   4. **Administration**
      - **a. Supplied** as 1-gram vials
      - **b. Dose.** 500 mg/m^2/week by IV infusion over at least 45 minutes

L. Pentostatin (2'-deoxycoformycin, dCF, covidarabine, Nipent)
   1. **Indications.** Hairy cell leukemia, lymphomas, and possibly cutaneous T-cell lymphoma
   2. **Pharmacology**
      - **a. Mechanism.** Antimetabolite. Inhibitor of adenine deaminase, an enzyme that is important for the metabolism of purine nucleosides. The mechanism of its antineoplastic effects is not firmly established.
      - **b. Metabolism.** The majority of dCF is excreted unchanged in the urine.
   3. **Toxicity**
      - **a. Dose-limiting.** Myelosuppression
      - **b. Common.** Immunosuppression; mild nausea and vomiting, diarrhea, altered taste; fatigue, fever
      - **c. Occasional.** Chills, myalgia, arthralgia; abnormal LFTs; keratoconjunctivitis, photophobia; renal failure
      - **d. Rare.** Hepatitis; pulmonary infiltrates and insufficiency
   4. **Administration**
      - **a. Supplied** as 10-mg vials
      - **b. Dose modification.** Reduce doses for renal impairment
      - **c. Dose.** 4 mg/m^2 IV infusion over 20 minutes with one or two liters of hydration every two weeks

M. Thioguanine (6-TG, aminopurine-6-thiol-hemihydrate)
   1. **Indication.** Acute granulocytic leukemia
   2. **Pharmacology**
      - **a. Mechanism.** Purine antimetabolite. After metabolic alteration into abnormal nucleotides, the drug is incorporated extensively into DNA, resulting in miscoding of transcription and DNA replication.
      - **b. Metabolism.** Thioguanine is not degraded by xanthine oxidase and, un-

like mercaptopurine, can be given in full doses with allopurinol. Clearance of the drug is primarily hepatic.

3. Toxicity
  a. Dose-limiting. Myelosuppression
  b. Common. Stomatitis, diarrhea
  c. Occasional. Nausea and vomiting, hepatic dysfunction, hepatic veno-occlusive disease; decreased vibratory sensation, unsteady gait

4. Administration
  a. Supplied as 40-mg tablets.
  b. Dose modification. Dose is reduced with impaired liver function.
  c. Dose
  (1) 100 mg/m^2 PO b.i.d. for 5 days *or*
  (2) 2–3 mg/kg PO daily until toxic effects are seen.

IV. Antitumor antibiotics

A. General pharmacology of antitumor antibiotics

  1. Antitumor antibiotics generally are drugs derived from microorganisms. They usually are cell cycle–nonspecific agents that are especially useful in slow-growing tumors with low growth fractions.
  2. They act by a variety of mechanisms. Several of these drugs interfere with DNA through intercalation, a reaction whereby the drug inserts itself between DNA base pairs. Intercalation with DNA prevents DNA replication and messenger RNA production, or both.
  3. Other drugs have other actions. For example, mitomycin C has alkylating activity. Bleomycin, which is cell cycle–phase specific, induces single-strand breaks in DNA and inhibits ligases (DNA repair enzymes).

B. Actinomycin D (Cosmegen, dactinomycin)

  1. Indications. Trophoblastic neoplasms, sarcomas, testicular carcinoma, Wilms' tumor
  2. Pharmacology
    a. Mechanism. Intercalates between DNA base pairs and prevents synthesis of messenger RNA; inhibits topoisomerase II
    b. Metabolism. Unknown; extensively bound to tissues, resulting in long half-life in plasma and tissue. Excreted in bile and urine as unchanged drug.
  3. Toxicity
    a. Dose-limiting. Myelosuppression
    b. Common. Nausea and vomiting (often worsening after successive daily doses and lasting several hours); alopecia, acne, erythema, desquamation, hyperpigmentation; radiation recall reaction. Drug is a vesicant that can cause necrosis if extravasated.
    c. Occasional. Stomatitis, cheilitis, glossitis, proctitis, diarrhea; vitamin K antagonism
    d. Rare. Hepatitis, anaphylaxis, hypocalcemia, lethargy
  4. Administration. Premedicate patients with antiemetics. Administer through a running IV infusion with extravasation precautions.
    a. Supplied as 0.5-mg vials.
    b. Dose modification. Reduce by 50 percent in the presence of renal or hepatic functional impairment.
    c. Dose
    (1) 0.25–0.60 mg/m^2 IV daily for 5 days every 3–4 weeks *or*
    (2) 1–2 mg/m^2 IV single dose every 3–4 weeks

C. Bleomycin (Blenoxane)

  1. Indications. Used as a single agent or in combination with other drugs (see Appendix A) for lymphomas, Hodgkin's disease, squamous cell carcinomas, testicular carcinoma, sarcomas, malignant effusions
  2. Pharmacology
    a. Mechanism. Binds to DNA, thereby inhibiting synthesis of DNA and, to a lesser extent, of RNA and proteins. Causes DNA strand cleavage by free radicals and inhibits DNA repair by a marked inhibition of DNA

ligase. Cell cycle G_2–phase specific; also active in late G_1, S, and M phases.

   b. Metabolism. Activated by microsomal reduction; bound to tissues but not to plasma protein; extensive degradation by hydrolysis in nearly all tissues. Both free drug and metabolic products are excreted into the urine.

  3. Toxicity

   a. Dose-limiting

    (1) Mild to severe shaking chills and febrile reactions are common (25% of patients), frequently within 4–10 hours of injection. However, they decrease in incidence and severity with subsequent administrations. An unusual anaphylaxislike reaction develops in one to eight percent of patients who have lymphomas.

    (2) Bleomycin pneumonitis with dyspnea, dry cough, fine moist basilar rales, interstitial radiographic changes, reduced diffusing capacity, hypoxia, and hypocapnia may be lethal. Pulmonary fibrosis and insufficiency occur in one percent of patients receiving cumulative doses less than 200 units/m^2, and in 10 percent of patients receiving larger doses (see Chap. 29, sec. **IV.A** for further details). Advanced age, underlying pulmonary disease, prior or concomitant radiotherapy to the chest, and prior exposure to bleomycin predisposes patients to pulmonary toxicity.

   b. Common

    (1) Sensitizes tumor and normal tissues to radiation

    (2) Dermatologic (50% of patients): hyperpigmentation of skin stretch areas (e.g., knuckles, elbows), hyperpigmented striae; hardening, tenderness, or loss of fingernails; hyperkeratosis of palms and fingers, scleroderma-like changes; skin tenderness, pruritus, urticaria, erythroderma, desquamation, alopecia

    (3) Anorexia, mucositis; a rancid smell ("like old gym socks") beginning about 10 seconds after injection.

   c. Occasional. Nausea, vomiting, unusual tastes; mild reversible myelosuppression, Raynaud's phenomenon, phlebitis, pain at injection site

  4. Administration. A 2-unit test dose is given before the first treatment followed by a 1–2-hour observation period to reduce the potential for cardiovascular collapse.

   a. Supplied as 15-unit (mg) vials

   b. Dose modification. The drug should not be given to patients with symptomatic chronic obstructive lung disease. It must be discontinued in patients who have erythroderma (continued treatment may lead to fatal exfoliative dermatitis). The drug must also be discontinued if there are symptoms or signs of interstitial lung disease. Routine pulmonary function tests are generally not helpful; some authorities recommend monitoring carbon monoxide diffusing capacity. Dosage should be reduced in patients with renal failure.

   c. Dose. Avoid cumulative dosage of greater than 400 units; some physicians limit the total dose to 300 units.

    (1) 10–20 units/m^2 IM, IV or SQ once or twice weekly (twice-weekly doses higher than 20 units each are likely to cause serious toxic reactions of the skin) *or*

    (2) 15–20 units/m^2 daily for 3–7 days by continuous infusion *or*

    (3) 60 units/m^2 dissolved in 100 ml of normal saline for intracavitary therapy

D. Daunorubicin (daunomycin, rubidomycin, Cerubidine)

  1. Indication. Acute leukemias

  2. Pharmacology. Anthracycline antitumor antibiotic. Essentially the same as doxorubicin. Active metabolite is daunomycinol.

  3. Toxicity. Same as doxorubicin. Daunorubicin may also cause precipitous fatal cardiomyopathy months after therapy has stopped; incidence becomes unacceptable after a total dose of 500–600 mg/m^2 has been given.

4. **Administration.** Same as doxorubicin. Use extravasation precautions.
   a. **Supplied** as 20-mg vials
   b. **Dose modification.** Same as doxorubicin
   c. **Dose.** 45–60 mg/m^2 IV daily for three days

E. **Doxorubicin** (Adriamycin, hydroxydaunorubicin, hydroxydaunomycin, Rubex)
   1. **Indications.** Effective in a large variety of tumors, usually in combination chemotherapy regimens (see Appendix A)
   2. **Pharmacology**
      a. **Mechanism.** Anthracycline antitumor antibiotic. Intercalates between DNA base pairs, forms free radicals, alters cell membranes, induces topoisomerase II-dependent DNA damage, inhibits preribosomal DNA and RNA. Cell cycle–phase nonspecific.
      b. **Metabolism.** Approximately 70 percent of the drug is bound to plasma proteins. Rapidly metabolized by the liver to other compounds, some of which are cytotoxic (including the active metabolite, doxorubicinol). The release rate from tissue binding sites is very slow compared to the capacity of the liver for metabolism; this results in relatively prolonged plasma levels of drug and metabolites.
      c. **Excretion.** Metabolites and free drug are extensively excreted in the bile. However, known elimination accounts for only 60 percent of the drug. The rate of drug elimination and its toxicity, thus, is rarely limited by liver function. Some chromogens are excreted through the kidney, occasionally imparting a red tinge to the urine.
   3. **Toxicity**
      a. **Dose-limiting**
         (1) Myelosuppression, particularly leukopenia, which reaches a nadir in 10–15 days and recovers within 21 days after administration.
         (2) Cardiomyopathy with congestive heart failure, which may be refractory, may result from repeated doses (see Chap. 29, sec. **VI.D** for further details). Monitoring the LVEF with radionuclide techniques is mandatory, particularly when the cumulative dose exceeds 300 mg/m^2 and when it exceeds 450 mg/m^2. Current data suggest that once the maximum cumulative dose has been reached, the drug can never be safely resumed. The drug should be discontinued if any of the following occurs:
            (a) Congestive heart failure.
            (b) Total cumulative dose of 550 mg/m^2 (450 mg/m^2 with a history of mediastinal irradiation).
            (c) ECG changes (sinus tachycardia, arrhythmias, flattened T waves, S-T segment depression, or voltage reduction).
            (d) Decreased LVEF to less than 50 percent or at least by 10 percent
      b. **Common**
         (1) Alopecia (nearly 100% of patients when administered as a bolus every 3–4 weeks, but minimal when the dose is divided and given weekly), nausea and vomiting (mild to severe), stomatitis (less common on intermittent single-dose schedule).
         (2) Adriamycin is a vesicant; extravasation of the drug results in severe ulceration and necrosis.
         (3) Sensitizes normal and malignant tissue to radiation. Previously irradiated skin sites may become erythematous and desquamate when the drug is started ("radiation recall reaction" can occur years after radiation was given).
      c. **Occasional.** Diarrhea; hyperpigmentation of nail beds and dermal creases, facial flush, flush along injected vein, skin rash; conjunctivitis, lacrimation; red-colored urine
      d. **Rare.** Activation of fibrinolysis, muscle weakness, fever, chills, anaphylaxis

4. **Administration.** The drug must be slowly pushed through a running IV line over 2–5 minutes using extravasation precautions or continuously infused through a central venous line. Rapid infusion may induce serious arrhythmias, flushing, or syncope. Protect drug from sunlight.
   a. **Supplied** as 10-, 20-, 50-, 100-, and 150-mg vials
   b. **Dose modification.** Adriamycin should not be given to patients with congestive heart failure from any cause. Previously, doxorubicin doses were reduced in the presence of hyperbilirubinemia, but there no longer appears to be justification for modification of drug dose for depressed liver function.
   c. **Dose**
      (1) 50–75 mg/m^2 IV bolus or continuous infusion over 2–4 days every 3–4 weeks
      (2) 30 mg/m^2 IV daily for three days every 3–4 weeks
      (3) 10–20 mg/m^2 IV weekly
   d. **Drug interaction.** The clearance of doxorubicin can be increased when coadministered with heparin.

F. **Idarubicin** (4-demethoxydaunorubicin, Idamycin)
   1. **Indications.** Acute leukemia
   2. **Pharmacology.** Anthracycline antitumor antibiotic. More lipophilic and better cell uptake than other anthracycline antibiotics; otherwise similar to doxorubicin. The active metabolite is 13-epirubicinol.
   3. **Toxicity.** Similar to doxorubicin. Myelosuppression is expected. Although idarubicin is less cardiotoxic than doxorubicin and daunorubicin, the same monitoring criteria apply.
   4. **Administration.** Slow intravenous injection over five minutes using extravasation precautions.
      a. **Supplied** as 5- and 10-mg vials
      b. **Dose modification.** Same as doxorubicin.
      c. **Dose.** 12 mg/m^2 IV daily for three days

G. **Mithramycin** (Mithracin, plicamycin)
   1. **Indication.** Refractory hypercalcemia (occasionally, multiple myeloma, chronic myelogenous leukemia).
   2. **Pharmacology**
      a. **Mechanism.** Osteoclast inhibitor, antitumor antibiotic. Cytotoxicity probably related to DNA intercalation and adlineation; inhibits DNA-dependent RNA synthesis without affecting DNA synthesis
      b. **Metabolism.** Unknown, eliminated in the urine (40%).
   3. **Toxicity.** Renal and hepatic damage are rare with dosage schedules used for hypercalcemia.
      a. **Dose-limiting.** Thrombocytopenia; coagulation defects may occur in the absence of thrombocytopenia and result in a severe hemorrhagic diathesis (usually with frequent doses).
      b. **Common.** Nausea, vomiting; hypocalcemia, hypophosphatemia, hypokalemia, hypomagnesemia, rebound hypercalcemia; abnormal LFTs (including prothrombin time); azotemia; skin and soft tissue necrosis if extravasated
      c. **Occasional.** Leukopenia, anemia; stomatitis, diarrhea; hyperpigmentation, acneiform rash; headache, dizziness, drowsiness, nervousness
      d. **Rare.** Toxic epidermal necrolysis, fever, lethargy, periorbital pallor
   4. **Administration.** Dose is dissolved in 50 ml 5% dextrose in half-normal saline and administered into a running IV using extravasation precautions.
      a. **Supplied** as 2.5-mg vials
      b. **Dose modification.** Mithramycin must be given cautiously to patients with hepatic or kidney dysfunction. The drug is withheld if studies show liver or renal damage, prolonged prothrombin time, serious thrombocytopenia, or normal or low calcium levels.
      c. **Dose for hypercalcemia.** 25 μg (0.025 mg)/kg IV every 3–7 days.

H. Mitomycin C (Mutamycin, mitomycin)
1. **Indications.** A variety of carcinomas
2. **Pharmacology**
   a. **Mechanism.** Antitumor antibiotic. After intracellular activation, functions as an alkylating agent. DNA cross-linking, DNA depolymerization, and free radical formation
   b. **Metabolism.** Widely distributed in tissues. Metabolized predominantly in the liver. Free drug (25%) and metabolites excreted in urine, but renal dysfunction does not significantly alter mitomycin elimination.
3. **Toxicity**
   a. **Dose-limiting.** Cumulative myelosuppression, which may be severe and prolonged (particularly thrombocytopenia)
   b. **Common.** Mild nausea and vomiting, anorexia; a vesicant drug that can cause necrosis if injected SQ (skin erythema and ulceration can occur weeks to months after administration and may appear at a site distant from the site of injection)
   c. **Occasional.** Alopecia, stomatitis, skin rashes, photosensitivity, pain at site of injection, phlebitis; hemolytic uremia-like syndrome (see Chap. 34, *Cytopenia*, **IV.C.** for details)
   d. **Rare.** Hepatic and renal (cumulative) dysfunction, paresthesias, blurred vision, fever; acute interstitial pneumonitis (especially when given with vinblastine)
4. **Administration.** Administer through a running IV infusion using extravasation precautions.
   a. **Supplied** as 5-mg, 20-mg, and 40-mg vials
   b. **Dose modification.** Reduce dose by 50 to 75 percent for patients who were previously treated with extensive irradiation or developed WBC less than $2000/\mu L$ with prior doses of mitomycin C.
   c. **Dose**
      (1) Single agent: $10–20$ mg/m^2 IV every $6–8$ weeks *or*
      (2) In combination: $5–10$ mg/m^2 IV every six weeks
      (3) For bladder instillation: $20–40$ mg every $1–2$ weeks

I. Mitoxantrone (Novantrone, dihydroxyanthracenedione, DHAD)
1. **Indications.** Breast cancer, lymphoma, acute leukemia.
2. **Pharmacology.** Mitoxantrone is in the anthracenedione class of compounds, which are analogues to the anthracyclines. Mechanism of action and routes of metabolism are similar but not identical to doxorubicin.
   a. **Mechanism.** DNA intercalation, single- and double-strand DNA breakage, inhibition of topoisomerase II.
   b. **Metabolism.** Metabolized by the liver. Excreted in the bile and urine as metabolites and unchanged drug.
3. **Toxicity.** Compared to the anthracyclines, mitoxantrone is associated with less cardiotoxicity, less nausea and vomiting, and decreased potential for extravasation injury.
   a. **Dose-limiting.** Bone marrow suppression
   b. **Common.** Mild nausea and vomiting, mucositis; alopecia (usually mild); blue discoloration of the urine, sclerae, fingernails, and over venous site of injection that may last 48 hours
   c. **Occasional.** Cardiomyopathy (most well-defined for patients who have previously received doxorubicin; appears to be less cardiotoxic than doxorubicin. Pruritus, LFT abnormalities, allergic reactions
   d. **Rare.** Jaundice, seizures, pulmonary toxicity
4. **Administration** as a 30-minute infusion; rarely causes extravasation injury if infiltrated
   a. **Supplied** as 20-, 25-, and 30-mg vials
   b. **Dose modification.** Hematologic
   c. **Dose** is $10–12$ mg/m^2 IV given every three weeks for solid tumors or daily for five days in combination with cytarabine for acute leukemia.

V. Plant alkaloids

A. General pharmacology of plant alkaloids

1. **Mitotic spindle inhibitors** are classically represented by vincristine and vinblastine. These drugs bind to microtubular proteins, thus inhibiting microtubule assembly (M-phase of the cell cycle) and resulting in dissolution of the mitotic spindle structure. Paclitaxel not only binds to microtubules but also promotes microtubule assembly and resistance to depolymerization, resulting in the production of nonfunctional microtubules.

2. **Topoisomerases** are enzymes that break and seal DNA strands. Camptothecin and its analogues (topotecan, CPT-11) are plant alkaloids that are specific inhibitors to topoisomerase I, interfering with the breakage-rejoining reaction by stabilizing a reversible enzyme-DNA cleavable complex and causing single-strand DNA breaks. Inhibitors of topoisomerases I and II include etoposide, teniposide, and drugs from other classes (amsacrine and the anthracycline antitumor antibiotics). By binding to DNA and topoisomerases, these drugs result in DNA damage that interferes with transcription and replication.

B. Etoposide (epipodophyllotoxin, VP-16, VP-16-213, Vepesid)

1. **Indications.** Testicular carcinoma, lung cancer, lymphoma, and a variety of other malignancies.

2. **Pharmacology**

   a. **Mechanisms.** Plant alkaloid, topoisomerase II inhibitor (see **A.2**). Inhibits mitosis; cell cycle–phase specific at G_2, late S, and M phases.

   b. **Metabolism.** Highly bound to plasma proteins; metabolized by the liver. Excreted in urine (40%) as intact and degraded drug; excretion of the remaining 60 percent is uncertain, biliary excretion accounts for only a small proportion.

3. **Toxicity**

   a. **Dose-limiting.** Neutropenia

   b. **Common.** Nausea and vomiting (with oral dosing, but uncommon with IV dosing); alopecia (usually mild); hypotension if rapidly infused

   c. **Occasional.** Anemia, thrombocytopenia, pain at injection site, phlebitis, abnormal LFTs, peripheral neuropathy

   d. **Rare.** Stomatitis, dysphagia, diarrhea, constipation, parotitis, rash, radiation recall reaction, hyperpigmentation; anaphylaxis, transient hypertension, arrhythmias; somnolence, vertigo, transient cortical blindness

4. **Administration.** Administer slowly over at least 30 minutes when given IV.

   a. **Supplied** as 50-mg capsules and 100-mg vials

   b. **Dose modification.** Administer with caution in the presence of renal dysfunction; reduce doses by 25 or 50 percent for creatinine clearance of less than 50 ml/min and less than 10 ml/min, respectively.

   c. **Dose**

      (1) 50 mg/m² PO daily for 21 days *or*

      (2) 50–120 mg/m² IV daily for 3–5 days

   d. **Drug interactions.** Calcium channel antagonists, such as verapamil, or methotrexate may increase cytotoxicity of VP-16.

C. Paclitaxel (Taxol)

1. **Indications.** Breast and relapsed ovarian carcinomas

2. **Pharmacology**

   a. **Mechanism.** Plant alkaloid (antimicrotubule agent); see **A.1**.

   b. **Metabolism.** Nearly totally protein bound and distributed well to body fluids (including effusions) with a plasma half-life of about five hours.

3. **Toxicity**

   a. **Dose-limiting**

      (1) **Neutropenia,** particularly in patients who were previously heavily treated or who receive cisplatin just prior to taxol

    (2) Hypersensitivity (3%) is manifested by cutaneous flushing, hypotension, bronchospasm, urticaria, diaphoresis, pain, or angioedema. Reactions usually develop within 20 minutes of starting the treatment; 90 percent of hypersensitivity reactions develop following the first or second dose.

    (3) Peripheral neuropathy, particularly in the higher dosage (>170 mg/m^2) schedules and in patients with concomitant etiologies for peripheral neuropathy. The distribution typically is "stocking-glove" and consists of dysesthesias, paresthesias, and loss of proprioception.

  b. Common. Alopecia (usually total and sudden within three weeks of treatment); thrombocytopenia (usually not severe); transient arthralgias and myalgias within three days of treatment (often requiring narcotics and ameliorated by nonsteroidal anti-inflammatory agents and prednisone), transient bradycardia (usually asymptomatic)

  c. Occasional. Nausea, vomiting, taste changes, mucositis (cumulative), diarrhea; atrioventricular conduction defects, ventricular tachycardia, cardiac angina; necrosis when extravasated

  d. Rare. Paralytic ileus, generalized weakness, seizures; myocardial infarction

4. Administration. Taxol should be given *before cisplatin* in combination regimens where both are administered. Patients who were heavily previously treated may require support with granulocyte-colony stimulating factor. Cardiac monitoring is recommended for patients taking cardiac medications or with a history of cardiac disease. Administer with extravasation precautions.

  a. Supplied as 30-mg vials

  b. Dose modification. Hematologic

  c. Dose. 135–175 mg/m^2 infused over 3–24 hours with the following premedications: dexamethasone, 20 mg PO given 12 and 6 hours before taxol; diphenhydramine, 50 mg IV, and ranitidine, 50 mg IV, are given 30 minutes prior to administering taxol.

D. Teniposide (VM-26, thenylidene-lignan-P, Vumon)

  1. Indications. Acute lymphoblastic leukemia

  2. Pharmacology

    a. Mechanism. Plant alkaloid; topoisomerase II inhibitor (see **A.2**)

    b. Metabolism. Virtually all of the drug is bound to protein. Systemic metabolism is significant, but metabolites have not been identified. Renal excretion is only a small fraction of its clearance.

  3. Toxicity

    a. Dose-limiting. Neutropenia

    b. Common. Thrombocytopenia, hypotension with too rapid an infusion

    c. Occasional. Nausea and vomiting, alopecia, abnormal LFTs, phlebitis

    d. Rare. Diarrhea, stomatitis; rash, anaphylaxis; azotemia; fever; paresthesias, seizures

  4. Administration. The drug is administered by slow IV infusion over at least 30 minutes

    a. Supplied as 50-mg vials

    b. Dose. 20–60 mg/m^2/day for five days or 100 mg/m^2 once or twice weekly

    c. Drug interactions. Anticonvulsants increase clearance of teniposide.

E. Vinblastine (Velban, vincaleukoblastine, Velsar, Alkaban)

  1. Indications. Lymphomas, testicular carcinoma, a variety of other cancers, histiocytosis X

  2. Pharmacology

    a. Mechanism. Plant alkaloids; see **A.1.** Binds to microtubular proteins. Inhibits RNA synthesis by affecting DNA-dependent RNA polymerases. Cell cycle–phase specific; it arrests cells at G(sub 2)-M interface.

    b. Metabolism. Highly bound to plasma proteins and to formed blood elements, especially platelets. Metabolized by the liver to active and inactive metabolites. Predominantly excreted in bile. Minimal free drug is recovered in urine.

3. **Toxicity**
   a. **Dose-limiting.** Neutropenia
   b. **Common.** Cramps or severe pain in jaw, pharynx, back or limbs following injection; local vesicant if extravasated
   c. **Occasional.** Thrombocytopenia, anemia
   d. **Rare.** Nausea, vomiting, diarrhea, mucositis, abdominal cramps, GI hemorrhage; acute interstitial pneumonitis (especially when administered with mitomycin C); ischemic cardiotoxicity

4. **Administration.** Administered by rapid infusion through the tubing of a running IV with extravasation precautions.
   a. **Supplied** as 10-mg vials
   b. **Dose modification.** Decrease dose by 50 percent for patients with serum bilirubin greater than 3.0 mg/dl.
   c. **Dose.** 5 mg/m^2 IV every one or two weeks; higher doses at three-week intervals are used for testicular carcinomas. As a continuous infusion, 1.7–2.0 mg/m^2/day is given over a 96-hour period.

F. **Vincristine** (Oncovin, Vincasar, leurocristine)
   1. **Indications.** A wide variety of malignancies
   2. **Pharmacology**
      a. **Mechanism.** Same as vinblastine
      b. **Metabolism.** Same as vinblastine
   3. **Toxicity**
      a. **A dose-dependent peripheral neuropathy** universally develops. Cranial nerves and the autonomic system may also be involved. The neuropathies usually reverse within several months. Jaw, throat, or anterior thigh pain occurring within hours of injection disappears within days and usually does not recur.
         (1) **Dose-limiting.** Severe paresthesias, ataxia, foot-drop (slapping gait), muscle wasting, cranial nerve palsies, paralytic ileus, obstipation, abdominal pain, optic atrophy, cortical blindness, seizures
         (2) **Not dose-limiting.** Mild hypoesthesia, mild paresthesias, transient jaw pain (and similar syndromes), loss of deep tendon reflexes
      b. **Common.** Tissue necrosis if extravasated, alopecia (20–40%)
      c. **Occasional.** Mild leukopenia (does not have significant effect on erythrocytes or platelets); rash, SIADH
      d. **Rare.** Nausea, vomiting, pancreatitis; fever
   4. **Administration.** Patients receiving vincristine should be given bulk laxatives routinely. Administered by rapid infusion using extravasation precautions.
      a. **Supplied** as 1-, 2-, and 5-mg vials
      b. **Dose modification.** Hepatic dysfunction; same as for vinblastine
      c. **Dose.** 1.0–1.4 mg/m^2 IV every 1–4 weeks (often limited to a one-time total dose of 2 mg in adults); continuous infusion regimens involve 0.5 mg/m^2/day for four days

G. **Vindesine** (Eldisine, desacetylvinblastine amide sulfate)
   1. **Indications.** Experimental for non-small cell lung cancer, leukemias, breast cancer, malignant melanoma
   2. **Pharmacology.** Same as vinblastine.
   3. **Toxicity.** Same as vinblastine, but alopecia is more common with vindesine. Neurotoxicity is same as for vincristine but is generally less severe.
   4. **Administration.** Same as vinblastine.
      a. **Supplied** as 10-mg vials
      b. **Dose modification.** Necessary for patients with hepatic dysfunction; same as for vinblastine
      c. **Dose.** 3–4 mg/m^2 IV every 1–2 weeks *or* 1.0–1.3 mg/m^2/day for 5–7 days repeated every three weeks.

VI. Other agents

A. L-Asparaginase (Elspar)

1. Indication. Acute lymphoblastic leukemia

2. Pharmacology

 a. Mechanism. This enzyme hydrolyzes asparagine into aspartic acid and, to a lesser extent, glutamine into glutamic acid. Leads to inhibition of protein synthesis. Kills cells that cannot synthesize asparagine by destroying extracellular asparagine stores. Cell cycle–specific for postmitotic G_1 phase.

 b. Metabolism. Plasma half-life (8–30 hours) is independent of dose. Metabolism is independent of hepatic and renal function. Only trace amounts are recovered in urine.

3. Toxicity

 a. Dose-limiting. Allergic reactions (including chills, urticaria, skin rashes, fever, laryngeal constriction, asthma, and anaphylactic shock) are the most frequent. Allergic reactions develop within one hour of dosing and are most likely to occur after several doses are given, particularly if the last dose was given more than one month previously and if the drug is administered IV rather than IM. Patients who respond to *Escherichia coli* asparaginase but develop allergic reactions may be treated relatively safely with another source of the enzyme.

 b. Common

  (1) Encephalopathy in 25 to 50 percent of patients. Lethargy, somnolence, and confusion tend to occur within the first few days of therapy, reverse after completion of therapy, and are rarely a cause for discontinuing treatment. Hemorrhagic and thrombotic CNS events occur later and are associated with the induced imbalances in the coagulation and fibrinolytic systems.

  (2) Nausea, anorexia, vomiting (60%)

  (3) Hepatitis (abnormal LFTs in more than 50% of treated patients, but rarely severe); pancreatitis (10%)

  (4) Coagulation defects associated with decreased synthesis of clotting factors, especially fibrinogen and antithrombin III (usually subclinical but may result in thrombosis or pulmonary embolism)

  (5) Prerenal azotemia (65%); a rise in BUN and blood ammonia levels not evidence of toxicity

  (6) Hyperglycemia

 c. Rare. Myelosuppression, diarrhea, severe renal failure, hyperthermia

4. Administration. Administer a small (2-unit) intradermal test dose to check for hypersensitivity. Epinephrine (1 mg, 1:1000), hydrocortisone (100 mg), and diphenhydramine (50 mg) should be readily available to treat anaphylaxis each time the drug is given.

 a. Supplied as 10,000-IU vials

 b. Dose modification. None for renal dysfunction. Use with caution for hepatic dysfunction or pancreatitis.

 c. Dose. Usually administered in combination with vincristine and prednisone at a dose of 6000 IU/m^2 IM three times weekly for nine doses

 d. Drug interactions. Asparaginase blocks the action of methotrexate and thus "rescues" from methotrexate toxicity

B. Estramustine (Emcyt)

1. Indications. Prostate cancer

2. Pharmacology. Classified as a hormone (effects are similar to estrogen) but also may be an antimicrotubule agent

3. Toxicity. Similar to estrogens (see **VII.F**)

4. Administration

 a. Supplied as 140-mg capsules

 b. Dose is 15 mg/kg/day in three divided doses taken on an empty stomach

C. Levamisole (Ergamisole)
   1. **Indications.** Adjuvant therapy for colon cancer in combination with 5-FU
   2. **Pharmacology**
      a. **Mechanism.** An antihelminthic drug that is believed to stimulate the immune system. Its mechanism of action for antitumor activity is unknown, however.
      b. **Metabolism.** Extensively metabolized by the liver. Only 5 percent of the drug is excreted unchanged in the urine.
   3. **Toxicity.** Levamisole was supposed to be nearly nontoxic, but experience has shown otherwise.
      a. **Dose-limiting.** Intolerance of the drug
      b. **Common.** Nausea; striking dysosmia and dysgeusia with exposure to city water (including sprinklers and showers)
      c. **Occasional.** Vomiting, flu-like syndrome, arthritis, edema; CNS hyperexcitation syndromes (agitation, confusion, nightmares, jitters, silliness, hyperalertness, headache, blurred vision, dysesthesias, tremors, tardive dyskinesia, hallucination, seizure)
      d. **Rare.** Alopecia, hematosuppression, dermatitis, conjunctivitis
   4. **Administration**
      a. **Supplied** as 50-mg tablets in packages of 36
      b. **Dose.** 50 mg t.i.d. PO for three days every two weeks given for one year with 5-FU
      c. **Drug interactions.** Antabuse-like reactions with alcohol; may increase blood levels of phenytoin and warfarin
D. Octreotide (Sandostatin, L-cysteinamide)
   1. **Indications.** Control of symptoms in patients with carcinoid syndrome, vasoactive intestinal peptide-secreting tumors (VIPomas), or cholera-like diarrhea caused by chemotherapeutic agents
   2. **Pharmacology**
      a. **Mechanism.** A long-acting analogue of somatostatin that inhibits the secretion of serotonin, VIP, gastrin, motilin, insulin, glucagon, secretin, and pancreatic polypeptide
      b. **Metabolism.** The elimination half-life is 1.5 hours and the duration of action is about 12 hours. Thirty percent of the drug is excreted unchanged in the urine.
   3. **Toxicity**
      a. **Dose-limiting.** Abdominal pain, vomiting, and loose stools
      b. **Dermatologic.** Injection site pain or other reactions, hair loss, rash, thinning of skin, hyperhidrosis
      c. **Occasional.** Hypoglycemia, hyperglycemia; hypertension, hypotension, thrombophlebitis, cardiac ischemia or failure; fat malabsorption, abnormal LFTs; visual disturbance, rhinorrhea, dry mouth, throat discomfort, prostatitis, chills, fever
      d. **Rare.** GI bleeding, cholelithiasis, hepatitis
   4. **Administration**
      a. **Supplied** as 1-ml ampules containing 0.05, 0.1, and 0.5 mg/ml
      b. **Dose.** 100–600 µg SQ in 2–4 divided doses
E. Suramin
   1. **Indications.** Investigational agent for prostate cancer
   2. **Pharmacology**
      a. **Mechanism.** Suramin is a glycosaminoglycan, an antitrypanosomal agent. Antitumor activity may be related to binding to growth factors and to other mechanisms.
      b. **Metabolism.** Totally bound to plasma proteins, especially albumin, and nearly all is excreted in the urine with an elimination half-life of 40–50 days.
   3. **Toxicity.** Life-threatening toxicities can usually be avoided by keeping the plasma concentrations below 300 µg/mL
      a. **Dose-limiting.** Thrombocytopenia

b. Neurotoxicity. Paresthesias, polyradiculoneuropathy (muscle weakness progressing to generalized flaccid paralysis)

c. Other. Leukopenia (mild), elevated clotting times, bleeding; adrenocortical insufficiency, hypocalcemia; nausea, vomiting, abnormal LFTs, metallic taste; nephrotoxicity; keratopathy, photophobia, blurred vision; fever, transient erythematous rash, pruritus

4. **Administration**
   a. **Supplied** as 1-gram vials
   b. **Dose.** 350 mg/m^2/day as a continuous IV infusion until plasma level reaches 250–300 μg/mL with two month periods off treatment

VII. Hormonal agents

A. Adrenocorticosteroids

1. **Indications.** Broad variety of oncologic problems that include the following:
   a. Component of combination chemotherapy regimens
   b. Symptomatic lymphangitic lung carcinomatosis
   c. Symptomatic brain metastases with or without cerebral edema
   d. Painful liver metastases
   e. Spinal cord compression
   f. Bilateral bronchial obstruction by tumor

2. **Toxicity and side effects** (usually associated with long-term therapy)
   a. Peptic ulcer disease
   b. Sodium retention (edema, heart failure, hypertension)
   c. Potassium wasting (hypokalemia, alkalosis, muscle weakness)
   d. Glucose intolerance, accumulation of fat on trunk and face, weight gain
   e. Proximal myopathy
   f. Personality changes including euphoria and psychosis
   g. Osteoporosis, aseptic hip necrosis
   h. Thinning and fragility of the skin
   i. Suppression of the pituitary-adrenal axis
   j. Susceptibility to infection

3. **Administration.** Patients receiving high doses of corticosteroids are given prophylactic oral antacid therapy. Methylprednisolone is preferred for patients with severe hepatic dysfunction.
   a. **Prednisone** (Deltasone, Orasone, and others)
      (1) **Supplied** as 1.0-, 2.5-, 5.0-, 10-, 20-, 25-, and 50-mg tablets and 1- and 5 mg/ml oral solutions.
      (2) **Dose.** 20–60 mg/m^2 PO daily
   b. **Methylprednisolone** (Medrol and others)
      (1) **Supplied** as 2-, 4-, 8-, 16-, 24-, and 32-mg tablets
      (2) **Dose.** 16–48 mg/m^2 PO daily
   c. **Dexamethasone** (Decadron, Hexadrol, and others)
      (1) **Supplied** as 0.25-, 0.5-, 0.75-, 1.0-, 1.5-, 2.0-, 4.0-, and 6.0-mg tablets; 1.0 mg/ml elixir; and 4-, 10-, 20-, and 24-mg vials
      (2) **Dose.** For cerebral edema from cancer, give 10 mg PO, IM, or IV initially, and then 4 mg every six hours; maintenance doses range from 8–96 mg/day.

B. Adrenocorticosteroid inhibitors

1. **Aminoglutethimide** (Cytadren, Elipten)
   a. **Indications.** Breast cancer, prostate cancer, Cushing's syndrome
   b. **Pharmacology**
      (1) **Mechanism.** An aromatase enzyme inhibitor that inhibits adrenocortical conversion of cholesterol to pregnenolone and blocks peripheral conversion of androgens to estrogens
      (2) **Metabolism.** 25 percent of drug is bound to plasma proteins. Metabolized by the liver. Excreted in the urine primarily as unchanged drug (50%).
   c. **Toxicity**
      (1) **Dose-limiting.** Adrenal insufficiency; postural hypotension (hypoaldosteronism)

(2) Common. Mild GI upset; transient maculopapular eruptions associated with fever (these remit in about four days without stopping the drug); transient fatigue; lethargy (resolves about six weeks after starting treatment)

(3) Occasional. Cerebellar signs, hypercholesterolemia, virilization, myalgia, fever, leg cramps

(4) Rare. Myelosuppression, desquamation, oral ulcers, hypothyroidism, lupus hepatitis-like syndrome

d. Administration

(1) Supplied as 250-mg tablets

(2) Dose. Start at 250 mg PO b.i.d. (with hydrocortisone, 100 mg/day) for two weeks. Then increase dose to 250 mg PO q.i.d., and decrease hydrocortisone to 10 mg in the morning and at noon and 20 mg at bedtime. The hydrocortisone prevents overriding of the adrenal blockade by inhibiting pituitary adrenocorticotropic hormone (ACTH) secretion. Occasionally a mineralocorticoid is also needed (fludrocortisone, 0.1 mg/day PO).

(3) Drug interactions. Aminoglutethimide induces the metabolism of warfarin, theophylline, digoxin, dexamethasone, and medroxyprogesterone; larger doses of these drugs may be needed.

2. Mitotane (o,p'-DDD, Lysodren)

a. Indications. Adrenal carcinoma, ectopic Cushing's syndrome

b. Pharmacology

(1) Mechanism. Causes adrenal cortical atrophy by inhibiting mitochondria; the exact mechanism is unknown. Blocks adrenocorticoid synthesis in normal and malignant cells. Aldosterone synthesis is not affected.

(2) Metabolism. Degraded slowly in the liver and extensively distributed in fatty tissues. Its action is antagonized by spironolactone; the two drugs should not be administered together. Metabolites are excreted in the bile and urine.

c. Toxicity

(1) Dose-limiting. Nausea and vomiting

(2) Common. Diarrhea, depression, lethargy, maculopapular rash, hypercholesterolemia

(3) Occasional. Orthostatic hypotension, hypertension; abnormal LFTs; irritability, confusion, tremors; shortness of breath, wheezing

(4) Rare. Permanent brain damage, myelosuppression, other dermatological problems, visual disturbances, hemorrhagic cystitis, fever

d. Administration. Plasma cortisol levels should be monitored periodically to assess the effectiveness of treatment and the possible development of adrenal insufficiency. Glucocorticoid and mineralocorticoid replacement therapy may be necessary.

(1) Supplied as 500-mg tablets.

(2) Dose modification. Reduce dose for patients with hepatic impairment.

(3) Dose. 4–6 gm PO daily in three divided doses; increase to 10 gm daily as tolerated.

C. Androgens

1. Indications (contraindicated in patients with prostate cancer). Breast carcinoma, short-range anabolic effect, stimulation of erythropoiesis, maintenance of libido in orchiectomized patients

2. Toxicity and side effects vary among preparations. Virilization, fluid retention, and hepatotoxicity, which is characterized by abnormal LFTs or cholestasis and is usually reversible, are frequent with certain preparations. May cause hypercalcemia in immobilized patients.

3. Administration

a. Testosterone cypionate (Depo-Testosterone)

(1) Supplied as 10-ml vials containing 50, 100, or 200 mg/ml

(2) Dose. 100 mg IM weekly; *or,* for orchiectomy patients, 200 mg IM every other week

b. Fluoxymesterone (Halotestin and others). Use with caution in patients with cardiac, hepatic, or renal disease.

(1) Supplied as 2-, 5-, and 10-mg tablets

(2) Dose. 10–40 mg/day in two or three divided doses

D. Antiandrogens (Eulexin, flutamide)

1. Indications. Prostate cancer

2. Pharmacology. Flutamide is an antiandrogen that inhibits androgen uptake or nuclear binding of androgens in target tissues. The drug is almost totally metabolized. The principal active metabolite (2-hydroxyflutamide) is metabolized by the liver, and half is excreted unchanged in the urine.

3. Toxicity

a. Common. Gynecomastia

b. Occasional. Galactorrhea, impotence, myalgia, nausea and vomiting

c. Rare. Hematosuppression, methemoglobinemia, diarrhea, abnormal LFTs

4. Administration

a. Supplied as 125-mg capsules

b. Dose. 250 mg t.i.d. PO, usually given in combination with luteinizing hormone–releasing hormone (LHRH) agonist analogues (see **VII.G**)

E. Antiestrogens (tamoxifen, Nolvadex)

1. Indication. Breast carcinoma.

2. Toxicity

a. Common. Thrombocytopenia (mild and transient), hot flashes, menstrual changes, uterine bleeding; lowered serum cholesterol (especially low-density cholesterol) while receiving tamoxifen

b. Occasional. Retinopathy or keratopathy (5%; reversible), cataracts; leukopenia, anemia; nausea, vomiting; hair loss (mild), rash; thrombophlebitis, thromboembolism; "tamoxifen flare" in first month of therapy

c. Rare. Abnormal LFTs; altered mental state; slightly increased occurrence of endometrial adenocarcinoma on prolonged use

3. Administration

a. Supplied as 10-mg tablets

b. Dose. 20 mg PO daily

F. Estrogens

1. Indications. Prostate and breast cancers

2. Toxicity

a. Nausea, feminization, uterine bleeding

b. Hypercalcemic flare in patients with breast cancer

c. Vaginal carcinoma in offspring if used during pregnancy

d. Painful gynecomastia (preventable in males with low dose breast irradiation)

e. Thromboembolic disorders (especially with doses >3 mg/day)

f. Abnormal LFTs, cholestatic jaundice (rare)

g. Chloasma, optic neuritis, retinal thrombosis; rash, pruritus

h. Fluid retention, hypertension, headache, dizziness, hypertriglyceridemia

i. Increased cardiovascular and cerebrovascular deaths in men with prostatic cancer

3. Administration

a. Diethylstilbestrol (DES)

(1) Supplied as 0.25-, 0.5-, 1.0-, and 5.0-mg tablets

(2) Dose

(a) Prostate carcinoma: 1–3 mg PO daily

(b) Breast carcinoma: 1–15 mg PO daily in divided doses

b. Diethylstilbestrol diphosphate (Stilphostrol)

        (1) Supplied as 250-mg ampules

        (2) Dose. 0.5–1.0 gm IV daily for five days

    c. Estramustine (Emcyt). See **VI.B.**

G. LHRH agonists (Leuprolide and others)

  1. Indications. Prostate (and possible breast) cancer

  2. Pharmacology. LHRH agonist analogues decrease serum levels of LH and follicle-stimulating hormone and result in castration levels of testosterone in men and of estradiol in women within two weeks of treatment.

  3. Toxicity and side effects

    a. Common. Hot flashes, decreased libido; impotence and gynecomastia in men; amenorrhea and uterine bleeding in women

    b. Occasional. Hypercholesterolemia, local discomfort at site of injection

    c. Rare. GI upset, rash, hypertension, azotemia, headache, depression

  4. Administration

    a. Leuprolide (Lupron)

      (1) Supplied as 3.75- and 7.5-mg vials; and a kit (14-mg multidose vial with syringes)

      (2) Dose. 7.5 mg of depot suspension IM or SQ monthly or 1 mg SQ daily

    b. Goserelin (Zoladex)

      (1) Supplied as 3.6-mg (pellet) in prefilled syringe

      (2) Dose. 3.6 mg SQ monthly

    c. Buserelin (Suprefact)

      (1) Supplied as 1 mg/ml (1000 µg/mL) injectable solution or nasal spray

      (2) Dose. By SQ injection: 500 µg SQ t.i.d. for first week, then 200 µg daily. By intranasal inhalation: 800 µg t.i.d. for one week, then 400 µg t.i.d.

H. Progestins

  1. Indication. Endometrial, breast, and renal carcinomas; or as an appetite stimulant

  2. Toxicity and side effects

    a. Menstrual changes, uterine bleeding, hot flashes, gynecomastia, galactorrhea

    b. Fluid retention, thrombophlebitis, thromboembolism

    c. Nervousness, somnolence, depression, headache

    d. Dermatologic (rare)

  3. Administration

    a. Medroxyprogesterone acetate (Provera, Depo-Provera)

      (1) Supplied as 10-mg tablets (Provera) or vials containing 400 mg/ml (Depo-Provera)

      (2) Dose

        (a) 1 gm IM weekly for six doses, then monthly *or*

        (b) 200–800 mg PO daily

    b. Megestrol acetate (Megace)

      (1) Supplied as 20- and 40-mg tablets

      (2) Dose. 40 mg PO q.i.d. for breast cancer and 80 mg q.i.d. for endometrial cancer; 160–1600 mg/day has been used as an appetite stimulant

VIII. Biologic therapies

  A. Hematopoietic growth factors have had a major impact on the ability to treat or defray chemotherapy-induced cytopenias. In vitro assays of hematopoiesis monitor the effects of colony-stimulating factors (CSFs) on burst-forming units (BFUs), or colony-forming units (CFUs) for erythrocytes (Es), granulocytes (Gs), macrophages (Ms), monocytes (Mos), megakaryocytes (Megs), and other blood cells.

    1. Erythropoietin (epoietin alpha, EPO, rhEPO, recombinant human erythropoietin, Epogen, Procrit). The administration of EPO can improve the hematocrit in some cancer patients, particularly those in need of red cell transfusions and with serum EPO levels that are not significantly elevated.

    a. Supplied as 2000-, 3000-, 4000-, and 10,000-units in 1-ml vials

    b. Toxicity. Hypertension, particularly with renal failure; shunt clotting in dialysis patients; allergic reactions (rare); possible thrombotic vascular events in patients with vascular disease (rare)

    c. Dose. For patients with chemotherapy-induced anemia: 150–300 units/kg SQ three times weekly (higher doses are not helpful). For patients with chronic renal failure or HIV-infection on zidovudine therapy: 50–100 units/kg SQ three times weekly to start; maintenance dose is 25 units/kg three times weekly. This therapy may decrease the transfusion requirement within 8–12 weeks of starting treatment; the target hematocrit is 30–33 percent.

2. Filgastrim (granulocyte colony-stimulating factor, G-CSF, Neupogen) stimulates CFU-G.

    a. Supplied as 300-μg (1 ml) and 480-μg (1.6 ml) vials.

    b. Toxicity. Transient bone pain (20% incidence) usually resolves without stopping treatment. Although splenomegaly is relatively common in patients receiving long-term therapy, it is rarely of clinical significance. Local inflammation at the injection site and mild LFT abnormalities may occur; other side effects are rare.

    c. Dose. 5 μg/kg/day SQ or IV for 7–14 days. Stop administration when the ANC exceeds 10,000/μl; the WBC decreases by 50 percent within 1–2 days. The dosage may be increased, but doses exceeding 10 μg/kg/day probably are not helpful.

3. Sargramostim (GM-CSF; Leukine, Prokine [yeast-derived]) and **molgramostim** (GM-CSF; Leukomax [*Escherichia coli*-derived]) stimulates CFU-GM and CFU-Meg.

    a. Supplied as 250- and 500-μg vials for sargramostim and 400-μg vials for molgramostim

    b. Toxicity. At low doses (5 μg/kg/day) side effects are similar to those caused by G-CSF. Fever, flu-like syndrome, and hypersensitivity reactions are more likely with GM-CSF preparations than with G-CSF. Diarrhea, asthenia, rash, malaise, and fluid retention (peripheral edema, effusions) may also occur. At transplantation doses (30 μg/kg/day or greater) a capillary-leak syndrome and its wide range of related side effects can occur.

    c. Dose. 250–1000 μg/m^2/day for 21 days have been administered in patients undergoing transplantation.

4. Other hematopoietic growth factors undergoing development

    a. Multi-CSF (IL-3) increases blood neutrophils and stimulates BFU-E, CFU-G, CFU-M, CFU-GM, CFU-Meg, and the pleuripotential CFU-GEMMo.

    b. PIXY-321 (GM-CSF/IL-3) stimulates CFU-GM, CFU-Meg, CFU-GEMMo, BFU-E, and BFU-Meg. It increases blood neutrophils in humans and blood neutrophils and platelets in primates.

    c. M-CSF (CSF-1) stimulates monocyte progenitors and activates and differentiates macrophages.

    d. Stem cell factor (also called kit ligand or mast cell growth factor) stimulates the size and number of all colonies in progenitor assays, including stem cells, megakaryocytes, mast cells, and melanocytes.

    e. "Thrombopoietin" (megakaryocyte growth and development factor) was recently discovered and stimulates CFU-Meg.

B. Immunotherapy

    1. Abbreviations. CTL (cytotoxic T lymphocyte), IL (interleukin), IFN (interferon), LAK (lymphokine-activated killer) cells, NK (natural killer) cells, MHC (major histocompatibility complex), TIL (tumor-infiltrating lymphocyte).

    2. Interferons

        a. Sources

            (1) IFN-α: Lymphocytes, macrophages, and other cells

(2) IFN-β: Fibroblasts and epithelial cells

(3) IFN-γ: Several lymphocyte subtypes after stimulation with antigen or mitogen (e.g., CD-4, CD-8, NK, or LAK cells)

b. Properties of IFN-α, -β, and -γ

(1) Antitumor activity for IFN-α and IFN-β, but not for IFN-γ

(2) Antiproliferative activity

(3) Inhibition of angiogenesis

(4) Regulation of differentiation

(5) Interaction with growth factors, oncogenes, other cytokines

(6) Enhancement of tumor-associated antigens

(7) Immunomodulation (NK cell activation, CTL activation, induction of MHC class I)

(8) Antiviral activity

c. Other properties of IFN-γ

(1) Antimicrobial activity mediated by monocytes and macrophages

(2) Regulation of lipid metabolism

(3) Immunomodulatory activity: activation of monocytes and macrophages, stimulation of MHC class II antigens, induction of B-cell immunoglobulin production, induction of IL-2 receptors

d. Clinical uses

(1) Response rates reported to be 75 to 90 percent in previously untreated patients: chronic myelogenous leukemia (chronic phase), hairy cell leukemia, myeloproliferative disorders, cutaneous T-cell lymphomas

(2) Response rates reported to be 40 to 50 percent in low-grade lymphomas, multiple myeloma

(3) Condylomata acuminata, non-A, non-B hepatitis, chronic granulomatous disease

e. Dose. A wide range of doses and schedules have been used, depending on the condition. From 2 to 10 to 36 million units/m^2 are given SQ for from 3–7 days weekly.

f. Toxicities (depend on dose and schedule of administration). Flu-like symptoms (75–100%) may be dose-limiting, develop in 1–2 hours, and peak 4–8 hours after injection. Malaise, headache, rashes (40–50%), GI complaints (20–40%), mild leukopenia or thrombocytopenia, elevated LFTs (30%), neurologic complaints, chronic fatigue (can be dose-limiting)

g. Supplied as

(1) IFN-α-2a (Roferon): 3, 6, and 36 million units/ml vials

(2) IFN-α-2b (Intron-A): 3, 5, 10, 25, and 50 million unit vials

(3) IFN-α-n1 (Wellferon): 8 to 12 million unit/ml vials

(4) IFN-α-n3 (Alferon): 5 million units/ml vials

(5) IFN-γ-1b (Actimmune): 3 million units/ml vials

3. IL-2 plays a major role in immune regulation. The primary action of IL-2 is to stimulate growth of activated T cells that bear IL-2 receptors. The binding of antigen in conjunction with IL-1 stimulates T cells to release IL-2, which signals further lymphocyte mitogenesis. Properties of the interleukins are summarized in Table 4-1.

a. Clinical uses. Approved by the Food and Drug Administration (FDA) for the treatment of metastatic renal cell carcinoma

b. Dose. 600,000–720,000 IU/kg every eight hours ("high dose") for five consecutive days for two cycles separated by 7–10 days. The course of treatment is repeated for patients who respond.

c. Toxicity. "High dose" therapy with IL-2 is highly toxic; it induces vascular permeability and promotes secretion of other lymphokines (such as IFN-γ) with their own sets of toxicities. These developments result in fluid retention and interstitial edema in several organ systems that appear to be reversible after administration of IL-2 ceases. "Low dose" IL-2 regimens are being investigated.

    d. Supplied as recombinant IL-2 (r-serHuIL-2, Aldesleukin, Proleukin) in 18 million IU vials

  4. Adoptive immunotherapy involves the transfer of TIL or LAK cells interacted with IL-2 to the host bearing the tumor. These cells have characteristics of non-MHC-restricted killer cells and are distinct from CTL and NK cells.

    a. CTLs destroy other lymphocytes that have acquired viral or tumor antigens. CTLs are stimulated by IFN and IL-2. The target cells must be of the same histocompatibility type as the cytotoxic T cell.

    b. NK cells (large lymphocytes with cytoplasmic granules) directly kill tumor cells. The activity and proliferation of NK cells are stimulated by a variety of lymphokines, including IFN and IL-2. The target cells need not be of the same histocompatibility type as the NK cells.

    c. LAK cells are collected by lymphocytapheresis and activated ex vivo by incubation with IL-2. Activated LAK cells acquire broad cytolytic activity against tumor cells.

    d. TIL can recognize tumor-associated antigens and accumulate in virtually all types of human tumors. TIL cultures can be readily established from most murine and human tumors. Administration of TIL with IL-2 appears to be 50–100 times more effective than LAK cells with IL-2. See sec. **D.1.**

    e. Clinical uses. Tumor regressions have been observed in 10 to 20 percent of patients with metastases from renal cancer, melanoma, and colorectal cancer.

  5. Monoclonal antibodies have the advantage of relative selectivity for tumor tissue and relative lack of toxicity. Major problems using them for therapy are technical and the development of human antimouse antibodies.

    a. Hybridomas. Mice, which are injected with live cancer cells, produce a large variety of lymphocyte clones, each of which has specificity for one antigen on the administered cancer cell. These lymphocytes are harvested from the spleen of the mouse and hybridized with a mouse myeloma cell, which then produces an antibody specific for each one of the original cancer cell antigens. These combined cells ("hybridomas") are separated into individual colonies, which produce a single type of antibody.

    b. Biologic effects. Monoclonal antibodies can attack certain cells directly (e.g., malignant lymphocytes exposed to a selective monoclonal antibody are lysed in the presence of complement). Various radioactive and chemotherapeutic agents can be conjugated to monoclones, which deliver these agents specifically to cancer cells. Plant toxins (e.g., ricin, abrin), bacterial toxins (*Pseudomonas* endotoxin A, diphtheria toxin), or ribosome-inactivating protein (RIP) can also be conjugated to monoclonal antibodies as **"immunotoxins."** Growth factors (e.g., IL, epidermal growth factor, tumor growth factor) can sometimes be used as carriers for toxins; these constructs are called **"oncotoxins."**

    c. Clinical uses

      (1) Imaging of tumors using radioisotope-labeled monoclones

      (2) Selectivity "purging" bone marrow of cancer cells

      (3) Treatment of tumors by conjugating substances

  6. Immune adjuvants, such as levamisole, BCG, H_2-receptor antagonists, retinoids, and thymic derivatives, are discussed with their related tumors.

 C. Differentiating agents induce cancer cells to mature along the expected pattern for the tissue of origin. Although a large number of agents have induced differentiation in vitro, the use of single agents to induce differentiation in vivo and regression of advanced cancer has been clinically disappointing; the singular exception is all-*trans*-retinoic acid in treating acute promyelocytic leukemia (see Chapter 25). Additionally, isoretinoin (13-*cis*-retinoic acid) has been effective in reversing oral leukoplakia and is being evaluated in various neoplasms of squamous epithelium. Many other agents showed promise and have been tested including 1,25-dihydroxyvitamin D_3, DMSO, cytosine arabinoside, phorbol esters, interferons, cyclic AMP analogues, and others.

D. Gene therapy can be defined as a therapeutic technique in which a functioning gene is inserted into a patient's cells to provide a gene or gene product that is missing, to provide a new gene or gene product, to modify the immune response, or to remove or inactivate an existing gene. With the explosion of scientific advances in this area, new possibilities for cancer therapy have emerged. Some possibilities are:

1. **Gene-modified TIL.** Although TILs can be specifically lytic, it appears that the secretion of cytokines such as IFN-γ and tumor necrosis factor (TNF) is the best correlate of the antitumor effectiveness of TILs. TILs depend on IL-2 for their continued survival. Clinical trials are underway using TIL transduced with the gene for TNF with the vision that transduction with the gene for IL-2 receptors may lessen the need for high doses of IL-2.

2. **Cytokine genes** have been introduced into a variety of animal tumors attempting to increase immunogenicity. Examples of genes that have been inserted include those for IL-2, IL-4, TNF, IFN-γ, and G-CSF.

3. **Antisense genes** may be injected in tumors attempting to block expression of oncogenes.

4. **Retroviral producer lines** may be injected into tumors attempting to introduce "suicide" genes into cancer cells.

5. **Bone marrow cells** are being subjected to gene modification attempting to increase resistance to chemotherapeutic agents.

E. Antisense oligonucleotides are short fragments of DNA that are complementary to the "sense" strand of mRNA. These molecules theoretically can inhibit the function of mRNA, which normally is translated into protein in the cytoplasm by ribosomes. If the protein is vital for cellular growth and reproduction, its inhibition could result in diminished cell viability. The use of antisense oligonucleotides are inhibitors of gene expression represents another genetically based therapeutic approach for cancer.

F. Circadian chronobiology. Three major biologic rhythms have been defined that correspond to the periodic changes in the environment: the solar day (circadian rhythm), the lunar month (circumtrigentan rhythm), and the year (circannual rhythm). Circadian rhythms are observable and reproducible for many biochemical and physiologic events in human beings, including activity, pulse, temperature, blood pressure, certain serum chemistry values, cell proliferation, tumor cell proliferation, and drug pharmacology. The suprachiasmatic nucleus of the hypothalamus appears to be the site of important circadian pacemaker cells in mammals. Data suggest that therapeutic effect may be maximized and toxicity minimized for cytotoxic drugs administered at selected times of day.

Table 4-1. Interleukins

Terminology		Growth factor activity		Other activities
Synonym	Molecule	Stimulates	Synergistic with	
Hematopoietin-1	IL-1		G-CSF GM-CSF	Costimulates B cells; Induces IL-2 production, IL-2 receptors, and other cytokines; Induces acute phase responses; Numerous immunologic activities
T-cell growth factor (TCGF)	IL-2	T cells, B cells, NK-cells, monocytes		Costimulates T cells and LAK cells; Stimulates TIL proliferation; Is chemotactic for T cells Costimulates B-cell proliferation and differentiation Stimulates Mo to become tumoricidal; Induces non-MHC restricted CTL killing; Induction/release of cytokines
Multi-CSF	IL-3	CFU-G, CFU-GM, CFU-GEMMo, CFU-M, CFU-Meg, BFU-E		
B-cell stimulating factor (BSF-1)	IL-4		EPO G-CSF IL-1	Costimulates IL-2-induced LAK; Activates B cells, T cells and M. Helps generation of CTL; Increases B-cell secretion of IgE and IgG_1; Decreases B-cell secretion of IgM, IgG_2 and IgG_3

Table 4-1 (continued)

Terminology		Growth factor activity		Other activities
Synonym	Molecule	Stimulates	Synergistic with	
B-cell growth factor (BCGF-II) T-cell replacing factor (TRF)	IL-5	B-cells eosinophils	GM-CSF or IL-3 to stimulate CFU-eos	Cofactor for CTL differentiation; Induces IL-2 receptor expression and release; Increases B-cell secretion of IgA and IgM
BSF-2	IL-6	Platelets in primates ($\pm$ IL-3)	IL-1, IL-3, GM-CSF	Increased in myeloma; Costimulates T cells; Induces acute phase responses; Induces B-cell differentiation; Induces mast cell differentiation in synergy with IL-3; Induces IL-2 production and CTL differentiation; Augments NK and LAK cytotoxicity; Enhances B-cell secretion of IgG; Enhances MHC class I expression
pBCGF	IL-7	B cells, T cells, NK cells, LAK cells	IL-2 to stimulate B cells and T cells	Induces LAK activity; Expands antitumor CTL; Enhances Mo secretion of cytokines and tumoricidal activity

PF4 superfamily Neutrophil chemotactic factor (NCF) T-cell factor (TCF) p40	IL-8		Chemotactic for neutrophils, basophils, T cells, B cells, and Mo
	IL-9	BFU-E, Meg cell line	Stimulates antigen-specific T-helper cell clones; Stimulates mast cell growth
Cytokine synthesis-inhibitor factor (CSIF)	IL-10	B cells, CD4 T cells, CD8 T cells, Mast cells	Costimulates proliferation of activated T-cells; Increases CTL precursors; Augments CTL activity; Suppresses IFN-γ production by macrophages
	IL-11	IL-3 to stimulate BFU-Meg and plasmacytoma	Stimulates T-cell dependent development of Ig-producing B cells
Cytotoxic lymphocyte-malnutrition factor/natural-killer stimulating factor (CLMF/NKSF)	IL-12	IL-2 to stimulate: LAK cells, NK cells, CD4 T cells, CD8 T cells, lymphoblasts	Stimulates antigen-activated CD4 and CD8-positive T cells (independent of IL-2); Stimulates IFN-γ secretion; Enhances NK activity

Key: CTL = cytotoxic T lymphocytes; EPO = erythropoietin; IFN = interferon; Ig = immunoglobulin; IL = interleukin; LAK = lymphokine-activated killer; MHC = major histocompatibility complex; NK = natural killer; TIL = tumor-infiltrating lymphocytes; BFU = burst-forming unit; CFU = colony-forming unit; CSF = colony-stimulating factor; E = erythrocyte; eos = eosinophil; G = granulocyte; M = macrophage; Meg = megakaryocyte; Mo = monocyte.

Sources: Adapted from S.A. Rosenberg, Principles and applications of biologic therapy. Chap. 17 in DeVita, V.T. Jr., Hellman, S., and Rosenberg, S.A. *Cancer, Principles & Practice of Oncology*, 4th edition. J.B. Lippincott, 1993; and Foon, K.A. The cytokine network. *Oncology* 7(12 Supp):11, 1993.

Symptom Care

Dennis A. Casciato

I. Pain

A. Background. The goal of chronic pain management in cancer patients is prevention or complete control of pain. The major impediments to this goal are ignorance and bias on the part of the physicians, nurses, patients, or patients' families. The first step in management should be directed toward relieving the physical cause of pain. Surgery, radiotherapy, or systemic therapy is selected depending on the site of involvement and the underlying disease.

   1. **Benign causes of pain.** Patients with neoplasms are likely to attribute every new pain to advancing cancer. Clear demonstration of nonmalignant causes of pain can both palliate the symptoms and reassure patients.

   2. **Placebos.** The use of placebos to evaluate whether the pain is "real" is not valid. Placebos are 50 percent as effective as the compared analgesic, whether it is aspirin or morphine. The conviction of the therapist about the potency of any drug is important to the placebo effect. Analgesia from placebos and opioids appears to have similar mechanisms involving endorphins.

   3. **Addiction.** Opioid tolerance and physical dependence are not the same as addiction. The possibility of addiction should never be considered a contraindication for the appropriate use of opioid analgesics, especially in patients with advanced cancer.

   4. **The mainstay of pain assessment** is patients' self-report of the pain history. Simple descriptive or numeric scales are helpful (e.g., a scale of 10). Have the patient keep time tables logging the presence or absence and location of pain and dose of analgesic taken.

   5. **Titration of analgesic dose to clinical response** is mandatory.

   6. **Ineffective analgesia.** The major reason for ineffective analgesia is insufficient doses of prescribed analgesics.

      a. Physicians largely underdose patients because of excessive concern about the dose and side effects of narcotics and fear of patient addiction.

      b. Patients are often reluctant to report pain because of concerns about distracting physicians from treatment of the underlying disease and fears that pain means the disease is worse.

      c. Patients may be reluctant to take prescribed narcotics because of concerns about becoming tolerant to pain medications or being thought of as an addict and worries about unmanageable side effects.

      d. Failure to control pain with *adequate analgesic therapy,* however, usually indicates the existence of factors other than focal tissue damage.

B. Non-narcotic analgesics

   1. **Acetaminophen** (Tylenol and others), 650 mg PO q.i.d., is nearly as effective as aspirin in both analgesic and antipyretic actions. Acetaminophen does not have the anti-inflammatory, ulcerogenic, or antiplatelet activities of aspirin.

   2. **Aspirin** is the standard against which other nonsteroidal anti-inflammatory drugs (NSAIDs) are compared. This analgesic is significantly more effective than placebo in patients with pain from cancer. Aspirin should not be used in patients with a history of the syndrome of nasal polyps and asthma, gastritis, peptic ulcer disease, or bleeding diathesis (including severe throm-

bocytopenia or concomitant use of anticoagulants). Aspirin can inhibit platelet aggregation for one week or more.

3. Other salicylates not associated with the antiplatelet activity of aspirin as they do not have the acetyl moiety include:
   a. Choline magnesium trisalicylate (Trilisate), 1000–1500 mg PO t.i.d.
   b. Choline salicylate (Arthropan), 870 mg PO q3–4h
   c. Magnesium salicylate (Doans, others), 650 mg PO q4h
   d. Sodium salicylate (generic), 325–650 mg PO q3–4h

4. Other NSAIDs may be especially useful for pain from bone metastases, paraneoplastic periostitis, or arthritis. These prostaglandin inhibitors should be given with the same precautions noted for aspirin (see **I.B.2**). They cost substantially more than aspirin. Choices from this class of drugs include:
   a. Carprofen (Rimadyl), 100 mg PO t.i.d.
   b. Diflunisal (Dolobid), 500 mg PO q12h
   c. Etodolac (Lodine), 200–400 mg PO q6–8h
   d. Fenoprofen calcium (Nalfon), 300–600 mg PO q6h
   e. Ibuprofen (several), 400–600 mg PO q6h
   f. Ketoprofen (Orudis), 25–60 mg PO q6–8h
   g. Ketorolac tromethamine (Toradol), 10 mg PO q4–6h
   h. Naproxen sodium (Anaprox), 275 mg PO q6–8h

C. Opioids alter patients' perception of pain and are the prototypical agents for central pain control. The differences among the opioids are grossly exaggerated; at effective doses, pain relief and side effects are similar. The "full agonist" opioids listed in Table 5-1 have increasing effectiveness with increasing doses and are not limited by a "ceiling." The doses are easily titrated. These agents do not reverse or antagonize other full agonists given simultaneously.

   1. Short-acting opioids
      a. Morphine sulfate (MS) remains the standard against which newer analgesics are measured. None of these agents is clinically superior for pain relief. MS is available in tablet, oral liquid, suppository, sustained-acting, and parenteral forms.
      b. Codeine (methylmorphine) is available alone and in several combinations with aspirin and acetaminophen. The effects of sedation, respiratory depression, and addictive potential are substantially less problematic for codeine than for morphine.
      c. Oxycodone (dihydrohydroxycodeinone) is well absorbed orally. It is available as 5.0-mg tablets alone and in combination with aspirin (Percodan) or acetaminophen (Percocet, Tylox).
      d. Hydromorphone (Dilaudid). The duration of action is only 1–2 hours for patients given small doses (2 mg) orally. As with other opioids, higher doses result in longer durations of effect.

   2. Long-acting opioids
      a. Controlled-release MS is the drug of choice for preventing chronic pain in patients with cancer (see **I.F**).
      b. Fentanyl transdermal patch (Duragesic) is a synthetic piperidine opioid analogue. The patch should be changed every three days (sometimes every two days). The peak analgesic effect is delayed 12–14 hours after applying and persists up to 24 hours after removing the patch.
      c. Methadone (Dolophine) has a primary half-life of 15 hours and a secondary half-life of 55 hours. This property leads to a high risk of cumulative toxicity. Methadone-induced respiratory arrest is sometimes preceded by increasing drowsiness and often develops as a sudden catastrophic event. Dose increments for methadone must be spaced several days apart. The authors usually do not recommend this drug for chronic pain in patients with cancer.
      d. Levorphanol (Levo-Dromoran) is equally effective orally and parenterally. The drug is longer acting and appears to be less likely than MS to cause nausea, vomiting, and constipation. The problem of delayed

Table 5-1. Commercial opioid products in the United States

Opioid analgesics [brand name]	Enteral form supplied as	Usual starting doses
SHORT-ACTING		
Codeine phosphate	15-, 30-, 60-mg (with ASA or AMP) tab	60 mg [0.5–1 mg/kg] q3–4h PO/SQ
Hydrocodone bitartrate		10 mg [0.2 mg/kg] q3–4h PO
[Anexsia 5/500, 7.5/650]	5.0-mg, 7.5-mg (+500- or 650-mg AMP) tab	
[Lorcet]	10.-mg (+650-mg AMP) tab	
[Lortab- 2.5/, 5/, 7.5/500]	2.5-, 5.0-, 7.5-mg (500 mg AMP) tab & liq	
[Lortab-ASA]	5.0-mg (+500-mg ASA) tab	
[Vicodin, Vicodin-ES]	5.0-mg, 7.5-mg (+500-mg AMP) tab	
Oxycodone HCl		10 mg [0.2 mg/kg] q3–4h PO
[Percodan]	4.5-mg (+325-mg ASA) tab	
[Percocet, Roxicet]	5.0-mg (+325-mg AMP) tab	
[Tylox, Roxicet 5/500]	5.0-mg (+500-mg AMP) tab	
[Roxicodone]	5.0-mg (+No ASA or AMP) tab	
Hydromorphone HCl		6 mg [0.06 mg/kg] q3–4h PO
[Dilaudid]	2-, 4-, 8-mg tab; 3-mg supp; 1-mg/ml (pint)	1.5 mg [0.015 mg/kg] q3–4h IV
[Hydrostat]	1-, 2-, 3-, 4-mg tab	
Morphine sulfate, immediate release		
[MSIR]	15- & 30-mg tab & cap	30 mg [0.3 mg/kg] q3–4h PO
[Roxanol, RMS]	5-, 10-, 20-, 30-mg supp	
[Roxanol, MSIR, OMS]	20-mg/ml (30 & 120 ml)	
[MSIR]	2- & 4-mg/ml (120 & 500 ml)	10 mg [0.1 mg/kg] q3–4h IV
LONG-ACTING		
Morphine sulfate, controlled release		
[MS Contin]	15-, 30-, 60-, 100-, 200-mg tab	30–120 mg [15–30 mg] q12h PO
[Oramorph]	30-, 60-, 100-mg tab	
Fentanyl	25-, 50-, 75- & 100-μg/hr patches (packs of 5)	25 μg/hr transdermal
[Duragesic]		
Levorphanol tartrate	2-mg tab	4 mg [0.04 mg/kg] q6–8h PO
[Levo-Dromoran]		2 mg [0.02 mg/kg] q6–8h IV
Methadone HCl	5- & 10-mg tab;	20 mg [0.2 mg/kg] q6–8h PO
[Dolophine]	1- & 2-mg/ml (500 ml)	10 mg [0.1 mg/kg] q6–8h IV

Key: AMP = acetaminophen; ASA = acetylsalicylic acid (aspirin).

accumulation for levorphanol is similar to that for methadone; the drug cannot be recommended for cancer pain prevention.

3. **Side effects of opioid analgesics** result mostly from their effect on the CNS and on smooth muscle tone.

   a. **GI effects** include constipation, nausea, vomiting, and biliary colic. Constipation is a universal concomitant of opioid therapy and is treated prophylactically (see **IV.A.3**).

   b. **Respiratory system.** Respiratory depression is a potentially life-threatening complication of narcotic overdose, but patients generally develop tolerance to the respiratory depressant effects of these agents. For subacute respiratory depression, withhold one or two opioid doses until symptoms resolve. For acute respiratory depression, administer **naloxone** (Narcan) slowly. Naloxone has no agonistic effects and produces no respiratory depression.

   To reverse narcotic-induced respiratory depression, the usual dose of naloxone is 0.4 mg (400 μg) every 3–5 minutes until respirations are 10–20 per minute. In patients on chronic opioid therapy, titrate the naloxone dose to improve respiratory function without reversing analgesia (e.g., 0.04–0.08 mg [40–80 μg] every 1–2 minutes). The reversal by naloxone lasts 20–40 minutes. If a patient took an overdose of methadone or levorphanol, the patient must be observed, and repeat doses of naloxone every few hours may be required for 24 to 72 hours.

   c. **CNS manifestations** include pupillary constriction, tremors, sedation, dysphoria, apprehension, apathy, mental confusion, hallucinations, and delirium. Narcotics may precipitate convulsions in patients with a medically controlled seizure disorder. Myoclonic jerks are problematic in patients on very high doses of MS (usually patients who are nearly refractory to its analgesic effect); try decreasing the dose by utilizing a variety of other analgesic techniques. For other CNS toxicities, decreasing the dose and increasing the frequency of administration of opioids, or administering caffeine, dextroamphetamine, or methylphenidate (Ritalin, 5–10 mg PO at breakfast and lunch) may help.

   d. **Other side effects**
      (1) **Genitourinary system.** Urinary urgency and urinary retention
      (2) **Cardiovascular system.** Orthostatic hypotension and sinus bradyarrhythmias
      (3) **Endocrine system.** SIADH; decreased release of adrenal corticotropic and gonadotropic hormones from the pituitary gland

4. **Drug interactions with narcotic analgesics**
   a. **Barbiturates** may result in increased CNS depression.
   b. **Phenothiazines** potentiate the analgesic effects of opiates.
   c. **Monoamine oxidase (MAO) inhibitors** should *not* be administered with narcotics because the combination may produce hypotension or hypertension, delirium, convulsions, respiratory arrest, or death. Examples of MAO inhibitors include procarbazine (Matulane, Natulan), phenelzine (Nardil), isocarboxazid (Marplan), tranylcypromine (Parnate), and pargyline (Eutonyl).
   d. **Curariform drugs** potentiate respiratory depression.
   e. **Rifampin** may precipitate withdrawal symptoms in patients taking methadone.

5. **Management of narcotic withdrawal.** The intensity of symptoms is usually inversely proportional to the duration of physical dependence. Symptoms develop within 2–48 hours after the last dose and usually peak at 72 hours. Opioid withdrawal is less life-threatening and dangerous compared to withdrawal from other classes of controlled drugs. Reassurance, education, and perhaps mild sedatives may well be all that is required for patients who develop physical dependence during hospitalization and who are not going to continue on the drugs. Small doses of clonidine, 0.05–0.1 mg PO t.i.d.

(or weekly skin patches of the drug) may reduce symptoms of withdrawal, especially tremors, hypertension, anxiety, and fevers.

D. Analgesics to be avoided

1. **Meperidine** (Demerol) is often prescribed in insufficient amounts and at intervals that are too long to maintain its pharmacologic effectiveness. Furthermore, repeated administration may result in CNS toxicity (tremor, confusion, seizures) due to accumulation of a toxic metabolite (normeperidine). High oral doses are required to relieve severe pain, and at effective analgesic doses, the risk of CNS toxicity increases.

2. **Propoxyphenes** (Darvon, Darvon-N) are usually ineffective; when effective, this is probably related to the acetaminophen content.

3. **Mixed agonist-antagonist drugs** are contraindicated in patients receiving opioid agonists because they may precipitate a withdrawal syndrome and increase pain. Examples of these agents are pentazocine (Talwin), butorphanol (Stadol), nalbuphine (Nubain), and denocine (Dalgan).

4. **Brompton's cocktail** has no analgesic benefit over using single opioid analgesics.

5. **Placebos.** See sec. **A.2.**

E. Administration of analgesics

1. **Starting treatment.** For mild to moderate pain, first use aspirin, acetaminophen, or an NSAID with or without adjuvant drugs (see **H**). When pain persists, *add* a short-acting opioid. If the peak effect does not last four hours, increase the dose rather than shortening the dosing interval. If pain continues or becomes moderate to severe, increase the opioid potency or dose.

2. **Dosage.** Inadequate dosage is the commonest cause of ineffectiveness. There is no maximum dosage of MS in patients with advanced cancer; the absolute milligram count is irrelevant.

3. **Route.** Opioids can be given orally, subcutaneously, rectally, transdermally (intranasally), intravenously, and into the epidural, subarachnoid, and intraventricular spaces of the cerebrospinal fluid (CSF). They should not be given intramuscularly in patients with chronic cancer pain because the injection causes pain and absorption of the drug is unreliable.

   When changing from the oral to the rectal route begin with the previous oral dose and titrate the dose upward frequently. When going from the oral route to parenteral route, use lower doses. The same is true when changing from the oral route to the subcutaneous, intramuscular, or intravenous route.

F. Treating constant pain in patients with advanced cancer. Develop a regimen that prevents pain rather than subdues it. Long-acting MS, particularly MS Contin, is the opioid of choice for cancer pain prevention. The analgesic effect of MS Contin peaks in 2–3 hours and lasts for 12 hours. The tablet should not be crushed, halved, or chewed, but can be administered rectally. MS Contin very rarely requires dosing more frequently than every 12 hours if adequate doses are given. Guidelines for pain prevention are as follows:

1. **Start with MS Contin** at a dose of 60–120 mg PO q12h (15–30 mg for small, frail opioid-naive patients). The starting dose depends on patient size, prior exposure to opioids, and the severity of pain. Doses should be taken on a regular basis ("by the clock"), but patients should not be awakened to receive drugs.

2. **Administer rapid-onset short-duration opioid agonists** (oral or parenteral) "as needed." Patients should not need to take more than 2–3 doses of short-acting opioids throughout the day for breakthrough pain; if so, increase the dose of the long-acting opioid.

3. **Give the appropriate dose,** which is the amount of opioid that controls pain with the fewest side effects. Depending on response and side effects, increase or decrease doses by 25 to 50 percent of the previous dose.

4. **Gradually taper opioids** when patients become pain-free as a result of other treatments to avoid withdrawal symptoms.

G. Parenteral administration of opioid analgesics should be reserved for patients who cannot tolerate the enteral routes or who are in acute pain crisis for which the rapid onset of action facilitates dose titration. Infusions of subcutaneous morphine may be given for their longer duration of action, but this becomes uncomfortable, particularly for emaciated patients. The intravenous route is preferred for patients who have inadequate subcutaneous tissue or who already have indwelling venous access devices.

1. **Patient-controlled analgesia (PCA)** using calibrated pump devices can be administered by either subcutaneous or intravenous routes. Boluses are used only to determine dose titration and to treat incident pains. Treatment in this manner is facilitated by using a computer-assisted drug-delivery system.

2. **Intravenous MS infusion.** Patients who have unremitting pain and who are expected to survive no longer than a few weeks may be treated with continuous, intravenous MS infusion. The starting dose is 5–10 mg/hr. The rate is increased until analgesia is attained or decreased if patients develop excessive drowsiness or respiratory depression.

3. **Infusion of MS into epidural or subarachnoid spaces** decreases systemic opiate exposure by stimulating opiate receptors at the spinal cord level and within the CNS. The analgesic effect of MS is amplified 5–10-fold by the epidural route and 50–100-fold by the subarachnoid route. This method is especially effective in patients with severe pain from bone metastases. Narcotic withdrawal symptoms, respiratory depression, and CNS depression appear to be rare with this treatment.

   These analgesic techniques, however, involve subarachnoid, epidural, or intraventricular infusion via implanted pumps or externalized catheters, and are invasive and expensive. They should be considered only for patients in whom aggressive local and systemic approaches have failed to adequately relieve pain or have been associated with intolerable toxicity. An intrathecal test dose of MS is given at least four days before implantation of a subarachnoid pump to gauge efficacy.

H. Adjuvant drugs in pain management

1. **Corticosteroids.** Peritumoral edema contributes to pain by pressure on or stretching of adjacent structures. Dexamethasone or prednisone may rapidly ameliorate headache from brain tumor or carcinomatous meningitis or liver pain from metastases stretching the liver capsule. Corticosteroids also improve mood and appetite and exert anti-inflammatory and antiemetic effects.

2. **Neuropathic pain syndromes,** particularly if the pains are lancinating or tic-like, can often be treated with tricyclic antidepressants alone or in combination with anticonvulsant drugs. These drug combinations are often effective in treatment of peripheral neuralgias, postherpetic neuralgia, and tic douloureux. Typical doses are:

   a. **Antidepressant drugs** (see sec. **H.3**)

   b. **Phenytoin** (Dilantin), 300–400 mg/day

   c. **Carbamazepine** (Tegretol), 400–800 mg/day

   d. **Valproic acid** (Depakene), 200–400 mg PO b.i.d. or t.i.d.

3. **Antidepressants** have innate analgesic properties, may potentiate the analgesic effect of opioids, and are useful for pain that has neuropathic or significant emotional components. Depressed patients may focus excessively on their pain. Treatment with a tricyclic antidepressant at bedtime may gradually improve the pain syndrome, although several weeks of therapy are required to produce an effect. The dose should be started low and increased slowly every few nights as long as no excessive morning sedation is present.

   a. **Nortriptyline** (Pamelor) has fewer sedative and anticholinergic side effects than amitriptyline. The starting dose is 25 mg PO h.s. (10 mg PO h.s. in frail patients); the dose is slowly escalated to 50–100 mg PO h.s.

   b. **Desipramine** (Desyrel), 100–300 mg PO h.s.

    c. Amitriptyline (Elavil), 75–150 mg/day PO h.s. Amitriptyline is the tricyclic with the largest track record for treatment of pain but has more side effects than other agents in the same class of drugs.

  4. Anxiolytic agents

    a. Benzodiazepines. Anxious or agitated patients often perceive anxiety as a painful sensation. Diazepam (Valium), alprazolam (Xanax), or lorazepam (Ativan) may be used if narcotic analgesics alone are not effective. These drugs should be avoided in patients with chronic brain syndrome and may produce paradoxical agitated, confusional states in some patients.

    b. Antihistamines, such as hydroxyzine (Atarax, Marax), 25–100 mg PO q.i.d., may be useful in the anxious patient as a mild anxiolytic agent with sedating, analgesic, antipruritic, and antiemetic properties.

    c. Haloperidol. Patients with chronic dementia may become agitated and confused when they develop pain. These patients often benefit from a regimen of haloperidol (Haldol), 1–3 mg/day with analgesics.

I. Behavioral modification for control of pain

  1. Operant conditioning is a method of symptom control that influences or changes behavior through manipulation of the consequences. Abnormal behavior associated with pain is not rewarded, but normal behavior is. The patient must also receive adequate analgesia for any actual pain.

  2. Hypnosis may help reduce or control pain in some patients, particularly when transiently uncomfortable therapy is necessary.

  3. Guided imagery. In this method, patients concentrate on what they imagine the tumor to be like inside the body and mentally try to make normal body defenses and antitumor therapy kill the tumor cells. Patients may also be told to focus on their pain and to imagine that it represents the body's attack on the tumor. Many patients gain an improved sense of well-being from this harmless technique, which may also be helpful for episodes of brief pain.

  4. Biofeedback and relaxation therapy may be useful for reducing tension and anxiety and have secondary salutary effects on pain.

  5. Cognitive distraction. Pain may be ameliorated by focusing attention on someone else or on something external. Television, radio, counting, praying, or repetition of simple statements (such as "I can cope") may be helpful for brief episodes of pain.

J. Physical methods of pain control

  1. Simple techniques that are useful for treating subacute and chronic pain include:

    a. Hot packs (avoiding burns) and **cold packs** (avoiding areas of poor circulation)

    b. Massage, pressure, vibration, and exercise

    c. Repositioning immobilized patients

    d. Immobilization for acute pain or for stabilization of compromised limbs

  2. Stimulation procedures

    a. Electric stimulation of specific areas may relieve pain. Transcutaneous stimulation is the simplest and safest method and has the most applications. The technique has been used primarily for neuritic types of pain (such as postherpetic neuralgia, amputation stump pain, phantom limb pain, and peripheral nerve injury), low back pain, and muscle tension syndromes. Dorsal column stimulation requires laminectomy and is rarely used in patients with chronic pain due to cancer.

    b. Acupuncture and acupressure do not appear to be effective for chronic cancer pain.

K. Neuroablative procedures require specially skilled anesthesiologists or neurosurgeons. Ablation of nerve tracts is accomplished with nerve section, radiofrequency lesioning, cryoanalgesia, or chemical neurolysis with 50–100% alcohol, 3–20% phenol, or hypertonic saline. Importantly, these techniques cause *reversible* nerve damage (i.e., pain will eventually return). Contraindications to most of these procedures are irreversible hemostatic defects, irreversible decreasing mental status, and long life expectancy.

1. **Nerve blocks** may be useful in patients with pain restricted to a single somatic nerve or adjacent nerves (e.g., postthoracotomy pain may be relieved by subcostal blocks). Short-acting local anesthetics are initially used to determine the location for a permanent procedure.

2. **Cordotomy** is the most useful procedure for patients with pain from cancer, particularly if the pain is unilateral and below the shoulder and if the expected survival is less than one year. Radiofrequency lesions to spinothalamic tracts of the spinal cord are generally placed at the C1-C2 level. Contralateral loss of superficial, deep, and visceral pain is produced in more than 75 percent of patients treated with percutaneous cordotomy.

   The duration of analgesia is limited to only a few months; there may also be a late development of incapacitating dysesthesia. In experienced hands, unilateral cordotomy is associated with low morbidity and mortality and minimal incidence of motor weakness and loss of bladder function. Common complications of bilateral cordotomy, on the other hand, include sleep apnea, fecal and urinary incontinence, loss of orgasm, and muscle weakness.

3. **Other neurolytic procedures**
   a. **Celiac plexus ablation** produces excellent results for upper abdominal visceral pain, particularly from cancers of the pancreas or stomach. It does not affect hepatic or splenic pain. In elderly patients in particular, percutaneous celiac plexus sympathectomy may be complicated by self-limited, severe hypotension, which resolves with liberal fluid administration.
   b. **Hypogastric plexus ablation** can be attempted for pelvic visceral pain. The procedure should not affect sphincter tone or lower extremity strength.
   c. **Spinal neurolysis** targets appropriate dorsal root ganglia. This procedure may be considered for unilateral chest wall pain or perineal pain.
   d. **Epidural corticosteroids** and hypertonic saline can be considered for vertebral body metastases, as well as for their more frequent use in pain from discogenic disease or spinal stenosis.

4. **Other neurosurgical procedures**
   a. **Medullary tractotomy** may be helpful in patients with intractable pain from head and neck cancers. Potential complications include diminished corneal reflexes, paresthesias, ipsilateral upper extremity ataxia, and contralateral body analgesia.
   b. **Cingulumotomy** is effective in patients with intractable pain caused by widespread cancer and emotional factors that make the pain intolerable. The procedure is directed at the intensity and unpleasantness of pain and does not interfere with intelligence, personality, or initiative.
   c. **Rhizotomy** requires laminectomy and thus severely restricts its usefulness in cancer patients with peripheral pain.
   d. **Glossopharyngeal nerve section** may be helpful in patients with glossopharyngeal neuralgia or pain in the faucial tonsil. The procedure may cause marked hypertension caused by interruption of the carotid sinus reflex.
   e. **Hypophysectomy** may relieve intractable pain caused by hormone-sensitive tumors. The procedure results in hypopituitarism and other problems.
   f. **Sympathectomy** is effective in several nonmalignant conditions, but does not relieve most cancer pain since the body wall is innervated by spinal nerves. Partial celiac plexus sympathectomy is useful, however, for pain from *pancreatic cancer* and should be considered at the time of laparotomy.

II. Oral symptoms
   A. **Stomatitis** can develop 2 to 10 days after treatment with many cytotoxic agents and during radiation to the head or neck. Resolution of symptoms usually occurs

2–3 weeks after completion of therapy but may persist longer. Sucking on ice chips or popsicles during the short infusion of certain cytotoxic agents (e.g., methotrexate) may prevent the development of stomatitis.

1. Symptoms and signs. Stomatitis is usually first noted by the patient as sensitivity to acid foods, such as citrus juice or hot food. Erythema and then aphthous ulcers develop. In severe cases, lesions progress to extensive ulceration and massive sloughing of the oral mucosa. The possibility of *Candida albicans* or herpesvirus infection should be excluded.

2. Treatment. The following measures may relieve symptoms:

   a. Foods that trigger the pain are avoided.

   b. Abstention from alcohol and tobacco.

   c. Sucking on popsicles and cold beverages.

   d. Rinsing the mouth frequently with baking soda mixed in water.

   e. Sipping 5–15 ml of viscous 2% lidocaine (Xylocaine) for 30 seconds before meals and as often as necessary.

   f. Sipping 2.5–5.0 ml of liquid hydrocodone (e.g., Lortab solution) or cocaine (1–2%).

   g. Swishing and expectorating commercial suspensions.

      (1) Ulcerease: Glycerine, sodium bicarbonate, and sodium borate

      (2) BAX: Lidocaine, diphenhydramine, sorbitol, and Mylanta

      (3) Stomafate: Sucralfate, Benylin syrup, and Maalox

B. Xerostomia is a complication of radiation therapy or radical surgery to the head and neck, of commonly used medications (such as antihistamines and opioids), and of mouth breathing. Treatment can consist of

1. Keeping something in the mouth (e.g., chewing gum).

2. Ensuring adequate intake of water and electrolyte solutions, such as Socco or Gatorade.

3. Sucking hard candies (e.g., Life Savers, cinnamon, lemon drops)

4. Frequent mouthwashing with cetylpyridinium (Cepacol)

5. Prescribing pilocarpine hydrochloride tablets (5–10) t.i.d. or q.i.d. Allow 8–12 weeks to assess effectiveness.

6. Applying a thin layer of petroleum jelly to the lips frequently. Alternatively, the application to chafed lips of "bag balm" (used for cow udders and obtainable from feed stores or veterinary supply houses) gives "amazing" results, according to irrefutable nurses.

7. Using commercial preparations of artificial saliva, such as Salivart or Xerolube sprays.

C. Abnormal taste is a common symptom in patients with cancer. Patients often complain of a metallic taste or of food not tasting right or being without taste. Loss of taste, specifically for red meat, is frequent. There may be a low threshold for bitterness (urea) or a high or low threshold for sweetness. Both chemotherapy and radiotherapy can aggravate loss of taste. Treatment possibilities are

1. Reducing the urea content of the diet by eating white meats, eggs, and dairy products.

2. Masking the bitter taste of urea-containing foods by marinating meats, using more and stronger seasonings, eating food at cold or room temperatures, and drinking more liquids.

3. Helping overcome general poor taste by eating foods that are tart (lemonade frozen in ice trays, pickles, vinegar) or which leave their own taste (fruit, lemon drops, hard candy).

4. Eliminating dental problems.

D. Halitosis. Treatment possibilities include:

1. Improving oral and dental hygiene

2. Ensuring adequate fluid intake

3. Using Cepacol mouthwash or Breath Assure capsules

4. For oropharyngeal malignancies, treating xerostomia (see sec. **II.B**) and using 10% hydrogen peroxide gargles (on awakening, p.c., and h.s.)

5. Treating oral candidiasis and other infections appropriately

E. Dysphagia

1. **Etiology.** Dysphagia may be caused by mechanical obstruction or neuromuscular defects and should be distinguished from odynophagia.

2. **Management.** After there is agreement about treatment and feeding goals, treatment possibilities include:

   a. **Dietary advice** regarding soft food.

   b. **Attempt to retard lumen constriction** with radiation or laser treatment of the tumor or intermittent bouginage with a blunt-tipped bougie. A trial of corticosteroids may also be given.

   c. **Endoprosthesis** (see Chap. 9, *Esophageal Cancer,* sec. **VI.B.2**). If the tube blocks, the patient should sip small amounts of water and, every 30 minutes, dilute hydrogen peroxide. Alternatively, the tube can be flushed with Coca Cola.

   d. **Reduce saliva production** when total obstruction produces sialorrhea and drooling with anticholinergics, irradiation of the salivary glands (400–1000 cGy), or alum mouthwashes.

III. Nausea and vomiting

A. Etiology

1. **Differential diagnosis.** Nausea and vomiting in cancer patients occur most often as a result of cytotoxic chemotherapy. Other causes include brain metastases, bowel obstruction, electrolyte imbalance (notably hypercalcemia), radiation therapy to the abdomen, and treatment with other drugs (narcotic analgesics, antibiotics).

2. **Cytotoxic drugs.** Drugs that are highly emetic include cisplatin, dactinomycin, anthracyclines, dacarbazine, nitrosoureas, nitrogen mustard, and high-dose cyclophosphamide (see Appendix B1). The mechanisms for nausea and vomiting from chemotherapy are poorly defined but appear usually to be mediated by the CNS; some drugs may have peripheral activity. Acute chemotherapy-induced vomiting typically occurs 1–2 hours after treatment and usually resolves in 24 hours. Subacute vomiting occurs 9–18 hours after giving chemotherapy (especially carboplatin or ≥ 700 mg/m^2 of cyclophosphamide. Delayed vomiting occurs 48–72 hours after giving cisplatin (especially with doses ≥ 100 mg/m^2) and diminishes in 1–3 days.

3. **Psychologic and behavioral factors** may induce or modify vomiting. Patients may vomit even before receiving chemotherapy (anticipatory vomiting) when the IV line is started, the syringe is seen, or even before leaving home on the day chemotherapy is scheduled. Emesis is more easily controlled, on the other hand, in patients with histories of chronic heavy alcohol use.

B. Management

1. **Prevention and treatment of vomiting.** It is best to prevent nausea and vomiting with adequate doses of antiemetics, particularly when drugs that are known to induce vomiting are used.

   a. **Serotonin receptor (5-HT3) antagonists** bind to type 3 receptors of serotonin (5-hydroxytryptamine, 5-HT) and are the drugs of choice to prevent emesis generated by highly emetic regimens. 5-HT3 blockers alone achieve complete abrogation of emesis in about 60 percent of patients and achieve major control of emesis in 75 percent of patients.

      (1) Dosage

      (a) Ondansetron (Zofran), 0.15 mg/kg IV every four hours for three doses, or 8 or 32 mg IV for one dose. Effectiveness is potentiated by dexamethasone.

      (b) Granisetron (Kytril), 10 μg/kg IV for one dose.

      (2) Side effects are mild headache, constipation, and transient transaminase elevations. Extrapyramidal side effects do not occur.

   b. **Metoclopramide** (Reglan), a procainamide derivative, acts both centrally (at the chemoreceptor trigger zone) and peripherally (by stimulating gastric and small bowel motility, thereby preventing gastric stasis and dilatation). This drug appears to have served a transitional role between the older agents and the newer 5-HT3 antiemetics.

    (1) Dosage: 1–3 mg/kg IV every two hours for 2–6 doses.

    (2) Side effects include mild sedation, dystonic reactions (especially in young patients), akathisia (restlessness), and diarrhea. The drug is given with lorazepam, diphenhydramine, and corticosteroids to prevent these complications.

  c. Phenothiazines are not as effective as 5-HT3 blockers or metoclopramide for patients who are given highly emetic cytotoxic agents.

    (1) Dosage: Prochlorperazine (Compazine), 10 mg IV or 25 mg PR q3–6h.

    (2) Side effects include sedation, orthostatic blood pressure changes, extrapyramidal dystonic reactions, and restlessness.

  d. Butyrophenones are potent inhibitors of the central pathways for vomiting; they have fewer cardiovascular side effects than phenothiazines. Other side effects are similar to the phenothiazines.

    (1) Haloperidol (Haldol), 1–3 mg PO or IM q2–4h for two or three doses.

    (2) Droperidol (Inapsine), 0.5 mg IV q4h as needed; dosage is increased to 0.75 to 1.0 mg IV if tolerance develops.

  e. Lorazepam (Ativan), 1 or 2 mg IV or sublingually (SL) q3–6h, is very useful in patients who are treated with cisplatin or who have refractory or anticipatory vomiting. The drug's amnesic effect and its ability to prevent or treat restlessness associated with metoclopramide are also helpful.

  f. Δ-9-tetrahydrocannabinol (THC) is the main active ingredient in marijuana and can relieve nausea and vomiting in some patients who do not respond to other antiemetic drugs. The drug should be prescribed cautiously for elderly patients and not at all for patients with cardiovascular or psychiatric illness.

    (1) Dosage is 2.5- to 10-mg PO q3–4h. THC is available as Marinol in 2.5-, 5.0- and 10-mg capsules.

    (2) Side effects include orthostatic hypotension, sedation, dry mouth, ataxia, dizziness, euphoria, and dysphoria. Maintaining a "high" is correlated with the antiemetic effect in younger patients.

  g. Corticosteroids are effective for treating chemotherapy-induced vomiting by themselves or with ondansetron. Recommended dosages are

    (1) Dexamethasone, 10–20 mg IV q4h for one or two doses

    (2) Methylprednisolone, 125 mg IV for one or two doses

2. Combination regimens to prevent emesis include

  a. 5-HT3 blockers plus a corticosteroid (with or without a phenothiazine)

  b. Metoclopramide plus a corticosteroid plus diphenhydramine plus lorazepam

3. Agents for treatment of nausea

  a. Antacids, which perhaps work by speeding gastric emptying

  b. Antihistamines. Promethazine (Phenergan), diphenhydramine (Benadryl), dimenhydrinate (Dramamine), and meclizine (Antivert) are given in dosages ranging from 12.5–50 mg/day PO q6h.

  c. Scopalamine (Transderm Scop), 1–6 patches for every three days

  d. Phenothiazines

    (1) Prochlorperazine (Compazine), 5–20 mg PO q4–6h

    (2) Thiethylperazine (Torecan), 10 mg PO t.i.d.

    (3) Chlorpromazine (Thorazine), 10–50 mg PO q4–6h

  e. Haloperidol (Haldol), 0.5–1.0 mg PO q4–12h

  f. Metoclopramide (Reglan), 10–20 mg PO q6–8h (if gastric stasis is suspected)

4. Delayed vomiting (see III.A.2), occurring 1–2 days after treatment, is most often seen following high doses of cisplatin and is difficult to treat. The following may be tried:

a. **Dexamethasone alone:** 8 mg b.i.d. PO for two days, then 4 mg b.i.d. for two days; *or,*

b. **Metoclopramide:** 0.5 mg/kg q.i.d. PO for two days with dexamethasone; *or*

c. **Ondansetron:** 4 or 8 mg t.i.d. to q.i.d. for three days with or without dexamethasone

5. **Anticipatory vomiting** is exceedingly difficult to palliate. Prevention of emesis when chemotherapy is first given is the best way to prevent anticipatory vomiting. Antiemetics should be prescribed generously and chemotherapy should be given as late in the day as possible. Symptoms may improve with

a. Sedatives, including antihistamines

b. Hypnosis by an experienced psychologist

c. Progressive muscle relaxation, which involves learning to relax by actively tensing and then relaxing specific muscle groups in a progressive manner.

d. Cognitive distraction (see **I.I.5**)

e. Relaxation techniques with guided imagery

f. Operant conditioning. For example, patients may be treated in an area and on a day different from their usual place and time.

IV. Colorectal symptoms

A. Constipation

1. **Etiology**

a. **Inactivity.** Prolonged bed rest, inadequate exercise, and neurologic problems resulting from spinal cord compression or cauda equina syndrome predispose to decreased motility of the bowel, hard stools, or impaction.

b. **Drugs.** Narcotic analgesics and vincristine are the most common offenders; others are calcium and aluminum antacids, anticholinergics, anticonvulsants, antidepressants, and abused laxatives or enemas.

c. **Metabolic abnormalities** include malignant hypercalcemia, hypokalemia, myxedema, and dehydration.

d. **Mechanical obstruction** of the bowel may be caused by fecal impaction, tumor, inflammatory strictures, or barium from contrast studies.

2. **Some preparations available** for the treatment of constipation in the United States are

a. **Bulk producers.** Psyllium mucilloid (Metamucil, Konsyl) must be taken with adequate liquids.

b. **Stool softeners**
   (1) Docusate sodium (Colace): 50- and 100-mg capsules
   (2) Docusate calcium (Surfak): 50- and 240-mg capsules
   (3) Mineral oil (Kondremul, Haley's MO); 30–120 ml daily

c. **Peristalsis stimulants**
   (1) Sennosides (Senokot): 8.6-mg tablet (or syrup)
   (2) Bisacodyl (Dulcolax): 5-mg tablet, 10-mg suppository, enema
   (3) Others: casanthrol, cascara sagrada, phenophthalein, castor oil

d. **Combinations**
   (1) Sennosides and docusate sodium (Senokot-S)
   (2) Casanthranol and docusate sodium (Peri-Colace)
   (3) Danthron and docusate sodium (Doxidan)

e. **Saline or osmotic laxatives** with or without cascara sagrada
   (1) Magnesium hydroxide (milk of magnesia): 15–30 ml PO h.s.
   (2) Magnesium citrate: 10-oz solution, tablets, suppositories
   (3) Sodium phosphates (Fleet Phospho Soda): PO or enema
   (4) Lactulose (Cephulac): 45–60 ml per dose
   (5) Polyethylene glycol (Go-LYTELY): 8 oz every 15 minutes
   (6) Diatrizoate meglumine (Gastrografin): 250 ml enema

3. **Prevention and management of narcotic-induced constipation.** Patients who are receiving regular dosages of narcotics (or vincristine) should be carefully questioned about bowel movements. They should be encouraged to drink liquids (i.e., water, prune juice, coffee) and to eat bran cereal daily.

However, these measures plus stool softeners are usually insufficient, and bulk producers are poorly tolerated. The combination of docusate plus senna extract in parallel increasing doses is recommended to prevent narcotic-induced constipation. Physicians should exercise caution; brand name preparations (e.g., Senokot-S, Peri-Colace) can cost 10 times more than generic preparations of these agents.

  a. Start all patients who take narcotic analgesics on two tablets of Senokot-S (or the equivalent) at bedtime. If no bowel movement occurs in any 24–48-hour period, increase the dosage to two, three, or four tablets b.i.d. or t.i.d. as needed.

  b. If no bowel movement occurs in any 48–72-hour period, add Dulcolax, 2 tablets PO h.s. (or to t.i.d. if needed).

  c. If no bowel movement occurs in any 72–96-hour period, give an osmotic or saline laxative (see **IV.A.2.e**).

  d. Clonidine, 0.1 mg PO b.i.d. to q.i.d., may be helpful for narcotic bowel. It can then be tapered when effective.

B. Rectal discharge

  1. Etiology. Rectal discharge may be caused by hemorrhoids, fecal impaction, tumor, radiation proctitis, and various rectal fistulae.

  2. Management. After addressing the primary cause, inflammation may be reduced with corticosteroid suppositories or enemas. The skin of the perineum and genitalia must be protected and kept clean (without soap) and dry.

V. Urinary symptoms

A. Dysuria

  1. Etiology. Inflammation of the urinary bladder or outlet.

  2. Management includes treatment of infection if present and

  a. Phenazopyridine (Pyridium), 100–200 mg PO t.i.d.

  b. Amitryptyline, 25–50 mg PO h.s. (especially for interstitial cystitis)

B. Bladder spasm

  1. Etiology. Vesicular irritation by cancer, postradiation fibrosis, indwelling catheter, cystitis, or anxiety.

  2. Management. Cystitis is treated with antibiotics, catheter change, and bladder irrigation if a urethral catheter is present. Drugs of choice are

  a. Flavoxate (Urispas), 200–400 mg PO q.i.d.

  b. Hyoscyamine sulfate

  (1) 0.125-mg tablets (Levsin), one or two tablets PO or SL q4h

  (2) 0.15-mg tablets (Cystospaz), one or two tablets PO q.i.d.

  (3) 0.375-mg sustained release capsules (Levsinex, Cystospaz-M), one capsule q12h

  c. Belladonna-opium suppositories (B & O Supprettes), one q4h

  d. Propantheline bromide (Pro-Banthine), 15 mg PO h.s. or b.i.d.

  e. Oxybutynin chloride (Ditropan), 5-mg PO t.i.d. or q.i.d.

  f. Blocks of the lumbar sympathetic plexus may be effective for the management of intractable bladder pain.

C. Urinary hesitancy

  1. Etiology. Malignant or benign prostate enlargement, infiltration of the bladder neck, presacral plexopathy, drugs, intrathecal block, bladder denervation by surgery, loaded rectum, inability to stand to void, and asthenia.

  2. Management. Address the specific causes; a urethral catheter may be necessary. Drugs that may be useful include:

  a. Terazosin hydrochloride (Hytrin), 1- to 10-mg PO h.s.

  b. Bethanecol (Urecholine), 10–30 mg PO b.i.d. to q.i.d.

D. Discolored urine may be caused by food or drugs and is of no concern, except for the anxiety provoked in the patient.

  1. Pink or red urine: Beets, blackberries, rhubarb; Adriamycin; phenolphthalein, senna, cascara, danthron (e.g., in Doxidan); deferoxamine (Desferal); chlorzoxazone (Paraflex); phenothiazines; phenazopyridine (Pyridium)

  2. Brown or black urine: Phenacetin, salicylate; metronidazole (Flagyl); nitrofurantoin, chloroquine, quinine quinacrine, sulfonamides (yellow-brown); L-dopa, methyldopa (Aldomet); iron dextran (Imferon)

   3. **Blue or green urine:** Methylene blue, food coloring and other dyes; riboflavin; indomethacin, amitryptyline, danthron, mitoxantrone

VI. Respiratory symptoms

A. Cough

   1. **Etiology.** The causes of cough are numerous.
   2. **Management**
      a. Recommend that patients stop smoking. The antitussive effect of abstinence may require four weeks, however.
      b. Antihistamines are given for postnasal drip, bronchodilators for bronchospasm, diuretics for heart failure, and antibiotics for infection. Antitumor therapy should be given if practical.
      c. Improve the efficacy of the cough by asking patients to sit up to cough, and consider physiotherapy and postural drainage.
      d. Mucolytics include
         (1) Water via humidifier
         (2) Inhalations of steam or compound benzoin tincture
         (3) Guaifenesin (Robitussin), potassium iodide (SSKI), acetylcysteine (Mucomyst)
      e. Antitussives include
         (1) Dextromethorphan (Robitussin-DM)
         (2) Benzonatate (Tessalon perles), 100 mg q4h
         (3) Scopolamine, 0.3 to 0.6 mg IM or SQ q4h, or Transderm Scop patches
         (4) Hydrocodone with phenyltoloxamine (Tussionex) or with homatropine (Hycodan). Both preparations contain 5 mg of hydrocodone per tablet or teaspoonful and are taken every 4–8 hours.
         (5) Other opioid analgesics, including morphine

B. Hiccups

   1. **Etiology.** Gastric distention, diaphragmatic irritation, phrenic nerve irritation, brain tumor, uremia, or infection.
   2. **Management.** The following suggestions are derived from personal experience and recommendations by Twycross and Lack.
      a. **Pharyngeal stimulation:** Two teaspoons of granulated sugar, two glasses of liquor, a cold key down the back of a hyperextended neck, a nasopharyngeal tube, and drinking a glass of cool water through a straw while plugging both the patient's ears with his or her fingers.
      b. **Reduction of gastric distention:** Nasogastric intubation, peppermint water (relaxes esophageal sphincter), or antiflatulents (simethicone).
      c. **Induction of hypercarbia** by breath-holding or using a rebreathing bag.
      d. **Central suppression of hiccup reflex** with chlorpromazine 25 mg IV.
      e. **Other helpful measures**
         (1) Metaclopramide, 10–20 mg PO q4h
         (2) Nifedipine, 10–20 mg PO q8h
         (3) Quinidine, 200 mg q.i.d.
         (4) Benzonatate (Tessalon perles), 100 mg q.i.d.
         (5) Atropine, 0.4–1.2 mg IV
         (6) Phrenic nerve crush has been used.

C. Preterminal dyspnea

   1. **Etiology.** Patients with terminal cancer and pulmonary insufficiency from any cause often have panic attacks when developing shortness of breath. They fear they will stop breathing and suffocate while asleep.
   2. **Management**
      a. **For respiratory panic,** calmly educate patients about breathing control and give diazepam PO.
      b. **For shortness of breath associated with tachypnea,** give morphine sulfate and corticosteroids PO.
      c. **For air hunger,** intravenous morphine sulfate and diazepam or lorazepam may be the only possible humane measures.

    d. For massive projectile hemoptysis, an occasional but fatal complication of lung cancer, give enough diazepam or morphine intravenously or rectally to render patients unconscious.

D. "Death rattle"
1. **Etiology.** Patients who are too weak to expectorate.
2. **Management.** Place patients in the semi-Fowler's position. Oropharyngeal suction may be used in unconscious patients for cosmetic purposes when staff or visitors are present. Scopolamine or atropine in dosages of 0.3–0.8 mg SQ q2–4h may be helpful.

VII. Skin problems

A. Pruritus

1. **Etiology.** Generalized pruritus can develop as a result of
   a. Scabies, dry flaky skin, or other primary skin conditions
   b. Biliary tract obstruction
   c. Paraneoplastic syndrome
   d. Cutaneous metastases or lymphomas
   e. Renal failure
   f. Psychiatric causes
   g. Iron deficiency, polycythemia vera, systemic mast cell disease
   h. Thyroid disease, hyperparathyroidism
   i. Hypersensitivity to drugs

2. **Management.** Control of the underlying cancer may relieve itching. Drugs suspected of causing hypersensitivity reactions should be stopped. Factors that increase the perception of pruritus include dehydration, heat, anxiety, and boredom.

   a. **Instructions to patients.** Patients should be told to avoid traumatizing the skin by alcohol rubs, woolen clothing, or frequent bathing. Excessive bathing, especially with detergents and hot water, results in dry skin, which causes itching in itself. The use of baby oil, olive oil, lanolin, bland creams, emollient creams, or petroleum jelly should be encouraged. The skin should be "oiled" after each bath or shower, blotting in the agent while toweling dry. The use of soap should be stopped and situations that result in increased sweating avoided.

   b. **Local therapy**
      (1) Bland cool compresses or calamine lotion
      (2) Vioform-Hydrocortisone cream b.i.d. or t.i.d. on inflamed areas
      (3) Electron beam radiotherapy is often effective in relieving pruritus from cutaneous lymphomas.
      (4) Biliary drainage procedures for obstruction.

   c. **Drug therapy**
      (1) Cyproheptadine (Periactin), 4–6 mg q6h
      (2) Antihistamines (see sec. **III.B.3.b**)
      (3) Diazepam (Valium), 5–10 mg b.i.d. or q.i.d.
      (4) Dexamethasone, 2 or 4 mg daily or b.i.d.
      (5) Methyltestosterone, 25 mg sublingually b.i.d., for cholestatic jaundice. The mechanism is unknown, but pruritus is frequently relieved.
      (6) Cholestyramine resin (Questran) is occasionally effective in patients with pruritus from biliary tract obstruction but causes severe constipation and malabsorption of foods and drugs.

B. Preventive skin care in dying patients is extremely important to their comfort. The following are recommendations of Twycross and Lack:

1. **Prevent decubiti by redistributing pressure**
   a. At home, obtain a camping mattress and fill it with water instead of air to create a waterbed.
   b. For wheelchairs, use an inflatable cushion or egg crate foam.
   c. Elbow and heel pads, sheepskin mats, self-adhering urethane foam, pillows, and bed cradles may be helpful.
   d. Turn or reposition patients frequently

2. **Provide optimal hydration and hygiene**
   a. Avoid soap on dry fragile skin, creams and ointments in intertriginous areas, and trauma (from restraints, tape, etc.).
   b. On normal skin, use mild soaps, pat dry, use gentle massage with bland cream, and use petroleum jelly on elbows and heels.
   c. On dry skin, use fine talc.
   d. On chafed areas, use silicone spray or Opsite.
   e. Change bed linen often.

C. **Hair loss**
   1. **Etiology.** Irradiation to the scalp and administration of certain cytotoxic drugs result in marked alopecia. Hair loss begins 2–3 weeks after these therapies are started. Hair usually regrows after therapy is discontinued. The relative risks of hair loss caused by chemotherapeutic agents are shown in Appendix B1.
   2. **Management**
      a. **Emotional support.** Patients need to be forewarned. Hair loss should be discussed openly and sympathetically and its importance compared to the potential benefits of therapy. Inform patients about the relative risks of the specific regimen for alopecia. Explain that hair loss is preceded by scalp itching or pain and that hair is often curly when it regrows.
      b. **Wigs** should be obtained as soon as hair loss becomes evident (or before). Complimenting patients' appearance in a wig (if sincere) aids in adjustment.
      Prescribe a "scalp prosthesis" for insurance carriers.
      c. **Other measures.** Suggest the use of hats and colorful scarves, soft-bristle brushes, mild shampoos, and satin pillow cases. Discourage the use of blow-dryers, hot rollers, and exposure of the scalp to the sun.

VIII. **Necrotic, malodorous tumor masses**
   A. **Pathogenesis.** Progressively growing tumor masses may erode through the overlying skin and ulcerate. The center of the mass becomes necrotic and develops a nauseating odor, which worsens if the mass becomes infected with anaerobic organisms. The stench makes it difficult for others to enter the room; patients become isolated from contact with others. Patients themselves often do not notice the odor.
   B. **Management**
      1. **RT.** Large masses that may invade the overlying skin should be irradiated to prevent skin breakdown.
      2. **Amputation** may be necessary for tumors that do not respond to RT or chemotherapy (e.g., an extremity that is ravaged with sarcoma or a breast with massive carcinoma).
      3. **Skin metastases** confined to one small area of the body may be amenable to local resection. However, recurrences are likely.
      4. **Chemotherapy or endocrine therapy** should be used appropriately for the primary tumor.
      5. **Local care**
         a. **Flushing.** Necrotic tumor masses and fistulas should be generously irrigated at least t.i.d. with large volumes of 3% hydrogen peroxide.
         b. **Silver nitrate,** 1% solution soaked in large gauzes may be applied to necrotic areas by a gloved operator every day or two to help reduce oozing and odor. Absorbed silver may cause renal damage.
         c. **Maggots** actually debride necrotic tissue. However, the sight of maggots in wounds is usually more than people can tolerate. Diethyl ether in generous amounts is applied to the tumor surface with 4- × 4-in gauze; the gauze is wrung out onto the lesion so it reaches the deeper ulcerated areas. Maggots rapidly recur if treatment with ether is stopped.
      6. **Measures to control odor**
         a. **Isolate** patients with malodorous tumors in private rooms. An outward facing fan is placed to blow air *out* of the window.

b. **Room deodorizers** should be used. The deodorant aromas should be changed every few days to avoid conditioning of the staff, who will soon identify the smell of the product with the rather thinly disguised stench of necrotic cancer.

c. **Metronidazole** (Flagyl), 250–500 mg q.i.d., may be helpful, particularly if anaerobic bacterial infection is present.

d. **Chloresium,** a 22% chlorophyll-copper complex in isotonic saline, is a true deodorizing agent and can be poured directly onto the necrotic tissues.

IX. Fever

A. **Causes.** The diagnosis of tumor-induced fever is one of exclusion. It may develop in the course of nearly any malignancy but is especially common in

1. Hodgkin's disease, malignant lymphomas, and myeloproliferative disorders
2. Retroperitoneal cancer
3. Metastatic cancer to the liver
4. Hepatocellular and renal cell carcinoma
5. Gastric and pancreatic cancers
6. Bone sarcomas

B. **Management**

1. Controlling the underlying tumor, when possible, is the most effective means of controlling fever from tumors.
2. Aspirin and acetaminophen may be alternated every two hours as necessary
3. Indomethacin, 25–50 mg PO t.i.d., is often helpful.
4. Corticosteroids may be helpful but are generally not necessary.

X. Obstructive lymphedema

A. **Etiology.** Lymphedema may be caused by the malignancy, its metastases, or its treatment (surgery or RT).

B. **Management.** If surgery, RT, and chemotherapy are not indicated

1. Prescribe diuretics such as Dyazide or Moduretic, one or two tablets daily; if ineffective, add a loop diuretic.
2. **Extremity pumps** (e.g., Lymphapres, a 12-chamber device that has replaced the Jobst pump) used b.i.d. may be helpful.
3. Use support stockings between pump applications.
4. Elevate the affected limb if the lower extremity is involved.
5. Consider the use of massage by a physical therapist, a compressive sleeve overnight, and dexamethasone (4 mg b.i.d.).

XI. Venous access problems

A. **Administering chemotherapy to patients with poor venous access**

1. **Switching to oral agents.** Many of the available chemotherapeutic agents are absorbed, although incompletely, when given orally. The oral route is useful if the need to attain predictable levels is not urgent.
2. **Difficulty finding veins** may be alleviated by several techniques:
   a. Hang the arms (wrapped in hot, moist towels, with tourniquets lightly applied) for 10 minutes below the level of the heart.
   b. Use a blood pressure cuff expanded halfway between systolic and diastolic pressures. Tight tourniquets are never helpful.
   c. Search other places to find veins, such as the upper arm or legs.
   d. Advise patients to drink plenty of liquids on the day before treatment and wear a sweater on the day of treatment to keep the arm warm.
   e. Place hot packs over the site prior to venipuncture.
3. **Vein training.** Patients with inaccessible veins are instructed to sit in a chair with the arms held below heart level and to squeeze tennis balls, Nerf balls or household sponges three times daily for 10 minutes or until fatigued. The arms may be wrapped periodically with warm, moist towels.
4. **Other methods** for securing venous access include arteriovenous fistula (see sec. **XI.C**) and right atrial Silastic catheters (see sec. **XI.E**).

B. **Heparin lock.** A plugged, short catheter may be used in patients requiring intermittent IV infusions. The catheter is flushed regularly with heparin.

C. An arteriovenous fistula may be established in patients who have inaccessible veins and a reasonably long expected survival. Administration of viscous solutions through the shunt promotes thrombosis.

D. Hypodermoclysis. Dehydration in patients with difficult venous access can be treated with parenteral fluids administered by clysis. A 21-gauge needle is inserted at a slight angle to the skin of the lateral thigh and then further inserted 1 to 2 in. into the subcutaneous tissue. One vial (150 units) of hyaluronidase (Wydase) is administered through the needle; the enzyme should not be infused into inflamed or cancerous areas. Ringer's lactate solution and mineral additives can then be given at a rate of 100 to 150 ml/hr.

E. Prolonged central venous catheterization. Polymerized silicone rubber (Silastic) catheters inserted into the right atrium via the cephalic vein can provide prolonged venous access for administering IV fluids, blood products, and drugs, and for sampling blood. Both external and subcutaneously implanted types are available.

1. A nonfunctioning catheter is usually the result of obstruction of the catheter tip by either the right atrial wall or a clot. Repositioning the patient usually dislodges the catheter from the atrial wall. A chest x-ray should be taken to evaluate the position of the catheter tip, if it is questionable.

a. Three ml of 1:1000 heparin should be injected into the line with a tuberculin syringe to provide extra pressure; replace the cap on the line and leave it in place for 15–60 minutes before flushing. Repeat the procedure four more times or until successful.

b. Urokinase, 5000 IU (Abbokinase Open-Cath) may also be tried if a clot is suspected.

c. An infusion of urokinase directly into the dysfunctional catheter may also successfully dissolve clots. The dose is 40,000 units/hour for 12 hours using a solution of 5000 units/ml. Patients should be observed for bleeding for 48 hours.

2. Complications. Catheter-related deaths are very rare. The most frequent problems are severing the catheter (if external), infections, and clotting. Differences in the incidences of documented infections between external catheters and subcutaneous ports are arguable; if infections do occur, they may be treated successfully with antibiotics without removing the catheter in the appropriate circumstances (see Chap. 35, sec. **II.G**). There are no differences in the incidence of clotting between external and subcutaneous catheter devices.

Factors that lead to early removal include persistent fever, entrance site infection, air leak, axillary or jugular or superior vena cava thrombosis, or pleural effusion (due to misplacement of the catheter into the pleural space). Pneumothorax may occur during placement of the catheter.

XII. Nutritional support

A. Mechanisms of malignant cachexia are poorly understood and are reviewed by Nelson et al (see *Selected Reading*). The characteristics of cancer cachexia that differ from starvation cachexia include equal mobilization of fat and skeletal muscle (rather than preferential mobilization of fat), normal or increased basal metabolic rate (rather than decreased), increased liver size and metabolic activity (rather than atrophy), normal or increased glucose turnover (rather than decreased), and increased protein breakdown (rather than decreased). Related factors include but are not limited to:

1. Metabolic abnormalities in cachexia of malignancy

a. Carbohydrates: Insulin resistance, glucose intolerance; increased gluconeogenesis, Cori cycle activity, glucose turnover, and serum lactase.

b. Fats. Decreased lipoprotein lipase; increased fatty acid mobilization and turnover, serum lipid levels, and glycerol turnover.

c. Proteins: Decreased skeletal muscle anabolism; increased skeletal muscle catabolism and protein turnover.

2. Decreased intake

a. Anorexia. Many tumors are associated with anorexia, typically manifested by an aversion to meat. Some patients experience decreased or altered sense of taste and smell.

b. Mechanical obstruction of any portion of the intestinal tract makes oral intake impossible. In advanced stages, tumors of the head and neck or ovary frequently make eating impossible.

c. Nausea and vomiting. See sec. III.

d. Diagnostic studies often require fasting; if such studies are not conducted efficiently, patients can become nutritionally compromised.

3. Increased losses

a. Biochemical abnormalities. See A.1.

b. Diarrhea. Severe diarrhea or malabsorption syndromes are associated with carcinoid syndrome, gastrinoma, medullary thyroid carcinoma, pancreatic carcinoma, small bowel lymphatic obstruction, excessive bowel resection, certain cytotoxic agents, and radiation enteritis.

c. Lactase deficiency is common in protein starvation and after some chemotherapies, making milk products unsuitable.

4. Natural history.
Increasing loss of body protein leads to progressively worsening anemia, hypoalbuminemia, hypotransferrinemia, loss of cell-mediated immunity, decreased work tolerance, decreased deep-breathing ability, increased risk of pneumonia, inability to ambulate, and then inability to sit up. Other signs include hair loss, scaling skin, brittle nails, and decubitus ulcer. Death occurs when 30 to 50 percent of body protein stores are lost.

B. Assessment of nutritional status.
Serial measurements of the following parameters provide prognostic information about the risk of sepsis and death:

1. Weight and serum albumin concentration. Substantial protein-calorie malnutrition is characterized by a recent loss of more than 10 percent of the stable preillness weight and by significant hypoalbuminemia (<3.0 gm/dl).

2. Transferrin (TF) has a half-life of about one week and more rapidly reflects changes in nutritional states (either improvement or deterioration) than albumin, which has a serum half-life of about three weeks. Serum TF is also less affected by factors that affect serum albumin concentration (i.e., hydration, infection, and position or activity).

3. Skin tests. Two or more of the following skin test antigens should give a positive intradermal reaction in an immunocompetent adult: tuberculin, mumps, *Candida,* and streptokinase-streptodornase.

4. Nutritional requirements. The healthy person requires 2000 to 2700 (25 cal/kg) calories per day distributed as follows: 15 percent protein (1 gm/kg body weight), 50 percent carbohydrate (3 gm/kg), and 35 percent fat (1 gm/kg). To achieve a positive nitrogen balance in cachectic patients, they require hyperalimentation with 2700–4000 calories and twice the recommended daily allowance for amino acids (protein equivalent) and essential nutrients.

C. Treatment of anorexia

1. Overview and fallacy. Progressive weight loss is part of the biology of progressive cancer. Realistically, nutritional therapy is useless if the tumor cannot be controlled. Yet, nutrition has a peculiar social mystique; "proper nutrition" is believed to be essential to the well-being of all patients, regardless of the underlying disease.

The patient and family can to some extent control dietary intake; this provides a sense of participating in treatment. However, bad diets or "health food" preparations at potentially toxic doses may further compromise the patient's nutritional status. A dying patient may be beleaguered by offers of food when he or she only desires a quiet, peaceful end.

2. Some measures that may be helpful in patients who fail to eat are

a. Use smaller, more frequent feedings.

b. A small helping looks better on a small plate; do not use large dinner plates.

c. Have food available whenever the patient is hungry.

d. Have the patient dress for meals and sit at the table, if possible.

e. Attend to stomatitis, dry mouth, and foul taste (see sec. II).

f. Vitamins may be used if not excessive. Vitamin C is ineffective therapy against tumors but is usually harmless unless substituted for proven therapy or if the doses ingested produce dysuria, diarrhea, or satiety.

g. Do not routinely weigh the patient.

3. **Appetite stimulants** that may be helpful include:

    a. Metoclopramide (Reglan), 10 mg PO before meals and h.s., may relieve anorexia, nausea, and early satiety, particularly when caused by dysmotility. Side effects include dystonic reactions and restlessness.

    b. Megestrol acetate (Megace), 40 mg PO q.i.d. Side effects include high cost, ankle edema, and hyperglycemia.

    c. Dexamethasone, 4 mg in the morning after food, particularly in patients who need an anti-inflammatory agent for pain control. Side effects include proximal myopathy (an indication for stopping the drug), fluid retention, and mental status changes.

    d. THC, 2.5–7.5 mg after breakfast and lunch, starting with the lower dose, which is then escalated. Side effects include dizziness, fluid retention, somnolence, and dissociation, particularly in the elderly.

    e. Other drugs

        (1) Hydrazine sulfate has not been shown to decrease anorexia.

        (2) Cyproheptadine (Periactin), 8 mg PO t.i.d., may mildly stimulate appetite but also cause sedation.

        (3) Antidepressants may be useful with anorexia due to depression.

4. **When cachexia supervenes,** Twycross and Lack recommend

    a. Dental relining improves chewing abilities and facial appearance

    b. An old photo helps the new caregivers recognize the essential humanness of the emaciated patient

    c. New photos of the patient with family, friends, and caregivers helps legitimize the value of this "new" person

    d. Educating the family about preventive care for new bony prominences and fragile skin

    e. At least one new set of well-fitting clothes, if affordable

D. Hyperalimentation in cancer patients. Nutritional deficiency leads to decreased immunocompetence, poor wound healing, and decreased tolerance to antitumor therapy. For cancer patients whose prognosis warrants nutritional support, enteral feeding (EF) or parenteral hyperalimentation (PH) may be given.

1. **Indications for EF. "If the gut works, use it."** Patients who have a functional GI tract but are unable to orally ingest adequate nutrients are candidates for EF. EF is far less expensive, more physiologic, and associated with fewer complications than PH.

2. **Indications for PH**

    a. The patient has a curable neoplasm but is likely to have a protracted recovery from treatment (such as extensive bowel resection), *or*

    b. The patient is cured of tumor but is awaiting surgical intervention and has residual nutritional problems (e.g., enterocutaneous fistulae), *or*

    c. The patient requires prolonged postoperative nasogastric suction (more than 4–7 days) for conditions that necessitate avoidance of oral intake

    d. Patients with severe malabsorption, vomiting, or diarrhea associated with cancer therapy.

3. **Contraindications for hyperalimentation**

    a. Contraindications for EF are intractable vomiting, upper GI bleeding, or intestinal obstruction.

    b. Hyperalimentation is not useful for patients with

        (1) Minimal nutritional deficits, *or*

(2) Weight loss caused by progressive cancer that is unlikely to respond to therapy, *or*

(3) Aggressive tumors that respond dramatically to therapy (e.g., lymphoma and small cell lung cancer)

c. PH given to patients receiving chemotherapy is associated with net harm. The mere presence of a central line and the lack of understanding of EF do not justify the use of PH. The average complication rate is about 12 percent (pneumothorax, thrombosis, and catheter-related septicemia), and no conditions can be defined in which such treatment appears to be of benefit. The routine use of PH for patients undergoing chemotherapy is strongly discouraged.

E. Enteral feeding provides liquid formula diets into the GI tract orally or by means of feeding tubes. More than 30 surgical techniques are available for tube enterostomy when needed. Percutaneous endoscopic placement, however, has the advantages of speed and lack of a surgical incision.

1. Preparations. Many enteral products are available, but a standard formula is usually sufficient for patients with an intact digestive system. Isotonic solutions that contain high nitrogen and a medium caloric density (1–2 kcal/ml) are satisfactory in 90 percent of patients (e.g., Osmolite HN, Isocal HCN). Preparations that contain a high concentration of amino acids are often unacceptable for patients with cancer-related meat aversion (e.g., Vivonex, Flexical). High-calorie preparations (e.g., Ensure-Plus, Magnacal) are often offered as caloric supplements but they are so rich that many patients refuse them.

2. Administration. Start tube feedings with a full strength solution at about 30 ml/hr. Increase the infusion rate to tolerance by increments of 10–25 ml/hr over 12–24 hours for 2–3 days.

3. Complications of EF

a. Frequent complications and corrections

(1) Vomiting and bloating: Reduce the flow rate.

(2) Diarrhea and cramping: Reduce the flow rate; dilute the solution; treat with an antidiarrheal drug; consider a different type of solution. Diarrhea is especially likely in patients who have been given broad-spectrum antibiotics.

(3) Hyperglycemia: Reduce the flow rate; give insulin.

(4) Edema: Usually requires no treatment; diuretics may be used.

(5) Offensive smell or taste: Add flavorings.

(6) Nasopharyngeal discomfort: Encourage the use of surgarless gum, gargling with warm water and mouthwash, topical anesthetics.

(7) Abnormalities of serum levels of sodium, potassium, calcium, magnesium, or phosphorus: adjust the formula's ingredients.

b. Infrequent complications and corrections

(1) Congestive heart failure: Administer fluids more slowly and treat cardiac decompensation.

(2) Fat malabsorption. Use low-fat formulas; add pancreatic enzymes.

(3) Elevated serum transaminase: Decrease carbohydrate content of formula

(4) Acute otitis media: Administer antibiotics; change nasogastric tube to other nostril.

(5) Clogged tube lumen: Flush with water or replace tube.

c. Rare complications that necessitate discontinuing therapy

(1) Aspiration pneumonia (unlikely to occur if the head of the bed is elevated to 45 degrees, volume overload is avoided, and the cough reflex is intact)

(2) Esophageal erosion from nasogastric tube

(3) Acute purulent sinusitis

(4) Hyperosmolar coma

Selected Reading

Pain

Cleeland, C. S. Pain and its treatment in outpatients with metastatic cancer. *N. Engl. J. Med.* 330:592, 1994.

Portenoy, R. K. Cancer pain: Pathophysiology and syndromes. *Lancet* 339:1026, 1992.

U.S. Department of Health and Human Services, Agency for Health Care Policy and Research. Clinical Practice Guideline Number 9. Management of Cancer Pain: Adults (AHCPR Publication No. 94-0593). U.S. Government Printing Office, 1994. (Patient booklet is AHPCR Publication No. 94-0595. Copies of either booklet may be obtained by calling 1-800-4-CANCER)

Central Lines

Groeger, J. S., et al. Infectious morbidity associated with long-term use of venous access devices in patients with cancer. *Ann. Int. Med.* 119:1168, 1993.

Haire, W. D., et al. Obstructed central venous catheters. Restoring function with a 12-hour infusion of low-dose urokinase. *Cancer* 66:2279, 1990.

Mueller, B. U., et al. A prospective randomized trial comparing the infectious and noninfectious complications of an externalized catheter versus a subcutaneously implanted device in cancer patients. *J. Clin. Oncol.* 10:1943, 1992.

Nutrition

Loprinzi, C. L., et al. Phase III evaluation of four doses of megestrol acetate as therapy for patients with cancer anorexia and/or cachexia. *J. Clin. Oncol.* 11:762, 1993.

McGeer, A. J., Detsky, A. S., and O'Rourke, K. Parenteral nutrition in patients receiving cancer chemotherapy. *Ann. Int. Med.* 110:734, 1989. (A position paper of the American College of Physicians)

Nelson, K. A., Walsh, D., and Sheehan, F. A. The cancer anorexia-cachexia syndrome. *J. Clin. Oncol.* 12:213, 1994.

Other Issues in Supportive Care

LeVeque, F. G., et al. A multicenter, randomized, double-blind, placebo-controlled, dose-titration study of oral pilocarpine for treatment of radiation-induced xerostomia in head and neck cancer patients. *J. Clin. Oncol.* 11:1124, 1993.

Levy, M. H., et al. Supportive care in oncology. *Curr. Probl. Cancer* 6:335, 1992.

Twycross, R. G., and Lack, S. A. *Therapeutics in Terminal Cancer*. London: Pitman, 1984. (Highly recommended for anyone caring for cancer patients)

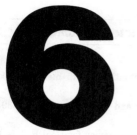

Psychosocial and Legal Aspects of Cancer Care

Barry B. Lowitz

When I thought I was learning to live, I was but learning to die.

LEONARDO DA VINCI

Psychosocial Issues

I. Psychological responses to the diagnosis of cancer tend to reflect premorbid mechanisms of coping and interacting. The presence of cancer disrupts virtually every aspect of the life of the patient and family. Premorbid psychiatric problems become intensified and "telescoped." Physicians and other health care personnel have an active role in helping patients and families to cope and function.

A. Common losses experienced by cancer patients

1. Loss of health and physical integrity (resulting from disease, disfigurement, and discomfort)
2. Loss of friends and loved ones (including separation to receive treatment, rejection by some friends or family members)
3. Inability to perform routine activities (such as self-care, job, and hobbies)
4. Loss of finances (resulting from cost of treatment and loss of job)
5. Loss of self-esteem
6. Loss of religious convictions ("What did I do wrong to deserve this?")

B. Common reactions

1. **Symptoms and signs.**
   a. **Hostility-anger** is the most common reaction and is typically manifested by displacement of anger about the disease onto doctors, relatives, and others. Patients and families frequently blame their current problems on mismanagement by previous health-care personnel.
   b. **Anxiety** is manifested by agitation, short concentration span, sleep problems, or compulsive behavior. It often worsens the subjective sensation of pain.
   c. **Guilt** may be manifested by blaming others for the illness. Patients or family members commonly ruminate over what they might have done to cause the illness. Family members often feel that if they had taken other actions, the illness would not have developed.
   d. **Entitlement** is manifested by petulant and demanding behavior. Patients feel that they deserve special treatment as compensation for their losses.
   e. **Compliance** with medical treatment develops when patients understand their disease and develop a sense of acceptance. Noncompliance is a regressive behavior that signals anxiety, depression, or unhealthy denial.
   f. **Depression** is an appropriate response if it is not severe. Depression is manifested by flat affect, insomnia, anorexia, withdrawal, and psychomotor retardation. Depression is often mistaken for dementia; establishing the differential diagnosis is essential to improve patients' ability to function.

      g. Dependency is a very common reaction to advanced malignancy and can immobilize patients.

      h. Psychoses that require pharmacologic intervention may develop.

C. Evaluation. Changes in behavior by either the patient or the patient's loved ones are the usual clues that problems exist. Assess the following:

    1. Emotional risk factors

      a. Prior emotional problems

      b. How the patient handled prior significant losses or hostilities (similar strategies will probably be used again)

      c. Presence of concomitant stresses

      d. Nature of interpersonal relationships

      e. Patient's attitude toward self

    2. Alterations in how a typical day is spent.

    3. Support given by family, friends, religious institution, employer, and others.

    4. The severity of depression. Determine specific concerns, such as financial or family problems, that result from the illness.

    5. Changes in sexual activity and interest.

D. Management

    1. General techniques. The physician should be a sympathetic listener who is open, understanding, and available. Specific attention should be directed as follows:

      a. Determine specific goals with the patient (e.g., travel, family events).

      b. Confront patients with depression or anxiety directly ("You look depressed"; "You look upset").

      c. Explain the medical problems clearly and consistently.

      d. Be flexible with therapeutic options, second opinions, and the patient's wishes.

      e. Denial may be a healthy psychological defense mechanism and should be supported if it does not interfere with the welfare of patients or their families.

      f. Patients and their families must be informed that sexual activities are not harmful and that cancer is not contagious. Many patients lose interest in sexual activity and require support from the physician; this is not abnormal, even in healthy people.

      g. Antidepressant medication can be very effective for sleep disorders, loss of interest, and unexplained fatigue. Unless medically contraindicated, an empirical trial of antidepressants for 4–6 weeks can be beneficial.

    2. Psychiatric consultation should be requested when the patient is extraordinarily difficult to manage. Expert consultation is essential when patients are immobilized by anxiety or depression, or are psychotic. Such consultations should seek psychiatric diagnoses, suggestions for behavior modification, and recommendations for psychopharmacologic therapy. The continued care of the patient, however, should remain in the hands of a member of the patient's established health care team.

II. Discussing diagnosis, treatment, and prognosis

A. General approach

    1. All patients need to be fully informed about their illness, its prognosis, and options for therapy. How to best inform a given patient depends on the patient's age, premorbid personality, economic situation, family or social factors, concomitant illnesses, and other determinants of his or her unique psychosocial makeup.

    2. The diagnosis of cancer should be presented to the patient as soon as tissue confirmation is obtained. The physician should meet the patient privately and allow enough time to discuss the diagnosis and answer questions. Care should be taken to *preserve eye contact* during this discussion.

    3. The physician's candor in discussion of the diagnosis creates trust and helps patients view further staging procedures as a positive approach to the disease.

4. Patients should be encouraged to regularly make a list of any general questions they or their families have and to bring this list to the next appointment.

5. Explanation of the diagnosis may have to be repeated. A patient often hears only what he or she wants or is ready to hear. Some will deny ever being told the diagnosis even when it is discussed several times. If such denial does not interfere with medical care or cause psychosocial problems, the patient need not be repeatedly confronted.

B. **Virtually all patients should be told the diagnosis.** Honest discussion removes the trauma of speculation. The diagnosis of cancer engenders a sequence of symptoms, complications, tests, treatments, and hospitalizations, that disrupt the patient's enjoyment of life. Time becomes precious. There are finances to plan, vacations to take, acquaintances to rekindle, things to be said, and dreams to fulfill. Life planning mandates patients' awareness of the diagnosis. Even patients with chronic brain syndrome probably should be told the diagnosis on the chance that they can comprehend at least part of what they are told.

C. **Common problems**

1. **Patients who deny the diagnosis** and want another opinion should be supported. The physician should tell these patients that they may want a second opinion and that their seeing another practitioner will not jeopardize the present relationship. The primary physician should offer to provide copies of all records for the second opinion doctor to review.

2. **Families who oppose the patients' knowing the diagnosis** should be answered honestly. Patients must be told regardless of the family's apprehension. The task then becomes dealing with the family's anxiety and assisting them in accepting the need for the patient to be fully informed. Certain cultures disdain having the elderly informed of the diagnosis of cancer; associated linguistic limitations may preclude the physician from accomplishing the above recommendations.

3. **Questionable ability to cope.** Some patients' ability to cope with the knowledge of the diagnosis may be legitimately questioned. A qualified mental health person may be able to assess the patient and help establish a way for the patient to be accurately informed and helped to cope with the stress.

4. **Passive patients**
   a. Patients who ask no questions at the time of diagnosis may also be denying facts. All patients should be asked directly for questions and be instructed to write them down for further discussion. It is important to briefly discuss the necessary diagnostic studies and management. Overly quiet patients should be encouraged to come back more frequently to avert poor follow-up or even suicide attempts.
   b. Patients who cooperate with therapy and ask few or no questions may want the physician and family to make the difficult decisions. Be certain that patients truly wish to have others involved in making decisions. Limit information for these patients to potentially unpleasant symptoms of therapy.

5. **Discussing the prognosis.** Rigid prognostication for a given patient is impossible. "The doctor gives me X months to live" is inappropriate for a patient to think or say. Doctors do not have "crystal balls" and realistically cannot set a "date for the execution." Doctors should avoid making guarantees and commitments that cannot be kept. The doctor should stress the variable course and unpredictability of disseminated cancer.

III. **Preparing patients for cancer treatment.** Most of the current technologies are complex, frightening, potentially mutilating, and toxic. Many difficult decisions must be made among unpleasant choices. The vast majority of patients and their families must actively participate in making these decisions.

A. **Organizations.** Patients who require ostomies (i.e., ileostomy, colostomy, or ureteral diversion) should be visited preoperatively by a stomal therapist and a member of one of the ostomy clubs. These clubs, while not technically oriented, are supportive of patients and families and can share patients' feelings and concerns. Laryngectomy patients can be similarly prepared by speech therapists and patient clubs that can be contacted through the American Cancer Society (ACS). Patients who require amputation may benefit from meeting with recovered amputees and physical therapists both before and after surgery. Patients with breast cancer may be helped by the ACS Reach for Recovery Program, which can help reinforce the goal of a return to normal function. The patients' spouse should be included as an active participant in all discussions of the disease and treatment.

B. RT. It is essential that the radiation therapist fully inform and prepare patients in advance concerning what to expect. The treatment environment (e.g., the "Radiation Hazard" signs, the whirring sound of a linear accelerator, and feeling isolated) should be described to help allay anxiety.

C. Chemotherapy. Patients who are to receive chemotherapy should be informed by the oncologist about the side effects, and frequency and duration of treatment. The patients' primary physician should be encouraging and hopeful.

IV. Social pressures affecting cancer treatment. Pressures from family members and well-meaning friends are dominant forces in management decisions affecting cancer patients. These forces often directly conflict with scientific standards of care and rational medical ethics. The physician may not be able to remedy the causes of the problems but can minimize their impact.

A. Patients' families and loved ones

1. **Children.** Even young children should be kept informed about what is happening to their loved ones. Children often fantasize and may think that something they did caused the illness. Emotional instability may be manifested as regressive behavior (such as loss of toilet training), night terrors, school problems, or other behaviors. If children are not informed, they may feel abandoned, isolated, and even more responsible. Professional counseling is necessary for many children. If the patient is close to death, the children should not be kept away. Frequent hospital visits are important both for the patients and the children.

2. **The concerned family.** Family members must be active participants in the care of the patient. A single family member or the patient should be appointed as spokesperson and should be educated about the patient's illness, the diagnostic plans, and the family's responsibilities. Concerned friends and family members often repeatedly ask the same questions, and a spokesperson can be a great help. Family conferences with the physician may alleviate that difficulty.

3. **The difficult family** may be identified by their having previously sought opinions from many different specialists, "none of whom were any good." Characteristically, they flatter, demand excessive consultations, and question treatment methods. If the physician tries to define limits, the family may respond by accusing him or her of insensitivity or may involve the physician in litigation. The root of these behaviors is often excessive panic or guilt. Some ways to handle these situations are

    a. **Do not be dogmatic** about the approach of past physicians. Families should be reassured that the past care was reasonable and appropriate (if it was); no two physicians do exactly the same things.

    b. **Family conferences** are helpful. The physician will not able to interact with each and every family member every time they have a question, but will be able to do so through an agreed upon spokesperson.

    c. **The patient is a victim** of such a family; the patient loses continuity of medical care to satisfy the panic or guilt of the family. If possible, talk this over with the patient directly. Most patients respond positively to the suggestion of bringing the family to the bedside in your presence and having the patient direct the family to change their behavior.

B. Disagreement between patient and family about management may involve cancer therapies, medical support, requests for other opinions, and so on. Two situations are commonly encountered in the practice of oncology: (1) The family wants the patient left alone to "die with dignity," and the patient wants to "keep fighting"; or, (2) the patient wants to be left alone and the family will not give up. These problems must be approached conjointly to avoid social, and possibly legal, disasters.

1. Present the options to patients in a private meeting or with the closest family members. Make it clear to patients that they must make the final decision.

2. When patients have reached a decision, have a conjoint meeting with them and their families to ensure that everyone knows and respects their wishes. It is important that patients state their wishes directly to the family in your presence. This protects families from having recriminations about doing too much or not enough later on, and makes it clear you are following the patient's informed direction. Such meetings should be documented in the patient's chart.

C. **When other opinions, experimental therapies, or more toxic therapies are sought**

1. **Second opinions** should be encouraged for all patients and families who broach the subject. A word of caution: The second opinion sometimes recommends an aggressive therapy of which you disapprove rather than a sound treatment approach that differs from yours. This disparity can lead to an endless chain of second opinions as patients agonize over the best decision. Although most physicians who give second opinions will respect your relationship with the patient, a few will libel you and actively condemn what you have done or are planning to do for the patient. An egocentric colleague or a tertiary care center that is "a bit short on patients" can be a risk for both the patient and you.

2. **Family members and well-meaning friends** often pressure patients into undertaking aggressive treatments that have not been adequately evaluated or have proven only marginally effective.

   a. These treatments are characteristically toxic and expensive, involve additional radiologic and laboratory studies to monitor the effects of therapy, and require additional medications to treat the side effects of the "breakthrough" therapy. When compared to a more standard approach, the combined diagnostic and therapeutic assault is not generally indicated. Unfortunately, patients are often made to feel that they owe it to their loved ones to "give it a chance."

   b. The physician must make it clear that the goal of treatment in patients with incurable cancer is palliation. Palliation means improvement of symptoms and function but does not mean reduction in size of an asymptomatic lesion or reduction in blood levels of a tumor marker. Highly toxic chemotherapy or aggressive or "innovative therapies" have little role in palliation. A gentle but direct approach is often necessary to keep patients out of harm's way.

3. **Management of patients participating in clinical trials**

   a. Experimental therapies that are organized as formal clinical trials stand in stark contrast to "creative oncology." Formal studies are approved by an Institutional Review Board, which protects human subjects who are undergoing experimental treatment. Such formal trials are the only valid method for determining the effectiveness or ineffectiveness of a new cancer treatment.

   b. Primary oncologists and primary care physicians should have an ongoing role with patients, during and after the experimental therapy. The primary doctors must have a copy of the protocol in the patients' chart.

   c. The side effects and cost of participating in a clinical trial must be weighed against the patient's hope that the treatment may prove effective.

D. **When families seek "quack" methods of cancer therapy**

1. **Seeking the cure.** Patients and their families often become desperate and

willing to try anything. They often fear conventional cancer therapies and may become convinced that the "medical establishment" is depriving them of a cure. Patients easily fall prey to quacks who may even be licensed physicians.

2. **Compromise.** Families or patients may seek unconventional therapy even while complying with conventional medical therapy. Unless the physician states his or her disapproval explicitly, families may think he or she approves. The physician should also state in advance that he or she will not accept that any improvement in the patient's condition results from the unacceptable modes of therapy. The physician should know which agents the patient receives as part of outside treatment; these agents may be actual antineoplastic drugs and their administration compounds the toxic reactions from other prescribed chemotherapy. If the patient prefers to completely abandon medical treatment, the physician should assure the patient and family that the physician will be available if needed.

3. **Confrontation.** The issue of cancer quackery must be confronted and fought with facts.
   a. Explain that increased morbidity occurs without competent, comprehensive medical supervision.
   b. Point out the excessive costs involved.
   c. Explain the reasons positive results occur with ineffective agents.
      (1) A small percentage of many tumor types regress spontaneously; these are the only results reported.
      (2) Patients who are "cured" by unproved methods often do not have cancer at all; biopsy specimens were never taken.
      (3) The disappearance of reversible, nonmalignant disease can look like a cancer response.
      (4) Some distributors of ineffective treatments use RT and chemotherapy in addition to the medically unacceptable remedy but ascribe responses to the latter.
   d. Explain that many unscrupulous entrepreneurs use psychological techniques to sell worthless products to desperate people who may be told such things as, "A powerful governmental agency (or the American Medical Association) is suppressing the use of a great cancer cure for reasons known only to themselves." The physician should acknowledge that although the legitimate medical profession does not have all the answers, this does not imply that someone else does.

E. **The media**
   1. **Journalism** can cause great harm to many individuals, but the harm to society of prior restraint or censorship of the media has been consistently proven far more dangerous.
   2. **Medical journalism.** Most people only know about an illness by what they hear from their physicians, other medical professionals, and the media. A journalist's job is to write news and not necessarily to provide information. A story that reports negative results for a therapy or insufficient testing of a therapy is information but not news, and such stories are rarely published. On the other hand, the excitement of a researcher who has found some positive early results or the happiness of a patient who appears to have benefited from an unusual therapy is very infectious for a journalist; such stories are frequently published. Furthermore, journalists are often "sitting on the door step" of research institutions. They often publish news articles about "breakthrough" treatments before they appear in medical journals or are appropriately evaluated by the research community. News is mistaken for information by most people, and the physician has a formidable job in helping patients to make informed decisions.
   3. **Media "breakthroughs"** are often embarrassing to the physician. Patients feel that any competent physician should "know these things." The best way to deal with this is to tell the patient directly that you are not familiar with the treatment but will find out more about it and help them evaluate

it. Most patients and families appreciate this kind of honesty. Those who do not are often medicolegal risks.

V. Interacting with the dying patient

A. The problem of methodology. Care of the dying patient requires artful methodology. Inexperienced doctors feel uncomfortable interacting with these patients, do not know what to say, and often avoid meaningful contact.

1. **We all die uniquely.** Each patient has unique fears or anxieties about death. However, many experts in thanatology have documented that patients are less afraid of death than of being abandoned.

2. **Emotional reactions in the dying patient** include denial and isolation, anger, bargaining, depression, and acceptance. There are, however, no regular and predictable stages of dying. Most patients fluctuate among these stages for varying periods of time, sometimes denying their illness, sometimes angry, sometimes depressed. The stage of acceptance, if ever present, is often transitory; when it does occur, it is usually brief, just before demise, and associated with the voluntary separation of patients from friends and relatives.

B. Techniques in thanatology. The role of the physician is to minimize the psychological discomfort of the patient. Since time is of the essence, a crisis intervention model can be employed.

Support defenses that tend to minimize the patient's discomfort.
Counteract harmful defenses.
Avoid isolating the patient.
Maintain an honest relationship to maximize patient trust.

1. **Provision of clinical data.** Knowing the disease's progress, details of laboratory and x-ray films, and discussing management plans help many patients gain some sense of control over their disease.

2. **Passive support.** There is little point in forcing discussions about death unless the patient shows anxiety, is depressed, or volunteers the subject. In-depth psychiatric analysis is also best avoided unless analysis itself is a useful defense for the patient.

3. **Support of attitude**
   a. Most people feel that a positive attitude is beneficial to their condition. Cancer patients often spontaneously adopt this view, and it should be supported by the physician. The risk is that when events turn for the worse, some people feel guilty that the change was their fault for not being able to maintain a positive attitude. The best intervention is to tell patients how well they have done, and that they probably would have fared much worse if they had a negative attitude.
   b. Some people may benefit psychologically and perhaps physically from relaxation techniques such as acupressure and muscle testing, mental imaging of their bodies destroying the tumors, self-hypnosis, and so forth. We actively encourage patients who want to try these methods of "holistic medicine" as long as they do not interfere with proven methods of treatment or endanger the patients' health.

4. **Support of hope.** Hope is never false. A positive attitude on the part of the physician provides comfort. Hopeful patients may spend more of their time thinking about living than about dying. Patients hope for more than just longer life: They hope to function well, be free of pain, and not be isolated from contact with other people or their physician. Even when the cancer ceases to respond to treatment, the physician can support these hopes.

5. **Discourage harmful defenses**
   a. **Anger out of control.** Patients who are frustrated about their disease often manifest anger toward family, friends, and medical personnel. This can also be a method that patients use to "protect" the family from loss and guilt; patients wrongly believe that if they are grumpy, they will not be missed as much. Confront the patient directly, "You have a right to be angry at your disease, but your family and I are on your side. We

all have to work together to treat your illness. Being angry with me [us] is not helping anyone." This technique may provide patients the defense of objectifying the disease as something separate from themselves.

   b. **Manipulative behavior** often reflects a pre-illness personality disorder but may be the only way the patients can avoid isolation. Physicians can often recognize manipulative behavior when they feel angry with these patients and feel guilty for feeling angry. Acceptable patient behavior must be defined in these circumstances. This definition and the consequences of unacceptable behavior should be discussed with the staff and the family.

   c. **The "hateful" patient** can present formidable problems in care. These patients make the staff angry by passive-aggressive behavior, accident proneness, manipulation of drug use, and by giving conflicting descriptions of their understanding of the disease and its treatment to various staff members. They tend to play people off against each other. These activities can be very destructive. It may be helpful to (1) refer the patient for counseling; (2) maintain a strictly technical relationship with the patient and place firm limits on physician availability; (3) confront the patient directly, "Your behavior makes it difficult for me to give you proper care;" note a few specifics. If there is no improvement, the patient probably should be instructed to find another physician. Be sure to document the reasons for referral in the medical records.

6. **Managing a patient's sense of isolation**
   a. **Physical isolation**
      (1) For patients who are left alone at home during the day and who call the doctor several times a week, recommend a day-care or occupational therapy center. Arrange for regular visits by the family.
      (2) Patients who are afraid not to be under continuous medical supervision should be asked directly if they have this concern. Arrange for hospice or nursing home care. Assure patients that nurses will contact the doctor for any problems.
      (3) If patients who have been stable seek acute medical admission, with or without objective evidence of worsening, this often represents a grave sign of imminent deterioration or of serious problems at home and is an absolute indication for acute hospital admission.

   b. **Psychosocial isolation**
      (1) **The garrulous patient.** Some patients talk incessantly at each visit and behave as if the doctor were their captive audience. If the physician defines and sticks to time limits for each visit, he or she is less likely to resent or isolate such patients.
      (2) **The depressed or agitated patient.** When patients appear depressed or anxious, confront the patient gently but directly, "You seem down today," or, "You seem upset." Encourage ventilation of feelings.
      (3) **The fearful patient.** The patient says, "I think I'm dying." The physician should ask if the patient is frightened or concerned about familial economic problems or the family's ability to cope after his death. The physician should ask if there is some way to help. Sometimes these questions allow the patient to focus on particular problems beyond the fears all share about death.

7. **When treatment options are expended**
   a. When little more can be done to control the tumor, patients should be informed of this and told that further therapy may only make them more ill. These patients should continue to be followed closely and solicitously even if they are not receiving specific anticancer treatment.
   b. Attention should then be focused on achieving goals other than tumor control such as relief of pain, control of other symptoms, and enjoyment of family life.
   c. Some patients express desire for chemotherapeutic agents after appro-

priate drugs have failed. Occasionally, drugs with some effectiveness may be used in doses too low to produce side effects for placebo effect; cost should be minimized and the family should be informed about the rationale for treatment.

8. When there is nothing to say

   a. Presence and interest are the most important commodities physicians have to offer in these settings. Soft touching, limited physical examination, and allowing the patient to speak freely may be comforting. Be a good listener and maintain eye contact. Personal feelings and sensitive words should be expressed. If the physician does not know what to say, he or she should either admit it to the patient or say nothing.

   b. Words are rarely helpful to conscious patients who are frightened and aware that they are about to die. Parenteral sedatives or narcotics may alleviate some anxiety, but merely being there and holding the dying patient's hand probably palliates the psychological discomfort of dying.

C. The team approach. A patient's dying can drain individual staff members. A team approach to the care of dying patients can diffuse the impact and benefit the patient. The responsibility for preventing patient isolation and monitoring patients' emotional reactions belongs to the nurse, psychologist, lay consultants, hospital team, families and friends, as well as to the physician. If a patient needs spiritual support, the clergy should be consulted. If there are estate problems or social problems, social services or attorneys should be consulted. It is important that one health care provider, usually the physician, is in charge to provide coordination and continuity.

VI. Physicians' reactions. Emotional problems in physicians, especially oncologists, frequently arise from regular exposure to death together with difficulty coping with their own aging and mortality. Physicians may wonder whether they will survive long enough to leisurely enjoy the fruits of many years of labor, recognition for their work, or be remembered for it after they die. These questions arise earlier in life for those taking care of dying people and may take on pathologic significance.

A. Signs of emotional problems in physicians include

   1. Feeling helpless in treating patients; feeling overwhelmed that few patients with advanced cancer can be cured
   2. Increasing feelings of guilt for not having been able to keep a patient alive; carrying a sense of inadequacy or depression
   3. Feeling hopeless about the prospects of cancer treatments
   4. Feeling remorse for unfulfilled dreams: working harder but starting to feel that medical practice has harmed enjoyment of life and medical altruism has been repaid by pain felt for sacrificing family, pleasures, and self
   5. Tending to buffer themselves from patients with house staff, colleagues, or a too-busy practice ("I cannot take it anymore")
   6. Becoming inappropriately aggressive or optimistic in therapy when it is evident that it will not benefit a patient; developing the "General complex" where physicians feel they are fighting a war against the unfairness of nature that they cannot win
   7. Feelings of chronic fatigue or exhaustion especially associated with inability to limit time and energy given to patient care

B. Acting on symptoms. These signs in physicians and other members of the health care team must be taken seriously because patients and staff can both be adversely affected. Positive action is required.

   1. A vacation or change in work milieu may be indicated. Vacation schedules should be compulsively kept; everyone, including thanatology personnel, needs some time for bereavement.
   2. Practice may have to be stopped altogether to preserve mental health.
   3. Psychiatric consultation should be sought for prolonged depression or anxiety, sleep disturbance, feeling that people are turning away, excessive consumption of alcohol or other drugs, or evidence of emotional impairment or chronic stress.

Legal Issues

I. Patients' rights to confidentiality
A. Work and cancer
1. Some employers discriminate against people with a history of cancer, many of whom are fully functional but without work. The physician can speak to discriminatory employers as long as the patient's right to professional confidentiality is preserved. Approval, signed by the patient, must be placed in the chart of each person that the physician speaks with about the patient's condition. An employer's medical liability can be eliminated if the patient signs a waiver.
2. Disabled people in the United States are now protected by "The Federal Americans with Disabilities Act." However, patients must understand their limitations, and the legislation does not coerce employers to allow workers to take unwarranted risks, nor expose others to danger resulting from patients' disabilities.

B. Driving automobiles and cancer.
In most states, the only exception to the right to confidentiality is reporting incompetence to drive a motor vehicle. Driving must be forbidden if patients are taking sedating drugs or have a disability severe enough to endanger public safety. Patients who persist in driving should be informed that physicians are obligated by law to file a report with the state department of motor vehicles.

II. Selling narcotic prescriptions.
Cancer patients who sell their narcotic prescriptions to drug abusers represent a serious problem. Patients may remain in pain if prescriptions are withheld, yet gain financial profit if the prescriptions are written.

A. Recognition.
These patients may be identified by a history of excuses for excessive refills. Other physicians also inadvertently prescribe drugs for the same patients.

B. Management
is difficult. All patients must be instructed that narcotic prescriptions are given only during regular work hours. A reasonable number of pills that will be prescribed at a given time should be defined.
1. Long-acting drugs, such as methadone, can be prescribed to be given by one designated person at recorded, scheduled times. Methadone has a relatively low value on the street markets.
2. Avoid prescribing narcotics that are pure (e.g., codeine alone). If such medications are required, prescribe smaller numbers of pills (without refills) more frequently.
3. Often even these measures fail to solve the problem. Local governmental drug authorities should be notified if drug abuse and sale are suspected.

III. Malpractice law suits.
Premiums for malpractice insurance, malpractice awards, attendant legal and court costs, and "defensive practice" represent about 2.5 percent of the cost of medical care in the United States.

A. Common physician errors and their prevention

> *Quality medical care almost always involves just being thorough and meticulous. On rare occasions, however, the physician may actually have to resort to thinking.*

1. **"Failure to diagnose"** in a timely way is the cause of the majority of successful plaintiff cases against physicians. Many of these cases relate to cancer. The "Seven Signs of Cancer" of the ACS are the most routinely missed in malpractice cases. Unbiopsied breast masses, anemias or blood in the stools from colon cancers, red cells in a routine urinalysis, and chest films with lesions found retrospectively taken in doctors' offices, without formal

reports in the chart from a board certified radiologist are the commonest causes of "failure to diagnose" cases.

If a physician is concerned about the possibility of cancer, the physician should document that he or she has made it clear to the patient that follow-up is necessary and that a specific date for follow-up has been made. Every call must be documented in the chart immediately after it is made, along with the date, time, and the physician's signature.

2. **Failure to do the obvious.** The more common oversights are simple to prevent by practicing sound, basic internal medicine. Failure to recognize fluid overload in hospitalized patients, to act on an unexplained temperature elevation, and to investigate chest pain or dyspnea appropriately account for a substantial number of lawsuits.

3. **Failure to refer to an appropriate specialist.** The classic and commonest examples are gynecologists who follow breast masses. Women with breast masses must be referred to a qualified surgeon without delay.

4. **Litigious patients and families** can sometimes be identified before problems start. Be wary of people who are inappropriately complimentary before they really get to know you. Look for narcissistic personality disorder in patients or families who give you a sense that they are entitled or tell you they heard you are the "top doctor" in your field.

B. **Prevention of law suits**

1. **Dated, detailed, handwritten, and signed documentation in the medical record** about every significant interaction that the physician has with the patient and family is the **sine qua non** for preventing law suits. Taped dictation is additive particularly if you put a written comment in the chart, "See dictated note for details." Such written records made close to the time of the interaction or procedure are considered the most reliable by the judicial system.

2. *Never, ever* go back and change or add to your notes or chart documentation such as informed consents, no matter how embarrassed you feel about a real error or oversight. Expert witnesses and attorneys almost never miss this virtual admission of negligence. Do not add notes to a chart that might be construed as self-serving.

3. **"Defensive medicine"** has almost no effect on preventing or prevailing in law suits. The best way to avoid doing unnecessary tests is to document that you have considered various diagnoses and possible tests, but that (use these exact words), "in my best clinical judgment, the risk of testing will cause more harm than the risk of missing a diagnosis that I consider unlikely."

4. **Keep patients and family** informed about why you are or are not proceeding with certain tests and treatments. Document these discussions in your notes.

5. **Discharge litigious patients or families** to a tertiary care center. It is helpful to let go of your ego and tell them that they need more sophisticated care than you know how to give. Even if this is not true, the patient feels, "Here's a really honest doctor who knows his or her limitations," and they walk away happy and you have saved yourself a headache.

C. **Some facts and tips on psychologically surviving a malpractice suit**

1. The defense (the doctor's malpractice company) wins the majority of cases that go to trial, even more so in jury trials and in smaller communities.

2. The *legal* standard of care in most areas requires that all personnel who came into contact in any manner with the patient be initially named in a law suit. If you are ancillary to the case, you will probably be dropped from the suit.

3. Most cases settle without trial because it is usually more profitable and less risky for the attorneys and liability carriers. The personal injury system is really just a business between attorneys and liability carriers. Most lawyers are so certain of a settlement that they do not start real case preparation until the trial is actually underway.

4. If you are deposed or do have to go to court, you are likely to encounter the standard inflammatory language of plaintiff attorneys who love to impugn you and try to push your buttons with such phrases as "malicious intent" and "egregious negligence." The more you appear to be cooperative and pleasant, the more the attorney appears out of line in saying nasty things about you. Don't "rent free space in your mind" to plaintiff's attorneys and become defensive or angry.

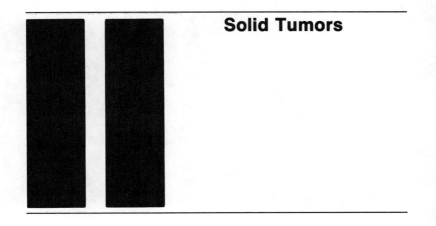

Solid Tumors

Head and Neck Cancers

Robert G. Parker,
Dale H. Rice, and
Dennis A. Casciato

General Principles

Head and neck cancers comprise a heterogeneous group of lesions. Tumors from various sites of origin have distinct behavior patterns and prognoses and require different management. Each primary site is considered separately following a discussion of common features.

I. **Epidemiology and etiology**
   A. **Incidence.** Primary head and neck malignant tumors constitute 5 percent of all newly diagnosed cancers in humans and result in approximately 16,000 deaths per year. One to three cases occur annually per 100,000 population in the United States. The incidence of squamous cell carcinoma is significantly higher in males (male:female ratio = 3 or 4:1).
   B. **Etiology.** Substantial alcohol intake and cigarette smoking are major risk factors for head and neck cancers. A variety of hereditary, environmental, occupational, and hygienic factors are of lesser importance. Conditions associated with increased incidences of specific head and neck cancers are *discussed in their respective sections.*
   C. **Multiple cancers.** Second primary cancers in the upper respiratory passage are present in about 5 percent of patients with head and neck cancers at the time of diagnosis. Eventually secondary cancers occur in 20 percent of all of these patients. This development is most frequent in patients who continue to consume alcohol and smoke cigarettes. The multiplicity of neoplasms suggests that the entire respiratory mucosa may be predisposed to develop malignant tumors, a so-called field defect. These patients may also develop cancers of the lung, pancreas, and other organs.

II. **Pathology and natural history**
   A. **Histology.** Squamous cell carcinomas constitute at least 95 percent of head and neck cancers except those in the hard palate and salivary glands. Minor salivary gland adenocarcinomas can occur throughout the upper aerodigestive tract. Sarcoma, melanoma, plasmacytoma, lymphoma, and tumors with other histologies are infrequently seen.
   B. **Metastases.** Head and neck cancers spread predominantly by local invasion of adjacent tissues and dissemination through lymphatic channels. Hematogenous dissemination, most commonly to the lungs, is a relatively late phenomenon.

III. **Diagnosis**
   A. **Common symptoms or signs**
      1. **Mass,** often painless
      2. **Mucosal ulcer,** often with mass
      3. **Localized (often referred) pain** in the mouth (teeth); throat, ear
      4. **Odynophagia or dysphagia**
      5. **Visual disturbances** related to cranial nerve palsies, proptosis, blindness
      6. **Hearing loss,** usually unilateral and often associated with serous otitis
      7. **Persistent unilateral "sinusitis,"** nasal obstruction, or bleeding
      8. **Unilateral tonsillar enlargement** in adults
      9. Five to ten percent of **white plaques (leukoplakia)** may be cancer in situ.

This condition must be differentiated from *Candida* infection (can be wiped off) and lichen planus (fine white lines often related to denture irritation).

B. Laboratory investigation. The pretreatment diagnostic evaluation of head and neck cancer must both document the extent of disease *and* exclude a coincident second primary cancer in the upper aerodigestive tract. A chest x-ray and a CT or MRI scan from the base of the skull to the thoracic inlet are included in the evaluation of location and extent of the cancer.

C. Endoscopy, which includes direct visualization of the nasopharynx, larynx, hypopharynx, cervical esophagus and proximal trachea, is useful for

1. **Documenting the presence, site, and extent of tumors** in the upper aerodigestive tract.
2. **Searching for other primary cancers** in patients with already recognized cancers in the upper aerodigestive tract.
3. **Evaluating cervical lymphadenopathy.** (A premature biopsy of the node can compromise both treatment and likelihood of cure if the origin is head and neck cancer.
   a. **Biopsy** of the suspicious node should be done only if
      (1) Thorough physical examination fails to reveal a primary tumor, *and*
      (2) CT or MRI examination does not disclose a primary tumor, *and*
      (3) Endoscopy fails to reveal a primary site (random "blind" biopsies of high-risk areas: nasopharynx, pharyngeal tongue, tonsillar fossa, and pyriform sinus may be performed in patients without obvious tumors), *and*
      (4) Fine-needle aspiration cytology fails to reveal the diagnosis
   b. **Specific criteria for endoscopy in patients** with cervical adenopathy
      (1) A node is firm and nontender or growing.
      (2) There is no evidence to suggest inflammatory disease (e.g., no response to a two-week course of antibiotics).
      (3) The patient is at high risk for cancer because the age is greater than 40 years or has a history of smoking and drinking.
      (4) No primary tumor is found on visual, digital, and mirror examination.

IV. Staging system and prognostic factors

A. Staging classification. The TNM-staging system for head and neck cancers is widely used.

Primary tumor (T)
T_0: No evidence of primary tumor
T_{IS}: Carcinoma in situ
T_{1-4}: See Table 7-1 for the specific features for each region involved

Cervical lymph nodes (N)
N_x: Nodes cannot be assessed
N_0: No regional lymph node metastasis
N_1: Single positive ipsilateral node less than or equal to 3 cm in diameter
N_{2A}: Single ipsilateral lymph node more than 3 cm but less than or equal to 6 cm
N_{2B}: Multiple ipsilateral lymph nodes but all less than 6 cm
N_{2C}: Bilateral or contralateral lymph nodes, but all less than 6 cm
N_3: Lymph nodes more than 6 cm

Distant metastases (M)
M_0: No (known) distant metastases
M_1: Distant metastases present

B. Stage groupings
Stage I $T_1 N_0 M_0$
Stage II $T_2 N_0 M_0$
Stage III $T_3 N_0 M_0$
$T_{1-3} N_1 M_0$
Stage IV $T_4 N_{0-1} M_0$
any T, N_{2-3}, M_0
any T, any N, M_1

Table 7-1. Classification of primary sites of head and neck tumors

Site	T_1	T_2	T_3	T_4
Lip, oral cavity, and oropharynx	≤2 cm	>2 and ≤4 cm	>4 cm	Invades adjacent structures[a]
Nasopharynx	One subsite	Invades more than one subsite	Invades nasal cavity or oropharynx	Invades skull or cranial nerves
Hypopharynx	One subsite	Invades more than one subsite or an adjacent site, without hemilarynx fixation	Invades more than one subsite or an adjacent site, with hemilarynx fixation	Invades adjacent structures[a]
Larynx: Glottis[b]	Limited to vocal cord(s); cords mobile; may involve commissure	Extends to supra- or subglottis or with impaired cord mobility	Vocal cord fixation	Extends beyond larynx
Larynx: Supraglottis	One subsite; cords mobile	Invades more than one subsite with normal cord mobility	Vocal cord fixation or invades postcricoid area, medial wall of piriform sinus or pre-epiglottic tissues	Extends beyond larynx
Larynx: Subglottis	Limited to subglottis	Extends to vocal cord(s) with normal or impaired cord mobility	Vocal cord fixation	Extends beyond larynx or through cricoid or thyroid cartilage
Maxillary sinus[c]	Limited to antral mucosa with no erosion of bone	Erosion of infrastructure including hard palate or nasal meatus	Invasion of cheek, posterior wall of sinus, floor or medial wall of orbit, or anterior ethmoid	Invades orbital contents or other adjacent structures[a]
Major salivary gland[d]	≤2 cm	>2 and ≤4 cm	>4 and ≤6 cm	>6 cm

[a] "Adjacent structures" include cortical bone, cartilage, deep (extrinsic) muscles of tongue, and skin and soft tissues of neck.

[b] The glottis includes the vocal cords, anterior commissure, and posterior commissure.

[c] The "suprastructure" includes the posterior bony wall and the posterior half of the superior bony wall; the "infrastructure" comprises the other bony walls.

[d] These T stages are separated into substage "a" for no local extension and substage "b" for local invasion of skin, bone, nerve, or soft tissue.

Source: Adapted from the *American Joint Committee for Cancer Staging and End-Results Reporting*, 1992.

C. Discordant clinical and pathological evaluation of stage. In some instances, biopsies of an apparently invasive cancer are interpreted as cancer in situ, cellular atypia, or dysplasia. This histologic interpretation requires additional biopsies, particularly at the margin of the gross tumor, because the initial biopsies may not have been representative of the lesion. If these biopsies are not conclusive, the entire gross tumor may be excised, if practical, for more complete examination. When an experienced clinician suspects a lesion to be an invasive cancer, it is important not to be deterred by initial inconclusive biopsies. Once the primary cancer has been positively identified, treatment planning can proceed based on likely extension of the tumor into adjacent tissues.

D. Prognostic factors

    1. Primary site. The site of origin of a cancer in the head and neck strongly influences the prognosis. For example, a cancer 1.0 cm in greatest dimension on a true vocal cord is more curable than a primary lesion of similar size arising subglottically or in the piriform sinus. However, the latter tumors usually are more extensive when diagnosed.

    2. Extent of tumor. The local extent of the primary tumor and metastases is a very important prognostic indicator. In the TNM staging system, the T (primary tumor) increases from T_1 to T_4 based on local tumor extent. Metastases to regional cervical lymph nodes are graded from N_1 to N_3 based on extent of involvement. Such regional node metastases, although seriously impacting on the prognosis, may not make the patient incurable. Distant metastases may be subgrouped according to anatomic site (i.e., M_1 (oss)-bone, M_1 (pul)-lung), and with rare exception, are indicative of incurability by current therapies.

    3. Histologic grade. Most cancers arising from the mucosa of the upper aerodigestive tract are epidermoid in character. These lesions usually are subdivided by grade ranging from well differentiated to poorly differentiated. Tumor grade correlates somewhat with biological behavior; less well differentiated primary cancers tend to grow more rapidly and be more locally or regionally extensive at the time of initial diagnosis.

V. Prevention

A. Abstinence. The limiting or elimination of alcohol and tobacco consumption (including chewing tobacco) remains the mainstay of prevention for most head and neck cancers.

B. Chemoprevention. Isoretinoin (13-*cis*-retinoic acid) can reverse severe oral leukoplakia. Continued maintenance therapy with attendant toxicity (rashes, conjunctivity, hypertriglyceridemia) is required to sustain the effect. Isoretinoin also appears to reduce the occurrence of second neoplasms in patients treated for primary head and neck squamous cell carcinomas; the drug does not prevent recurrence of the original neoplasm, however.

VI. Management. Prior to commitment for therapy of all patients, there should be input from members of a dedicated multidisciplinary group that includes a surgeon, radiation oncologist, medical oncologist, diagnostic imaging specialist, pathologist, and dentist. Patients must be frequently examined after treatment. Recurrent or persistent tumors usually can be recognized within two years of initial treatment.

A. Surgery

    1. General principles

        a. The **primary cancer** should be removed with tumor-free margins of normal tissues. Cosmesis is secondary to adequate resection. Tumor extension into bone requires sophisticated partial resection, when appropriate, or complete resection, followed by an insertion of a prosthesis.

        b. Preservation of function (i.e., swallowing or speech) is a prime consideration.

        c. A **primary resection** for proven or suspected metastases to cervical lymph nodes should involve en bloc removal of all lymph nodes and adjacent normal tissues. This may be a "radical neck dissection" or a partial neck dissection. Less extensive dissections include removal of tumor-involved lymph nodes that do not adequately respond to primary irradiation.

d. Fulguration of primary or metastatic cancer in the head and neck usually is inappropriate.

2. Surgical procedures

  a. Composite resections are usually performed for cancers of the oral cavity and oropharynx. This procedure involves the en bloc resection of the primary lesion, part of the mandible (if closely adjacent to the tumor or necessary for closure), and the cervical lymph nodes. Small lesions of the oral cavity can occasionally be treated with a more limited, mandible-sparing procedure.

  b. Neck dissection definitions and indications vary among surgeons.

    (1) A classic radical neck dissection (RND) removes en bloc all tissue from the mandible to the clavicle, from the anterior border of the trapezius to the midline strap muscles, and between the superficial layer of the deep cervical fascia (platysma) and the deep layer of the deep cervical fascia. Among the resected structures are the sternocleidomastoid muscle, internal jugular vein, and the eleventh cranial (accessory) nerve.

    (2) A modified radical neck dissection spares certain structures, usually the eleventh cranial nerve or the sternocleidomastoid muscle. It is usually reserved for the treatment of patients with clinically negative cervical lymph nodes, planned postoperative neck irradiation, or minimal tumor in neck nodes.

    (3) A partial neck dissection results in only partial removal of the lymph nodes. In its extreme, a partial neck dissection involves removal of only a solitary nodal mass.

3. Complications of radical surgery

  a. Cosmetic and functional deformity

  b. Speech impediment or loss

  c. Aspiration pneumonia

  d. Shoulder or arm weakness, paresthesias, and pain with RND

B. RT

  1. General principles. The intent of irradiation of head and neck cancers is long-term or permanent local-regional tumor control. The possibility of cure is directly related to the extent of tumor at the time of treatment. RT can control cancers arising in the head and neck with preservation of an intact anatomic part and consequently with preservation of function and cosmesis.

    a. The **volume** at the primary tumor site, which requires high-dose irradiation, must include a margin outside of all cancer cells and so is comparable to that which would be removed surgically. Anatomic barriers, such as bone and peripheral nerves, may be a greater deterrent to surgical removal than to irradiation. Thus cancers arising in the mucosa of the nasopharynx or posterior pharyngeal wall usually are irradiated by choice because of anatomic barriers. In other primary sites, such as the vocal cord and retina, the extreme morbidity of loss of voice or sight associated with obtaining a tumor-free margin surgically usually makes RT preferable.

    b. The **anatomic sites** of actual or likely spread of cancer, such as the regional lymph nodes, frequently are included in continuity with the primary tumor site, whether the treatment be surgery or irradiation. The primary and high-risk sites may be treated simultaneously or consecutively by the same or different methods.

    c. Large **total doses** (i.e., 6500–7500 cGy) of radiations, approaching the tolerance of normal tissues, usually are required to eradicate squamous cell carcinomas arising in the mucosa of the head and neck. Occasionally, the usual daily dose of 180–200 cGy may be delivered at less than 24-hour intervals (accelerated fractionation) or several smaller increments may be used every 24 hours (hyperfractionation).

 d. Postoperative RT. After the removal of all grossly detectable cancer, doses of 4500–6000 cGy result in a very high frequency (90–95%) of tumor control with few detectable sequelae.

 Advantages of this sequence include an appraisal of tumor extent that is unaltered by irradiation and performance of surgery in unirradiated tissue with possibly fewer technical problems and more rapid healing. Such planned use of RT should begin as soon as wound healing permits.

 e. Preoperative RT may be attempted when the initial gross extent of tumor makes resection problematic. Such planned preoperative radiation plus resection must be distinguished from unplanned surgery at varying intervals after high-dose, curative RT has failed to control the cancer. Such attempted surgical rescue is associated with increased morbidity related to late radiation-induced tissue changes.

2. Adverse effects of RT. The frequency and severity of sequelae of RT are related to the specific sites and tissue volumes irradiated, the condition of the normal tissues prior to irradiation, the total dose and incremental doses, the pattern of application, the quality of the radiations, concurrent disease and use of medications, and philosophy of the physicians and patients.

 a. Acute, self-limiting sequelae

  (1) Skin and conjunctival "reactions" include erythema, discoloration, and rarely superficial ulceration.

  (2) Epilation may be followed by regrowth of hair of a different density and even color.

  (3) Mucositis can result in dysphagia when the oral cavity, hypopharynx, or cervical esophagus is involved.

  (4) Edema may lead to hoarseness when the endolarynx is involved.

  (5) Xerostomia is secondary to irradiation of the salivary glands with high total doses. The possibility of secondary dental caries, usually at the gumline, may be greatly reduced by the maintenance of good oral hygiene and use of fluoride gel. The return of salivation may be incomplete. The alteration or loss of taste usually completely recovers before the return of salivation.

  (6) Lhermitte's syndrome, consisting of "electric shocklike" sensations in the upper or lower limbs precipitated by flexion of the neck, results from irradiation of the cervical spinal cord to relatively high doses.

  (7) Serous otitis media may follow irradiation of the middle ear. This clears spontaneously.

 b. Chronic sequelae

  (1) Myelopathy of the cervical spinal cord is the most dreaded long-term sequelae. This condition follows exposure to very high doses (less than 1% incidence at 6000 cGy in 200-cGy daily increments).

  (2) Necrosis of the mandible is infrequent and can be nearly eliminated by careful irradiation techniques and good dental care.

  (3) Ulceration of soft tissue is a rare long-term consequence and usually is related to irradiation to a high total dose in conjunction with surgery.

  (4) Cataracts may follow irradiation of the lens. This sequela usually can be avoided by careful technical application. This development is more frequent in elderly individuals and those with diabetes. Cataracts due to irradiation can be successfully treated surgically.

C. Chemotherapy. Patients with disseminated head and neck cancers usually die within six months. Several chemotherapeutic agents measurably shrink recurrent or disseminated head and neck cancers, but the duration of response is short (usually <2 months). Many nonrandomized pilot studies and early reports have shown impressive response rates. Responses to chemotherapy are greatly influenced by tumor grade and extent, and the significance of the response is affected by the patient's nutritional status, performance status, and comorbid conditions. Cytotoxic drugs do not improve survival. A few generalizations about cytotoxic agent therapy for head and neck carcinomas can be made.

1. **Single agents.** Methotrexate, bleomycin, carboplatin, cisplatin, and 5-fluorouracil are the most active single agents, each achieving significant tumor reduction in 15–30 percent of patients.
2. **Method of administration.** Intraarterial perfusion of drugs provides no benefit compared to IM or IV routes.
3. **Combination chemotherapy regimens** are not consistently superior to single agents. The most useful combination regimen to date is cisplatin and 5-fluorouracil (PF); adding another drug to this combination has not improved results. The dosages in PF, which are given every 21–28 days, are:
   Cisplatin, 100 mg/m^2 IV on day 1, *and*
   5-fluorouracil, 1000 mg/m^2/day as a 120-hour infusion
4. **Laryngeal carcinoma.** Sequential chemotherapy and definitive RT is effective for achieving laryngeal preservation in a high percentage of patients with advanced cancer. Randomized trials have not been completed, and the precise contribution of chemotherapy to this benefit is uncertain.
5. **Postoperative adjuvant chemotherapy** may benefit selected subgroups, which are not well-defined. These subgroups may include patients who have oral cavity tumors (especially small bulk disease) and those who achieved a response to preoperative chemotherapy. For head and neck cancers as a whole, postoperative adjuvant chemotherapy decreases the occurrence of distant metastases and may increase survival in high-risk groups but has no effect on disease-free survival or overall survival.
6. **Preoperative (neoadjuvant) chemotherapy** (with or without surgery or RT)
   a. Neoadjuvant chemotherapy can result in tumor regression in 60–90 percent and in complete responses (CRs) in 20–25 percent of patients with locally advanced head and neck cancers, many of which have been pathologically documented. Patients with CRs have better survival than nonresponders or those with partial responses, but this is not a valid statistical comparison.
   b. A response to chemotherapy predicts that those patients will respond further to RT. RT may be enough additional therapy for those who achieve a CR with chemotherapy (i.e., surgery may not be necessary).
   c. The appropriate sequence of chemotherapy, RT, and surgery has not been well-defined.
   d. The frequency of subsequent distant metastases is decreased when chemotherapy is given, but no improvement in survival results.
7. **Local recurrence and metastatic disease.** Combination chemotherapy with PF achieves response rates of about 45 percent (reported range: 10–75%). The highest response rates are seen in tumors originating in the oral cavity and nasopharynx. No combination improves survival rates.

D. **Treatment of the primary cancer**
1. **T_{1-2} cancer at the primary site.** Small malignancies usually can be treated by either RT or surgery with equal success. The choice of modality depends on the tumor's location, accessibility, histologic grade and the patient's vocation, health, and treatment preference. Tumors of high grade often are best treated with RT. Deeply invasive tumors and tumors adjacent to or invading bone are often best managed surgically. **Postoperative RT is indicated** when
   a. The cancer is histologically identified at or near the surgical margins.
   b. The cancer is poorly differentiated.
   c. There is extensive involvement of the lymphatics by tumor.
   d. Many cervical lymph nodes contain cancer or the tumor extends through the capsule of the node into surrounding tissues.
2. **T_{3-4} cancer at the primary site.** The management of T_3 lesions usually should combine surgery with preoperative or postoperative RT. Neither sequence has been demonstrated to be clearly superior. If surgery is not considered feasible, patients may be treated with either high-dose RT alone or RT preceded by or followed by chemotherapy. The addition of chemotherapy

to RT is still being investigated. It has often resulted in an improved response rate but with increased morbidity and no improvement in median survival.

E. Treatment of cervical lymph nodes is determined by the site and extent of the primary tumor, the proposed treatment modality for the primary lesion, and the N staging of the cervical nodes.

1. **Patients without enlarged cervical lymph nodes** have an incidence of tumor-containing nodes as high as 60 percent. Exceptions to this high incidence include vocal cord cancers and paranasal sinus cancers, small lip cancers, and low-grade salivary gland malignancies. For most other head and neck cancer sites, the homolateral cervical nodes should be treated with either RT or a modified RND, even if not grossly tumor-bearing.

2. **Patients with enlarged cervical lymph nodes**
   a. **RND** usually is performed whenever the primary site is treated surgically. **RND should be followed by RT if**
      (1) Any node is larger than 3.0 cm in greatest dimension.
      (2) Multiple nodes are involved.
      (3) The primary tumor is poorly differentiated.
      (4) The tumor extends through the capsules of the nodes.
   b. **RT** usually is the treatment of choice for primary carcinomas (or lymphomas) of the nasopharynx, pharyngeal tongue, soft palate, or tonsillar region or when the tumor-involved nodes cannot be resected. **RT should be followed by modified RND** if
      (1) The tumor-enlarged nodes do not completely grossly respond.
      (2) The tumor-involved nodes were initially unresectable but become resectable.
      (3) The tumor-involved nodes are unchanged or become enlarged after 6–8 weeks of RT.

F. Persistent tumor. When a cancer reappears at the previously treated primary site, it results from incomplete destruction of all tumor cells. Although this often is called recurrence, it is actually regrowth of a persistent tumor. If a discrete new tumor arises separately from a previously treated primary site, it represents a new or second cancer. Surgery usually is the treatment of choice to salvage RT failures. Surgical failures often can be salvaged by irradiation or additional surgery.

G. Supportive care

1. **Adequate nutrition** can be maintained by diet supplements between meals, nasoesophageal or gastrostomy tube feedings, or hyperalimentation.

2. **Opportunistic infections** frequently occur in debilitated patients during therapy and must be treated. Oral candidiasis is the most common infection in head and neck cancer patients (see Chap 35, sec. **VI.B**).

3. **Dental care**
   a. All patients who are likely to receive high doses of radiation to the oral cavity, including a portion of the mandible, or to the salivary glands should have a dental consultation prior to therapy.
   b. Fluoride gel treatment during and after the period of RT reduces dental problems.
   c. Dentures should not be worn during RT and for a period of 6–9 months after its completion. These dentures should have a soft lining and not result in local sites of pressure.

4. **Psychological support**
   a. Reiterate the appropriateness and necessity of particular treatments.
   b. Explain postsurgical reconstruction and rehabilitation.
   c. Reinforce patient avoidance of alcoholic beverages and tobacco.
   d. Emphasize the maintenance of good oral hygiene.
   e. Emphasize the importance of long-term follow-up.

VII. Special clinical problems

A. Increasing induration of neck or facial tissues in a previously irradiated area may indicate persistent cancer. If involved by carcinoma, the skin is usually tense, brawny, and purplish in color, often fixed to the underlying tissues or bone, and usually associated with an enlarging mass. Occasionally, no discrete masses are palpable, but the involved tissues are firm to stony hard. In contrast, postradiation induration is usually flat, smooth, and confined to areas of high dose. A biopsy often is hazardous. Treatment can usually be undertaken using clinical criteria without tissue diagnosis.

B. Residual ulcers. A residual ulcer is occasionally found after RT of a large tumor and usually represents uncontrolled cancer. It may also represent an incompletely healed site of eradicated disease. If the lesion does not heal after 8–12 weeks, a biopsy may be indicated.

C. Unsightly cosmetic facial defects pose major problems for both patients and those who must interact with them. Health professionals should combine a professional, detached view of physical defects with compassion.

D. Massive facial edema is an occasional end-stage problem in advanced head and neck cancer and is usualy caused by venous or lymphatic obstruction in the neck or mediastinum. These patients usually die of cerebral edema, hemorrhage, or inanition.

E. Arterial rupture with exsanguination may result from tumor erosion through the carotid or other major arteries and is usually rapidly fatal. RT should be attempted in patients with tumor adjacent to a major vessel. It may locally control the tumor and stimulate fibrosis and healing to avert or delay this disaster.

F. Airway obstruction can be a cause of death for patients with untreated or uncontrolled cancer of the upper respiratory passages.

   1. Emergency tracheostomy may be required in patients with a severely compromised upper air passage (e.g., stridor) prior to treatment.

   2. Prednisone, 40–60 mg/day PO, may provide temporary relief for some patients when other modalities have been ineffective. Patients who cannot swallow can receive methylprednisolone, 40 mg SQ.

   3. Antibiotics for the treatment of superimposed infection may relieve airway or swallowing difficulties and reduce accompanying foul odors.

   4. Chemotherapy may be used in patients who have already received maximum tolerable doses of radiation in an attempt to achieve tumor reduction.

G. Inability to swallow may be a complication of uncontrolled head and neck tumors. Alimentation by gastrostomy tube or IV therapy is probably not warranted in patients whose cancer is refractory to RT and chemotherapy, because prolonged survival may be accompanied by advancing cancer with airway obstruction, facial edema, or intractable pain.

H. Infection occurs in some patients with bulky, necrotic tumors. The infection may be associated with fever, pain, or swelling, and may be caused by normal mouth flora. Sometimes symptomatic relief can be obtained using a broad-spectrum antibiotic (e.g., metronidazole).

Specific Head
and Neck Cancers

The relative occurrence, sex predominance, most common site, and histology of the constituents of head and neck cancers are compared in Table 7-2.

I. Lip (sites: vermilion border and mucosal surfaces)

   A. Natural history

      1. Risk factors include smoking, long-standing hyperkeratosis, sun and wind exposure, chronic irritation, and xeroderma pigmentosum.

      2. Presentation. Ninety-five percent occur on the lower lip. The presenting sign or symptom usually is a recurrent scab, sore, blister, or ulcer with or without a mass.

      3. Lymphatic drainage. First to submental and submaxillary nodes, and then to upper anterior cervical (jugular) and intraparotid nodes. Lymphadenopa-

Table 7-2. Features of head and neck cancers by site of origin

Primary tumor	Most common site	Relative occurrence	Cervical lymph node metastases at time of presentation
Lip*	Lower lip (90%)	15%	5%
Oral cavity*	Tongue (lateral border)	20%	40%
Oropharynx*	Tonsillar region	10%	80% for tonsillar fossa and base of tongue 40% for other sites
Hypopharynx*	Pyriform sinus	5%	80%
Larynx*	True vocal cord	25%	<5% for early glottic 35% for other sites
Nasopharynx*	Roof	3%	80%
Nasal cavity and paranasal sinuses	Maxillary antrum	4%	15%
Salivary glands	Parotid (80%)	15%	25%

* At least 97 percent are squamous cell carcinomas.

thy is seen in 5–10 percent of patients at presentation and is related to the size of the primary cancer.
B. Differential diagnosis
  1. Keratoacanthoma is a self-limiting, endophytic, exophytic lesion of sun-exposed skin that may mimic squamous cell carcinoma. However, it arises rapidly and resolves spontaneously within months.
  2. Infected hyperkeratosis
  3. Leukoplakia
  4. Syphilitic chancre
C. Treatment of primary lesions. Since lip carcinoma is often detected early, it is equally curable by surgery, various irradiation techniques, or chemosurgery. Therefore the choice of therapy is determined by the condition of tissues, expected cosmetic results, patient's age, comfort, and convenience, and treatment costs. Treatment modalities are as follows:
  1. **Leukoplakia, severe dysplasia, and small carcinoma in situ.** Vermilionectomy (lip shave).
  2. **T_1 and T_{IS} (lesion ≤1 cm).** RT or surgical excision.
  3. **T_{1-4} (lesion >1 cm).** RT is cosmetically preferred, but excision and reconstruction give similar curative results.
  4. **Commissure involvement.** RT is cosmetically and functionally preferable if the commissure is involved.
D. Treatment of regional nodes
  1. **Clinically negative neck.** Observe or irradiate the first echelon of nodes in large or poorly differentiated primary tumors.
  2. **Clinically positive neck.** Modified RND with or without contralateral suprahyoid dissection. Postoperative RT is given based on the findings of RND.
E. Recurrences. Most treatment failures occur locally.
  1. **Surgical failures** are best treated with RT or additional surgery and RT failures with surgery.
  2. **Delayed neck dissections** for subsequently appearing cervical metastases do not appear to affect survival.
F. Local tumor control rate exceeds 90 percent for cancers up to 3 cm and is 75 to 80 percent for larger cancers.

II. Oral cavity (sites: floor of mouth, oral tongue, buccal mucosa, gingiva, retromolar trigone, hard palate)

A. Natural history

1. **Risk factors** include smoking, excessive consumption of alcohol, poor oral hygiene, prolonged focal denture irritation, betel nut chewing, and syphilis.

2. **Presentation.** Most oral cavity cancers first appear as a painless ulcer or mass. If symptomatic, patients complain of local pain; difficulty chewing, swallowing, eating, or speaking; or that dentures do not fit well.

3. **Lymphatic drainage** involves the upper jugular and submandibular nodes. The likelihood of bilateral adenopathy increases as the lesion approaches the midline. Lymphadenopathy occurs in about 40 percent of patients at presentation.

B. Diagnosis. Obtain x-ray films of the chest and mandible to detect distant metastases and bone erosion or mental nerve foramen enlargement (an indication of perineural infiltration); panarex views of the mandible are preferred.

C. Treatment of primary lesions

1. **Oral tongue and floor of mouth carcinoma**

   a. **Very small lesions** (≤ 1 cm). Surgical excision, interstitial RT, or external RT through the peroral cone; the neck is not treated electively.

   b. **T_{1-2} lesions.** Surgery, if location allows a wide excision without functional deformity; or, combination external and interstitial RT. The choice between surgery and RT is made according to the patient's health, psychological, social, and occupational factors.

   c. **Extensive lesions.** RT alone or combination RT and surgical resection. Surgery (alone or with RT) is preferred when there is mandibular invasion or attachment, verrucous carcinoma, or for treating unreliable patients.

   d. **Local tumor control rate** exceeds 90 percent for T_1 and T_2 primary cancers.

2. **Gingiva and hard palate carcinoma.** Most tumors of the upper gingiva and hard palate are salivary gland adenocarcinomas. Gingival and palatal lesions involve bone early on. Surgery is usually the preferred treatment.

   a. **Early lesions.** Surgery.

   b. **Advanced lesions.** Surgery and RT.

   c. **Local tumor control.** Small tumors are usually locally controlled. The control rate of T_4 lesions is about 40 percent.

3. **Buccal mucosa carcinoma**

   a. **T_1 lesions.** Surgery or RT.

   b. **T_{2-3} lesions.** RT.

   c. **T_4 lesions.** Surgery and RT, if feasible.

   d. **Local tumor control rate** exceeds 90 percent for T_1 lesions but drops to 50 to 60 percent for extensive tumors.

4. **Retromolar trigone carcinoma**

   a. **Early lesion.** Surgery.

   b. **Advanced lesion** (usually involves bone). Surgery, often with RT.

   c. **Local tumor control.** Most T_{1-2} tumors are controlled.

D. Treatment of regional nodes

1. **Clinically negative neck**

   a. **T_1 primary.** Observe if the patient is reliable and the lesion is low grade.

   b. **T_{2-4} primary or the lesion is high grade**

      (1) If primary lesion is treated surgically, perform elective RND.

      (2) If primary lesion is treated with RT, treat nodes with RT.

      (3) If primary lesion is treated with both modalities, the cervical nodes can be treated with either modality.

2. **Clinically positive neck**

   a. If the primary lesion is treated surgically, do RND.

   b. If the primary lesion is treated with RT, radiate the neck and do modified or partial RND for residual enlarged nodes or nodes originally larger than 3 cm.

c. If the cervical lymphadenopathy is fixed, begin treatment with RT. If the nodes become mobile during RT, do a neck dissection after 5000 cGy. If the nodes remain immobile, complete the full course of RT.

3. Indications for neck irradiation after RND

a. Multiple tumor-containing nodes, *or*

b. Node greater than 3 cm or tumor extends outside capsule, *or*

c. High-grade malignancy

III. Oropharynx (sites: posterior surface of anterior tonsillar pillar, faucal arch, tonsillar fossa, soft palate, pharyngeal tongue [including vallecula], pharyngeal walls)

A. Natural history

1. Presentation

a. Cancers arising in the pharyngeal tongue may be clinically silent until quite extensive. The lesion may be entirely submucosal and recognizable only by induration.

b. Tonsillar and pharyngeal tongue tumors frequently are initially recognized by nodal metastases.

c. Symptoms include odynophagia (referred), local pain, otalgia, dysphagia, and trismus (an indication of deep infiltration of muscle by tumor).

2. Lymphatic drainage. Lesions of the pharyngeal tongue and tonsillar fossa metastasize to the upper jugular nodes. The incidence of nodal metastases at the time cancer is detected varies with the primary site.

B. Diagnosis. These lesions can be visualized and are palpable. A CT scan or MRI of the neck is helpful to detect masses in the tongue and vallecula and to visualize a pharyngeal wall mass, abnormal thickening, or enlarged lymph nodes.

C. Treatment of primary lesions

1. Soft palate carcinoma. Forty to fifty percent of patients have cervical nodal metastases at the time of diagnosis.

a. **Small lesions.** Usually RT.

b. **Large lesions.** RT alone is preferred, since extensive surgical resection can result in compromise of ability to speak and swallow.

c. **Local tumor control rate** is 80 to 90 percent for T_{1-2} tumors and 75 to 80 percent for T_3–T_4 tumors.

2. Tonsillar region carcinoma. Nodal metastases are detected in 70 percent of patients at the time of diagnosis.

a. **Early lesions.** Surgery (composite resection with RND) or RT.

b. **Advanced lesions.** Surgery and RT.

c. **Local tumor control rate** exceeds 85 percent for T_1–T_2 cancers, 50 to 75 percent for T_3 cancers, and 25 percent for T_4 cancers.

d. **Approximate five-year survival.** Invasion of the pharyngeal tongue or trismus markedly decreases likelihood of a cure.

Stage	Five-year survival (%)	Nodes	Five-year survival (%)
T_{1-2}	70	All N_0	80
T_{3-4}	20	All N_1	45
		All N_3	10

3. Anterior tonsillar pillar carcinoma (may be included in oral cavity carcinoma) is better differentiated histologically and has less of a propensity for early metastasis than other oropharyngeal sites.

a. **Early lesions.** Surgery or RT.

b. **Advanced lesions,** particularly if deeply infiltrative or involving the base of tongue or bone, are treated with surgery or combined surgery and RT.

c. **Local tumor control rate** exceeds 85 percent for T_{1-2} cancers.

4. Pharyngeal tongue carcinoma. Lymphadenopathy is detected in 80 percent of patients at presentation and is bilateral in nearly one half.

a. **Early lesions** (uncommon). Surgery or RT.

      b. Advanced lesions (across the midline). RT alone since the alternative of total glossectomy in unacceptable to most patients.

      c. Local tumor control rate is about 75 percent for T_1 cancers, 60 percent for T_3 cancers, and 15 percent for T_4 cancers.

  5. Pharyngeal wall carcinoma. Most lesions that extend well onto the posterior wall are not curable by surgery.

      a. Early lesions. RT.

      b. Advanced lesions. Combined RT and surgery.

      c. Local tumor control rate ranges from 30 to 50 percent for T_{2-3} cancers; T_1 cancers are rare.

D. Treatment of regional nodes. Since most of the cancers of this region require RT as primary or adjuvant therapy, RT rather than surgery is commonly used in the treatment of cervical node metastases.

  1. N_0 and N_1. If surgery is used to treat the primary site, then RND is done; if RT is used to treat the primary, then RT is used for the neck.

  2. N_{2A}. Similar to N_0 and N_1, but RND is often required for residual disease.

  3. N_{2B}. RT, followed by modified RND.

  4. N_{3A}. RT and RND, if possible.

  5. N_{3B}. Treat each side individually.

  6. Indications for RT after RND

      a. Multiple tumor-containing nodes, *or*

      b. Node greater than 3 cm or tumor perforating the capsule, *or*

      c. High-grade pathology

E. Follow-up of oropharyngeal carcinoma. Careful and frequent follow-up visits are essential because of

  1. Surgical salvage of RT failures can be successful.

  2. Incidence of subsequent second malignancies is 5 to 10 percent.

IV. Nasopharynx

A. Natural history. Nasopharyngeal tumors comprise a variety of histologies. The approximate incidence of specific types is as follows: 85 percent epithelial tumors (either moderately to poorly differentiated squamous cell carcinoma or its lymphoepithelial variant [Schmincke or Regaud tumor]), 10 percent lymphomas, and 5 percent other histologic types (undifferentiated carcinoma, melanoma, plasmacytoma, angiofibroma of childhood).

  1. Presentation. Nasopharyngeal tumors spread directly through the pharyngeal space to the structures in or near the cavernous sinus and the foramina of the middle cranial fossa (including the gasserian ganglion and its branches). Destruction in the parasphenoid bones and nerve compression can result in severe pain and nerve palsy. Cranial nerve VI, which passes around the brain stem and along the cavernous sinus, is usually the first nerve to be affected, resulting in a lateral rectus muscle paresis.

      a. Common symptoms and signs. Enlarged neck nodes, headache, epistaxis, nasal obstruction (often unilateral), unilateral decreased hearing secondary to eustachian tube obstruction, sore throat (inferior extension), and pain on neck extension.

      b. Retrosphenoidal syndrome usually starts with the sixth cranial nerve and subsequently involves the second through sixth cranial nerves. Symptoms include unilateral ophthalmoplegia, pain, ptosis, trigeminal neuralgia, and unilateral weakness of muscles of mastication.

      c. Syndrome of the retroparotid space results from nodal compression of the ninth through twelfth cranial nerves and sympathetic nerves at the base of the skull. Symptoms include difficulties with swallowing, taste, salivation, and respiration; weakness of the trapezius, sternocleidomastoid muscles, homolateral tongue, and soft palate; and Horner's syndrome.

  2. Lymphatic drainage. Because the tumor is relatively anaplastic and the nasopharynx has a rich lymphatic network, these carcinomas may spread to lymph nodes when the primary tumor is small.

      a. First involved are the retropharyngeal and lateral pharyngeal nodes, followed by the upper cervical nodes. Involvement of the high, posterior cervical nodes is characteristic.

   b. Lymphadenopathy is present in 80 percent of patients at presentation; 50 percent is bilateral.

B. Diagnosis. Carefully examine regional lymph nodes. Rhinoscopy, indirect nasopharyngoscopy, and triple endoscopy are performed. A CT scan or MRI of the base of the skull, pharynx, and neck is essential.

C. Treatment of primary tumors

   1. RT alone (bilateral) is used for both the primary tumor and the regional nodal metastases.

   2. Surgery is not feasible because of the inadequacy of the surgical margins at the base of the skull and the frequent involvement of the retropharyngeal and cervical nodes bilaterally.

D. Treatment of regional nodes. RT is the treatment of choice. Neck dissection is reserved for adenopathy that persists or regrows after irradiation in patients with apparently controlled primary tumors.

E. Gross reappearance of the cancer at the primary site can be retreated with additional external beam RT or the placement of a removable radioactive source in the nasopharynx. Such retreatment is only moderately successful and may often produce long-term side effects.

F. Local tumor control exceeds 90 percent for T_{1-3} primary cancers. Control of cervical adenopathy by RT is equally successful for N_0-N_{3A} disease.

V. Larynx

A. Natural history. Although cancer of the larynx represents only 2 percent of the total risk of cancer in humans, it is the most frequent head and neck cancer except for skin cancer. There is a direct etiological relationship to cigarette smoking. Alcohol ingestion probably is less important as an etiologic agent than for other head and neck cancers. The clinical presentation depends on the primary site and extent of the cancer. Tumors arising from the true vocal cords, which are usually diagnosed when smaller, are less likely to infiltrate surrounding tissues or to metastasize to regional lymph nodes than are tumors arising subglottically or supraglottically.

   1. Presentation. Persistent hoarseness is the usual presenting symptom for patients with cancers arising on the true vocal cords (glottis). At other primary sites sore throat with dysphagia or nonpainful, regional adenopathy may develop.

   2. Lymphatic drainage

   a. Glottic (true vocal cord) carcinomas. The true vocal cords are devoid of lymphatics. Therefore cervical node metastases develop only when the tumor has extended to adjacent structures.

   b. Supraglottic carcinomas. This group includes tumors arising from the suprahyoid epiglottis, infrahyoid epiglottis, false vocal cords, ventricles, arytenoids, and aryepiglottic folds, which are drained by a rich lymphatic network. Approximately 40–50 percent of these patients develop regional adenopathy involving the upper (subdigastric) or middle internal jugular nodes.

   c. Subglottic carcinomas. These tumors arise from an arbitrarily defined "structure" extending caudad from 5 mm below the free margin of the vocal cord (inferior limit of the vocalis muscle) to the lower margin of the cricoid cartilage. Lymphatics, which are sparse, extend through the cricothyroid membrane to the pretracheal (Delphian) nodes or the lower internal jugular nodes.

   3. Curability is related to the site of origin, ranging from most curable to least curable as follows: true vocal cord cancers; tumors arising from the false cords, epiglottis, ventricles, aryepiglottic folds; tumors arising in the subglottis are infrequently controlled.

B. Diagnosis

   1. Studies. Indirect laryngoscopy, performed during deep breathing and phonation, can determine the mobility of the vocal cords and arytenoids. Direct laryngoscopy facilitates biopsy and may provide better visualization of the ventricles and subglottic larynx. CT and MRI are useful to determine tumor extent, particularly when the thyroid cartilage and pre-epiglottic space are involved.

2. Differential diagnosis

a. Hyperkeratosis

b. Laryngocele

c. Polyps (which appear as glistening, pedunculated masses)

d. Papillomas (which are white, grapelike growths)

C. Treatment of primary lesions

1. Principles

a. The **overriding requirement** for treatment is preservation of the patient's life, voice, and swallowing reflex. These considerations have led to the increasing use of more limited surgical procedures combined with RT or RT alone.

b. **Salvage (total) laryngectomy** is usually required for patients in whom more conservative treatments fail.

c. **Deeply infiltrative tumors** are more difficult to evaluate because of accompanying distortion and edema. Laryngectomy is therefore favored in many of these patients.

d. **Sequential chemotherapy and definitive RT** is effective for achieving laryngeal preservation in a high percentage of patients with advanced cancer in both glottic and supraglottic lesions without compromising overall survival. It is not known, however, whether administering higher doses of RT alone would achieve the same result.

e. **Sequelae of therapy**

(1) Total laryngectomy necessitates tracheostomy and loss of normal voice. About 50 to 70 percent of patients develop satisfactory esophageal speech.

(2) RT of the larynx is rarely associated with painful chondritis and edema of the laryngeal structures.

2. Glottic carcinoma

a. **Treatment of primary tumor**

(1) T_{is}. RT or "cord-stripping" for focal areas of disease.

(2) T_{1-2}. RT is preferable to surgery (either cordectomy or vertical laryngectomy). Involvement of the arytenoid or more than one-third of the opposing cord is a contraindication to hemilaryngectomy. Postoperative RT is given following hemilaryngectomy if the tumor is close to the surgical margins.

(3) T_3. Lesions that fix the true vocal cords can be divided into two groups: relatively smaller lesions, which respond to irradiation (local control is 50–60% with possible surgical salvage) and extensive tumors (bilateral, compromised airway) that require surgery and usually postoperative RT.

(4) T_4. Total laryngectomy and RT.

b. **Treatment of persistent or recurrent disease**

(1) Surgery for RT failure. The surgical salvage rate for early glottic cancer is about 85 percent.

(2) RT or total laryngectomy for failure of partial laryngectomy or cordectomy.

(3) RT for failure of total laryngectomy. Salvage rates are poor. (RT usually should be used as a postoperative adjuvant.)

c. **Tumor control**

(1) T_1. Greater than 90 percent with RT and approaches 100 percent with surgical salvage.

(2) T_2. Seventy-five to eighty-five percent with RT and approaches 90–100 percent with surgical salvage.

(3) T_3. Sixty to sixty-five percent with RT and 75 percent with surgery plus RT. Ultimate control of 80–85 percent with surgical sal-

vage. Sixty to sixty-five percent voice preservation with primary RT.

  (4) T_4. Forty to forty-five percent with laryngectomy. Up to 50 percent with RT and surgical salvage.

3. Supraglottic carcinoma (epiglottis, aryepiglottic fold, vallecula, arytenoid, ventricle, false cord)

  a. Treatment of primary tumor

   (1) T_1. RT or supraglottic resection.

   (2) T_{2-3}. RT frequently controls exophytic cancers. Surgery, which is reserved for RT failures, is favored for infiltrative disease or lesions involving the base of the epiglottis or false cords. Surgical procedures include supraglottic or total laryngectomy.

   (3) T_4. Surgery and RT.

  b. Indications for postoperative RT

   (1) Bulky or infiltrating lesions, *or*

   (2) Close or positive operative margins, *or*

   (3) Multiple positive lymph nodes, *or*

   (4) Deep connective tissue, thyroid cartilage, or perineural involvement, *or*

   (5) Poorly differentiated histology

  c. RT treatment failures usually require total laryngectomy. The surgical salvage rate is 80 percent for RT failures.

  d. Local tumor control rates are 90 to 95 percent for T_{1-2} cancers, about 80 percent for T_3 cancers, and 40 to 50 percent for T_4 cancers.

4. Subglottic carcinoma

  a. Early lesions. RT or total laryngectomy.

  b. Advanced lesions. Total laryngectomy and RT.

  c. Approximate five-year survival without evidence of disease is less than 25 percent.

D. Treatment of regional nodes. Glottic carcinomas are treated without neck dissection, unless cervical nodes are palpable (<10%). Supraglottic and infraglottic carcinomas usually require some form of cervical node therapy. Clinically positive nodes are generally managed with RND.

VI. Hypopharynx (pharyngeal walls, pyriform sinus, postcricoid pharnyx)

A. Natural history

  1. Presentation. Odynophagia, dysphagia, and otalgia are common presenting symptoms. Late clinical findings include cough, aspiration pneumonia, hoarseness, and neck masses.

  2. Direct extension. These tumors behave aggressively with early direct extension; they are usually detected in an advanced stage.

  3. Lymphatic drainage involves the retropharyngeal and midjugular nodes. Lymphadenopathy is present in 80 percent of patients at presentation.

B. Diagnosis. Indirect laryngoscopy, direct laryngoscopy, and CT scan or MRI of the neck are performed.

C. Treatment of primary lesions

  1. Pyriform sinus tumors

   a. Small, exophytic lesions (particularly in upper pyriform sinus). RT.

   b. Other early T_{1-2} lesions. Total or partial laryngectomy, and partial or total pharyngectomy and RT combined.

   c. T_{3-4} lesions. Laryngopharyngectomy and RT. If inoperable because of involvement of the posterior pharyngeal wall or massive neck disease, treat with RT alone.

  2. Posterior pharyngeal wall tumors. RT alone.

  3. Persistent or recurrent disease. Salvage is poor.

D. Treatment of regional nodes

  1. Clinically negative neck. Prophylactic RT or RND.

  2. Clinically positive neck. Combined RND and RT.

E. Tumor control. Many T_{1-2} cancers can be locally controlled. The likelihood of control of cervical node metastases varies with the size and number of nodes.

VII. Nasal cavity and paranasal sinuses

A. Natural history. Although cancers often involve both the nasal cavity and paranasal sinuses at the time of diagnosis, it is important to separate those cancers limited to the nasal fossa from those arising in the sinuses. Most tumors of the nasal cavity and paranasal sinuses are squamous cell carcinomas. Some adenocarcinomas, sarcomas, plasmacytomas, lymphomas, minor salivary gland tumors, and esthesioneuroblastomas also occur.

1. **Presentation.** Symptoms and signs often mimic inflammatory sinusitis and include local pain, tenderness, toothache, bloody nasal discharge, loosening of teeth, and interference with fit of dentures. Other symptoms are visual disturbances, proptosis, nasal obstruction, trismus, and a bulging cheek mass that can ulcerate through the skin and palate.

2. **Lymphatic drainage** involves the retropharyngeal, submaxillary, and upper anterior and posterior cervical nodes. At the time of presentation, lymphadenopathy is present in 15 percent of patients who have early disease and in more patients with advanced disease.

B. Diagnosis

1. **Studies.** Rhinoscopy, endoscopy, sinoscopy, and CT scan or MRI of the involved structures are performed. Bone destruction on radiographs is the hallmark of malignancy, although it can also occur in certain benign conditions (e.g., papilloma, osteomyelitis).

2. **Differential diagnosis**
   a. Inverting papilloma of the nasal cavity
   b. Destructive mucocele of the sinus

C. Treatment of primary lesions

1. **Paranasal sinuses**
   a. **Surgery** is usually indicated because of the frequency of osseous involvement. The desire to obtain a wide margin beyond the tumor is tempered by a reluctance to produce serious sequelae. If disease extends through the orbital wall, orbital exenteration is performed. Reconstructive and cosmetic surgery using prosthetic devices is often necessary.
   b. **RT** is nearly always necessary because the resection margins are often minimal or positive and the neoplasm is frequently of high grade.

2. **Nasal cavity tumors**
   a. **Early lesions.** RT is preferable if surgery will produce a deformity. Surgery is favored if bone is destroyed or if the lesion is a sarcoma.
   b. **Advanced lesions.** Combined surgical resection and RT is most commonly used. RT alone is used for lymphomas, plasmacytomas, rhabdomyosarcomas, lethal midline granuloma, malignant histiocytosis, and esthesioneuroblastoma. Adjuvant chemotherapy is used for rhabdomyosarcoma. Ewing's sarcoma, and osteogenic sarcoma.
   c. **Local tumor control rate** approaches 100 percent for stage I tumors.

3. **Nasal vestibule carcinomas**
   a. **Early lesions.** RT is preferable if surgery will produce a deformity.
   b. **Advanced lesions.** RT alone.
   c. **Recurrent or persistent disease after RT.** Surgery, cryosurgery, chemosurgery, and laser surgery have all been advocated.
   d. **Local tumor control rate** exceeds 90 percent for small tumors.

4. **Ethmoid sinus carcinoma.** Surgery and RT. Approximate five-year survival rate is 30 percent.

5. **Frontal and sphenoid sinus carcinomas.** RT alone. Results are dismal.

6. **Maxillary antrum carcinoma.** Fenestration prior to surgical extirpation provides tissue biopsy, decreases tumor bulk via curettage, and allows for drainage of necrotic debris during treatment. Treatment is as follows:
   a. **Early lesions.** Surgery alone.

      b. Advanced lesions. Surgery with either pre- or postoperative RT.

      c. Very advanced lesions. Chemotherapy initially, then surgery and RT.

      d. Unresectable disease. Chemotherapy and high-dose RT.

      e. Recurrences. Surgery or RT or chemotherapy, alone or in combination, is used. Salvage is very poor.

      f. Approximate five-year survival is 60 percent for patients with T_{1-2} lesions and 30 to 40 percent overall.

D. Treatment of regional nodes

  1. T_{1-2}, N_0. No treatment.

  2. T_{3-4}, N_0. Prophylactic upper neck RT.

  3. **All N_{1-3}.** If surgery is part of the management of the primary lesion, then RND is done. If RT is being used primarily, then partial neck dissection might still be necessary for initial large or residual tumors.

E. Sequelae. Most failures are local. Subsequent cosmetic surgery or prosthetic reconstruction should await healing and a reasonable likelihood of local control. Delayed homolateral cataract may follow RT.

VIII. Salivary glands

A. Natural history. The parotid gland accounts for 80 percent of the salivary gland neoplasms in adults. Approximately 75 percent of parotid tumors are benign. In contrast, nearly half of tumors arising in the submaxillary or minor salivary glands are malignant.

  1. Histology of malignant tumors

    a. Mucoepidermoid tumors (high and low grade)

    b. Adenoid cystic carcinoma (high and low grade; also called cylindroma)

    c. Undifferentiated carcinoma

    d. Malignant mixed tumors (epithelial and mesenchymal components)

    e. Adenocarcinoma

    f. Squamous cell carcinoma (considered to be high grade)

    g. Acinic cell tumors

    h. Malignant lymphoma

  2. Presentation. Most malignant salivary gland tumors appear as a painless swelling. Local pain (particularly pain along the distribution of an adjacent nerve) and development of nerve palsy are highly indicative of malignancy.

  3. Tumor spread. The malignant neoplasms tend to spread by direct extension and infiltration, but high-grade tumors also metastasize distantly or to regional nodes. Adenoid cystic carcinomas (cylindromas) tend to infiltrate along nerve trunks; they may recur months or years after initial therapy. Pulmonary metastases from adenoid cystic cancers often have an indolent course; the diagnosis may not be established until years after treatment of the primary tumor.

  4. Lymphatic drainage

    a. Parotid gland tumors metastasize to intraparotid, submaxillary, and upper cervical nodes.

    b. Submaxillary gland tumors metastasize to subdigastric, submaxillary, and upper jugular nodes.

B. Diagnosis

  1. Studies. A CT scan or an MRI should be obtained.

  2. Differential diagnosis. Most salivary gland swellings are due to inflammation or ductal obstruction. The intraparotid lymph nodes receive afferent lymphatic drainage from the skin of the face, scalp, ear, and buccal mucosa. Symptoms and signs to differentiate benign from malignant parotid masses are shown in Table 7-3.

C. Treatment of parotid gland carcinoma. Wide surgical excision (total parotidectomy) is the standard treatment. However, there is a tendency to use less radical surgery in combination with postoperative RT to spare the facial nerve while decreasing the possibility of local recurrence. Early data indicate that fast neutron irradiation is more effective than conventional photon irradiation.

Table 7-3. Differential diagnosis of parotid gland masses

Characteristic	Benign	Malignant
Growth rate	Slow, steady	Usually rapid
Pain	Rare	Often present
Tenderness	Occasional	Frequent
Seventh nerve palsy	Absent	Often present (nearly pathognomonic)
Consistency	Cystic to rubbery	Very hard
Attachment	Mobile	Fixed to muscle or skin
Trismus	Absent	Present when deeply invasive
Lymph nodes	Absent unless infected	Occasionally present

1. **Treatment according to tumor grade**
   a. **High-grade or large malignant tumors with facial nerve involvement.** Total parotidectomy with facial nerve resection *and* RND, usually with RT
   b. **High-grade or large malignant tumors without facial nerve involvement.** Same as **a** but possibly with no resection or only partial resection of the facial nerve *and* postoperative RT
   c. **High-grade tumors, superficial lobe, without facial nerve involvement.** Same as **a**, *or* superficial lobectomy and postoperative RT
   d. **Low-grade tumors.** Same as **a, b,** and **c** but without prophylactic RND
2. **Postparotidectomy sequelae**
   a. Facial nerve palsy
   b. Auriculotemporal syndrome of gustatory sweating
3. **Use of radiotherapy**
   a. **Postoperative RT** is generally given to the tumor site if
      (1) The tumor is high grade, *or*
      (2) Resection margins are positive or close, *or*
      (3) Tumor is peeled off the facial nerve or there is histologic evidence of perineural involvement, *or*
      (4) Tumor invades deeply, *or*
      (5) Tumor excision is for recurrence
   b. **Curative RT** is attempted only if patient is unresectable or medically inoperable.
   c. **Recurrent benign tumors.** RT is advocated after reexcision (or after the initial treatment if the resection margins are positive).
4. **Chemotherapy** (see **D**).
D. **Treatment of submaxillary gland carcinoma**
   1. **Surgery.** Wide resection of contents of submaxillary space (including connective tissue and nerves, surrounding muscle, and periosteum) with RND.
   2. **Postoperative RT** indications are similar to those for the parotid gland.
   3. **Chemotherapy** for salivary gland cancers has not been extensively investigated. Adriamycin, fluorouracil, and methotrexate used alone or in combination occasionally result in substantial tumor response.
E. **Results of treatment**
   1. **Malignant salivary gland tumors**
      a. **Local control rate.** Overall, 75 percent; high-grade and squamous cell carcinoma, 30 percent; low-grade carcinoma, 80 percent.
      b. **Survival rate.** Recurrences can occur 10 or 15 years after treatment. Therefore, five-year survival statistics are not reliable.

   2. Benign mixed tumors have a recurrence rate of 25 percent after lumpectomy and 2 percent after lobectomy. One fourth of recurrences are malignant.

Selected Reading

Department of Veterans Affairs Laryngeal Cancer Study Group. Induction chemotherapy plus radiation compared with surgery plus radiation in patients with advanced laryngeal cancer. *N. Engl. J. Med.* 324:1685, 1991.

DeVita, V. T., Jr., Hellman, S., and Rosenberg, S. A. (eds.). *Cancer: Principles and Practice of Oncology* (4th ed.). Philadelphia: Lippincott, 1993.

Ensley, J., et al. The impact of conventional morphologic analysis on response rates and survival in patients with advanced head and neck cancers treated initially with cisplatin-combination chemotherapy. *Cancer* 57:711, 1986.

Hong, W. K., et al. Prevention of second primary tumors with isoretinoin in squamous-cell carcinoma of the head and neck. *N. Engl. J. Med.* 323:795, 1990.

Jacobs, C., Makuch, R. Efficacy of adjuvant chemotherapy for patients with resectable head and neck cancers. A subset analysis of the head and neck contracts program. *J. Clin. Oncol.* 8:838, 1990.

Khafif, R. A., et al. Elective radical neck dissection in epidermoid cancer of the head and neck. A retrospective analysis of 853 cases of mouth, pharynx, and larynx cancer. *Cancer* 67:67, 1991.

Laramore, G., et al. Adjuvant chemotherapy for resectable head and neck cancer: Report on intergroup study 0034. *Int. J. Radiat. Oncol. Biol. Phys.* 23:705, 1992.

Million, R. R., and Cassissi, N. J. *Management of Head and Neck Cancer* (2nd ed.). Philadelphia: Lippincott, 1994.

Perez, C. A., and Brady, L. W. (eds.). *Principles and Practice of Radiation Oncology* (2nd ed.). Philadelphia: Lippincott, 1992.

Pfister, D., Strong, E., and Harrison, L. Larynx preservation with combined chemo- and radiotherapy in advanced head and neck cancer. *J. Clin. Oncol.* 9:830, 1991.

Rooney, M., et al. Improved complete response rate and survival in advanced head and neck cancer after three-course induction therapy with 120-hour 5-FU infusion and cisplatin. *Cancer* 55:1123, 1985.

Vokes, E. E. (editor). Head and neck cancer. *Semin Oncol.* 21:279, 1994 (entire issue).

Zidan, J., et al. Multidrug chemotherapy using bleomycin, methotrexate, and cisplatin combined with radical radiotherapy in advanced head and neck cancers. *Cancer* 59:24, 1987.

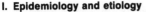

Lung Cancer

Hassan J. Tabbarah,
Barry B. Lowitz, and
Robert B. Livingston

I. Epidemiology and etiology

A. Incidence. Lung cancer is the most common visceral malignancy and accounts for roughly one-third of all cancer deaths. Annually there are 172,000 new cases in the United States, and the incidence is increasing.

B. Etiology

1. **Smoking.** Scientific studies have conclusively proved that smoking cigarettes is a major cause of lung cancer; the risk of lung cancer in smokers is 30 times greater than in nonsmokers. Smoking cigars or pipes doubles the risk of lung cancer compared to the risk in nonsmokers. Passive smoking probably increases the risk of lung cancer about twofold, but because a proportion of the risk associated with active inhalation is about 20-fold, the actual risk is quite small.

   a. The risk of lung cancer is related to **cumulative dose,** which for cigarettes is quantified in "pack-years." One in seven persons who smoke more than two packs per day will die of lung cancer. The incidence of death from lung cancer begins to be above that of the nonsmoking population at 10 pack-years (Table 8-1).

   b. **Following the cessation of smoking,** the risk steadily declines, approaching but not quite reaching that of nonsmokers after 15 years of abstinence for patients who smoked for less than 20 years. The risk is reduced for patients who smoked for more than 20 years but never approaches that of nonsmokers.

   c. The risk of the major cell types of lung cancer is increased in smokers. Some adenocarcinomas, especially in women, are unrelated to smoking, as are most tumors belonging to the bronchoalveolar carcinoma subtype.

2. **Asbestos** is causally linked to malignant mesothelioma. Asbestos exposure also increases the risk of lung cancer, especially in smokers (three times greater risk than smoking alone). Thus the risk of lung cancer in smokers who are exposed to asbestos is increased 90-fold.

3. **Radiation exposure** may increase the risk of small cell lung cancer in both smokers and nonsmokers.

4. **Other substances** associated with lung cancer include arsenic, nickel, chromium compounds, chloromethyl ether, and air pollutants.

5. **Lung cancer** is itself associated with an increased risk of another lung cancer occurring both synchronously and subsequently.

6. **Other lung diseases.** Lung scars and chronic obstructive pulmonary disease are associated with an increased risk of lung cancer. Scleroderma is associated with alveolar carcinoma.

II. Pathology and natural history

A. Small cell carcinoma (20% of lung cancers). Small cell lung cancer (SCLC) comprises several histologic subtypes: oat cell, polygonal cell, lymphocytic, and spindle cell. The natural histories of these subtypes are virtually identical.

1. **Location.** More often central or hilar (95%) than peripheral (5%).

2. **Clinical course.** Patients with SCLC often have widespread disease at the time of diagnosis. Rapid clinical deterioration in patients with chest masses often indicates SCLC.

Table 8-1. Cigarette smoking and the lifetime risk of lung cancer

Consumption (pack-years)	Risk of lung cancer (%)
20	1
60	5
90	8
100	13
120	20
>135	33

Source: Adapted from B. Cady, et al., History taking for cancer detection. In *Cancer. A Manual for Practitioners* (5th ed.). Boston: American Cancer Society, 1978. P. 6.

   a. Hematogenous metastases commonly involve the brain, bone marrow, or liver. Pleural effusions are common.
   b. Relapse after RT or chemotherapy occurs in the sites initially affected as well as in previously uninvolved sites.
 3. Associated paraneoplastic syndromes (Hypercalcemia occurs rarely, even in the presence of extensive bony metastases.)
   a. SIADH (most common)
   b. Hypercoagulable state (common)
   c. Ectopic ACTH syndrome (uncommon)
   d. Eaton-Lambert syndrome (myasthenic syndrome) (occasional, but rarely seen with any other tumor)
   e. Gynecomastia
 B. Squamous cell carcinoma (25–30% of lung cancers)
   1. Location. More often central (80%) than peripheral (20%).
   2. Clinical course. Compared to other kinds of lung cancers, squamous cell lung cancers are most likely to remain localized early in the disease and to recur locally following either surgery or RT.
   3. Associated paraneoplastic syndrome
   a. Hypercalcemia resulting from ectopic production of parathyroid hormone-related peptide (PTH-RP) is the more frequent syndrome.
   b. Hypertrophic osteoarthropathy (occasional).
   c. Hypercoagulable state.
 C. Adenocarcinoma and large cell carcinoma (50–60% of lung cancers). Adenocarcinoma is the most common cell type occurring in nonsmokers, especially young women. However, the majority of cases are smoking-associated.
   1. Location. These tumors appear most often as peripheral nodules (70%).
   2. Clinical course. More than 50 percent of patients with adenocarcinoma, apparently localized as a peripheral nodule, have regional nodal metastases. Adenocarcinomas and large cell carcinomas have similar natural histories and spread widely outside the thorax by hematogenous dissemination, commonly involving the bones, liver, and brain.
   3. Associated paraneoplastic syndromes
   a. Hypertrophic osteoarthropathy
   b. Hypercoagulable state
   c. Hypercalcemia due to PTH-RP or cytokines (HHM)
   d. Gynecomastia (large cell)
 D. Uncommon tumors of the lung
   1. Bronchial carcinoids may present with local symptoms from airway obstruction, ectopic ACTH production, or carcinoid syndrome (see Chap. 15, sec. **II**).
   2. Cystic adenoid carcinomas ("cylindroma") are locally invasive cancers, which can metastasize to other areas of the lung and to distant sites (see Chap. 19, sec. **VI**).

Table 8-2. Sites of lung cancer metastases by cell type

Metastatic site	Approximate frequency (%)			
	Squamous	Large cell	Adenocarcinoma	Small cell
Mediastinal lymph nodes	30	40	40	95
Liver	30	30	45	50
Brain	20	30	30	40
Bone	25	40	40	35
Bone marrow	5	–	–	30

   3. Carcinosarcomas are large lesions that have a tendency to remain localized and are more often resectable than other lung malignancies.
   4. Mesotheliomas are caused by exposure to asbestos and occur in the lung,
   pleura, peritoneum, or tunica vaginalis or albuginea of the testis. A history
   of asbestos exposure of any duration at any time is prima facie evidence
   that it caused the mesothelioma. Although mesothelioma is still uncommon,
   the incidence is increasing.
      a. Histopathology. Mesotheliomas consist of several histologic variants:
      sarcomatous, epithelioid, and others that have the histologic appearance
      of adenocarcinoma. The latter type can be distinguished from other ade-
      nocarcinomas by the absence of mucin staining and the loss of hyal-
      uronic acid staining following digestion by hyaluronidase.
      b. Clinical course. The diffuse (usual) form of mesothelioma spreads rap-
      idly over the pleura and encases the lung. It may develop multifocally
      and invade the lung parenchyma. Distant metastases are not common
      and usually occur late in the course. Liver, brain, and bone may be
      involved, especially if there is a sarcomatous pattern.
   E. Sites of metastases. The frequencies of involvement of various organ systems
   by metastases from the four most common histologic subtypes of lung cancer
   are indicated in Table 8-2.
III. Diagnosis. If non–small cell lung carcinoma (NSCLC) is diagnosed, the subsequent
evaluation is directed to two questions: **resectability** and **operability.** Is the tumor
resectable with the potential for cure? Can the patient tolerate an operation that
involves all or part of a lung? The suggested sequence for the evaluation of possible
lung cancer is as follows:

Step 1   History, physical examination, and routine laboratory studies.
Step 2   If cancer is found or strongly suspected, look for evidence of metastases.
          Studies are selected according to abnormalities found in step 1.
Step 3   If there is no evidence of metastatic disease, proceed with either of the
          following:
             Workup of solitary pulmonary nodule (see sec. **III.D**), *or*
             Workup of other clinical presentations (see sec. **VI.A**)
Step 4   Proceed with surgery for medically operable patients who have clinically
          resectable disease.

   A. Symptoms and signs
      1. Symptoms. A history suggestive of lung cancer includes smoking, new or
      changing cough, hoarseness, hemoptysis, anorexia, weight loss, dyspnea,
      unresolving pneumonias, chest wall pain, and symptoms of paraneoplastic
      syndromes.
         a. Patients with apical cancers (Pancoast's tumor) may have paresthesias
         and weakness of the arm and hand, and Horner's syndrome (ptosis, mio-

sis, and anhidrosis caused by paralysis of the cervical sympathetic nerves).

   b. Evidence of metastatic disease includes bone pain; neurologic changes; jaundice, bowel and abdominal symptoms with a rapidly enlarging liver, subcutaneous masses; and regional lymphadenopathy.

   2. Physical findings. Physical examination should be performed with the concept that evidence of metastases precludes thoracotomy with curative intent. Particular attention should be paid to the head and neck for concomitant cancers; to lymph node areas in the supraclavicular fossa, neck, and axilla for metastases; and to the abdomen for organomegaly.

B. Laboratory studies

   1. Radiographs

   a. Chest x-ray. If a mass is found, old x-ray films should be obtained for comparison. Persistent infiltrates, particularly in the anterior segments of the upper lobes, are suggestive of cancer.

   b. CT scan of the mediastinum for the staging of lung cancer has been reported to have an overall accuracy of 70 percent. Mediastinal lymph nodes are considered abnormal when larger than 1.5 cm in diameter and normal when smaller than 1.0 cm; nodes between these two limits are indeterminate. CT scan of the thorax is superior to chest x-ray and MRI. CT scanning provides information about extent and invasion of the primary tumor and presence of pleural effusion as well as information about lymph node status. If a 1.5-cm limit is used to call a node abnormal, sensitivity is relatively poor, but specificity is excellent. Conventional tomography is reported to be superior to CT in assessing hilar adenopathy.

   2. Pursuit of abnormalities found on preliminary evaluation. In the absence of abnormalities evident from history, physical examination, and routine blood studies, the studies listed below are likely to be normal.

   a. Bone scan in all patients with SCLC. In NSCLC, a bone scan is obtained if there is bone pain, elevated alkaline phosphatase, hypercalcemia or evidence of stage III disease.

   b. Bone x-ray (plain film) of painful areas.

   c. Endocrine evaluation if there is abnormal electrolyte profile consistent with a paraneoplastic syndrome (see Chap. 27).

   d. Spinal MRI for patients who have suspected epidural metastases in the spinal canal or suspected lung cancer with back pain or brachial plexopathy.

   e. Abdominal CT should probably be performed in all patients except those with clinical stage I squamous carcinoma or with otherwise obvious stage IV disease.

   f. Brain CT or MRI should be obtained as part of routine staging for patients with SCLC, which is associated with an 8–10 percent incidence of neurologically asymptomatic brain metastases. These studies are not recommended for staging patients with NSCLC in the absence of clinical signs.

C. Obtaining pathologic proof of lung cancer. The diagnosis of lung cancer must be proved histologically. The only possible exceptions to this are certain patients who have superior vena cava obstruction when such verification would endanger life (see Chap. 29, section **I.C**). Pursuit of the diagnosis should stop with the least invasive procedure that gives histologic proof of malignancy or unresectability.

   1. Sputum cytology, which was once routine practice, has been largely replaced by the flexible fiberoptic bronchoscope. Even repeated sputum cytology is positive in only 60 to 80 percent of centrally located neoplasms and 15 to 20 percent of peripheral ones.

   2. Flexible fiberoptic bronchoscopy should be performed in all but the smallest and most peripheral lesions. Two-thirds of all cancers can be seen. Additional ones are evident only as extrinsic bronchial narrowing, which may be diagnosed through the bronchoscope by transbronchial biopsy.

3. **Bone marrow aspiration and biopsy.** We recommend bone marrow examination only for patients with apparently limited disease SCLC or apparently resectable NSCLC but with one of the following:
   a. Elevated serum LDH, *or*
   b. Significant anemia or leukoerythroblastic blood smear, *or*
   c. Increased serum alkaline phosphatase values, *or*
   d. Questionable bone scan results
4. **Suspicious cutaneous nodules** are biopsied in the absence of other obvious distant metastases.
5. **Lymph nodes.** Enlarged, hard, peripheral lymph nodes in the absence of other obvious distant metastases are biopsied. Blind biopsy of nonpalpable supraclavicular nodes is positive for cancer in less than 5 percent of cases. The finding of granuloma in lymph nodes can be misleading; some patients have cancer concomitant with sarcoidosis or granulomatous infections.
6. **Mediastinoscopy** is useful for
   a. *Routine* preoperative staging (radiologic assessment alone of the mediastinum is inadequate).
   b. Medically tenuous patients in whom positive findings would eliminate an unnecessary thoracotomy.
   c. Patients with mediastinal masses, negative sputum cytology, and negative bronchoscopy.
   d. Evaluation of lymphadenopathy. On rare occasions, a patient with a peripheral lung cancer may have mediastinal node enlargement due to nonmalignant causes. With central lesions, hyperplastic nodes related to postobstructive infection are not uncommon. Mediastinoscopy may permit the patient to be considered for curative resection.
7. **Percutaneous and transbronchial needle biopsy.** If cancer is found by these techniques and medical resectability is assumed, mediastinoscopy or thoracotomy inevitably follow in the absence of evidence of metastatic disease. If cancer is suspected and the needle biopsy reveals a granuloma, the cancer may have been missed. *Whatever the result, the patient would have undergone an unnecessary invasive procedure.* The authors do not advocate these techniques for the diagnosis of lung cancer or pulmonary nodules in otherwise operable patients. They may, however, be necessary for inoperable patients with negative bronchoscopy.

D. **Evaluation of the solitary pulmonary nodule** requires a diagnostic strategy that maximizes the chance of detecting cancer and minimizes the chance of performing a needless thoracotomy if the nodule is benign. *The diagnostic approach must be individualized.* The flow diagram (Fig. 8-1) provides guidelines for the diagnosis of the solitary pulmonary nodule. Facts that should be considered include

1. **Characteristics that define a solitary pulmonary nodule** are
   a. A peripheral lung mass measuring less than 6 cm in diameter.
   b. The patient is asymptomatic with respect to the nodule.
   c. Physical examination is normal.
   d. CBC and liver function tests are normal.
2. **Calcification** of the nodules has little bearing on the diagnostic approach. Calcified nodules are more likely to be malignant unless the pattern is circular, crescentic, or completely and densely calcified.
3. **Risk that a solitary pulmonary nodule is malignant**
   a. **According to age**
      (1) Under 35 years: less than 2 percent
      (2) 35 to 45 years: 15 percent
      (3) Over 45 years: 30 to 50 percent
   b. **According to tumor volume doubling time (DT)**
      (1) DT of 30 days or less: less than 1 percent

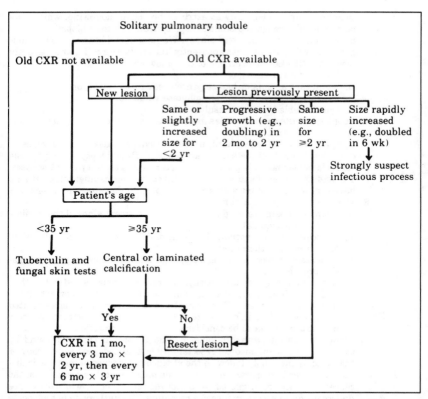

Fig. 8-1. Guidelines for approaching the solitary pulmonary nodule. CXR = chest roentgenogram; mo = months; yr = years.

      (2) DT of 30 to 400 days: 30 to 50 percent
      (3) DT greater than 400 days: less than 1 percent
    c. According to smoking history. The risk of a solitary nodule being cancerous in a smoker compared to nonsmoker is not known. The incidence is generally higher for smokers in the older age group.
   4. Needle biopsies of solitary pulmonary nodules are falsely negative in 15 percent of cases and are not recommended (see **III.C.7**).
IV. Staging system and prognostic factors (T = primary tumor; N = regional lymph nodes; M = distant metastases) The TNM system is applied primarily to NSCLC.

Stage   **Extent**
T_X Primary tumor cannot be assessed or tumor proven by the presence of malignant cells in sputum or bronchial washings but not visualized roentgenographically or bronchoscopically
T_0 No evidence of primary tumor
T_{IS} Carcinoma in situ
T_1 A tumor that is 3.0 cm or less in greatest dimension, surrounded by lung or visceral pleura, and without evidence of invasion proximal to a lobar bronchus at bronchoscopy (i.e., not in the main bronchus)
T_2 A tumor within a lobar bronchus at least 2.0 cm distal to the carina with any of the following features: more than 3.0 cm in greatest dimension, invasion into visceral pleura, or associated with atelectasis or obstruc-

tive pneumonitis that extends to the hilar region but does not involve the entire lung.

T_3 A tumor of any size that directly invades chest wall (including superior sulcus tumors), diaphragm, mediastinal pleura, parietal pericardium; or involves the main bronchus less than 2 cm distal to the carina but not the carina; or has associated atelectasis or obstructive pneumonitis of the entire lung.

T_4 A tumor of any size with invasion of the mediastinum heart, great vessels, trachea, carina, esophagus, or vertebral body; or the presence of malignant pleural effusion

N_X Regional lymph nodes cannot be assessed
N_0 No demonstrable metastasis to regional lymph nodes
N_1 Metastasis to ipsilateral or peribronchial ipsilateral hilar including direct extension
N_2 Metastasis to ipsilateral mediastinal or subcarinal lymph nodes
N_3 Metastasis to contralateral mediastinal lymph nodes, contralateral hilar lymph nodes, ipsilateral or contralateral scalene or supraclavicular lymph nodes

M_0 No (known) distant metastases
M_1 Distant metastasis present

Stage Grouping	TNM Stage	Median Survival (NSCLC)	5-year Survival (NSCLC)
Stage I	$T_1N_0M_0$	60+ months	80%
	$T_2N_0M_0$	60+ months	40–50%
Stage II	$T_1N_1M_0$	29 months	30–40%
Stage IIIA	$T_3N_0M_0$	26 months	20–30%
	$T_3N_1M_0$	16 months	15–20%
(operable)	$T_{1-3}N_2M_0$	22 months	15–30%
Stage IIIA (inoperable)	$T_{1-3}N_2M_0$ (N_2 multiple levels)	10 months	
Stage IIIB (inoperable)	Any TN_3M_0, or T_4 any N M_0	10 months	
Stage IV	Any T any N M_1	6–9 months	

A. Disease extent—inoperable. Lung cancer that was not previously irradiated and is confined to one hemithorax (limited disease) has a better prognosis than extensive disease (metastases or recurrences after RT). Median survival for untreated patients is shown in Table 8-3.

B. Performance status (PS) has direct bearing on patient survival and should be accounted in studies evaluating treatment modalities for lung cancer. Criteria for assessment of functional PS are described on the inside of the back cover. Patients who feel well and have few symptoms of disease survive longer than ill patients. Median survival time according to PS and disease extent in untreated lung cancer patients is presented in Table 8-3.

Table 8-3. Median survivals of untreated lung cancer patients

Performance status (%)*	Limited disease (weeks)	Extensive disease (weeks)
10–40	10	2
50–70	20	10
80–100	30	20

*Karnofsky performance scale (see inside back cover).
Source: Abstracted from M. Zelen, Keynote address on biostatistics and data retrieval. *Cancer Chemother. Rep.* 4:31, 1973.

Table 8-4. Tumor spread detected by mediastinoscopy

Cell type	Tumor spread detected (%)	Ipsilateral only (%)	Contralateral or bilateral (%)
All cell types	50	40	60
Well-differentiated squamous cell	15	70	30
Large cell or adenocarcinoma	65	40	60
Small cell	70	30	70

C. **Tumor histology.** Survival is not greatly influenced by cell type if PS and extent of disease are taken into account. However, patients with SCLC have debility and extensive disease more often than those with the other cell types. A few patients with very indolent but unresectable squamous lung cancer may live for several years. The probability that mediastinoscopy will detect tumor spread (and its attendant poor prognosis) in patients with potentially resectable tumors, as it is related to the histopathology, is shown in Table 8-4.

D. **Oncogenes.** *Suppressor oncogene* alterations are common in NSCLC and are associated with a poor prognosis; mutated p53 (17p) oncogene occurs in 50 percent of patients with NSCLC and 100 percent with SCLC. *Dominant oncogene* overexpression (*c-myc,* K-*ras, erb* B2) is uncommon but is associated with a poor prognosis.

V. **Prevention and early detection**

A. **Prevention** is the best way to control lung cancer. More than 90 percent of patients with lung cancer would not have developed the disease if they had not smoked. Every smoking patient should be advised of the enormous risks. Several ongoing studies are evaluating the role of retinoids and other compounds in preventing secondary tumors.

B. **Early detection** of lung cancer by screening high-risk populations with chest x-ray and sputum cytology has not been clearly demonstrated to improve survival rates. The role of chest x-rays is currently being reevaluated. New antibody tests and fluorescent bronchoscopy are also under study.

VI. **Management**

A. **NSCLC—deciding whether to resect.** Once histologic proof of lung carcinoma is obtained, resectability is determined by the histopathology and extent of the tumor and by operability according to the overall medical condition of the patient. Age and mental illness per se are not factors in deciding operability. Approximately 50 percent of patients with NSCLC are potentially operable. About 50 percent of tumors in operable patients are resectable (25% of all patients) and, approximately 50 percent of patients with resectable tumors survive 5 years (12% of all patients, or 25% of operable patients).

1. **Signs of unresectable lung cancer**
   a. Distant metastases, including metastases to the opposite lung
   b. Persistent pleural effusion, with or without malignant cells (a parapneumonic effusion that clears and may permit subsequent resection).
   c. Superior vena cava obstruction
   d. Involvement of the following structures:
      (1) Supraclavicular or neck lymph nodes (proved histologically)
      (2) Contralateral mediastinal lymph nodes (proved histologically)
      (3) Recurrent laryngeal nerve
      (4) Tracheal wall
      (5) Mainstem bronchus less than 2 cm from the carina (some surgeons consider this resectable)

2. **Cardiac status.** The presence of uncontrolled cardiac failure, uncontrolled arrhythmia, or a recent myocardial infarction (within 3–6 months) makes the patient inoperable.

3. **Pulmonary status.** The patient's ability to tolerate resection of part or all of a lung must be determined. The presence of pulmonary hypertension or of abnormalities on certain pulmonary function tests makes the patient inoperable.

   a. **Clinical observation.** Any patient who can walk up a flight of stairs without stopping and without severe dyspnea is likely to tolerate a pneumonectomy.

   b. **Routine pulmonary function tests.** Arterial blood gases and spirometry should be obtained on all patients before surgery. Pulmonary function tests must be interpreted in the light of optimal pulmonary toilet and patient cooperation. The patient with test abnormalities should be considered for therapy with bronchodilators, antibiotics, chest percussion, and postural drainage before inoperability is concluded. The following results suggest inoperability:

   (1) A $PaCO_2$ that is greater than 50 mm Hg or a PaO_2 that is less than 50 mm Hg, *or*

   (2) Forced vital capacity (FVC) less than 40 percent of predicted value, *or*

   (3) Maximum voluntary ventilation (MVV) less than 50 percent of predicted value, *or*

   (4) Forced expired volume at one second ($FEV_{1.0}$) less than or equal to 1.0 L.

   c. **Special pulmonary function tests**

   (1) **The quantitative perfusion lung scan** is done when patients with impaired pulmonary function are suspected of not being able to tolerate excision of lung tissue. The $FEV_{1.0}$ is measured before the scan. The percentage of blood flow to each lung is calculated from the results of the scan. The percentage of flow in the noncancerous lung is multiplied by the $FEV_{1.0}$, giving a measure of the anticipated postoperative $FEV_{1.0}$. Pneumonectomy is contraindicated if the calculated postoperative $FEV_{1.0}$ is less than 700 ml because the patient is likely to develop refractory cor pulmonale and respiratory insufficiency.

   (2) **Pulmonary artery pressure** is measured in cases in which clinical evaluation suggests inoperability but the patient still wants an operation. The patient is inoperable if the pulmonary artery pressure is greater than 35 mm Hg at rest or becomes greater than 35 mm Hg with exercise or after occlusion of the pulmonary artery in the lung to be resected.

B. **NSCLC: Management of operable disease**

   1. **Surgery.** Surgical resection of the primary tumor is the treatment of choice for patients who can tolerate surgery and who have stage I, stage II, or certain types of localized stage III NSCLC. The selection of the operative procedure varies with the surgeon's criteria for patient selection, the extent of disease, and the patient's ventilatory function. Definition of nodal involvement during surgical resection is mandatory to determine prognosis and to evaluate the results of treatment; the anatomic boundaries of 13 nodal stations have been described.

   A multicenter study of contemporary operative mortality due to lung surgery documented the following death rates within 30 days of operation: pneumonectomy 7.7 percent, lobectomy 3.3 percent, and segmentectomy or wedge resection 1.4 percent. Advanced age, weight loss, coexisting disease, reduced FEV, and more extensive resection are significant risk factors.

   a. **Incomplete resections** are rarely, if ever, indicated.

   b. **Segmentectomy or lobectomy** is used for peripheral tumor without

Table 8-5. Management of NSCLC: Stages IIIA and IIIB

Survival	RT alone	RT and chemotherapy
Median	9–10 months	14 months
1 year	40–45%	55%
2 year	10–15%	25–40%
3 year	2–10%	15–20%

gross lymph node involvement or transgression of a fissure. Lobectomy is the procedure of choice in patients whose lung function permits it. Conservative resection appears to be associated with a significant increase in local recurrence rate.

c. **Bilobectomy, sleeve lobectomy, or pneumonectomy** with or without lymph node dissection is used for other tumors.

2. **Pancoast tumor.** RT should be employed as the preliminary treatment for Pancoast tumors ($T_3N_0M_0$, stage IIIA) prior to surgical resection of the primary tumor and involved chest wall.

3. **Adjuvant therapy.** Since the majority of patients undergoing complete resections for lung cancer relapse and die within 2 years of resection, adjuvant therapies are indicated for patients with hilar or mediastinal lymph node metastases.

   a. **Stage I.** Postoperative adjuvant RT or chemotherapy offer no survival benefit, do not increase the time to relapse, and are not recommended.

   b. **Stage II or IIIA squamous cell carcinoma** that was completely resected. Adjuvant RT reduces local recurrence but does not improve survival. Thoracic irradiation is not recommended until local problems develop.

   c. **Stage II or IIIA adenocarcinoma and large cell carcinoma.** Adjuvant chemotherapy with a regimen such as CAP (see Appendix A1) for disease that was completely resected is associated with fewer recurrences, a delay in the time to recurrence, and improved survival. The median survival may be prolonged by about 7–24 months, and the 5-year survival is increased (about 30%).

   d. **Surgical margins and highest nodal station.** Adjuvant combination chemotherapy and RT for patients with positive resection margins or with tumor in the highest resected mediastinal lymph nodes reduces local relapse rates but has only a small impact on survival rate. Adjuvant therapy is generally not recommended in these patients.

C. **NSCLC: Management of inoperable disease**

1. **Resectable but inoperable.** RT should be the primary treatment for medically inoperable but resectable patients. The overall survival rate at five years is about 20 percent (one-half the rate of that for a comparable group of patients treated surgically), depending on the size of the primary tumor. The sterilization rate ranges from 25 to 50 percent for small tumors.

2. **Stages IIIa, IIIb.** The standard treatment in the past for these patients has been RT, with modest evidence of survival benefit and palliation in the majority. RT resulted in a median survival of nine months, two-year survival of 10 to 15 percent, and five-year survival of 5 percent (worse in IIIb). Recent data indicate a survival advantage at one, two, and three years for the use of combined modalities in this setting (chemotherapy plus RT with or without surgery); the two-year survival has been reported to be 25 to 40 percent. Both sequential and concurrent chemotherapy and irradiation may be employed. Cisplatin/vinblastine and cisplatin/etoposide (PE) (see Appen-

dix A1) are the usual drug combinations. Table 8-5 compares the results of treatment.

Patients who receive "neoadjuvant" chemotherapy with or without irradiation initially often become resectable. Whether performance of resection adds to the result obtained is as yet unknown. However, a recent prospective, randomized study documented increase in median survival in those patients who received preoperative chemotherapy: 26 months versus 8 months with surgery alone.

3. **Stage IV.** Fully ambulatory patients have modestly increased survival, and symptoms are often palliated by the use of cisplatin or carboplatin-containing chemotherapy. At present, no definitive evidence indicates that combinations are superior to either of the platinum drugs used alone. Patients who are less than fully ambulatory receive little benefit from presently available chemotherapy, and supportive care alone is usually appropriate in this group.

D. **SCLC: Management**
   1. **Limited stage (I, II, III).** Less than 5 percent of patients with SCLC have stage I–II disease. About 40 percent, however, have disease that is clinically confined to the hemithorax and draining regional nodes at presentation (stages IIIa and IIIb).
      a. **Combined therapy.** The available data indicate that these patients should receive both chemotherapy and RT to the chest. If given concurrently as induction, combined modalities yield a median survival of 18 months and five-year survival of 20 to 25 percent.
      b. **Prophylactic brain irradiation** is reported to decrease the rate of brain metastases. The use of this treatment is controversial because of the ocurrence of post-RT leukoencephalopathy and the doubtful increase in survival when compared to patients who are treated only if and when brain metastases develop.
   2. **Extensive stage.** The fully ambulatory patient with extensive disease will have a good response to combination chemotherapy (PE or cyclophosphamide/adriamycin/vincristine [CAV], or alternation of PE and CAV). Only 15 to 20 percent of such patients, however, achieve CR. The median survival of fully ambulatory patients is about one year, but survival beyond two years is unusual. See Appendix A1 for drug dosages and other regimens.

   Patients who are less than fully ambulatory may be appropriate candidates for CAV/PE. These patients should be considered as well for trials with new chemotherapeutic agents, as their period of benefit from "standard" regimens is generally only a few months.

VII. **Special clinical problems**
   A. **Positive sputum cytology with a negative chest x-ray** (stage $T_XN_0M_0$) and no other evidence of disease is an occasional problem, usually occuring in screening programs. Patients should be examined by CT scan of the chest and fiberoptic bronchoscopy with selective washings. Bronchial washings may not be helpful in localizing the malignancy, because multiple sites may have tumors or suspected dysplastic change.
      1. When these measures fail to identify a lesion, patients must be informed that the likelihood that they have a cancer too small to be detected is high. Such patients should be followed with monthly chest x-rays and should be strongly advised to stop smoking. Repeated sputum cytology is not helpful if the original cytology findings were class 5 and laboratory errors were not suspected.
      2. The cytologic discovery of an unequivocal small cell cancer in the absence of other findings should be confirmed by repeat sampling and solicitation of a second pathologist's opinion at another institution. Once the diagnosis is confirmed, patients should be treated with chemotherapy.
   B. **Air-fluid level** revealed by chest x-ray is a normal finding in patients who have undergone pneumonectomy but represents an abscess or bronchopleural fistula in patients who have undergone lobectomy. Patients with bronchopleural fistula

may have a cough that produces copious amounts of serosanguineous fluid. These patients may be in immediate danger of drowning in their secretions; closed tube thoracotomy, which may be followed by open drainage, is required.

Selected Reading

Davis, S., et al. A prospective analysis of chemotherapy following surgical resection of clinical stage I–II small cell lung cancer. *Am. J. Clin. Oncol.* 16:93, 1993.

Dillman, R. O., et al. A randomized trial of induction chemotherapy plus high dose radiation versus radiation alone in stage III non-small cell lung cancer. *N. Engl. J. Med.* 323:940, 1990.

Eddy, D. M. Screening for lung cancer. *Ann. Intern Med.* 111:232, 1989.

Einhorn, L. H. Neoadjuvant therapy of stage III non–small cell lung cancer. *Ann. Thorac. Surg.* 46:362, 1988.

Elias, A. Chemotherapy and radiotherapy for regionally advanced non–small cell lung cancer. *Chest* 103(Suppl):362s, 1993.

Feld, R. Adjuvant chemotherapy with cyclophosphamide, doxorubicin and cisplatin in patients with completely resected stage I non–small cell lung cancer. *J. Natl. Cancer Inst.* 85:299, 1993.

Flehinger, B. J., et al. The effect of surgical treatment on survival from early lung cancer. *Chest* 101:1013, 1992.

Green, M. New adjuvant strategies for the management of resectable non–small cell lung cancer. *Chest* 103(Suppl):352s, 1993.

Johnson, D. H., et al. Thoracic radiotherapy does not prolong survival in patients with locally advanced, unresectable non–small cell lung cancer. *Ann. Intern Med.* 113:33, 1990.

Mountain, C. F. Lung cancer staging classification. *Clin. Chest Med.* 14:43, 1993.

Mountain, C. F. Surgery for stage IIIa-N2 non–small cell lung cancer. *Cancer* 73: 2589, 1994.

Rosell, R., et al. A randomized trial comparing preoperative chemotherapy plus surgery with surgery alone in patients with non–small cell lung cancer. *N. Engl. J. Med.* 330:153, 1994.

Schaake-Koning, C., et al. Effects of concomitant cisplatin and radiotherapy on inoperable non-small cell lung cancer. *N. Engl. J. Med.* 326:524, 1992.

Skarin, A. T. Analysis of long-term survivors with small cell lung cancer. *Chest* 103(Suppl):440s, 1993.

Smith, I. E., et al. Carboplatin, etoposide, and ifosfamide as intensive chemotherapy for small cell lung cancer. *J. Clin. Oncol.* 8:899, 1990.

9

Gastrointestinal Tract Cancers

Hassan J. Tabbarah

Cancers of the gastrointestinal tract account for 20 percent of all new visceral cancers and 22 percent of cancer deaths in the United States. The frequency and mortality of cancers of the various gastrointestinal organs are shown in Table 9-1. In several other countries, gastrointestinal cancers are an even more significant health problem.

Esophageal Cancer

I. Epidemiology and etiology
   A. **Epidemiology.** The incidence of esophageal cancer is noted in Table 9-1.
      1. Esophageal cancer is the foremost malignancy in the Bantu of Africa. South Africa, Japan, China, Russia, Scotland, and the Caspian region of Iran also have relatively high incidences.
      2. Occupations at risk include waiters, bartenders, metal workers, and construction workers.
   B. **Etiology**
      1. **Carcinogens**
         a. **Long-term use of tabacco and alcohol** increases the incidence of esophageal cancer.
         b. **Native beer of the African Bantu** contains zinc and nitrosamines, which may be carcinogenic.
         c. **Dietary carcinogens**
            (1) Plants growing in soil deficient in molybdenum reduces their content of vitamin C and cause hyperplasia of esophageal mucosa, a precursor of cancer.
            (2) Elevated nitrates in the drinking water and soup kettles that concentrate the nitrate.
            (3) Food containing fungi: *Geotrichum candidum* (pickles, air-dried corn), *Fusarium* sp., and *Aspergillus* sp. (corn).
            (4) Bread that is baked once a week and eaten when moldy *(G. candidum)*.
            (5) Dried persimmons, a rough food that injures the esophageal mucosa when eaten (China).
      2. **Predisposing factors**
         a. Tylosis palmaris et plantaris (hyperkeratosis of the palms and soles) is a rare genetic disease that is transmitted as a mendelian dominant (nearly 40% develop esophageal cancer).
         b. Lye stricture (up to 30%).
         c. Esophageal achalasia (30%).
         d. Esophageal web (20%).
         e. Plummer-Vinson syndrome (sideropenic dysphagia, 10%).
         f. Short esophagus (5%).
         g. Peptic esophagitis (1%).
         h. Other conditions associated with esophageal cancer
            (1) Patients with head and neck cancer

Table 9-1. Occurrence of gastrointestinal cancers in the United States (1994)

Primary site	Proportion of gastrointestinal tract cancers		
	Frequency of new cases (%)	Frequency of cancer death (%)	Male-female ratio
Esophagus	5	8	8:3
Stomach	11	12	3:2
Small bowel	1	1	1:1
Colon	46	40	1:1
Rectum	18	6	1:2
Liver and biliary tract*	7	11	1:1*
Pancreas	12	22	1:1
TOTAL	100	100	1:1

*Approximately 20% are primary liver cancers, 35% bile duct cancers, and 45% gallbladder cancers. The male-female ratio is 5:2 for liver and bile duct cancers and 1:5 for gallbladder cancer.
Note: Gastrointestinal tract malignancies account for approximately 233,000 new cancers and 121,000 cancer deaths annually.

       (2) Patients with celiac disease
       (3) Chronic esophagitis without Barrett's esophagus (see sec. **II.A**)
       (4) Thermal injury to the esophagus because of drinking boiling hot tea or coffee (Russia, China, and Middle East)

II. Pathology and natural history
    A. Histology. Squamous cell tumors constitute 98 percent of esophageal cancers in the upper and middle esophagus; the remainder are adenocarcinomas and rare sarcomas, small cell carcinomas, or lymphomas. In the lower esophagus, adenocarcinoma is slightly more common and may arise from esophageal continuation of the gastric mucosa (Barrett's esophagus) or may represent extension of a gastric adenocarcinoma.
    B. Location of cancer in the esophagus
      1. Cervical: 10 percent
      2. Upper thoracic: 40 percent
      3. Lower thoracic: 50 percent
    C. Clinical course. Esophageal cancer is highly lethal; more than 90 percent of patients die of the disease. Approximately 75 percent present initially with mediastinal nodal involvement or distant metastasis. Death is usually caused by local disease that results in inanition or aspiration pneumonia.

III. Diagnosis
    A. Symptoms and signs. Dysphagia is the most common complaint. Patients become unable to swallow solid foods and eventually liquids. Symptoms rarely develop until the esophageal lumen is greatly narrowed and metastasis has occurred. Pain may or may not be present. Physical findings other than cachexia or hepatomegaly are rare.
    B. Diagnostic studies
      1. Preliminary studies include physical examination, CBC, LFTs, chest x-ray, and barium esophagogram. If an esophagogram abnormality or history suggests carcinoma, esophagoscopy is performed. Brushings are obtained and lesions biopsied.
      2. CT scan staging predicts invasion or metastases with an accuracy rate of more than 90 percent for the aorta, tracheobronchial tree, pericardium, liver, and adrenal glands; 85 percent for abdominal nodes; and 50 percent for paraesophageal nodes.
      3. Endoscopic ultrasound (EUS) is more accurate than CT in assessing tumor depth and paraesophageal nodes.

IV. Staging system and prognostic factors. A TNM staging classification is available. Long-range survival is achieved only in patients with tumors that involve less than 5 cm of the esophagus and have neither obstruction nor extraesophageal spread $(T_1N_0M_0)$. Patients with esophageal cancer rarely meet these criteria. Most patients die of their disease within 10 months of diagnosis. The five-year survival rate is less than 10 percent despite all efforts at treatment.

V. Screening and early detection. In China, mass screening utilizes "the Chinese balloon" (a long, small caliber stomach tube with a balloon covered with nylon netting on the distal end). This balloon is passed into the stomach, inflated, and then withdrawn the entire length of the esophagus; cells for cytologic study are trapped in the nylon net. In the United States, screening for esophageal cancer is not effective but patients with higher risk may undergo periodic upper endoscopy.

VI. Management. The aggressiveness of surgical treatment and RT is highly varied among institutions.

A. Resection of primary tumor. Results of surgical resection in cancer of the esophagus are poor. The operative mortality is about 15 percent. In the United States the five-year survival in patients undergoing tumor resection is less than 10 percent. Aggressive surgery, however, may be justified for some patients with lesions in the lower half of the esophagus.

In China, the five-year survival is 85 percent for early cancer and 35 percent for moderately advanced disease. This high five-year survival must be interpreted with caution, because esophageal cancer is an indolent disease at the outset and may require 10 years before it takes an aggressive course.

B. Palliating an obstructed esophagus can be accomplished by several procedures and permit enteral nutrition.

   1. Laser therapy may relieve obstruction and bleeding. Endoscopic laser therapy has less than 1 percent mortality rate but may require prior mechanical dilatation. Although successful laser therapy may require multiple endoscopic sessions, it can be done on an outpatient basis, and its overall cost is still much less than the cost of palliative surgery.

   2. Endoprosthesis. At least 17 devices are available for esophageal intubation. Approximately 15 percent of patients with malignant esophageal obstruction are candidates for tube placement. The tube may be introduced with a pusher tube, which is either loaded onto a bougie or over an endoscope. The latter method permits visualization of the obstructed lumen. The success rate is 90 to 97 percent.

   a. Advantages of tube placement are ability to swallow saliva, pleasure of oral alimentation, relief from pulmonary aspiration of esophagopulmonary fistula, independence from physician or hospital for constant care, and ability to spend time with family and friends in comfort.

   b. Contraindications to placement of endoprosthesis are carcinoma less than 2 cm below the upper sphincter, limited life expectancy (<6 weeks), and uncooperativeness.

   c. Complications include perforation, dislocation, tumor overgrowth, reflux stricturing, pressure necrosis, foreign body obstruction, bleeding, and failure of intubation. The complication rate (early and late) is 10 to 25 percent.

   3. Feeding gastrostomy is not advisable because it does not palliate dysphagia, does not abolish troublesome saliva and secretions, does not increase life expectancy, and has its own morbidity and mortality.

   4. Colonic interposition to bypass the obstructed segment is associated with high mortality from the procedure itself and is not recommended.

C. Combined modality therapy

   1. Preoperative (neoadjuvant) chemoradiation therapy. 5-FU and cisplatinum combined with radiation therapy (RT, 3000–3600 cGy) in patients with squamous cell carcinoma or adenocarcinoma of the thoracic esophagus have been reported to result in higher response rates and longer median survival at the cost of increased toxicity. The overall median survival of the patients who underwent esophageal resection was 23 months, and 20 percent of patients who received chemoradiation achieved CRs (no evidence of cancer in the resected specimens). The apparent increases in survival, however, have not been confirmed in a randomized study. Furthermore, the survival rates were the same for complete responders and partial responders who underwent surgery, and the survival rates at two years and beyond were also the same for patients who refused (or were denied) surgery and those who underwent esophagectomy. Therefore, preoperative neoadjuvant chemoradiation cannot be recommended at the present time.

2. **Primary therapy without surgery.** In a prospective, randomized trial of patients with squamous cell or adenocarcinoma of the thoracic esophagus, combined modality treatment (5-FU/cisplatin plus 5000 cGy) resulted in improved median survival (9 months versus 12.5 months) when compared to RT alone (6400 cGy). The patients receiving the combined modality experienced decreased local and distant recurrences, but significantly more toxicity, much of which was serious or life-threatening. Only half of the patients received all the planned cycles of chemotherapy. Thus combined modality therapy may be considered only in younger patients with good performance status.

D. Advanced disease
   1. **RT** has provided long-range survival for some patients with lesions of the cervical esophagus. It may sustain esophageal patency for a period of time and is useful for treating symptomatic metastases.
   2. **Chemotherapy** is not useful for either controlling or palliating esophageal cancer. The responses using single agents (15–20%) are usually partial and of brief duration (2–5 months). Combination chemotherapy, usually including cisplatin, is associated with reported response rates ranging from 15 to 80 percent, a median duration of response of seven months, and substantial toxicity. Higher response rates, however, do not translate into significant benefit for these patients, and the outcome remains poor. The author recommends using single agents if chemotherapy is contemplated.

Gastric Cancer

I. Epidemiology and etiology
A. Incidence. The prevalence and death rates of gastric carcinoma have been markedly and significantly decreasing in all regions of the world and in all age groups by about 2 to 7 percent per year. Dietary factors and improvement in food storage are believed to be the major factors causing this decline. Improvements include reduction in toxic methods of food preservation (such as smoking and pickling), a decline in salt consumption, greater use of refrigeration, and increased consumption of fruits and vegetables. Mortality from gastric cancer is highest in East Asia (Hong Kong, Japan, and Singapore) and lowest in the United States. Of interest, the Nordic and Western European countries have incidence rates two to three times higher than the United States. The incidence remains high in Japan but decreases in the offspring of Japanese immigrants to the United States. The average age of onset is 55 years.

B. Etiology
   1. **Diet.** Gastric cancer has been linked with the ingestion of red meats, cabbage, spices, fish, salt-preserved or smoked foods, and alcohol; low fat and protein consumption; and low intake of vitamins A and E. Selenium dietary intake may be inversely proportioned to the risks of gastric cancer but not of colorectal cancer.
   2. ***Helicobacter pylori* infection** is associated with an increased risk of gastric adenocarcinoma and may be a cofactor in the pathogenesis of non-cardiac gastric cancer. *H. pylori* was detected in 65 percent of patients with gastric cancer but in only 38 percent of the patients with cancer located at the gastric cardia.

3. **Heredity and race.** African, Asian, and Hispanic Americans have a higher risk of gastric cancer than whites. The highest rates of gastric cancer death in the Western world are found in Chile, Costa Rica, Argentina, and Colombia. In contrast, rates from Ecuador, Guatemala, Honduras, and Mexico are comparable or lower than those in the United States. Gastric cancer is still prevalent in whites of low socioeconomic class.

4. **Pernicious anemia, achlorhydria, and atrophic gastritis.** Pernicious anemia carries a low risk of adenocarcinoma; the carcinoma is usually discovered years later. Cancer-oriented screening and follow-up in pernicious anemia are mandatory for medicolegal reasons.

5. **Previous gastric resection.** Gastric stump adenocarcinomas have hypochlorhydria (with male predominance), dysplasia of gastric mucosa, elevated gastrin levels, and a poor prognosis. Two meta-analyses support this increased risk, with a latency period of 15 to 20 years.

6. **Mucosal dysplasia** is graded from I–III with grade III showing marked loss in cell differentiation and increased mitosis. The finding of high-grade dysplasia by experienced pathologists in two separate sets of endoscopic biopsies is considered to be a marker of gastric cancer. The significance of metaplasia remains controversial.

7. **Other risk factors.** Gastric cancer is more common in males, older individuals (>50 years of age), and persons with blood group A.

II. Pathology and natural history

A. Histology and classification.
Approximately 95 percent of gastric cancers are adenocarcinomas. Five percent are leiomyosarcomas, lymphomas, carcinoids, squamous cancers, or other rare types.

1. **Useful characteristics for gastric cancer**

   a. **Histologic classification (Lauren):** diffuse, intestinal, and mixed types. This classification has proved to be the most useful for adenocarcinomas because the two major types (diffuse and intestinal) represent groups of patients with differing ages, sex ratios, survivals, epidemiology, and apparent origin. Studies have shown that "diffuse" histology affects younger patients with slight predominance among women. Diffuse histology occurred in 50 percent of all cases and 55 percent of unresectable cases.

   b. **Clinical classification (gross anatomy).** Superficial (superficial spreading), focal (polypoid, fungate, or ulcerative), and infiltrative (linitis plastica) types.

   c. **Japanese Endoscopic Society (JES) classification.** Type I (polypoid or mass-like), type II (flat, minimally elevated or depressed), and type III (cancer associated with true ulcer).

2. **Location of cancers.** Distally located cancers are considered to be epidemic in nature and related to dietary variation, whereas proximal cancers and diffuse histology are endemic. It is believed that the decline in incidence of distal tumors in the United States has unmasked the endemic variety.

   a. **Distal location:** 40 percent

   b. **Proximal:** 35 percent

   c. **Body:** 25 percent

B. Clinical course.
Gastric carcinoma spreads by the lymphatic system and blood vessels, by direct extension, and by seeding of peritoneal surfaces. The ulcerative and polypoid types spread through the gastric wall and involve the serosa and draining lymph nodes. The scirrhous type spreads through the submucosa and muscularis, encasing the stomach, and in some instances spreading to the entire bowel. Widespread metastatic disease may affect any organ, especially the liver, lung (may be lymphangitic), peritoneum, supraclavicular lymph nodes (Virchow's node), left axillary lymph nodes (Irish's node), and the umbilicus (Sister Joseph nodule). Sclerotic bone metastases, carcinomatous meningitis, and metastasis to the ovary in women (Krukenberg's tumor) or rectal shelf in men (Blumer's shelf) may also occur.

C. Associated paraneoplastic syndromes
1. Acanthosis nigricans (55% of cases that occur in malignancy are associated with gastric carcinoma)
2. Polymyositis, dermatomyositis
3. Circinate erythemas, pemphigoid
4. Dementia, cerebellar ataxia
5. Idiopathic venous thrombosis
6. Ectopic Cushing's syndrome or carcinoid syndrome (rare)

III. Diagnosis
A. Symptoms and signs.
Gastric cancer often progresses to an advanced stage before symptoms and signs develop. Symptoms of advanced disease include anorexia, early satiety, distaste for meat, weakness, and dysphagia. Abdominal pain is present in approximately 60 percent of patients, weight loss in 50 percent, anemia in 40 percent, and a palpable abdominal mass in 30 percent. The abdominal pain is similar to ulcer pain, is gnawing in nature, and may respond initially to antacid treatment but remains unremittent. Hematemesis occurs uncommonly; when present, other diagnoses should be suspected (bleeding is seen more often with gastric sarcomas).

B. Diagnostic studies
1. **Preliminary studies** include CBC, LFTs, upper GI barium studies, and chest x-ray.
2. **CT of abdomen** is very useful for assessing the extent of disease. At celiotomy, however, 50 percent of patients are found to have more extensive disease than predicted by CT.
3. **EUS** is up to six times more accurate in staging the primary gastric tumors than CT, but differentiation between benign and malignant changes in the wall is often difficult. EUS is useful in imaging the cardia, which may be difficult to evaluate by CT.
4. **Endoscopy.** The combination of flexible upper GI endoscopy with biopsy of visible lesions, exfoliative cytology, and brush biopsy is able to detect more than 95 percent of gastric cancers. Biopsy of a stomach lesion alone is accurate in only 80 percent of cases. Positive gastric cytology with no endoscopic or x-ray abnormalities indicates superficial spreading gastric cancer.

C. Differential diagnosis and gastric polyps.
The differential diagnosis of gastric cancer includes peptic gastric polyps, ulcer, leiomyoma, leiomyoblastoma, glomus tumor, malignant lymphoma (and pseudolymphoma), granulocytic sarcoma, carcinoid tumors, lipoma, fibrous histiocytoma, and metastatic carcinoma. Gastric polyps rarely undergo malignant transformation (3% after seven years), but many contain independent carcinoma.
1. **Inflammatory gastric polyps** are not true neoplasms. They are usually located in the pyloroantrum and are associated with hypochlorhydria but not with carcinoma.
2. **Hyperplastic gastric polyps** (Ménétrier's polyadenome polypeux) are the most common polyps (75%). Randomly distributed throughout the stomach, these polyps are usually small and multiple. Coexisting carcinoma is present in 8 percent of cases.
3. **Adenomatous polyps** are usually located in the antrum of the stomach and are frequently single and large. Coexisting carcinoma is present in 40 to 60 percent of patients.
4. **Villous adenomas** rarely occur in the stomach but are more often malignant.
5. **Polyposis syndromes**
   a. **Familial gastric polyposis** presents with multiple gastric polyps but no skin or bone tumors. The gastric wall is usually invaded with atypical carcinoma.
   b. **Familial colonic polyposis** is associated with gastric involvement in over 50 percent of patients. The gastric polyps are adenomatous, hyperplastic, or of the fundic gland hyperplasia type. Gastric carcinoma and carcinoid tumor may occur.

IV. Staging and prognostic factors

A. Staging system.
A TNM system has been developed for gastric cancer that accounts for degree of penetration into the stomach wall, the presence of lymph involvement (whether adjacent or distant) and distant metastases. Unfortunately, the current TNM system does not recognize the location of the tumor within the stomach, the number of lymph nodes rather than their location relative to the stomach, the histologic type (Lauren's classification), the pattern of growth (linitis plastica), or whether all disease could be resected (and if so, the type of resection).

B. Prognostic factors.
Previously, data using *three grave prognostic signs* (serosal involvement, nodal involvement, and tumor at the line of resection) have shown that if no signs of these are present, the five-year survival is 60 percent, and if all are present, the five year survival is less than 5 percent.

1. **Stage.** Multivariate analysis indicated that stage (see **A**), invasion, and lymph node involvement are the most significant prognostic factors. The most important prognostic determinant appears to be the number of positive lymph nodes. Interestingly, patients with one to three lymph nodes involved with metastasis have as good a prognosis as those without nodal involvement.

2. **Clinical classification.** Survival is better with superficial than with focal and worst with infiltrative types of cancer.

3. **JES classification.** Survival is better with type II (flat) than with type III (associated with ulcer) and worst with type I (polypoid).

4. **Grade.** Tumors with high histologic grade have a poor prognosis.

5. **Flow cytometry.** The median disease-free survival is 18 months for patients with diploid tumors and 5 months with aneuploid tumors. Aneuploid tumors constitute 96 percent of gastroesophageal junction-cardia carcinomas and only 48 percent of body-antrum tumors. Women are more likely to have diploid tumors.

6. **Nature and extent of resection.** Survival is better with curative resection versus palliative resection, distal gastrectomy versus proximal gastrectomy, and subtotal gastrectomy versus total gastrectomy.

V. Screening and early detection.
Early detection of gastric cancers is clearly improved with relentless investigation of persistent upper GI symptoms. In Japan, the use of a gastrocamera resulted in an early detection of gastric cancer. Gastric cancer, which was detected in 0.3 percent of those screened, was associated with 95 percent five-year survival (50% of the patients had involvement of mucosa and submucosa only). Screening for gastric cancer is not recommended, however, in the United States.

VI. Management

A. Surgery

1. **Curative resection.** Subtotal gastrectomy with adequate margins of grossly uninvolved stomach (3–4 cm) and regional lymph node dissection is the treatment of choice for gastric cancer. Total gastrectomy is not superior to subtotal gastrectomy for achieving cures and should be used only when indicated by the local extent of the disease. More extensive lymphatic dissection (e.g., of the celiac lymph nodes), omentectomy, and splenectomy are no longer advisable. Patients with gastric cancer who have no obvious signs of metastatic disease are *usually non-resectable if one or more of the following clinical findings are present.*
   a. Palpable abdominal mass
   b. Severe anemia (hemoglobin <10 gm/dl)
   c. Significant weight loss (>10% of body weight)

2. **Palliative resections** are performed to rid patients of infected, bleeding, obstructed, necrotic, or ulcerated polypoid gastric lesions. For these purposes, a limited gastric resection may suffice. Palliative resections, as compared to more extensive resections, may result in improved median survival, mostly because of reduced morbidity and mortality associated with limited surgery.

3. **Vitamin B$_{12}$ deficiency** develops in all patients who undergo total gastrectomy within six years and in 20 percent of patients who undergo subtotal gastrectomy within 10 years.

B. Chemotherapy

1. **Adjuvant chemotherapy.** The responsiveness of gastric cancer to chemotherapy given before resection is unexpectedly striking, but the impact of these responses on survival remains uncertain.

   a. **Systemic adjuvant chemotherapy.** Nearly all trials involving 5-FU in combination with other agents (doxorubicin, mitomycin, or cytarabine) as adjuvant therapy have failed to show any benefit. A recent meta-analysis of data from 14 trials published since 1980 on adjuvant chemotherapy after resection of gastric cancer versus surgery alone concluded that postoperative chemotherapy cannot be considered standard treatment.

   b. **Intraperitoneal adjuvant therapy.** As the resection site is the most common place for recurrence of gastric cancer, intraperitoneal chemotherapy is being advocated in certain centers.

      (1) **Perioperatively:** Intraperitoneal mitomycin (50 mg) given in Japan was associated with significantly higher survival than untreated patients. Side effects are mild and well tolerated.

      (2) **Postoperatively:** Intraperitoneal cisplatin and 5-FU followed by systemic 5-FU or 5-FU and mitomycin is being evaluated. Side effects are mainly neutropenia and sclerosing encapsulating peritonitis (late toxicity).

2. **Chemotherapy for advanced disease.** Single agents produce low response rates. Combination regimens produce higher response rates but are more toxic and more costly. Cisplatin has been increasingly used in new combinations that also yield higher response rates, but the incidence of important toxic events exceeds 10 percent. The reported response rates are approximately 20 percent for 5-FU alone and 10 to 50 percent for combination chemotherapy; the median survivals range from 5 to 11 months. After nearly two decades of using combination chemotherapy, including mitomycin, Adriamycin, epirubicin, methotrexate, nitrosoureas, or cisplatin, there is little evidence that any of these drugs add to the results obtained from 5-FU alone.

C. RT

1. **Localized disease.** RT alone has not proved useful for gastric cancer. RT (4000 cGy in four weeks) in combination with 5-FU (15 mg/kg IV on the first three days of RT), however, appears to improve survival over RT alone in patients with localized but unresectable cancers.

2. **Advanced disease.** Gastric adenocarcinoma is relatively radioresistant and requires high doses of radiation with attendant toxic effects to surrounding organs. RT may be useful for palliating pain, vomiting due to obstruction, gastric hemorrhage, and metastases to bone and brain.

Colorectal Cancer

I. Epidemiology and etiology

A. Incidence. Colorectal cancer is the second most common cause of cancer mortality after lung cancer. However, both the incidence and the mortality rates have begun to decline after they peaked in 1985. The incidence of colorectal cancer reflects the population's current geographic location and not the country of origin. In the United States, cancer of the colorectum is more common in the East than the West and in the North than the South.

The risk of developing colorectal cancer increases with age, but 3 percent of colorectal cancers occur under the age of 40. The incidence is 19 per 100,000 for those under 65 years of age and 337 per 100,000 among those over 65 years of age. Annually, an estimated 149,000 new cases of colorectal cancer develop and an estimated 56,000 persons die of the disease. In the United States an individual has 5 percent lifetime risk of developing colorectal cancer.

B. Etiology. Multiple forces drive the transformation of colorectal mucosa to cancer. Inheritance and diet both are critical, but the extent of their independence as variables remains unknown.

  1. Polyps. The main importance of polyps is their well-recognized relationship to colorectal cancer. The evolution to cancer is a multistage process that proceeds through mucosal cell hyperplasia, adenoma formation, and growth and dysplasia, to malignant transformation and invasive cancer. The development of colorectal adenomas and carcinomas probably involves both environmental and genetic factors. Environmental carcinogens appear to act on a genetically susceptible mucosa, causing cellular proliferation. Oncogene activation and chromosomal deletion then lead to adenoma formation, growth with increasing dysplasia, and invasive carcinoma.

   a. Types of polyps. Histologically polyps are classified as neoplastic or non-neoplastic. Non-neoplastic polyps have no malignant potential and include hyperplastic polyps, mucous retention polyps, hamartomas, lymphoid aggregates, and inflammatory polyps. Neoplastic polyps (or adenomas) have malignant potential and are classified according to the World Health Organization system as tubular, tubulovillous, or villous adenomas depending on the presence and volume of villous tissue.

   b. Frequency of polyp types. Approximately 70 percent of polyps removed at colonoscopy are adenomas, 75 to 85 percent of which are tubular (no or minimal villous tissue), 10 to 25 percent are tubulovillous (<75% villous tissue), and fewer than 5 percent are villous (>75% villous tissue).

   c. Dysplasia may be classified as mild, moderate, or severe. However, it is preferable to classify dysplasia into only two grades: low and high. Terms like "carcinoma in situ," "intramucosal carcinoma," or "focal carcinoma" should be avoided to prevent misinterpretation that may lead to overtreatment. Approximately 6 percent of adenomas have severe dysplasia and 4 percent have invasive carcinoma at the time of diagnosis.

   d. The malignant potential of adenomas correlates with increasing size, the presence and the degree of dysplasia in a villous component, and the patient's age. Small colorectal polyps (<1 cm) are not associated with increased occurrence of colorectal cancer; the incidence of cancer, however, is increased 2.5- to 4-fold if the polyp is large (>1 cm) and 5- to 7-fold in patients who initially had multiple polyps. The study of the natural history of untreated polyps larger than 1 cm showed that the risk of progression to cancer is 2.5 percent at 5 years, 8 percent at 10 years, and 24 percent at 20 years. The time to malignant progression depends on the severity of dysplasia: 3.5 years for severe dysplasia and 11.5 years for mild atypia.

   e. Management of polyps. Because of the adenoma-cancer relationship and the evidence that resecting adenomas prevents cancer, newly detected polyps should be excised and additional polyps should be sought. The incidence of synchronous adenomas in patients with one known adenoma is 40 to 50 percent. Most polyps discovered during colonoscopy can be completely removed by snare polypectomy and the entire specimen submitted for histopathologic examination. Polyps less than 1 cm in diameter may be missed on the initial colonoscopy. The 1993 recommendations of the American College of Gastroenterology for the management of colorectal polyps are discussed in Bond, et al (see Selected Reading).

   f. Intestinal polyposis syndromes. Table 9-2 summarizes familial polyposis syndromes and their histology distribution, malignant potential, and management (see sec. **V** for discussion of the potential benefit of anti-inflammatory drugs).

  2. Diet. Excess intake of fat or calories or low intake of fiber (fruits, vegetables,

Table 9-2. Polyp syndromes and colorectal cancer

Disease	Histology	Distribution of polyps	Malignant potential	Associated manifestations	Age for education	Age for FOB test	Age for colonoscopy[a]	Surgery
Discrete polyps and colon cancer	Few AP	Colon	High	None	—	≥45 years	≥45 years	Same as for general population
Hereditary discrete common polyps and colorectal cancer	AP	Proximal colon	High	Lynch syndrome #1[b]	30–35 years	30–35 years, then semiannually	35 years, then every 2 years	Same as for general population
Hereditary nonpolyposis colorectal cancer ("cancer family syndrome")	AP → AC	Colon cancer proximal to splenic flexure	High	Lynch syndrome #2[b]	Teens	None (endoscopic surveillance)	Full colonoscopy at 25 years, then every 2 years until 35 years, then yearly	Subtotal colectomy[c]
Familial colon cancer	AP	Proximal colon, may be distal	High	None	30–35 years	30–35 years, then semiannually	35 years, then every 2 years	Same as for general population
FAP and Gardner's syndrome	Scattered AP → AC	Usually colon; also stomach and small bowel	High	See footnote[d]	Preteens	None (endoscopic surveillance)	10 years, then yearly[e]	Prophylactic subtotal colectomy[c,f]
FAP and Turcot's syndrome	Scattered AP → AC	Colon	High	Central nervous system tumors	Preteens	None (endoscopic surveillance)	Same as for Gardner's syndrome	Same as for Gardner's syndrome[c]

				Skin tumors		None (endoscopic surveillance)	Same as for Gardner's syndrome	Same as for Gardner's syndrome[c]
FAP and Oldfield's syndrome	Scattered AP → AC	Colon	High	Skin tumors	Preteens	None (endoscopic surveillance)	Same as for Gardner's syndrome	None
Peutz–Jeghers syndrome	Hamartomas of muscularis mucosa	Stomach, small bowel, colon, and ovary	Low	Buccal and cutaneous pigmentation	Preteens	≥45 years	≥45 years	None
Generalized gastrointestinal juvenile polyposis	JP	Stomach, small bowel, and colon	Low	None	Preteens	None	≥45 years	None
Juvenile polyposis coli of infancy	JP	Stomach, small bowel, and colon	None	Protein-losing enteropathy	Preteens	None	No special indications	None
Cronkhite-Canada syndrome	JP	Stomach, small bowel, and colon	None	Protein-losing enteropathy, alopecia, nail dystrophy, and hyperpigmentation	Adults	None	No special indications	None

Key: AP = adenomatous polyps; AC = adenocarcinoma; FAP = familial adenomatous polyposis; FOB = fecal occult blood; JP = juvenile (retention) polyps.

a Colonoscopy should be repeated every 6 months or every year if polyps or other abnormalities are present.

b Lynch described two syndromes of hereditary colorectal cancer (Lynch, H. T. The surgeon and colorectal cancer genetics. Arch. Surg. 125:699, 1990.)
Lynch syndrome #1: Autosomal dominant inheritance with susceptibility to early onset of colorectal cancer proximal to the splenic flexure in the absence of diffuse polyps.
Lynch syndrome #2: Most of the features of syndrome #1 with excess incidences of carcinomas of the endometrium, ovary, kidney, ureter, bladder, bile duct, and small bowel and of lymphoma.

c Prophylactic colectomy should be considered if 5 to 10 adenomatous polyps are present or if polyps recur.

d Epidermoid cysts, fibromas, desmoids, dental and osseous abnormalities, intra- and retroperitoneal fibrosis, ampullary carcinoma, and tumors in other glandular structures.

e Follow with ophthalmoscopy for associated congenital hypertrophy of the retinal pigment epithelium.

f Or, total colectomy with pouch reconstruction. Nonsteroidal anti-inflammatory drugs decrease the number and size of polyps (see Colorectal Cancer. sec. V.B.3).

and grains) increases the risk of colorectal cancer. Interestingly, a study on 8000 Japanese-Americans who were followed for over 20 years showed that an increase in serum cholesterol level was associated with a decreased risk for colon cancer, particularly of the ascending colon, but not rectal cancer. The higher incidence of rectal and sigmoid cancer in men may be related to their greater consumption of alcohol.

3. **Inflammatory bowel disease**
   a. **Ulcerative colitis** is a clear precursor of colon cancer. Approximately 1 percent of colorectal cancer patients have a history of chronic ulcerative colitis. The risk for the development of cancer in these patients varies inversely with the age of onset of the colitis and directly with the extent of colonic involvement and duration of active disease. The cumulative risk is 3 percent at 15 years, 5 percent at 20 years, and 9 percent at 25 years.

   The **recommended approach** to the increased risk of colorectal cancer in ulcerative colitis has been annual colonoscopy to determine the need for total proctocolectomy in patients with extensive colitis of more than eight years' duration. This strategy is based on the assumption that dysplastic lesions can be detected before invasive cancer has developed. A recent analysis of prospective studies concluded that immediate colectomy is essential for all patients diagnosed with dysplasia (high-grade or low-grade). Most importantly, the analysis demonstrated that the diagnosis of dysplasia does not preclude the presence of invasive cancer. The diagnosis of dysplasia has inherent problems with sampling of specimens and with variation in agreement among observers (as low as 60%, even with experts in the field).

   b. **Crohn's disease.** Patients with colorectal Crohn's disease have an increased risk of colorectal cancer but the risk is less than those with ulcerative colitis. The risk is increased about 1.5 to 2 times.

4. **Genetic factors**
   a. **Family history** may signify either a genetic abnormality or shared environmental factors. About 15 percent of all colorectal cancers occur in patients with a history of colorectal cancer in first-degree relatives.
   b. **Gene changes.** Specific inherited (adenomatous polyposis coli gene) and acquired genetic abnormalities (*ras* gene point mutation, *c-myc* gene amplification; allele deletion at specific sites at chromosomes 5, 17, and 18) appear to be capable of mediating steps in the progression from normal to malignant colonic mucosa. About half of all carcinomas and large adenomas have associated point mutations, most often in the K-*ras* gene. Such mutations are rarely present in adenomas smaller than 1.0 cm. 17p- is demonstrated in three-quarters of all colorectal carcinomas and 5q- in more than one-third of colonic carcinoma and large adenomas (see Appendix C3 for terminology). The genes responsible for familial adenomatous polyposis, which are called MCC (mutated in colorectal cancer) genes, were isolated recently and were found to segregate with the 5q chromosome region.
   c. **Tumor location.** Proximal tumors appear to represent a more stable form of the disease and may arise through the same mechanisms that underlie inherited nonpolyposis colon cancer. Distal tumors show evidence of greater genetic instability and may develop through the same mechanisms that underlie polyposis-associated colorectal cancer.

5. **Smoking.** Men and women smoking during the previous 20 years have three times the relative risk for small adenomas (<1 cm) but not for larger ones. Smoking more than 20 years was associated with a 2.5 relative risk for larger adenomas.

6. **Other factors.** Personal or family history of cancer in other anatomic sites (such as breast, endometrium, and ovary) increases the risk of developing colorectal cancer. Exposure to asbestos (e.g., in brake mechanics) increases the incidence of colorectal cancer 1.5 to 2 times. Recent data indicate that

human papillomavirus infects the columnar mucosa of the colon and may cause benign and malignant neoplasia.

II. Pathology and natural history

A. Histology. Adenocarcinomas constitute 98 percent of colorectal cancers above the anal verge. Cancers of the anal verge are squamous cell carcinomas. Carcinoid tumors cluster around the rectum and cecum and spare the rest of the colon.

B. Location. Two-thirds of colorectal cancer occurs in the left colon and one-third in the right colon. Approximately 20 percent of colorectal cancers develop in the rectum. Rectal tumors are detected by digital rectal examination in 75 percent of cases. Nearly 3 percent of colorectal adenocarcinomas are multicentric, and 2 percent of patients develop a second primary tumor in the colon.

C. Clinical presentation. The common clinical complaints of patients with colorectal cancer relate to the size and location of the tumor. Right-sided colonic lesions result in abdominal pain, bleeding, and weight loss rather than in colonic obstruction, and the pain is usually dull and ill-defined. Left-sided lesions lead to changes in bowel habits, bleeding, gas pain, decrease in stool caliber, constipation, increased use of laxatives, and colonic obstruction.

D. Clinical course. Metastases to the regional lymph nodes are found in 40 to 70 percent of cases at the time of resection. Venous invasion is found in up to 60 percent of cases. Distant metastases occur most frequently in the liver and lung, followed by the adrenals, ovaries, and bone. Metastases to the brain are rare. Rectal cancers are three times more likely to recur locally than proximal colonic tumors. Nearly half of deaths from colorectal cancer are caused by local recurrence (obstruction, perforation, peritonitis, sepsis, bleeding, and uremia), and the other half are related to visceral metastases.

III. Diagnosis

A. Diagnostic studies. Approximately 85 percent of patients diagnosed with colorectal cancer can undergo surgical resection. Some patients may have a poor general medical condition that precludes surgical intervention. Others may have incurable cancer but may benefit from palliative resection to prevent obstruction, perforation, bleeding, and invasion to adjacent structures. Once the clinical diagnosis of colorectal cancer is made, several diagnostic and evaluation steps should be taken.

1. **Biopsy confirmation** of malignancy is important. If an obstructing lesion cannot be biopsied, brush cytology may be feasible and important.

2. **General evaluation** includes a complete physical examination with digital rectal examination, CBC, LFTs, CEA, and chest x-ray.

3. **CT** with contrast of the abdomen and pelvis may identify liver or intraperitoneal metastases.

4. **Endoscopy or barium enema** is indicated to assess the entire colonic mucosa; about 3 percent of patients have synchronous colorectal cancers. Because measurement of tumors in the sigmoid colon or upper rectum by flexible endoscopy is not always reliable, rigid sigmoidoscopy is necessary to assess the exact location of the tumor and to ensure that the tumor does not require a low anterior resection.

5. **EUS** significantly improves the ability to assess preoperatively the local extent of the large bowel tumors, especially rectal tumors. The accuracy rate is 95 percent for EUS, 70 percent for CT, and 60 percent for digital rectal examination. In rectal cancer, the combination of EUS to assess tumor extent and digital rectal examination to determine mobility should enable both precise planning of surgical treatment and definition of those patients who may benefit from chemoradiation.

B. Biologic markers

1. **CEA** is the best known marker for monitoring colorectal cancer disease status and for detection of early recurrence and liver metastases. CEA is too insensitive and nonspecific to be valuable for screening of colorectal cancer (see Chap. 1, sec. **III.D.2.b**). However, elevation of serum CEA levels does correlate with histologic differentiation, stage of the disease, and vis-

ceral involvement. Although serum CEA concentration is an independent prognostic factor, its value lies in serial monitoring after surgical resection.
2. **New markers,** such as CA 19-9 (see Chap. 1, sec. **III.D.5.b**), may be of value in monitoring recurrences and complement CEA. Monoclonal antibodies (anti-CEA, anti-TAG-72) may be also useful in immunohistologic chemical staining of tissues.

IV. Staging and prognostic factors
A. Staging system.
Although an approved TNM system exists, the **Astler-Coller modification of the Dukes system** is most widely used for colorectal cancer.

Stage	Description	Five-year survival
A	Limited to mucosa, negative nodes	90–100%
B_1	Extension into muscularis propria, negative nodes	65–85%
B_2	Extension through entire bowel wall, negative nodes	60–70%
B_3	Extension into adjacent organs, negative nodes	55–65%
C_1	Positive nodes, lesion limited to muscularis propria	40–50%
C_2	Positive nodes, lesion through entire bowel wall	25–35%
C_3	Positive nodes, tumor invasion of adjacent organs	0–20%
D	Distant metastatic disease (median survival)	6–12 mo

B. Prognostic factors
1. **Stage** is the most important prognostic factor (see **IV.A**).
2. **Histologic grade** significantly influences survival regardless of stage. Patients with well differentiated carcinomas (grades 1 and 2) have a better five-year survival than poorly differentiated carcinomas (grades 3 and 4).
3. **The anatomical location** of the tumor seems to be an independent prognostic factor. For equal stages, patients with rectal lesions have a worse prognosis than colon lesions, and transverse and descending colon lesions result in poorer outcomes than ascending or rectosigmoid lesions.
4. **Clinical presentation.** Patients who present with bowel obstruction or perforation do worse than patients who present with neither of these problems.
5. **Chromosome 18.** The prognosis of patients with an allele loss of chromosome 18q is significantly worse than those with no allelic loss. The survival of patients with stage B disease is the same as stage A when there is no allelic loss and the same as with stage C when there is allelic loss. These observations may prove to be helpful in selecting patients with stage B disease for adjuvant therapy.

V. Screening and prevention
A. Screening.
The National Cancer Institute (NCI), the American College of Surgeons, the American College of Physicians, and the ACS recommend that asymptomatic individuals who are 50 years of age and older have a sigmoidoscopy examination (preferably flexible) every three to five years. An annual digital rectal examination is recommended by the ACS and NCI for individuals 50 years of age and older, but the arguments for this practice are not strongly substantiated. Screening colonoscopy of individuals with family history of colorectal cancer in first-degree relatives should begin at age 40.

The value of testing fecal occult blood (FOB) for screening remains controversial. A study involving 21,756 patients (age 40 and older) showed a significantly higher survival and a lower cancer mortality with borderline significance in those persons who had sigmoidoscopy and FOB tests as compared to those who had sigmoidoscopy only.

B. Prevention.
The management of patients with ulcerative colitis is discussed in sec. **I.B.3.a.**
1. **Periodic sigmoidoscopy** identifies and removes precancerous lesions (polyps) and reduces the incidence of colorectal cancer in individuals who undergo colonoscopic polypectomy.
2. **Diets** that are high in fiber and low in fat or contain calcium supplements or both may deter polyp progression to cancer.

3. **NSAIDs.** In a randomized, double-blind, placebo-controlled study of patients with familial polyposis, the NSAID sulindac at a dose of 150 mg b.i.d. significantly decreased the mean number and mean diameter of polyps as compared with those given placebo. The size and number of the polyps, however, increased three months after the treatment was stopped but remained significantly lower than at baseline. Recent data further suggest that the use of NSAIDs (aspirin or sulindac) reduces the formation, number, and size of colorectal polyps and reduces the incidence of colorectal cancer, whether familial or nonfamilial.

VI. Management

A. **Surgery** is the only universally accepted curative treatment for colorectal cancer. Curative surgery should excise the tumor with wide margins and maximize regional lymphadenectomy while preserving functions. For lesions above the rectum, right hemicolectomy, transverse colectomy, left hemicolectomy, or sigmoidectomy is performed. Subtotal colectomy and ileoproctostomy may be advisable for a patient with potentially curable colon cancer and with adenomas scattered in the colon and with a family history of colorectal cancer in first-degree relatives.

1. **Arterial supply.** Excision of a tumor in the right colon should include the right branch of the middle colic artery as well as the entire ileocolic and right colic artery. Excision of a tumor at the hepatic or splenic flexure should include the entire distribution of the middle colic artery.

2. **Avoidance of permanent colostomy** has been encouraged by the knowledge that 5 cm of tumor-free margin is not necessary, especially for tumors with average histologic differentiation. With the emergence of new surgical techniques (stapling), preservation of the GI integrity without the need for a permanent colostomy is possible.

3. **Rectal tumors** may be treatable by primary resection and more distal anastomosis, usually without even a temporary (anastomosis protective) colostomy, if the lower edge is above 8 cm from the anal verge in a woman or above 9–10 cm from the anal verge in a man. Treatment options for rectal tumors include

   a. **Middle and upper rectum** (6–15 cm): Anterior resection of rectum

   b. **Lower rectum** (0–5 cm): Coloanal anastomosis, with or without a pouch, transanal excision, transsphincteric and parasacral approaches, diathermy, primary radiation therapy, or abdominal-perineal (AP) resection.

4. **Obstructing tumors** in the right colon are usually managed by primary resection and primary anastomosis. Obstructing tumors in the left colon are managed with initial decompression (proximal colostomy) followed by resection of the tumor and deferred closure of the colostomy. Recent trends, however, are toward extending resection and primary anastomosis to include obstructing tumors in the transverse, descending, and even sigmoid colon.

5. **Perforated colon cancer** requires initial excision of the primary tumor and a proximal colostomy followed later by reanastomosis and closure of the colostomy.

B. **Adjuvant therapy**

1. **Adjuvant chemotherapy for stage C colon cancer** (lymph node involvement) with 5-FU plus levamisole have reduced the incidence of recurrence by 41 percent ($P < 0.001$) in three large prospective, randomized trials. This treatment improves the 5-year survival rate from 50 to 62 percent and reduces cancer-related deaths by 33 percent. It is not clear, however, whether this improvement represents a truly increased cure rate or a delayed recurrence and cancer death. After a median follow-up of five years, the decrease in recurrence and improvement in survival have persisted. Currently, various regimens involving levamisole or leucovorin are being tested in clinical trials.

a. **5-FU and levamisole** are begun simultaneously 3–5 weeks after surgery:
   (1) **Dosage**
      5-FU, 450 mg/m^2 by rapid IV injection daily for five days, then weekly for 48 weeks starting at 28 days; *plus*
      Levamisole, 50 mg PO t.i.d. for three days every two weeks for one year.
   (2) **Chemistry abnormalities.** The side effects of this combination includes elevation of serum alkaline phosphatase in 40 percent of patients, and, less often serum aminotransferase and bilirubin. These abnormalities are sometimes associated with a rising CEA level and with fatty liver, as demonstrated by CT or biopsy. Such changes are consequential only because they raise the question of hepatic metastasis; otherwise they are reversible.
   (3) **Neurotoxicity** is documented in 5 percent of patients and manifested by cerebellar signs and symptoms of impaired thinking. In severe instances, MRI has shown changes characteristic of leukoencephalopathy, which usually return to normal after therapy has been discontinued.
b. **Other regimens.** Preliminary results of studies using the combination of 5-FU and leucovorin in different dosages have demonstrated a decrease of the recurrence rate by 30 to 35 percent (see Appendix A1).

2. **Adjuvant therapy for rectal cancer.** Because of the anatomical characteristics and close proximity of pelvic organs to the rectum, surgeons cannot achieve wide, tumor-free margins during the resection of rectal cancer. Almost 50 percent of recurrences in rectal cancer occur in the pelvis. Numerous randomized, controlled studies of both preoperative and postoperative RT have demonstrated no improvement in survival; at best there has been a small decrease in the rate of local recurrence.

   Recently, two new regimens using RT in combination with 5-FU (used as a radiosensitizer) resulted in a significant reduction in the rates of local recurrence, distant metastasis, cancer-related deaths, and all deaths. Apparently the addition of 5-FU (given either by rapid injection or by continuous intravenous infusion throughout the period of radiation) to RT was crucial for the marked reduction in the local recurrence of rectal cancer. The addition of a nitrosourea to the regimen did not improve the results. Two adjuvant therapy regimens are effective in stage B2 and C rectal cancer.
   a. **Regimen A** is begun 22–70 days after surgery.
      (1) 5-FU, 500 mg/m^2 by rapid IV injection daily for five days starting on days 1 and 28.
      (2) RT, 5040 cGy in 180-cGy fractions for five days weekly for six weeks, begun on day 56 after the initiation of 5-FU therapy.
      (3) 5-FU, 500 mg/m^2 by rapid IV injection daily for three days, begun simultaneously with RT, and repeated on the first three days of the last week of RT.
      (4) 5-FU, 400 mg/m^2 by rapid IV injection daily for five days beginning one month after RT and repeated in four weeks but at a dose of 500 mg/m^2 daily for five days.
   b. **Regimen B.** Same as above except that when administered with RT (see a.(3)), 5-FU is given by continuous infusion throughout the period of radiation at a dose of 225 mg/m^2/day.

C. **Follow-up.** About 85 percent of all recurrences are evident within three years after surgical resection. High preoperative CEA levels usually revert to normal within six weeks after resection.
   1. **Clinical evaluation.** After curative surgical resection, patients are seen at three-month intervals for two years, at six-month intervals for three years, and annually thereafter. Patients who had an anterior resection for rectal cancer should have a sigmoidoscopy at each visit.
   2. **Chest x-rays** should be performed on all patients annually.

3. **Colonoscopy.** Patients who presented with obstructing colon lesions should have colonoscopy three to six weeks after surgery to ensure the absence of a neoplastic lesion in the remaining colon. The purpose of endoscopy is to detect a metachronous tumor, suture line recurrence, or colorectal adenoma. Suture line recurrence in the colon can be treated with curative resection, but suture line recurrence in the rectum is notoriously non-resectable. In the absence of obstruction, colonoscopy is performed one year after surgery and, if negative, at two- to three-year intervals theratfer.

4. **Rising CEA levels** call for further studies to identify the site of recurrence. These studies include CTs of the abdomen, pelvis, and chest, and other studies as dictated by symptoms. If pelvic recurrence of a rectal cancer is suspected, MRI may be more helpful than CT.

D. **CEA-based "second look" laparotomies** have not been evaluated in prospective, randomized trials. Retrospective studies of patients undergoing laparotomy for asymptomatic elevations of CEA levels have showed that 60 percent of patients were potentially resectable, about 55 percent of those patients were actually resectable with curative intent, and about 60 percent of the latter developed recurrence. Only 10 to 12 percent of patients undergoing laparotomy remained alive and disease-free. This small percentage of success must be viewed against the 10 to 12 percent of patients in whom tumor could not be found at the second look operation. Thus, although CEA-directed surgery may benefit some individuals, the author does not recommend its routine use.

E. **Management of isolated recurrence.** Early detection and surgical resection of isolated intrahepatic or pulmonary recurrence may be curative or result in improved survival. Resection of isolated hepatic metastasis that involves one lobe of the liver may result in a 30 percent five-year survival. Resection of isolated pulmonary metastasis may result in five- and ten-year survival rates of 40 percent and 20 percent, respectively.

F. **Management of advanced colorectal cancer**

1. **Chemotherapy.** The two most commonly used chemotherapeutic agents are fluorouracil and floxuridine alone or in combination with leucovorin. Combinations with other drugs (methotrexate, cisplatin, biological response modifiers) also have been used.

   a. **Biochemical modulation of 5-FU with leucovorin.** The combination of 5-FU and leucovorin increases the activity as well as the toxicity of 5-FU and results in significant improvement in regression rate and survival. The partial response rate is approximately 35 percent. The dose-limiting toxicities are diarrhea, mucositis, and hematosuppression. Regimens currently being used with essentially the same response rate involve low-dose or high-dose leucovorin given weekly or for five days every 4–5 weeks (see Appendix A1).

   b. **Continuous IV infusion of 5-FU** changes the toxicity profile from hematologic to predominantly mucositis when compared to bolus administration. Three randomized trials, however, have showed that continuous infusion of 5-FU using an ambulatory infusion pump, as compared to rapid injection, does not result in improved survival.

   c. **Hepatic arterial infusion** does not result in improved survival or palliation for patients with colorectal cancer that has metastasized to the liver compared to intravenous treatment.

2. **RT** may be used as the primary and only treatment modality for a small, mobile rectal tumor, or in combination with chemotherapy adjuvantly for resected rectal tumors (see above). RT in palliative doses relieves pain, obstruction, bleeding, and tenesmus in about 80 percent of cases. In addition, RT is effective in relieving pain caused by extensive liver metastasis (the dose to the liver should not exceed 2200 cGy to prevent hepatic necrosis).

Anal Cancer

I. Epidemiology and etiology

A. Incidence. Anal cancers constitute one to two percent of large bowel cancers and most commonly develop in patients 50 to 60 years of age. Cancer of the anal canal is more frequent in women than in men (female-male ratio is 2:1), but cancer of the anal margin is more frequent in males. During the last decade, however, the incidence of anal canal cancer in men younger than 35 years of age has increased, and the gender ratio is reversed in this age group.

B. Etiology. In the majority of patients with carcinoma of the anus, no etiologic factor has been identified.

1. **Diseases associated with anal cancer** include prior irradiation, anal fistulae, fissures, chronic local inflammation, hemorrhoids, Crohn's disease, lymphogranuloma venereum, condylomata acuminata, carcinoma of cervix, and carcinoma of the vulva.

2. **Infectious agents.** The human papillomavirus is a prime suspect to be a causative agent for anal cancer (see Chap. 36, sec. **V.D.2**). Although HIV has been suggested as a causative agent, anal tumors are extremely rare in IV drug abusers. Other associated infections include herpes simplex virus type 2, *Chlamydia trachomatis* in women, and gonorrhea in men.

3. **Immune suppression.** Kidney transplant patients have a 100-fold increase in anogenital tumors.

4. **Cigarette smoking** is associated with an eightfold increase in the risk of anal cancer.

5. **Anal receptive intercourse** in men but not in women is strongly associated with anal cancer at a risk ratio of 33. Studies have shown that the incidence of anal cancer (squamous and transitional cell carcinomas) is six times greater in single men than in married men. Single women are not at an increased risk.

II. Pathology and natural history

A. Anatomy. The anal canal is a tubular structure 3–4 cm in length. The junction between the anal canal and perineal skin is known as the anal verge (Hilton's line). The pectinate (or dentate) line is located at the very center of the anal canal. The lining of the anal canal is composed of columnar epithelium in its upper portion and keratinized and nonkeratinized squamous epithelium in its lower portion. Intermediate epithelium (also known as "transitional" or "cloacogenic" epithelium, which resembles bladder epithelium) lines a middle zone (0.5 to 1 cm in length) that corresponds to the pectinate line. Anal tumors appear to originate near the mucocutaneous junction and grow either upward into the rectum and surrounding tissue or downward into the perineal tissue.

B. Lymphatics. Some of the upper lymphatics of the anus communicate with those of the rectal ampulla that lead to the sacral, upper mesocolic, and paraortic lymph nodes. The lower lymphatics communicate with those of the perineum that lead to the superficial inguinal lymph nodes.

C. Histology. Squamous cell carcinoma accounts for 63 percent of cases; transitional cell (cloacogenic) carcinoma, 23 percent; and mucinous adenocarcinoma, 7 percent (often with multiple fistulous tracts). Basal cell carcinoma (2%) is curable either by local excision or irradiation. Paget's disease (2%) is a malignant neoplasm of the intraepidermal portion of the apocrine glands. Malignant melanoma (2%) usually begins at the pectinate line and progresses as single or multiple polypoid masses; the prognosis is poor and depends on tumor size and depth of invasion. Other forms include small cell carcinoma (very rare but extremely aggressive), verrucous carcinoma (a polypoid neoplasm closely related to giant condyloma acuminata), Bowen's disease, embryonal rhabdomyosarcoma (infants and children), and malignant lymphoma (in patients with AIDS).

III. Diagnosis

A. Symptoms. Bleeding occurs in 50 percent of patients, pain in 40 percent, sensation of a mass in 25 percent, and pruritus in 15 percent. About 25 percent of patients are asymptomatic.

B. Physical examination should include digital anorectal examination, anoscopy, proctoscopy, and palpation of inguinal lymph nodes. Anorectal examination may have to be performed under sedation or general anesthesia in patients with severe pain and anal spasm.

C. Biopsy. An incisional biopsy is necessary and preferable to confirm the diagnosis. Excisional biopsy should be avoided. Suspicious inguinal lymph nodes should be biopsied to differentiate inflammatory from metastatic disease. Needle aspiration of these nodes may establish the diagnosis; if aspiration is negative, surgical biopsy should be performed.

D. Staging evaluation should include physical examination, chest x-ray, and LFTs. Pelvic CT and endoscopic ultrasound of the anal canal may be useful.

IV. Staging and prognostic factors

A. Staging system. The TNM staging system may be used. Anal margin tumors are staged as for skin cancer. The T stage of anal canal tumors is determined by size and by invasion into adjacent organs:

T_x: Primary tumor cannot be assessed

T_{IS}: Carcinoma in situ

T_1: Tumor ≤2 cm in greatest dimension

T_2: Tumor >2 cm but ≤5 cm in greatest dimension

T_3: Tumor >5 cm in greatest dimension

T_4: Tumor of any size that invades adjacent organ or organs (e.g., vagina, urethra, bladder [involvement of sphincter muscle *alone* is *not* classified as T_4])

B. Prognostic factors

1. TNM stage. Patients with T_1 cancer (lesions <2 cm (T_1) in diameter) have a significantly better prognosis than those with larger lesions. Five-year survival rates are more than 80 percent for patients with T_1 and T_2 cancers and less than 20 percent for those with T_3 and T_4 cancers. The survival is poor even with aggressive therapy for lesions larger than 6–10 cm in diameter. In a multivariate analysis, T stage was the only significant independent prognostic factor for anal cancers. Metastasis to lymph nodes also results in a poor outcome.

2. Other factors

a. Histology. The histologic type (i.e., cloacogenic versus epidermoid) has not been found to be prognostically relevant. Keratizing carcinoma is associated with a better outcome than nonkeratizing cancers. Patients with mucoepidermoid carcinoma and small cell anaplastic carcinoma have a worse prognosis.

b. Symptoms. Asymptomatic patients do better than symptomatic patients. Symptoms are usually directly related to the size of the tumor.

c. Tumor grade. Patients with low-grade tumors have a better five-year survival rate than patients with high-grade tumors (75% versus 25%, respectively). DNA ploidy may or may not have prognostic significance.

V. Prevention and early detection. Early detection depends on the patient's and physician's awareness of the disease, the presence of risk factors, and the histologic examination on all surgical specimens, even those removed from minor anorectal surgery. Yearly anoscopy may be indicated in high-risk patients. Anal examination should be performed routinely in patients with cervical and vulvar cancer.

VI. Management. Chemotherapy and RT are the primary therapeutic modalities for anal carcinoma. AP resection is now used as salvage treatment for chemoradiation-resistant disease (i.e., patients who fail to respond or who relapse after a CR). Because anal cancer is a rare tumor, most reports contain a small number of patients accrued over several years; randomized studies do not exist.

A. Combined chemoradiation therapy is the primary treatment of choice for anal carcinoma. The combination of RT and chemotherapy resulted in higher rates of both local control and survival (82%) and preserved anal function when compared to surgery. The administration of a high dose of RT reduced the incidence of persistent carcinoma and eliminated the need for surgical lymphadenectomy. The RT dose, the number of chemotherapy cycles required to improve local control rate, and the role (if any) of invasive restaging after completion of therapy remain controversial.

1. **Primary therapy.** External beam RT appears to be superior to interstitial implants. RT doses greater than 5000 cGy do not appear to be necessary. Using mitomycin C (MMC) plus 5-fluorouracil (5-FU) with RT is superior to 5-FU alone with RT. The combination of these two drugs with RT is superior to RT alone. RT regimens vary among institutions; 5-FU is given by continuous IV infusion in each case. Two useful regimens are

   a. **Radiation Therapy Oncology Group (RTOG).**
   MMC: 10 mg/m^2 IV bolus (day 2)
   5-FU: 1000 mg/m^2/24 hrs by continuous IV infusion (days 2–4 and days 28–32)
   RT: 170 cGy/day between days 1 and 28;
   Total dose: 4500–5000 cGy

   b. **National Tumor Institute (Milan)**
   MMC: 15 mg/m^2 IV bolus (day 1)
   5-FU: 750 mg/m^2/24 hrs by continuous IV infusion (days 1–5)
   RT: 180 cGy/day for two weeks with a two-week rest;
   Total dose: 5400 cGy (in patients with locally advanced disease, the boost dose is increased but the total dose does not exceed 6000 cGy)

2. **Follow-up therapy.** Additional six-week cycles of chemotherapy with MMC and 5-FU are given depending on tumor control or treatment toxicity. Full-thickness biopsy at the original tumor site is performed six to eight weeks after the completion of therapy. Patients are examined at three-month intervals for the first year and six-month intervals thereafter. AP resection is performed for biopsy-proven carcinoma during the followup period.

B. Surgery alone. Wide, full-thickness excision is sufficient treatment for discrete, superficial, anal margin tumors and results in 80 percent five-year survival unless the tumor is large and deep. AP resection of the anorectum as the exclusive treatment for anal canal tumors and large anal margin tumors results in only a 55 percent five-year survival rate.

Pancreatic Cancer

I. Epidemiology and etiology

A. Incidence. In the United States, the incidence of pancreatic cancer is 9 cases per 100,000 population and has not changed since 1973. Blacks are more frequently affected with an incidence of 15 per 100,000. Annually there will be 27,000 new cases of pancreatic cancer with a male to female ratio of 1:1. The disease is rare before the age of 45 years but its occurrence rises sharply thereafter.

In India, Kuwait, and Singapore, the rate is less than 2 per 100,000. In Japan the incidence has risen sharply from 2 to 5 per 100,000 in the past 20 years.

B. Etiology and risk factors. The cause of pancreatic cancer remains unknown but several factors are associated with its occurrence.

1. **Cigarette smoking** is the most prominent risk factor for pancreatic cancer with a relative risk of at least 1.5. The risk increases as the level of cigarette smoking increases and the excess risk levels off 10–15 years after cessation of smoking. The risk is ascribed to tobacco-specific nitrosamines.

2. **Diet.** A high intake of fat, meat, or both increases the risk, whereas the intake of fresh fruits and vegetables appears to have a protective effect.

3. **Partial gastrectomy** appears to result in a two to five times higher than expected incidence of pancreatic cancer 15–20 years later. The increased formation of N-nitroso compounds by bacteria that produce nitrate reductase and proliferate in the hypoacidic stomach has been proposed to account for the increased occurrence of gastric and pancreatic cancer.

4. **Cholecystokinin.** Pancreatic cancer has been induced experimentally by long-term duodenogastric reflux, which is associated with increased chole-

cystokinin levels. Some clinical evidence suggests that cholecystectomy, which also increases the circulating cholecystokinin, may increase the risk of pancreatic cancer.

5. **Diabetes mellitus** has been found in 13 percent of patients with pancreatic cancer and in only 2 percent of the controls. Experimental studies have shown that the diabetic state enhances the growth of pancreatic carcinoma. Diabetes mellitus that occurs in patients with pancreatic cancer is characterized by marked insulin resistance that appears to decline after tumor resection. Islet amyloid polypeptide, a hormonal factor secreted by pancreatic beta cells, reduces insulin sensitivity in vivo and glycogen synthesis in vitro, and may be present in elevated concentrations in patients with pancreatic cancer who have diabetes.

6. **Tropical and hereditary pancreatitis** are associated with pancreatic cancer, but other forms of pancreatitis are not.

7. **Toxic substances.** Occupational exposure to 2-nephthylamine, benzidine, and gasoline derivatives appear to increase the risk of pancreatic cancer by a factor of five. Prolonged exposure to DDT and two DDT derivatives (ethylan and DDD) is reported to result in a fourfold to sevenfold increased risk for pancreatic cancer.

8. **Socioeconomic status.** Pancreatic cancer occurs in a slightly higher frequency in populations of lower socioeconomic status.

9. **Coffee.** Analysis of 30 epidemiologic studies showed that only one case control study and none of the prospective studies confirmed a statistically significant association between coffee consumption and pancreatic cancer.

10. **Idiopathic deep vein thrombosis** is statistically correlated with the subsequent development of mucinous carcinomas (including the pancreas), especially among patients in whom venous thrombosis recurs during follow-up.

11. **Dermatomyositis and polymyositis** are associated with an increased risk of pancreatic cancer and other cancers.

12. **Tonsillectomy** has been shown to be a protective factor against the development of pancreatic cancer, an observation that has been described for other cancers as well.

II. Pathology

A. **Primary malignant tumors** of the pancreas involve either the exocrine parenchyma or the endocrine islet cells (the latter are discussed in Chap. 15, sec. **VI**). Nonepithelial tumors (sarcomas and lymphomas) are very rare. Ductal adenocarcinoma makes up 75 to 90 percent of malignant pancreatic neoplasms: 57 percent occur in the head of the pancreas, 9 percent in the body, 8 percent in the tail, 6 percent in overlapping sites, and 20 percent of unknown anatomic subsite. Uncommon but reasonably distinctive variants of pancreatic cancer include adenosquamous, oncocytic, clear cell, giant cell, signet ring, mucinous, and anaplastic carcinoma. Anaplastic carcinomas often involve the body and tail rather than the head of pancreas. Reported cases of pure epidermoid carcinoma (a variant of adenosquamous carcinoma) probably are associated with hypercalcemia. Cystadenocarcinomas have an indolent course and may remain localized for many years.

B. **Metastatic tumors.** Autopsy studies show that for every primary tumor of the pancreas, four metastatic tumors are found. The most common tumors of origin are the breast, lung, cutaneous melanoma, and non-Hodgkin's lymphoma.

C. **Genetic abnormalities.** Mutant c-K-ras genes have been found in most specimens of human pancreatic carcinoma and their metastases.

III. Diagnosis

A. **Symptoms.** Most patients with pancreatic cancer are symptomatic at the time of diagnosis. Predominant initial symptoms include abdominal pain (80%), anorexia (65%), weight loss (60%), early satiety (60%), xerostomia and sleep problems (55%), easy fatigability (45%); weakness, nausea or constipation (40%); depression (40%), dyspepsia (35%), vomiting (30%), hoarseness (25%); taste change, bloating or belching (25%), dyspnea, dizziness or edema (20%), cough, diarrhea, hiccup or itching (15%); and dysphagia (5%).

B. Clinical findings. At presentation patients with pancreatic cancer have cachexia (44%), serum albumin less than 3.5 gm/dl (35%), palpable abdominal mass (35%), ascites (25%), or jaundice (20%). Metastases are present to at least one major organ in 65 percent of patients, to the liver in 45 percent, to the lungs in 30 percent, and to the bones in 3 percent. Carcinomas of the distal pancreas do not produce jaundice until they metastasize and may remain painless until the disease is advanced. Occasionally, acute pancreatitis is the first manifestation of pancreatic cancer.

C. Paraneoplastic syndromes. Panniculitis-arthritis-eosinophilia syndrome that occurs with pancreatic cancer appears to be caused by the release of lipase from the tumor. Dermatomyositis; polymyositis; recurrent, idiopathic deep vein thrombosis; and Cushing's syndrome have been reported to be associated with cancer of the pancreas.

D. Diagnostic studies

1. **Ultrasonography (US).** Abdominal US is technically adequate in 60 to 90 percent of patients, is noninvasive, safe, and inexpensive. US can detect pancreatic masses as small as 2 cm, dilatation of the pancreatic and bile ducts, hepatic metastases, and extrapancreatic spread. Intraoperative US facilitates surgical biopsy and may detect unsuspected metastases in 50 percent of patients.

2. **CT** is neither operator-dependent nor limited by air-containing abdominal organs, as is US. CT is favored over US because it can also demonstrate retroperitoneal invasion and lymphadenopathy, both of which are not well detected by US. A pancreatic tumor must be at least 2 cm in diameter to become visible. "Dynamic CT" with continuous infusion of intravenous contrast is the best test for assessing the size of the tumor and its extension. At least 20 percent of pancreatic tumors believed to be resectable may not be detectable by CT.

3. **MRI** has no demonstrated advantage over CT in the diagnosis and staging of pancreatic cancer.

4. **Endoscopic retrograde cholangiography (ERCP)** is the mainstay in the differential diagnosis of the tumors of the pancreatobiliary junction, 85 percent of which originate in the pancreas (about 5% each in the distal common bile duct, ampulla, and duodenum). Ampullary and duodenal carcinoma can be easily visualized and biopsied with ERCP. The pancreatogram typically shows the pancreatic duct to be encased or obstructed by carcinoma in 97 percent of cases.

   It may be difficult to distinguish between pancreatic cancer and chronic pancreatitis because both diseases share clinical and radiologic characteristics. Pancreatic duct stricture usually does not exceed 5 mm in chronic pancreatitis; strictures longer than 10 mm (especially if irregular) indicate pancreatic cancer. Cytologic examination of cells in samples of pancreatic juice obtained during ERCP with secretin stimulation has been reported to be highly specific for the diagnosis of carcinoma and 85 percent sensitive. Brush biopsy of the pancreatic stricture (when possible) increases the diagnostic yield.

5. **EUS.** Prospective studies showed that EUS is more accurate than standard US, CT, and ERCP for diagnosis, staging, and predicting resectability of pancreatic tumors. Angiography, CT, and US were of limited value for lesions less than 3 cm, whereas EUS detected 100 percent of them. EUS can detect tumors smaller than 2 cm; ERCP cannot. The additional information obtained from EUS has been reported to result in a major change in the clinical management in one-third of patients and aid in the clinical decision in three-quarters of them.

   The present limitations of EUS include a short optimal focal range of only 4 cm, the inability to reliably differentiate focal chronic pancreatitis from carcinoma, and the inability to differentiate chronic lymphadenitis from metastatic lymph node involvement.

6. **Percutaneous fine-needle aspiration cytology** is safe and reliable, with a

reported sensitivity of 55 to 95 percent and no false-positive results for the diagnosis of pancreatic cancer. This procedure should be performed for histologic confirmation on all patients with unresectable or metastatic disease unless a palliative surgical procedure is planned. Needle aspiration cytology distinguishes adenocarcinoma from islet cell tumors, lymphomas, and cystic neoplasms of the pancreas that are less aggressive and do not have a cystic appearance on CT or ultrasound.

The drawbacks to percutaneous aspiration biopsy include the potential tumor seeding along the needle tract, an increase in intraperitoneal spread, and a negative biopsy result that does not exclude the diagnosis of malignancy. Furthermore, early and smaller tumors are most likely to be missed by this technique.

7. **Angiography** is excellent for assessing major vascular involvement but is not very useful in determining the size and location of tumor (pancreatic cancer is hypovascular).

8. **Laparoscopy** can demonstrate extrapancreatic involvement in 40 percent of patients without demonstrable lesions on CT.

9. **Tumor markers.** No currently used serum marker is sufficiently sensitive or specific to be considered reliable for screening of pancreatic cancer.

   a. **CA 19-9** is widely used for the diagnosis and follow-up of patients with pancreatic cancer but is not specific for pancreatic cancer (see Chap. 1, sec. III.D.5.b).

   b. **CEA** is of minimal value in pancreatic cancer.

   c. **Testosterone-dihydrotestoserone ratio** is normally about 10 and is reported to be less than 5 in over 70 percent of men with pancreatic cancer. A low testosterone-dihydrotestosterone ratio is present in a higher percentage of stage I pancreatic cancer and is less sensitive but more specific than CA 19-9 level for the diagnosis of pancreatic cancer.

IV. Staging and prognostic factors

A. **Staging system.** The TNM system is most commonly used. T_1 and T_2 tumors are potentially resectable tumors. T_1 is tumor localized to the pancreas, and T_{1a} is tumor less than 2 cm in diameter. T_2 indicates that there is a limited direct extension into the duodenum, bile duct, or stomach. T_3 indicates advanced direct extension that is incompatible with surgical resection.

B. **Preoperative evaluation.** Identifying patients with unresectable pancreatic tumor or with metastasis or vessel involvement would spare many patients a major operation. Operative mortality and morbidity for pancreatic surgery remain high, except in specialized centers. Modern diagnostic methods have reduced unnecessary laparotomies from 30 percent to 5 percent and have increased the resectability rate from 5 percent to 20 percent. Accuracy in determining resectability prior to exploration has become even more important because of the availability of effective decompression of biliary obstruction endoscopically without laparotomy.

   CT, angiography, and laparoscopy assess different aspects of resectability and are complementary. In general, if one of these studies is positive, the resectability rate is about 5 percent, whereas if all are negative, the resectability rate is 78 percent. Gross nodal involvement is usually associated with other signs of unresectability and may be identified by CT.

C. **Prognostic factors.** Fewer than 20 percent of patients with cancer of the pancreas survive the first year, and only 3 percent are alive five years after the diagnosis.

   1. **Resectable disease.** The five-year survival of patients whose tumors were resected is poor; the reported range is 3 to 25 percent. The five-year survival is 30 percent for patients with small tumors (2 cm or less in diameter), 35 percent for patients with no residual tumor or patients in whom the tumor did not require dissection from major vessels, and 55 percent for patients without lymph node metastasis.

   2. **Nonresectable or metastatic disease.** The median survival of patients with such disease is 2 to 6 months. Performance status and the presence of

four symptoms (dyspnea, anorexia, weight loss, and xerostomia) appear to influence survival; patients with the higher performance status and the least number of these symptoms lived the longest.

V. Management

A. Surgery.
Only 5 to 20 percent of patients with pancreatic cancer have resectable tumors at the time of presentation. The remaining require some form of palliation for the relief of jaundice, duodenal obstruction, or pain.

1. **Surgical procedures**
   a. **Pancreaticoduodenal resection** (Whipple's procedure or a modification) is the standard operation. This implies that only cancer involving the head of pancreas is resectable.
   b. **Modified Whipple's with preservation of pylorus,** which is currently a more commonly used operation in the United States, has resulted in a significant reduction of postgastrectomy syndrome with no decrease in survival.
   c. **Whipple's operation combined with extensive lymph node dissection,** which is used in Japan, has not resulted in better survival.
   d. **Regional pancreatectomy** confers no survival advantage.
   e. **Total pancreatectomy** does not yield better results, produces exocrine insufficiency and brittle diabetes mellitus, and should not be performed.

2. **Surgical mortality and morbidity.** The mortality rate from pancreatic resection is less than 5 percent when the operation is performed by expert surgeons, who are relatively few in number. Nationally, however, the surgical mortality rate is approximately 18 percent. The major complication rate is 20 to 35 percent and includes sepsis, abscess formation, hemorrhage, and pancreatic and biliary fistulae.

3. **Relief of obstructive jaundice** by surgical biliary bypass (cholecystojejunostomy or choledochojejunostomy) is very effective, but the average survival is five months and the postoperative mortality rate in large collected series is 20 percent. Jaundice can be relieved endoscopically by the placement of stents with a success rate up to 85 percent, a procedure-related mortality of 1 to 2 percent, and significant reduction in the length of hospitalization and recovery. Randomized trials showed no difference in survival between endoscopic stent placement and surgical bypass, but patients treated with stents had more frequent readmissions for stent obstruction, recurrent jaundice, and cholangitis.

B. Adjuvant therapy
appears to be a reasonable approach for the rare patient who has undergone curative resection and has no lymph node metastasis. Only one prospective randomized study (completed by the Gastrointestinal Study Group) showed that RT and 5-FU following a curative Whipple's procedure improved survival. In that study, the median survival was 20 months for patients treated adjuvantly, and 3 of 21 patients survived five years or more. For patients not treated adjuvantly, the median survival was 11 months and only 1 of 22 patients survived five years. The five-year survival was 40 percent for patients with no lymph node involvement and less than 5 percent for patients with lymph node metastasis.

C. Therapy for locally advanced disease

1. **External beam RT combined with 5-FU** (15 mg/kg IV on the first three days of RT) significantly improves survival as compared to RT alone (10 months versus 5.5 months).

2. **Intraoperative RT** delivered to a surgically exposed tumor by an electron beam through a field-limiting cone may increase the median survival to 13 months with excellent local control (5% of patients have lived 3–8 years). Intraoperative RT relieves pain in 50 to 90 percent of patients.

D. Chemotherapy for metastatic disease.
5-FU has a response rate of 20 percent in pancreatic cancer. Other drugs with reported activity include mitomycin, streptozocin, and ifosfamide. With one exception, all randomized studies showed that median survival in patients receiving chemotherapy has not been significantly better than in patients given supportive therapy alone. In one study in

the United Kingdom, tamoxifen resulted in a slightly longer survival, but the difference between the treated and monitored group was not statistically significant. LHRH agonists and antagonists are being evaluated.

E. **Neuroablation for pain control.** The pain caused by pancreatic cancer can be extremely distressing and frequently requires the use of large doses of narcotics, particularly sustained-release morphine (see Chapter 5, sec. I). **Chemical splanchnicectomy** *should be performed at the time of operation* in nonresectable cases. Either 6% phenol or 50% alcohol (25 ml is injected on each side of the celiac axis) is used. This procedure results in relief of pancreatic cancer-related pain in over 80 percent of patients. **Percutaneous chemical neurolysis** of the celiac ganglion, which may be attempted in patients who did not have an intraoperative splanchnicectomy or were not explored, is reported to be equally effective. Transient postural hypotension may occur. Celiac plexus block may be repeated if initially unsuccessful.

Liver Cancer

I. Epidemiology and etiology

A. **Incidence.** Liver cancer is the most common neoplasm and most common cause of cancer death in the world, including Africa and Asia. One million deaths due to hepatocellular carcinoma (HCC) occur each year worldwide. In the United States, 16,000 new cases of cancer of the liver and biliary passages will develop annually. HCC is two to three times more common in males than in females.

B. **Conditions predisposing to HCC**

1. **Hepatitis B virus (HBV).** High titers of hepatitis B surface antigen (HBsAg) and core antibody (HBcAb) are frequently found in patients with HCC. HBsAg was found in the serum of 50 to 60 percent of patients with HCC and in 5 to 10 percent of the general population. In the United States, HCC is increased by 140-fold in HBsAg carriers. Anti-HBcAb was found in 90 percent of black South African and 75 percent of Japanese patients with HCC, as compared to 35 percent and 30 percent of matched controls, respectively. When HCC develops the patient usually has had chronic HBV infection for three to four decades. The risk factors for the development of HCC in HBsAg carriers are the presence of cirrhosis; family history of HCC; increasing age; male sex; Asian or African race; cofactors (such as alcohol, aflatoxin, and perhaps smoking); and the duration of the carrier state. In the Far East, HBV is transmitted vertically from mother to infant in the first few months of life; in Africa, HBV is transmitted horizontally.

2. **Cirrhosis.** HCC very often develops in a cirrhotic liver. Autopsy studies showed that 60 to 90 percent of HBsAg-positive subjects have associated cirrhosis and 20 to 40 percent of patients with cirrhosis have HCC. Studies show that in Taiwan, the annual estimated incidence of HCC is 0.005 percent in HBsAg-negative patients, 0.25 percent in HBsAg-positive patients, and 2.5 percent in HBsAg-positive patients with liver cirrhosis (500 times higher than in HBsAg-negative patients). In France, the development of HCC in the presence of alcoholic cirrhosis was nearly always associated with HBV infection, and alcoholism was thought to hasten the development of HCC. In Italy, the prevalence of HCC in individuals with cirrhosis was nearly 7 percent with a yearly crude incidence of 3 percent; hepatitis C virus chronic infection was the cause of cirrhosis in 45 percent of these patients.

3. **Hepatitis C virus (HCV)** infection is a risk factor for the development of HCC. Apparently HCV induces cirrhosis and to a lesser extent increases the risks for patients with cirrhosis. HCV infection acts independently of HBV infection, alcohol abuse, age, and gender. The ratios for HCC risk factors in patients with chronic liver disease, adjusted for age, sex, and other factors, are as follows:

   a. Risk ratio 6–7-fold: Age 60 to 69 years, HBsAg positive

   b. Risk ratio 4-fold: High titer anti-HBcAb, anti-HCV positivity
   c. Risk ratio 2-fold: Presence of liver cirrhosis, currently smoking
4. **Aflatoxin.** Aflatoxin has been proven to be a potent hepatocarcinogen in experimental animals and human beings. For example, the daily intake of aflatoxin in Mozambique is four times greater than in Kenya, and the incidence of HCC is eight times greater.
5. **Mutations of tumor suppressor gene p53** have been reported in 50 percent of patients with HCC. These mutations are correlated both with geographic areas where the ingestion of aflatoxin is common and with the prevalence of HBV infection.
6. **Sex hormones.** The risk for liver cell adenomas and HCC is increased in women who have used oral contraceptives for eight or more years. Although liver cell adenomas regress with discontinuation of oral contraceptives in the majority of cases, adenomas must be considered premalignant. Close and prolonged follow-up is necessary for women who use oral contraceptives. HCC has also been observed in patients with long histories of androgen administration.
7. **Cigarette smoking, alcohol intake, diabetes, and insulin intake.** A study performed in Los Angeles showed that in non-Asian populations that have a low risk for HCC, cigarette smoking, heavy alcohol consumption, and diabetes mellitus, especially with insulin administration, appear to be significant risk factors for HCC.
8. **Other factors.** A relatively small number of HCCs develop in patients with various other diseases. The most common of these are alpha$_1$-antitrypsin deficiency, tyrosinemia, and hemochromatosis. Phlebotomy therapy can deplete hepatic iron and induce regression of hepatic fibrosis but does not prevent the development of HCC in hemochromatosis. Clonorchiasis, vinyl chloride exposure, and administration of thorium dioxide or methotrexate are also associated with the development of HCC.

II. **Pathology and natural history**
  A. **Pathology**
   1. **Liver cell adenoma** has low malignant potential. True adenomas of the liver are rare and occur mostly in women taking oral contraceptives. The majority of adenomas are solitary; occasionally multiple (10 or more) tumors develop in a condition known as liver cell adenomatosis. These tumors are smooth encapsulated masses and do not contain Kupffer cells. Patients are usually symptomatic; hemoperitoneum occurs in 25 percent of cases.
   2. **Focal nodular hyperplasia (FNH)** has no malignant potential. FNH occurs with a female-male ratio of 2:1. The relationship of oral contraceptives to FNH is not as clear as for hepatic adenoma; only one-half of patients with FNH take oral contraceptives. FNH tumors are nodular, not encapsulated, but do contain Kupffer cells. Patients are usually asymptomatic; hemoperitoneum rarely occurs.
   3. **HCC** may present grossly as a single mass, multiple nodules, or as diffuse liver involvement; these are referred to as "massive," "nodular," and "diffuse" forms. The growth pattern microscopically is trabecular, solid, or tubular, and the stroma, in contrast to bile duct carcinoma, is scanty. A rare sclerosing or fibrosing form has been associated with hypercalcemia. Fibrolamellar carcinoma, another variant, occurs predominantly in young patients without cirrhosis, has a favorable prognosis, and has no elevation of serum alpha fetoprotein levels. In the United States almost half of HCCs in patients under 35 years of age are fibrolamellar, and over half of them are resectable.
   4. **Bile duct adenomas** are solitary in 80 percent of cases and may grossly resemble metastatic carcinoma. Most are less than 1 cm in diameter and are located under the capsule.
   5. **Biliary cystadenoma and cystadenocarcinoma.** Benign and malignant cystic tumors of biliary origin arise in the liver more frequently than in the extrahepatic biliary system.

Table 9-3. Differential diagnosis of hepatocellular carcinoma (HCC) versus adenocarcinoma

Characteristics	HCC	Adenocarcinoma[a]
Clinical features		
Sex predilection	Males	None
Presence of cirrhosis	Common	Exceptional
Preferential spread	Through veins	Through lymphatics
Pathologic features		
Gross features	Soft and hemorrhagic	Hard and whitish
Main growth pattern	Trabecular	Glandular
Growth at tumor margin	Replacement	Often sinusoidal
Fibrous stroma	Minimal[b]	Often prominent
Microscopic features		
Tumor cell nucleus		
Intranuclear inclusions	Common	Uncommon
Prominent nucleolus	Typical	Often
Tumor-cell cytoplasm	Often abundant; eosinophilic, granular, or clear	Variable
Hyaline globules	Occ present	Rare
Mallory bodies	Occ present	Absent
Bile	Occ present	Absent
Mucin	Absent	Often present
Hepatocyte dysplasia	May be present	Absent
Immunohistochemistry		
Copper, copper-binding protein	Often present	Absent
α-fetoprotein	Often present	Occ present (metastases)
Polyclonal CEA (canalicular)	Often present	Absent
Monoclonal CEA (cytoplasmic)	Rarely present	Often present
Hepatocyte cytokeratins only	Often present	Other cytokeratins present
Erythropoiesis-associated	Often present	Absent

Key: Occ = occasionally; CEA = carcinoembryonic antigen.
[a] Adenocarcinoma = cholangiocarcinoma and metastatic adenocarcinoma.
[b] The fibrolamellar and sclerosing variants of HCC are exceptions as they contain prominently fibrous stroma.
Adapted from Sternberg, S. S. (ed.). *Diagnostic Surgical Pathology* (2nd ed.). New York: Raven Press, 1994. P. 1543.

6. **Bile duct carcinoma** (cholangiocarcinoma; see Chap. 9, *Extrahepatic Bile Duct Cancer*). Malignant tumors of intrahepatic bile ducts are less common than HCC and have no relation to cirrhosis. Mixed hepatic tumors with elements of both HCC and cholangiocarcinoma do occur; the majority of these cases are actually HCC with focal ductal differentiation. Table 9-3 depicts the clinical and pathologic differences between HCC, bile duct carcinoma, and metastatic adenocarcinoma.

B. **Natural history.** Most patients die of hepatic failure and not from distant metastases. The disease is contained within the liver in only 20 percent of cases. HCC invades the portal vein in 35 percent of cases, hepatic vein in 15 percent, contiguous abdominal organs in 15 percent, or vena cava and right atrium in 5 percent. HCC metastasizes to the lung in 35 percent of cases, abdominal lymph nodes in 20 percent, thoracic or cervical lymph nodes in 5 percent, vertebrae in 5 percent, and kidney or adrenal gland in 5 percent.

   C. Associated paraneoplastic syndromes include fever, erythrocytosis, gynecomastia, hypercalcemia, hypoglycemia, and virilization (precocious puberty).

III. Diagnosis

   A. Symptoms and signs. Pain in the right subcostal area or on top of the shoulder from phrenic irritation is common. Severe symptoms of fatigue, anorexia and weight loss, and unexplained fever are not uncommon. Many patients have vague abdominal pain, fever, and anorexia for up to two years before the diagnosis of carcinoma is made. Hemorrhage into the peritoneal cavity is often seen in patients with HCC and may be extensive and fatal. Ascites may be present and is of ominous prognosis. Any sudden deterioration in a patient with known liver disease or with positive HBsAg should raise the suspicion of HCC.

   B. Diagnostic studies

      1. LFTs may be normal or elevated and are affected by liver cirrhosis. Elevated serum bilirubin and LDH values and lowered serum albumin are associated with a poor survival. Serum gamma-glutamyl transferase (GGT) isoenzyme II (out of eleven isoenzymes) was positive in 90 percent of patients with HCC. GGT-II was negative in most patients with acute and chronic viral hepatitis or extrahepatic tumors, in pregnant women, and in healthy controls. GGT-II was found to be valuable for the detection of small or subclinical HCC.

      2. Biopsy of liver nodules. Some authors believe that percutaneous liver biopsy carries a high risk and has little or no role in the workup of liver tumors, while others believe that it can be performed without any significant risk. Nevertheless, liver biopsy is needed to establish the diagnosis and may be obtained either at operation or percutaneously.

      3. Serum α-FP is often elevated in patients with HCC but can also be elevated in patients with benign chronic liver disease (see Chap. 1, sec. **III.D.2.a**). In patients with liver cirrhosis and no HCC, serum α-FP may be normal or elevated with values ranging from 30 to 460 ng/ml (median: 30–70). In patients with HCC, the serum α-FP concentrations may range from 30 to 7000 ng/ml (median: 275). Measurement of α-FP fractions L_3, P_4, and P_5 (different sugar-chain structures) may allow the differentiation of HCC from cirrhosis in some cases. It may also be predictive for the development of HCC during follow-up of patients with cirrhosis.

      4. Radiologic studies

         a. US. HCC is usually well circumscribed, hyperechogenic, and associated with diffuse distortion of the normal hepatic parenchyma. Metastatic deposits are usually hyperechogenic but may be hypoechogenic.

         b. CT. HCC typically appears as an area of low attenuation on CT. Lesions may occasionally be isodense with normal hepatic parenchyma, however. Metastatic tumors with low attenuation (close to the density of water) include mucin-producing tumors of the ovary, pancreas, colon, and stomach and tumors with necrotic centers, such as sarcomas. Mucin-producing metastases may have near normal attenuation values because of diffuse microscopic calcifications within the tumor.

         c. MRI has been reported to be superior to CT scanning and US for the detection of liver tumors. Cost and availability are important factors in the selection of diagnostic methods.

         d. Selective hepatic, celiac, and superior mesenteric angiography can confirm portal vein involvement, define the arterial supply, and identify vascular lesions that are as small as 3 mm in diameter. Intra-arterial epinephrine injection can differentiate normal hepatic arteries from tumor vessels, which do not constrict because of the absence of smooth muscles in their walls.

         e. Radionuclide scans

            (1) Liver-spleen scan. All primary and metastatic liver tumors, except for FNH and regenerating nodules, are devoid of Kupffer cells and appear as "cold" areas in liver scans. However, the liver-spleen scan has now been replaced by US and CT.

(2) Gallium scan of liver may be able to differentiate primary hepatic tumors from metastatic carcinoma because gallium is taken up by the HCC.

IV. Staging and prognostic factors

A. Staging. The initial step is to establish whether the HCC is resectable. Unresectability may be determined either at exploratory laparotomy or by CT, MRI, or angiography. Unresectable disease includes bilobar or four-segment hepatic parenchymal involvement, portal vein thrombus, and vena caval involvement with tumor or tumor thrombus. Metastatic disease includes involvement of regional lymph nodes, which is proven by biopsy at surgery. Liver failure or portal hypertension alone does not contraindicate surgery.

B. Prognostic factors. The number of liver lesions and the presence of vascular involvement are the most significant determinants. Neither the presence nor the degree of AFP elevation has any prognostic importance. The prognostic factors that relate to survival in patients with resectable HCC are

1. **Number, size, and location of liver lesions.** The five-year survival for patients with a solitary tumor is 45 percent and 15 to 25 percent for those with multiple liver lesions. The five-year survival is 40 to 45 percent for patients with small tumors (2–5 cm) and 10 percent for patients with tumors larger than 5 cm. Patients without cirrhosis with tumors located in the left lobe of the liver or in the right inferior segments (anteriorly or posteriorly) have the best prognosis.

2. **Vein involvement.** All patients with gross tumor thrombi involving the portal vein or hepatic vein die within three years, whereas the five-year survival for patients with no vascular involvement of any kind is 30 percent.

3. **Extent and type of resection.** The five-year survival for patients undergoing curative resection is 55 percent compared to 5 percent for those undergoing noncurative resections. The five-year survival is 85 percent for hepatic lobectomy, 50 percent for subsegmentectomy, and 20 percent for wedge enucleation. In patients with resected HCC, the liver is the site of disease recurrence in 90 percent of cases.

4. **Hepatic reserve.** Patients who have better hepatic reserve, as determined by retention rate of indocyanine green dye at 15 minutes, have better survival.

V. Prevention and early detection

A. Prevention. Avoidance of the risk factors for HCC is difficult in those parts of the world where socioeconomic conditions are poor and where HBV infection is endemic.

1. Almost four billion people (75% of the world population) live in areas of intermediate or higher prevalence for HBV. Infections with HBV and HCV can be treated with interferons, although prevention of initial infection is preferable. Protection against HBV, if attempted, is best done in infancy. In the United States, vaccination with recombinant HBsAg is recommended for health workers in contact with blood, for persons residing for more than six months in areas that are highly endemic for HBV, and for all others at risk.

2. Steps should be taken to reduce the high levels of aflatoxin food contaminations that exist in many areas of Asia and southern Africa, as has been done in the Western world.

B. Early detection. Two recent reports describe attempts for early detection of HCC in patients with liver cirrhosis. A study from Italy shows that patients with persistently elevated serum α-FP have a higher incidence of HCC (3% per year) than those with fluctuating levels. This screening program did not appreciably increase the rate of detection of potentially curable liver tumors, however. In a study from Japan, higher percentages of α-FP L_3, P_4, and P_5 fractions allowed the differentiation of HCC in some cases.

VI. Management

A. Liver anatomy. The liver is anatomically divided into four lobes: a larger right lobe, which is separated from a smaller left lobe by the attachment of the falciform ligament, and two small lobes (the quadrate lobe on the anterior inferior aspect and the caudate lobe). Practical surgical anatomy divides the liver into nearly equal halves, and each half is divided into two segments. The right half is divided into anterior (ventrocranial) and posterior (dorsocaudal) segments. The left half is divided into medial and lateral segments by a visible left sagittal accessory fissure. Each of the four segments is subdivided into superior and inferior subsegments. The French literature labels the eight liver subsegments with Roman numerals.

B. Localized and resectable HCC. Only 10 percent of HCCs are resectable with solitary or unilobar hepatic lesions at the time of diagnosis. The survival in resectable lesions depends on the prognostic factors discussed in section **IV.B.** In the United States, the median survival following surgical resection is approximately 22 months for patients with cirrhotic livers and 32 months for patients with normal livers (range: 2 months to 15 years). The perioperative morbidity is minimal and is slightly higher in the cirrhotic group. Morbidity includes subphrenic abscess, subhepatic abscess, pneumothorax, and wound infection. Total hepatectomy with orthotopic liver transplantation is of limited benefit except in the rare patient with unresectable nonmetastatic fibrolamellar HCC.

C. Localized and nonresectable disease

1. **Preoperative multimodality treatment followed by surgery.** At Johns Hopkins University, preoperative external beam radiation therapy (2100 cGy in 300-cGy fractions) and chemotherapy (both 15 mg/m^2 of Adriamycin and 500 mg/m^2 of 5-FU given on days 1, 3, 5, and 7 of RT) resulted in greater than 50 percent tumor reduction in all patients. Most patients also received radiolabeled polyclonal antiferritin immunoglobulin conjugate with [131]iodine. The actuarial five-year survival, the types of operative procedures performed, and the complication rates for patients with initially unresectable tumors who received preoperative chemoradiation therapy were similar to the five-year survival rates of patients with initially resectable tumors.

2. **Chemoradiation therapy.** Conformal (three-dimensional) radiation therapy and intra-arterial fluorodeoxyuridine appear to produce a durable response rate and good median survival (19 months) in patients with nondiffuse HCC.

3. **Transcatheter arterial embolization (TAE)** of unresectable HCC using a mixture of gel foam powder and contrast media with or without chemotherapeutic drugs has been used with some success. TAE also may be used preoperatively to reduce intraoperative bleeding or as a palliative measure in patients with far advanced HCC. Reports of delayed formation of gallstones following TAE suggest that elective cholecystectomy may be advisable at the time of partial hepatectomy.

4. **Ethanol injections.** Percutaneous intralesional installation of absolute ethanol under US guidance has a reported five-year survival of nearly 80 percent. Groups of Japanese investigators have found that this technique yields a better survival than surgery, even for resectable lesions.

D. Nonresectable and metastatic disease

1. **Tamoxifen.** About 40 percent of patients with HCC have estrogen receptor protein in the cell cytosol. Large tumors are commonly estrogen receptor-negative. In a prospective, randomized study, tamoxifen (30 mg/day) resulted in a significant improvement in 12-month survival.

2. **Recombinant interferon-α-2a,** 50 million IU/m^2 IM three times a week, resulted in a significant improvement in median survival and more objective tumor regression as compared to the no-treatment group in a recent randomized, placebo-controlled study from China.

3. **Systemic chemotherapy** has a response rate of 20 percent and does not impact on median survival (3–6 months). Adriamycin as a single agent or

in combination with other drugs has been used. Mitoxantrone is as effective as Adriamycin but with less toxicity.

Gall Bladder Cancer

I. Epidemiology and etiology

A. Incidence. Primary gall bladder carcinoma (GBC) is the most malignant tumor of the biliary tract and the fifth most common cancer of the digestive tract. GBCs were found in 1 to 2 percent of operations on the biliary tract.

B. Risk factors. The etiology of GBC remains unknown. The reported risk factors are

  1. **Sex.** The female-male ratio is 3:1 to 4:1. Acalculous carcinoma is also more common in women.
  2. **Race.** The incidence of GBC is doubled in southwest American Indians, who also have a two- to threefold greater incidence of cholelithiasis.
  3. **Older age.** The mean age for the occurrence of GBC is 65 years; the disease is very rare before age 40.
  4. **Chronic cholecystitis and cholelithiasis** are associated with the development of GBC in 50 percent and 75 percent of cases, respectively. Calcification of the wall of the gallbladder (porcelain gallbladder) increases the risk of GBC by 10 to 60 percent. Previous operations on the biliary tract (including cholecystostomy) antedate GBC by a mean of 16 years (range: 1–50 years). Thus malignant degeneration does not require the presence of gall stones.
  5. **Benign neoplasms.** Both inflammatory and cholesterol polyps are associated with appreciable risk. Papillary and nonpapillary adenomas of the gall bladder may contain carcinoma in situ. Malignant transformation is rare, however.
  6. **Ulcerative colitis** increases the risks of extrahepatic biliary cancer by a factor of 5 to 10; 15 percent of these cancers occur in the gall bladder.
  7. **Carcinogens.** Rubber industry employees have a higher incidence and earlier onset of GBC.

II. Pathology and natural history

A. Pathology. Most GBCs are adenocarcinomas showing varying degrees of differentiation. The mucus secreted by this cancer is typically of the sialomucin type in contrast to the sulfomucin type secreted by the normal or inflamed mucous-secreting glands. Other types of GBC include adenoacanthoma, adenosquamous carcinomas, and undifferentiated (anaplastic, pleomorphic, sarcomatoid) carcinomas. Some adenocarcinomas have choriocarcinoma-like elements and others have morphology equivalent to small cell carcinoma.

B. Natural history. GBC has a propensity to involve the liver, stomach, and duodenum by direct extension. The common sites of metastasis are the liver (60%), adjacent organs (55%), regional lymph nodes (35%), peritoneum (25%), and distant visceral organs (30%).

C. Clinical presentation. GBC may present as one of the following clinical syndromes:

  1. **Acute cholecystitis** (15% of patients). These patients appear to have less advanced carcinoma, a higher rate of resectability, and longer survival.
  2. **Chronic cholecystitis** (45%)
  3. **Symptoms suggestive of malignant disease** (e.g., jaundice, weight loss, generalized weakness, anorexia, or persistent right upper quadrant pain) (35%)
  4. **Benign nonbiliary manifestations** (e.g., gastrointestinal bleeding or obstruction) (5%)

III. Diagnosis

A. Symptoms. The lack of specific symptoms prevents detection of GBC at an early stage. Consequently, the diagnosis is usually made unexpectedly at the time of surgery, because the clinical signs commonly mimic benign gall bladder disease. Pain is present in 75 percent of patients; jaundice, anorexia, or nausea and vomiting in 45 percent; weight loss or fatigue in 30 percent; and pruritus or abdominal mass in 15 percent.

B. Physical examination. Certain combinations of symptoms and signs may suggest the diagnosis, such as an elderly woman with history of biliary symptoms that have changed in frequency or severity. A right upper quadrant mass or hepatomegaly and constitutional symptoms suggest GBC.

C. Laboratory examination. Elevated serum alkaline phosphatase was present in 65 percent of patients, anemia in 55 percent, elevated bilirubin in 40 percent, leukocytosis in 40 percent, and leukemoid reaction in 1 percent of patients with GBC. The association of elevated alkaline phosphatase without elevated bilirubin is consistent with GBC; approximately 40 percent of these patients have resectable lesions.

D. Radiologic examination
   1. **Abdominal US** is abnormal in approximately 98 percent of patients. Cholelithiasis, thickened gall bladder wall, a mass in the gallbladder or a combination of these are the most common findings. US is diagnostic of GBC in only 20 percent of cases, however.
   2. **CT** of the abdomen may be diagnostic in 50 percent of patients.
   3. **Percutaneous transhepatic cholangiography** (PTHC) is abnormal in 80 percent of cases and diagnostic in 40 percent.
   4. **ERCP** is abnormal in approximately 75 percent of cases and diagnostic in 25 percent.

IV. **Staging and prognostic factors**
   A. Staging. There are two commonly used staging systems: the American Joint Commission to Cancer Staging (AJCC) system (stages 0–IV) and Nevin system (stages 1–5).
   Stage I: An intramuscular lesion or muscular invasion unrecognized at operation and later discovered by the pathologist.
   Stage II: Transmural invasion.
   Stage III: Lymph node involvement.
   Stage IV: Involvement of two or more adjacent organs, or more than 2 cm invasion of liver, or distant metastasis.

   B. Prognostic factors. The overall median survival of patients with GBC is six months. After surgical resection only 27 percent are alive at one year, 19 percent at three years, and 13 percent at five years. Stage of the disease is the most significant prognostic factor. The five-year survival following surgical resection is 65 to 100 percent for stage I, 30 percent for stage II, 15 percent for stage III, and 0 percent for stage IV. Poorly differentiated (higher grade) tumors and the presence of jaundice are associated with poorer survival. Ploidy patterns do not correlate with survival.

V. **Prevention.** Cholecystectomy has been recommended to prevent GBC. For every 100 gallbladders removed, there is one patient with GBC. However, the overall mortality of cholecystectomy is also approximately 1 percent (including patients with diabetes and gangrenous gallbladder as well as patients with cholangitis or gallstone pancreatitis).

VI. **Management.** Despite the improvement of diagnostic capabilities, better perioperative care, and more aggressive surgical approach, GBC remains a terminal illness in most patients.
   A. Cholecystectomy is the only effective treatment. The best chance for long-term survival is the serendipitous discovery of an early cancer at the time of cholecystectomy. Radical cholecystectomy or resection of adjacent structure has not resulted in better survival.
   B. RT appears to have no added benefit in the adjuvant setting. RT may be useful as a primary treatment (without surgical resection) using either external-beam RT alone or external-beam RT plus iridium 192 implants. RT may relieve pain in a small number of patients.
   C. Chemotherapy. The data on adjuvant systemic chemotherapy are anecdotal.

5-FU-based combinations are most commonly used, but the response rates are poor.

Extrahepatic Bile Duct Cancer

I. Epidemiology and etiology

A. Epidemiology. Bile duct carcinomas (BDCs, cholangiocarcinomas) are rare and occur with equal frequency in males and females at the average age of 60 years. Tumors arising from the intrahepatic bile ducts are discussed with liver cancers. BDC accounts for less than one-third of biliary tract cancer; GBC is the most common type. Half of patients with BDC have undergone cholecystectomy for cholelithiasis.

B. Etiology and risk factors. An increased incidence of BDC has been reported in patients with Crohn's disease, choledocholithiasis, cystic fibrosis, chronic long-term ulcerative colitis, sclerosing cholangitis, and *Clonorchis sinensis* infestation. The incidence is also reportedly increased in patients with congenital anomalies of the intrahepatic and extrahepatic bile ducts (e.g., cysts, congenital dilatation of the bile ducts, choledochal cyst, Caroli's disease, congenital hepatic fibrosis, polycystic disease, abnormal pancreaticocholedochal junction).

II. Pathology

A. Histology. Malignant tumors of the bile ducts are usually adenocarcinoma. Microscopically, BDCs generally extend to 1 to 4 cm beyond the gross margin of the tumor. Multiple foci of carcinoma in situ may be noted. Other malignant tumors that involve the bile ducts include anaplastic and squamous carcinomas, cystadenocarcinomas, primary malignant melanoma, leiomyosarcoma, carcinosarcoma, and metastatic tumors (particularly breast cancer, myelomas, and lymphomas). See *Liver Cancer,* **II.A.4–6.**

B. Location. BDCs are divided anatomically into those that arise from the upper third of the biliary tract, including the hilum (50–70% of all tumors); the middle third (10–25%); the lower third (10–20%); and the cystic duct (<1%). Tumors found near the junction of the right and left hepatic duct (Klatskin tumor) are usually small and may be inconspicuous at laparotomy. Adenocarcinomas located in the right and left hepatic ducts or common hepatic duct are frequently scirrhous, constricting, diffusely infiltrating, or nodular and may mimic sclerosing cholangitis or stricture. Adenocarcinomas of the common bile duct or cystic duct are more often fungating and may have a better prognosis. Carcinoma of the cystic duct is rare, and distention of the gallbladder occurs before jaundice becomes apparent.

III. Diagnosis

A. Symptoms. Jaundice is present in 90 percent of patients. Abdominal pain, weight loss, fever, malaise, or hepatomegaly occurs in 50 percent of cases. Patients with proximal tumors in the upper third of the biliary tract usually have symptoms twice as long as those with tumors in the lower third. Ascites, spider angiomas, and splenomegaly are seen in less than 3 percent of patients.

B. Laboratory studies

1. **Serum chemistries.** Serum bilirubin greater than or equal to 7.5 mg/dl is found in 60 percent of cases, alkaline phosphatase greater than twice normal in 80 percent, and elevation of transaminase and prothrombin time in 25 percent.

2. **Tumor marker.** Serum CA 19-9 is elevated in 90 percent of patients.

3. **Radiologic examination**

   a. **Abdominal US** shows dilatation of the common bile duct or intrahepatic biliary ducts.

   b. **CT** may reveal a mass and suggest the site or origin of carcinoma.

   c. **PTHC** is the most specific test for proximal bile duct lesions.

   d. **ERCP** is the best diagnostic test for distal bile duct tumors.

      e. Angiography and portovenography are useful in determining the extent of the disease for the preoperative evaluation of resectability.

IV. Staging and prognostic factors

A. Staging. All patients should be initially staged so that those individuals with unresectable tumors are not subjected to needless surgery. If PTHC shows that the tumor extends into the parenchyma of both the right and left lobes of the liver, the tumor is unresectable, and no surgery is performed. If angiography shows encasement of the main portal vein or hepatic artery, the tumor is also unresectable. If, however, the tumor extends into only one lobe or there is involvement of one branch of the portal vein or hepatic artery, then surgical exploration is considered with the possibility of adding hepatic lobectomy to the hepatic duct resection. The criteria (Blumgart's) for unresectability are

1. Bilateral intrahepatic duct involvement.
2. Entrapment of the main trunk of the portal vein.
3. Bilateral invasion of the branches of the portal vein or hepatic artery.
4. Ductal involvement in the contralateral lobe.

B. Prognostic factors. The poor prognostic variables with statistical significance are mass lesion, cachexia, poor performance status, serum bilirubin greater than or equal to 9 mg/dl, multicentric disease, hilar or proximal sites, high tumor grade, sclerotic histology, liver invasion, lymph node involvement, and advanced stage.

V. Management

A. Surgical resection is the only treatment that may result in long-term survival. In specialized medical centers approximately 45 percent of patients who are explored undergo complete resection with no gross tumor left behind, 10 percent have an incomplete resection, and 45 percent are not resectable. Tumors in the middle and distal ducts have a higher resectability rate than tumors in the proximal ducts, which have a maximal resectability rate of 20 percent. The median survival of patients whose tumors are resected for cure is 11 to 33 months, and the five-year survival is approximately 12 percent. The 30-day operative mortality may be as high as 25 percent. The high postoperative complication rate includes wound infection, cholangitis, liver abscess, subphrenic abscess, pancreatitis, and biliary fistulae.

B. Adjuvant therapy has been advocated to reduce the high incidence of local recurrence (up to 100%), but it does not appear to improve survival after curative resection. The role of adjuvant RT remains unclear. Cholangiocarcinoma is radiosensitive but bile duct tolerance to radiation is limited. The complications of RT include biliary and duodenal stenosis.

C. Biliary tract bypass

1. **Surgical biliary tract bypass** is carried out predominantly in those patients whose tumors are found to be unresectable at operation. Biliary-enteric anastomosis is usually performed using roux-en-y jejunal loop. The operative mortality ranges from 0 to 30 percent and the median survival varies from 11 to 16 months. The theoretical advantage of operative drainage is the decreased potential for recurrent cholangitis.
2. **Surgical stenting.** T-tube or U-tube catheters can be passed through the obstruction. A T-tube is hard to replace when it becomes clogged. The advantage of a U-tube is that both of its ends are externalized separately, making replacement easy when the tube becomes obstructed. The 30-day mortality for operative stenting varies from 10 to 20 percent.
3. **Endoscopic stenting** has two advantages: a decreased morbidity and no creation of external fistulization. This method is more successful with distal bile duct tumors and is associated with a 30-day mortality of 10 to 20 percent.
4. **Percutaneous stenting** to provide drainage, either as externalized stent or an endoprosthesis, is associated with a 30-day mortality of 15 to 35 percent.

D. Other methods of treatment

1. **Liver transplant** is not considered appropriate because of the high incidence of local recurrence.

2. **RT** appears to have some effect on the tumor size and may relieve jaundice in patients without biliary stenting. RT may be used (usually with biliary stenting) either as primary treatment or as adjuvant therapy. Conventional external beam RT has the advantage of giving a moderately high dose of radiation (5000–6000 cGy) to a relatively large volume of tissue and is more effective in treating bulky tumor masses. Implantation with iridium 192 seeds (effective radius of 1 cm from the seeds) delivers high-dose RT to localized residual disease after surgical resection or may provide palliation to patients with bile ducts obstructed by tumor. The typical dose with iridium 192 seeds is 2000 cGy.

3. **Chemotherapy** is of no benefit. 5-FU is ineffective with a response rate of 8 percent. Combinations of 5-FU with nitrosoureas showed no better responses.

Cancer of the Ampulla of Vater

I. **Pathology.** Carcinoma of the ampulla of Vater is a papillary neoplasm arising in the last part of the common bile duct where it passes through the duodenum. Distinction between true ampullary tumor and periampullary tumors originating in the duodenal mucosa or pancreatic ducts is important because the periampullary cancers have a poor prognosis. The differentiation may be made by examination of the mucins they produce. Ampullary cancer produces sialomucins, whereas periampullary cancers produce sulfated mucins.

II. **Staging system and prognostic factors.** The TNM staging system is now used to stage ampullary cancer. The prognosis of patients with ampullary carcinoma is better than cancer arising in any other site in the biliary tree. Pancreatic invasion and lymph node metastasis are the two most important prognostic factors. Five-year survival is in excess of 50 percent when no nodal metastasis and no invasion of the pancreas have occurred. Nodal metastasis, which is directly related to the size of the tumor, occurs much more frequently in patients with tumors larger than 2.5 cm.

III. **Management.** Surgery is the only curative treatment modality for ampullary carcinoma. Pancreaticoduodenal resection (Whipple's procedure or a modification) is the surgical procedure of choice. The five-year survival ranges from 5 to 55 percent depending on lymph node involvement, invasion of the pancreas, and histologic differentiation. Ampullectomy (local ampullary excision) performed on poor-risk patients with apparently localized disease is associated with a 10 percent five-year survival.

Selected Reading

Esophageal Cancer

Forastiere, A. A., et al. Preoperative chemoradiation followed by transhiatal esophagectomy for carcinoma of the esophagus: Final report. *J. Clin. Oncol.* 11:1118, 1993.

Herskovic, A., et al. Combined chemotherapy and radiotherapy compared with radiotherapy alone in patients with cancer of the esophagus. *N. Engl. J. Med.* 326: 1593, 1992.

Kelsen, D. P. (ed.). Esophageal cancer. *Semin. Oncol.* 21 (4):401, 1994 (entire issue).

Pritikin, J., et al. Endoscopic laser therapy in gastroenterology. *West. J. Med.* 157:48, 1992.

Silk, Y., and Nava, H. Endoprosthesis for malignant esophageal stricture. *Contemp. Surg.* 36:11, 1990.

Tio, T. L., et al. Endosonography and computed tomography of esophageal carcinoma. *Gastroenterology* 96:1478, 1989.

Gastric Cancer

Atiq, O. T., et al. Phase II trial of postoperative adjuvant intraperitoneal cisplatinum and fluorouracil and systemic fluorouracil chemotherapy in patients with resected gastric cancer. *J. Clin. Oncol.* 11:425, 1993.

Cady, B., et al. Gastric adenocarcinoma: A disease in transition. *Arch. Surg.* 124:303, 1989.

Hagiwara, A. Prophylaxis with carbon-absorbed mitomycin against peritoneal recurrence of gastric cancer. *Lancet* 339:629, 1992.

Hermans, J., et al. Adjuvant therapy after curative resection for gastric cancer: Meta-analysis of randomized trials. *J. Clin. Oncol.* 11:1441, 1993.

Ichikura, T., et al. Comparison of the prognostic significance between the number of metastatic lymph nodes and nodal stage based on their location in patients with gastric cancer. *J. Clin. Oncol.* 11:1894, 1993.

Sugarbaker, P. H., et al. Rationale for integrating early post-operative intraperitoneal chemotherapy in the surgical treatment of gastrointestinal cancer. *Semin. Oncol.* 6:83, 1989.

Sundt, T. M. III, et al. Ménétrier's Disease. A trivalent gastropathy. *Ann. Surg.* 208:694, 1988.

Colorectal Cancer

Bernstein, C. N., et al. Are we telling patients the truth about surveillance colonoscopy in ulcerative colitis. *Lancet* 343:71, 1994.

Bond, J. H., et al. Polyp guideline: Diagnosis, treatment and surveillance for patients with nonfamilial colorectal polyps. *Ann. Intern. Med.* 119:836, 1993.

DeCosse, J. J., et al. Colorectal cancer: Detection, treatment and rehabilitation. *Cancer* 44:27, 1994.

Giardiello, F. M., et al. Treatment of colonic and rectal adenomas with sulindac in familial adenomatous polyposis. *N. Engl. J. Med.* 328:1313, 1993.

Jen, J., et al. Allelic loss of chromosome 18q and prognosis in colorectal cancer. *N. Engl. J. Med.* 331:213, 1994.

Lennard-Jones, J. E., et al. Precancer and cancer in extensive ulcerative colitis: Findings among 401 patients over 22 years. *Gut* 31:800, 1990.

Moertel, C. G., et al. Fluorouracil plus levamisole as effective adjuvant therapy after resection of stage III colon carcinoma: A final report. *Ann. Int. Med.* 122:321, 1995.

Moertel, C. G., Chemotherapy for colorectal cancer. *N. Engl. J. Med.* 330:1136, 1994.

Peleg, H., et al. Aspirin and nonsteroidal anti-inflammatory drug use and the risk of subsequent colorectal cancer. *Arch. Intern. Med.* 154:394, 1994.

Sandler, R. S., et al. Smoking, alcohol and risk for colorectal cancer. *Gastroenterology* 104:1445, 1993.

Winawer, S. J., et al. Prevention of colorectal cancer by colonoscopic polypectomy. *N. Engl. J. Med.* 329:1977, 1993.

Anal Cancer

Doci, R., et al. Combined chemoradiation therapy for anal cancer. A report of 56 cases. *Ann. Surg.* 215:150, 1992.

Johnson, D., et al. Carcinoma of the anus treated with primary radiation therapy and chemotherapy. *Surg. Gynecol. Obst.* 177:329, 1993.

Jones, R. D., et al. Changes in the radiation treatment of cancer of the anus in Glasgow. *Br. J. Radiol.* 66:797, 1993.

Martenson, J. A. Jr., and Gunderson, L. L. External radiation therapy without chemotherapy in the management of anal cancer. *Cancer* 71:1736, 1993.

Melbye, M., et al. High incidence of anal cancer among AIDS patients. The AIDS/Cancer Working Group. *Lancet* 343:636, 1994.

Pancreatic Cancer

Cameron, J. L., et al. Factors influencing survival after pancreaticoduodenectomy for pancreatic cancer. *Am. J. Surg.* 161:120, 1991.

Ekbom, A., et al. Pancreatitis and pancreatic cancer: A population-based study. *J. Natl. Cancer Inst.* 86:625, 1994.

Gastrointestinal Study Group. Further evidence of effective adjuvant combined radiation and chemotherapy following curative resection of pancreatic cancer. *Cancer* 59:2006, 1987.

Gudjonsson, B. Cancer of the pancreas 50 years of surgery. *Cancer* 60:2284, 1987.

Haddock, G., and Carter, D. C. Aetiology of pancreatic cancer. *Br. J. Surg.* 77:1159, 1990.

Permert, J., et al. Islet amyloid polypeptide in patients with pancreatic cancer and diabetes. *N. Engl. J. Med.* 330:313, 1994.

Prandoni, P., et al. Deep vein thrombosis and the incidence of subsequent symptomatic cancer. *N. Engl. J. Med.* 327:1128, 1992.

Singh, S. M., Longmire, W. P. Jr., and Reber, H. A. Surgical palliation for pancreatic cancer. The UCLA experience. *Ann. Surg.* 212:132, 1990.

Snady, H. Endoscopic ultrasonography: An effective new tool for diagnosing gastrointestinal tumors. *Oncology* 6:63, 1992.

Warshaw, A. L., et al. Preoperative staging and assessment of resectability of pancreatic cancer. *Arch. Surg.* 125:230, 1990.

Liver Cancer

Ellis, L. M., et al. Current strategies for the treatment of hepatocellular carcinoma. *Curr. Opin. Oncol.* 4:741, 1992.

Gyorffy, E. J., et al. Transformation of hepatic cell adenoma into hepatocellular carcinoma due to oral contraceptive use. *Ann. Intern. Med.* 110:489, 1989.

Lai, C. L., et al. Recombinant interferon-alpha in inoperable hepatocellular carcinoma: A randomized controlled trial. *Hepatology* 17:389, 1993.

Robertson, J. M. Treatment of primary hepatobiliary carcinoma with conformal radiation therapy and regional chemotherapy. *J. Clin. Oncol.* 11:1286, 1993.

Sato, Y., et al. Early recognition of hepatocellular carcinoma based on altered profiles of alpha-fetoprotein. *N. Engl. J. Med.* 328:1802, 1993.

Simonelti, R. G., et al. Hepatitis C virus infection as a risk factor for hepatocellular carcinoma in patients with cirrhosis. *Ann. Intern. Med.* 116:97, 1992.

Sitzmann, J. V., and Abrams, R. Improved survival for hepatocellular cancer with combined surgery and multimodality treatment. *Ann. Surg.* 217:149, 1993.

Tsukuma, H., et al. Risk factors for hepatocellular carcinoma among patients with chronic liver disease. *N. Engl. J. Med.* 328:1797, 1993.

Venook, A. P. Treatment of hepatocellular carcinoma: Too many options. *J. Clin. Oncol.* 12:1323, 1994.

Gall Bladder Cancer

Chao, T. C., and Greager, J. A. Primary carcinoma of the gallbladder. *J. Surg. Oncol.* 46:215, 1991.

Donohue, J. H., et al. Carcinoma of the gallbladder. Does radical resection improve outcome? *Arch. Surg.* 125:237, 1990.

Silk, Y. N., et al. Carcinoma of the gallbladder. The Roswell Park experience. *Ann. Surg.* 210:751, 1989.

Extrahepatic Bile Duct Cancer

Blumgart, L. H. *Surgery of the Liver and Biliary Tract,* vol. 2. Edinburgh, New York: Churchill Livingstone, 1988. Pp. 829–51.

Cameron, J. L., et al. Management of proximal cholangiocarcinoma by surgical resection and radiation therapy. *Am. J. Surg.* 159:91, 1990.

Magistrelli, P., et al. Changing attitudes in the palliation of proximal malignant biliary obstruction. *J. Surg. Oncol.* 3:151, 1993.

Nagorney, D. M., et al. Outcomes after curative resection of cholangiocarcinoma. *Arch. Surg.* 128:871, 1993.

Strom, B. L., et al. Pathophysiology of tumor progression in human gallbladder: Flow cytometry, CEA, CA 19-9 levels in bile and serum in different stages gallbladder disease. *J. Natl. Cancer Inst.* 81:1575, 1989.

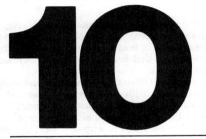

Breast Cancer

Charles M. Haskell and
Dennis A. Casciato

I. Epidemiology and etiology
A. Incidence
1. Breast cancer is the most common lethal neoplasm in women. The ACS has estimated that breast cancer will comprise 32 percent of all new malignant neoplasms and 18 percent of deaths from cancer in women. The annual incidence of breast cancer in the United States increases dramatically with age (5 per 100,000 at age 25, rising to 150 per 100,000 at age 50 and over 200 per 100,000 by age 75).
2. The incidence of male breast cancer is about 2.5 per 100,000. Fewer than 1 percent of all breast cancer cases occur in men.

B. Etiology. Breast cancer is the result of mutations in one or more **critical genes.** Two genes in women on chromosome 17 have been implicated. The most important gene is called BRCA1 (at 17q21); the other is the p53 gene (at 17p13). A third gene is the BRCA2 gene on chromosome 13. A fourth gene implicated in the etiology of breast cancer is the androgen receptor gene, found on the Y chromosome. Mutations of the latter gene have been associated with several cases of male breast cancer but not female breast cancer. Implicated in the etiology of breast cancer is the androgen receptor gene, found on the Y chromosome. Mutations of this gene have been associated with several cases of male breast cancer but not female breast cancer.

The best established etiologic agent in breast cancer is exposure to **radiation.** This presumably works by inducing critical mutations in BRCA1 or perhaps a related gene that is yet to be discovered. A viral etiology has also been postulated but never proved in humans.

Complex experimental and epidemiologic evidence points strongly to the influence of **hormones** and **diet** in the pathogenesis of breast cancer. The variation of incidence of breast cancer in different populations is highly correlated with consumption of dietary fat, dietary sugar, or parity in 75 percent of cases affecting postmenopausal women and in about 50 percent of cases affecting premenopausal women.

1. **Diet.** Diets in Western countries typically have a high content of fat and sugar. The dietary contents of both fat and total calories independently strongly correlate with the incidence of breast cancer. Women from Western countries have about six times the risk of breast cancer as do women from Asian or underdeveloped countries. The risk of breast cancer increases progressively with age except in countries with low-fat diets where the risk is stabilized or decreased in older women. The risk changes accordingly when populations move from a low-risk country to a high-risk country and adopt the dietary habits of the new country. However, it is likely that the impact of diet on breast cancer incidence occurs at an early age, such as in childhood or adolescence. Currently no data in humans prove that changing from a high-fat diet to a low-fat diet later in life reduces the risk of breast cancer.
2. **Hormones.** There is ample evidence implicating hormones in the etiology of breast cancer, but the role of individual hormones is uncertain. High prolactin levels are clearly related to the development of breast cancer in animal models, but epidemiologic evidence is conflicting, and a causative relationship between prolactin and breast cancer has not been proved in

human beings. Estrogens, either alone or in combination with progestins in various oral contraceptive preparations, are also of concern. Short-term studies have shown no increased risk of breast cancer from oral contraceptives, whereas other studies suggest that long-term use may increase the risk of breast cancer in young women.

3. **Links between diet and hormones.** Differences in estrogen and prolactin levels in female populations correlate with differences in dietary fat; that is, high-fat diets are associated with increased hormone secretion. Furthermore, obesity is associated with increased adrenal production of androstenedione, which is converted to estrogens in adipose tissue; this source of production and conversion continues after menopause. Finally, tumor-promoting steroid hormones are also fat-soluble and likewise may be accumulated in breast tissue. Whichever hormones, biochemical pathways, or physiologic interactions are most operative, links between diet and hormones and the development of breast cancer are clearly present.

4. **Hereditary breast cancer.** Familial aggregations of breast cancer occur in about 18 percent of cases, but only about 5 percent of cases can be considered truly familial based on extended pedigree analysis. Most of these are due to mutations in the BRCA1 and BRCA2 genes. The disease tends to occur at an earlier age and to be bilateral in patients with familial breast cancer. It can also be associated with carcinomas developing in other organs (especially the colon, ovary, or uterus), or with other rare cancers (sarcomas, brain, leukemia, adrenal glands) as part of the Li-Fraumeni syndrome associated with mutations in the p53 gene. Familial transmission can occur through either the maternal or paternal germ line as an autosomal dominant trait. In such families, the lifetime risk of females developing breast cancer is at least 50 percent.

C. **Risk factors for breast cancer**
   1. **High-risk factors** (threefold or more increase)
      a. **Age** (more than 40 years old).
      b. **Previous cancer in one breast,** especially if it occurred before menopause.
      c. **Breast cancer in the family.** Increased occurrence of breast cancer is seen in mothers, daughters, and sisters particularly, but also in aunts, cousins, and grandmothers. Mothers, daughters, and sisters of women who develop bilateral or unilateral breast cancer before menopause have a higher risk of developing breast cancer.
      d. **Hyperplasia with atypia.** Most forms of benign breast disease do not predispose patients to the subsequent development of breast cancer. This is especially true of "fibrocystic disease." Women with proliferative disease of the breast with atypical hyperplasia (atypia) have an increased risk of developing breast cancer (fivefold increase), however. The risk of atypia is greater in patients with a strong family history of breast cancer (11-fold increase).
      e. **Parity.** Women who are nulliparous or who were first pregnant after the age of 31 years are three to four times more likely to develop breast cancer than those who complete the first pregnancy before the age of 18.
      f. **Lobular carcinoma in situ** carries a 30 percent risk of invasive cancer.
      g. **Risk factors in men.** Klinefelter's syndrome, gynecomastia, and family history of male breast cancer.
   2. **Intermediate risk factors** (1.2- to 1.5-fold increase)
      a. Menstruation history of
         (1) Early menarche
         (2) Late menopause
      b. Oral estrogens (see sec. I.B.2) in women
      c. History of cancer of the ovary, uterine fundus, or colon
      d. Diabetes mellitus
      e. Use of alcoholic beverages
   3. **Factors known to decrease risk**

   a. Asian ancestry
   b. Term pregnancy before age 18 years
   c. Early menopause
   d. Surgical castration before the age of 37 years
   4. Factors having no effect on risk (previously thought to be risk factors):
   multiparity, lactation, and breast feeding.

II. Pathology and natural history

   A. Histology may influence treatment decisions, but the stage of disease is usually
   more important. Poorly differentiated tumors (high-grade) have a worse prognosis than well-differentiated (low-grade) tumors. Inflammatory carcinoma has a
   very poor prognosis, irrespective of stage. For patients with negative nodes, a
   group of "special tumor types" is associated with a better prognosis (typical
   medullary, mucinous, papillary, and pure tubular types). For early disease without lymph node involvement (stage I), the five-year survival rate is about 80
   percent for invasive ductal carcinomas and 90 to 95 percent for invasive lobular,
   comedocarcinomas, and colloid carcinomas.

   1. Ductal adenocarcinoma (78%) tends to be unilateral. Invasive ductal carcinoma can occur with and without scirrhous components; nearly all male
   breast cancer is of this type. Noninvasive ductal adenocarcinoma (sometimes called ductal carcinoma in situ or intraductal carcinoma) usually occurs without forming a mass because there is no scirrhous component.

   2. Lobular carcinoma (9%). About half of the cases of lobular carcinoma are
   found in situ without any sign of local invasion (this disease is considered
   premalignant by some authorities and has been termed "lobular neoplasia").
   Lobular carcinoma is associated with an increased risk of bilateral breast
   cancer (about one-third of cases). The classic form of the disease (including
   the alveolar and mixed variants) is frequently bilateral, but otherwise it
   has a somewhat better prognosis than infiltrating ductal carcinomas. The
   solid and signet ring cell variants have a worse prognosis than infiltrating
   ductal carcinoma because of a high propensity to metastasize as a diffuse
   or finely nodular infiltrate in the retroperitoneum with prominent desmoplastic (fibrotic) reaction. Taking all forms of invasive lobular carcinoma
   as a group, the overall prognosis is about the same as for infiltrating ductal
   carcinoma.

   3. Special types with a good prognosis (10%). Pure papillary, tubular, mucinous, and typical medullary carcinomas. Adenocystic carcinomas may
   qualify as well, but they are sufficiently rare for this to be uncertain.

   4. Comedocarcinoma (5%). Ducts packed with small cell tumor and central
   debris.

   5. Medullary carcinoma (4%). Undifferentiated cells with a heavy lymphocytic infiltrate.

   6. Colloid carcinoma (3%). Duct is blocked with inspissated carcinoma cells
   and proximal cysts develop.

   7. Inflammatory carcinoma (1%). Poorest prognosis. Lymphatics become
   packed with tumor leading to breast and skin changes that mimic infection.

   8. Paget's disease of the breast. Unilateral eczema of the nipple; always
   associated with ductal carcinoma in women. Prognosis is good if detected
   before a mass is present.

   B. Mode of spread. Breast cancers spread by contiguity, lymphatic channels, and
   blood-borne metastases. The most common organs involved with symptomatic
   metastases are regional lymph nodes, skin, bone, liver, lung, and brain.

   C. Lymph node metastases
   1. Axillary lymph node metastases are present in 55 to 70 percent of patients
   at the time of diagnosis. Clinically normal axillae have histologic evidence
   of metastases in 40 percent of patients.

   2. Axillary dissections lead to removal of an average of 15 to 20 lymph nodes
   (range of 0–80). The prognosis depends on the number of histologically
   positive nodes found and is independent of the number of nodes removed.

3. The number of nodes found to contain tumor increases by up to 30 percent with meticulous serial sectioning.
4. Tumors that grow fast are more likely to metastasize to lymph nodes than tumors that grow slowly.
5. Tumor size is closely associated with the presence of axillary metastases.

Tumor size (cm)	Patients with four or more positive lymph nodes (%)
<1	25
1–2	35
2–3	50
>3	55–65

6. Internal mammary nodes have evidence of tumor in 26 percent of patients with inner quadrant lesions and 15 percent with outer quadrant lesions. Mammary node metastases rarely occur in the absence of axillary node involvement.

D. Natural history. *Breast cancer is a heterogeneous disease, which grows at very different rates in different patients and is often a systemic disease at the time of initial diagnosis.* Evidence for this statement is as follows:

1. **The tumor doubling time of breast cancer.** A 1-cm breast tumor contains about 10^9 cells and has undergone 30 of the 40 doublings that will occur before the patient dies. The tumor doubling time (TDT) of primary breast cancer varies from 25 to 200 days for early lesions, but in advanced disease the TDT may exceed 500 days. Thus, a 1-cm tumor may have been present for 2 to 17 years prior to diagnosis. Biochemical measurements of aneuploidy and rapid cell division predict for early recurrence and early death.

2. **Prognosis is influenced by biochemical markers**
   a. Endocrine tissues contain receptors for critical hormones. Receptors for estrogen (ER) and progesterone (PgR) should be routinely assessed in breast cancer specimen because they are useful in choosing therapy (see sec. **VI.D.1**) and their presence predicts for a better prognosis.
   b. Numerous biochemical changes in breast cancer tissue can influence prognosis, including HER-2/*neu*, cathepsin-D, heat shock protein, nm23, p53, pS2, and PCNA. This area continues to undergo investigation.

3. **Local measures have only a limited effect on survival.** Untreated patients have a median survival of 2.5 years. Patients treated with mastectomy or RT have an improved survival expectancy over untreated patients. However, they continue to die at a faster rate than age-matched controls for the first 20 years after treatment. Whatever the cause of death, 75 to 85 percent of patients with a history of breast cancer have evidence of the tumor at autopsy.

4. **Removal of a primary tumor does not substantially alter the risk of metastases.**
   a. Distant metastases are present in two-thirds of breast cancer patients at the time of diagnosis.
   b. Variation in local therapies (radical, modified radical, or simple mastectomies with or without RT) does not alter survival results.
   c. Patients with axillary lymph node metastases have a high rate of relapse with distant metastases despite apparently complete removal of all local tumor.
   d. Breast cancer that recurs locally is associated with distant metastases in 90 percent of cases.

5. **Regional lymph nodes are harbingers of systemic disease and not barriers to tumor spread.**
   a. Removal of axillary nodes at surgery does not affect the frequency of recurrence, the development of distant metastases, or survival rates.
   b. Half of all patients with four or more positive axillary nodes have clinical evidence of metastatic disease within 18 months.
   c. The 10-year survival rate is about 65 percent for patients without axil-

Table 10-1. Nipple discharges

Type of discharge	Frequency	Approximate chance of cancer
Milky	1%	Negligible
Purulent	5%	Negligible
Multicolored and sticky	10%	Negligible
Serous	35%	5%
Serosanguineous	30%	15%
Bloody	25%	20%
Watery	5%	50%

lary node metastases, 40 percent with one to three positive nodes, and 15 percent with four or more positive nodes.

E. Associated paraneoplastic, metabolic, and neoplastic problems
  1. **Nonmalignant conditions** that may be associated with breast cancer
    a. Dermatomyositis (breast cancer is the most commonly associated malignancy, and treatment of the cancer has been associated with resolution of dermatomyositis)
    b. Acanthosis nigricans
    c. Cushing's syndrome (rare)
    d. Paraneoplastic neuromuscular disorders
    e. Hypercalcemia (only in the presence of metastases)
    f. Hemostatic abnormalities (rare)
  2. **Second malignancies** in patients with breast cancer
    a. Ovarian cancer, especially in familial breast cancer
    b. Colorectal carcinoma
    c. Meningioma

III. Diagnosis
  A. Physical findings and differential diagnosis
    1. **Breast lumps** are detectable in 90 percent of patients with breast cancer and constitute the most common sign on history and physical examination. The typical breast cancer mass has a **dominant character** and tends to be solitary, unilateral, solid, hard, irregular, nonmobile, and nontender.
    2. **Spontaneous nipple discharge** through a mammary duct is the second most common sign of breast cancer. Nipple discharge develops in approximately 3 percent of women and 20 percent of men with breast cancer, but is a manifestation of benign disease in 90 percent of patients. Discharge in patients more than 50 years old is more likely to represent cancerous rather than benign conditions. The character of nipple discharge is quite helpful in establishing a diagnosis (Table 10-1).
      a. **Discharges treated medically.** Milky discharges are galactorrhea, purulent discharges are due to infection, and multicolored or sticky discharges represent duct ectasia. These types of discharge are rarely associated with cancer. Duct ectasia (comedomastitis) appears as burning, itching, and pain associated with palpable subareolar, tortuous, tubular swellings.
      b. **Discharges treated surgically.** Serous, serosanguineous, bloody, or watery discharges may represent intraductal papilloma (usually characterized by nipple discharge without a mass), cysts, or cancer; surgical exploration is imperative.
    3. **Other presenting manifestations** include skin changes, axillary lymphadenopathy, or signs of locally advanced or disseminated disease. A painful breast is a common symptom but is usually a result of something other than

the cancer. Paget's carcinoma appears as unilateral eczema of the nipple. Inflammatory carcinoma appears as skin erythema, edema, and underlying induration in the absence of infection.

    4. Benign lesions resembling breast carcinoma

        a. Lumps. Fibrous tumors, lymphadenitis, calcified fibroadenomas, myoblastomas, posttraumatic fat necrosis, residual inflammatory masses, complex cysts, plasma cell mastitis (sequelae of duct ectasia)

        b. Nipple discharges (see 2)

        c. Skin and nipple changes. Inflammatory diseases, superficial thrombophlebitis (Mondor's disease)

B. Evaluation after discovery of a suspected mass

    1. Biopsy. Any new or previously unevaluated breast mass in any woman of any age that has a "dominant" character must be biopsied without delay.

        a. Skinny-needle aspiration cytology may be performed if both technical and cytopathologic expertise are available. The method is easy, quick, and safe. "Seeding tumor cells along the needle track" is not a consideration in breast cancer. The sensitivity in diagnosing malignancy has been reported to be 90 to 95 percent, with almost no false-positives (98% specificity).

        b. Excisional biopsy. The NIH Consensus Development Program recognizes a two-step procedure as the current standard practice. A diagnostic biopsy specimen should be studied with permanent histologic sections before definitive treatment alternatives are discussed with the patient. The exception to this practice would be for a patient who insists on mastectomy immediately; these patients should undergo complete staging procedures before the biopsy is undertaken.

            (1) Patients should be informed that most breast lumps are benign, but the possibility of cancer is real.

            (2) The biopsy should excise the tumor if it is small.

            (3) Fresh tissue should be sent for ER, PgR, and histologic evaluation.

    2. Cyst aspiration. Patients with a soft, rounded, movable mass are likely to have a cyst that can be managed with aspiration. Local anesthetics may distort the ability to feel if a mass has resolved after aspiration and should therefore be avoided. After aspiration has been attempted, it is necessary to obtain a biopsy specimen under the following circumstances:

        a. No fluid can be aspirated.

        b. Fluid is aspirated, but a mass remains palpable.

        c. The fluid is bloody.

        d. The mass recurs at a two-week follow-up examination.

        e. The cytology examination of the fluid reveals malignancy; these patients require definitive cancer treatment.

    3. Mammography detects 85 percent of breast cancers. Although 15 percent of breast cancers cannot be visualized with mammography, 45 percent of breast cancers can be seen on mammography before they are palpable. A normal mammographic result must not dissuade the physician from obtaining a biopsy of a suspicious mass.

        a. Clear indications for mammography

            (1) Evaluation of suspected benign or malignant breast disease, including an assessment of apparently normal breast tissue in patients with a dominant mass

            (2) Evaluation of the contralateral breast in patients with documented breast cancer

            (3) Follow-up of patients with prior breast cancer

            (4) Follow-up of patients with premalignant breast disease (gross cystic disease, multiple papillomatosis, lobular neoplasia, and severe atypia)

        b. Other possible indications for mammography

            (1) Evaluation of breasts that are difficult to examine

            (2) Workup of metastatic adenocarcinoma from an unknown primary

(3) Evaluation of patients at high risk for breast cancer (especially patients with prior breast augmentation with silicone and patients with a strong family history of breast cancer)

(4) Screening for breast cancer (see sec. **V.B**).

c. **Mammographic signs of malignancy** (sensitivity approximately 75% and specificity almost 90%)

(1) Calcium deposits, unless in a mulberry (fibroadenoma) or curvilinear (cystic disease) pattern

(2) Mammary duct distortion or asymmetry

(3) Skin or nipple thickening

(4) Breast mass

IV. Staging system and prognostic factors

A. Staging system. The standard staging system for breast cancer is the TNM system (Table 10-2). Importantly, regional disease (stage III) is now separated into operable (IIIA) and inoperable disease (IIIB). "Relative survival" rates for each of the stage groupings are also shown in Table 10-2.

B. Prognostic factors and approximate survival

1. Clinical stage

Clinical stage	Five years (%)	Ten years (%)
0	>90	90
I	80	65
II	60	45
IIIA	50	40
IIIB	35	20
IV and inflammatory breast cancer	10	5

2. Histologic involvement of axillary lymph nodes (survival rates shown are for those not treated with adjuvant chemotherapy)

Axillary lymph nodes	Five years (%)	Ten years (%)
None positive	80	65
1–3 positive nodes	65	40
>3 positive nodes	30	15

3. Tumor size

Size of tumor (cm)	Ten years (%)
<1	80
3–4	55
5–7.5	45

4. Hormone receptors. Patients with ER-positive tumors appear to have longer survivals compared to patients with ER-negative tumors.

V. Prevention and early detection

A. Prophylactic mastectomy can be considered only for very high-risk groups. Even "total mastectomy" can leave breast tissue behind, so there is no guarantee that breast cancer will truly be prevented by mastectomy.

1. Prophylactic simple mastectomy and reconstructive surgery can be considered for

a. **Patients with benign breast disease and a family history of bilateral, premenopausal breast cancer** (see sec. I.C.1.c). These patients need to have biopsies done frequently on suspected masses, but the results usually prove to be benign. The morbidity of repeated biopsies may be offset by a definitive procedure. The patient must be informed that even a "total" mastectomy leaves residual breast tissue in situ, so it does not guarantee prevention of later breast cancer.

b. **Patients with a previous history of breast cancer and fibrocystic disease in the remaining breast.**

c. **Patients with lobular carcinoma in situ.**

2. Age for prophylactic mastectomy. The appropriate age is not well defined.

Table 10-2. Postoperative-pathologic staging system for breast cancer

TNM classification			Stage grouping		Relative survival[a]	
Primary tumor (T)	Lymph nodes (N)	Distant metastases (M)	Stage[b]	TNM classification	3-year	6-year
T_0: No demonstrable tumor in breasts	—	M_0: Absent	—	—	—	—
T_{IS}: Noninvasive carcinoma in situ or Paget's disease of the nipple	N_x: IAN unknown	M_1: Present	0	T_{IS} N_0 M_0	100%	98%
T_1: Greatest dimension: ≤2 cm	N_0: IAN negative		I	T_{IS} N_x M_0	98%	95%
T_{1a} ≤0.5 cm	N_1: IAN positive but not fixed;		IIA	T_1 N_0 M_0	95%	84%
T_{1b} >0.5, ≤1 cm	N_{1a}: None >0.2 cm[b]		IIB	T_0 N_1 M_0	84%	66%
T_{1c} >1.0, ≤2 cm	N_{1b}: Any >0.2 cm			T_1 N_1 M_0		
T_2: Greatest dimension: >2 cm and ≤5 cm	N_2: IAN positive and fixed		IIIA	T_2 N_0 M_0	68%	49%
T_3: Greatest dimension: >5 cm	N_3: Ipsilateral internal mammary lymph node metastases			T_2 N_1 M_0		
T_4: Any size with[c]:	Any status		IIIB	T_3 N_0 M_0	64%	46%
T_{4a}: Extension to chest wall				T_{0-2} N_2 M_0		
T_{4b}: Skin ulceration, edema nodules				T_3 N_{1-2} M_0		
T_{4c}: Both T_{4a} and T_{4b}			IV	T_4 Any N M_0	34%	15%
T_{4d}: Inflammatory carcinoma				Any T N_3 M_0		
Any size				Any T Any N M_1		

Key: IAN = ipsilateral axillary nodes.

[a] Relative survival rates according to stage of disease are adapted from data obtained from more than 50,000 patients by the National Cancer Institute between 1983 and 1987.

[b] The prognosis of patients with N_{1a} is similar to that of patients with N_0.

[c] Skin dimpling and nipple retraction do not affect staging classification. Inflammatory carcinoma of the breast is characterized by diffuse, brawny induration of the skin with an erysipeloid edge, usually with no underlying palpable mass.

Source: Adapted from the *American Joint Committee for Cancer Staging and End-Results Reporting,* 1992.

Such patients should be apprised of the risks involved, followed carefully, and be prepared to consider prophylactic mastectomy after they reach 30 years of age.

B. Screening women for breast cancer is controversial because the long-term survival advantage of detecting small lesions early on is not established. The most aggressive recommendations for screening are those of the ACS. They are briefly summarized here for reference.

   1. **Monthly self-examination** for all women more than 20 years of age. Premenopausal women should perform the examination five days after the end of the menstrual cycle; postmenopausal women should examine themselves on the same day each month.

   2. **Physical examination** by a physician every three years for women between 20 and 40 years of age and annually for women over 40 years of age.

   3. **Mammography.** Current mammographic techniques using dedicated film screen equipment expose the breast to 0.02 cGy for a two-view study; xeromammography increases this dose two- to threefold. An exposure of 1.0 cGy is expected to increase the risk of breast cancer by six cases per million population.

      a. Annual mammograms have been demonstrated to reduce breast cancer mortality in women over 50 years of age.

      b. The ACS recommends a mammogram as a baseline for women 35 to 39 years old, and mammograms every 1 to 2 years for women 40 to 49 years old, and yearly for women age 50 and older.

      c. The NCI makes no recommendations for mammographic screening before age 50, but does recommend annual mammography after age 50.

VI. Management

A. Pretreatment staging procedures

   1. **Clinical stages I and II**

      a. CBC, LFTs, calcium and phosphorous levels

      b. Chest x-ray film

      c. Mammography

      d. Bone scan or liver scan are not indicated unless signs, symptoms, or biochemical tests suggest an abnormality.

   2. **Clinical stages III and IV**

      a. Same as for stages I and II (see sec. **VI.A.1.a–c**)

      b. Liver scan (usually by CT)

      c. Bone scan (routine) with plain film correlation

      d. Bone marrow aspiration if there is unexplained cytopenia or leukoerythroblastic blood smear

B. Limited local disease: stages I and II.

There is no clearcut survival difference between total mastectomy with axillary node dissection ("modified radical mastectomy") and limited surgery ("tylectomy" or "total gross removal" or "quadrantectomy") followed by definitive radiation therapy for the local treatment of breast cancer. In some cases there are distinct medical reasons for choosing one form of local therapy over the other and the patient should be so informed. However, the ultimate choice of therapy is strongly influenced by the personal values and fears of the individual patient and the final choice is hers. The physician's primary responsibility is to help the patient decide by carefully describing the advantages and disadvantages of each treatment strategy. In either case, the Reach for Recovery Program of the ACS may facilitate the rehabilitation of the patient after the completion of primary therapy. Controversy surrounds the question of adjuvant therapy for presumed micrometastatic tumor in patients with stage II disease and in selected cases with other risk factors predicting a poorer prognosis (e.g., ER-negative disease and highly undifferentiated tumors).

   1. **Total mastectomy with axillary node dissection (modified radical mastectomy)** is currently the standard surgical procedure for patients who choose surgery as their only local treatment. Removal of the axillary nodes is of both therapeutic and staging value. It is generally unnecessary to use

adjunctive RT after this procedure unless there are large numbers of axillary lymph nodes involved by tumor or extensive lymphatic vascular invasion.

a. Contraindications to surgery. Patient cannot tolerate operation.

b. Advantages of mastectomy

   (1) This is the most efficient and reliable way to control local tumor, and it eliminates residual breast tissue that is at risk of developing a new primary neoplasm.

   (2) If adjuvant chemotherapy is needed later, it is much easier to give after surgery than after RT.

c. Disadvantages and complications of mastectomy

   (1) Cosmetic deformity (can be largely corrected by reconstruction or managed by the use of a prosthesis)

   (a) Indications for breast reconstruction include the availability of adequate skin and soft tissue for a reasonable cosmetic result and realistic expectations on the part of the patient.

   (b) Contraindications for breast reconstruction include inflammatory carcinoma, the presence of extensive radiation damage to the skin from prior treatment, unrealistic expectations on the part of the patient, and the presence of comorbid diseases that render surgery dangerous.

   (2) Lymphedema (about 5%); nerve damage (rarely significant)

2. **RT following limited surgery** involves the total gross removal of tumor by surgery (lumpectomy), an axillary node dissection for staging purposes, and then a protracted course of RT, which takes about six weeks. Most of the radiation is given as megavoltage gamma irradiation to the entire breast (about 4500–5000 cGy), and the remainder is given as a boost to the area of the biopsy (1000–2000+ cGy by electron beam or ^{192}iridium implants).

a. Contraindications to limited surgery plus RT

   (1) Multicentric carcinoma in the breast (a relative but not absolute contraindication).

   (2) Original carcinoma not visualized by mammography (a relative contraindication that relates to the need to follow these patients for local recurrence after RT).

   (3) Large, pendulous breasts (poor cosmesis).

   (4) Paget's disease (relative contraindication).

   (5) Very extensive intraductal (in situ) carcinoma in the original biopsy or reexcision specimen with positive or uncertain margins. This predicts for a high rate of local recurrence after RT (about 25%).

b. Advantages of limited surgery plus RT

   (1) Cosmetic appearance.

   (2) Retention of breast.

c. Disadvantages and complications of limited surgery plus RT

   (1) The retained breast can be a site of recurrent breast cancer or a new primary neoplasm. Careful follow-up with physical examination and mammography is therefore mandatory. Local recurrence mandates mastectomy.

   (2) RT is protracted and may be complicated by skin erythema, ulceration, inflammatory fibrosis of the breast, radiation pneumonitis or pericarditis, rib fractures, or delayed carcinogenesis.

3. **Adjuvant therapy: rationale.** Most women with invasive carcinoma of the breast have a systemic disease in which "micrometastases" have already occurred by the time of initial treatment with surgery or radiation therapy. Since the available forms of systemic therapy are only palliative when used at the time of definite metastatic disease, "adjuvant" therapy has been given immediately after local treatment with the intent of curing the patient of residual micrometastases and is now a standard part of medical practice.

Table 10-3 summarizes the results of a "meta-analysis" of 75,000 women treated with chemotherapy, endocrine therapy, or both. This population comprised 90 percent of patients ever entered into 133 randomized trials

Table 10-3. Meta-analysis of adjuvant therapy for breast cancer

Analyzed treatment group	Control group	Number of patients	Effect on overall survival: reduction in annual odds of death from any cause[a] (% ± SD)
Patients aged <50 years			
TAM alone	Nil	2216	17 ± 10[b]
TAM + CT	CT	6362	3 ± 5
CT alone	Nil	2976	27 ± 6
CT + TAM	TAM	386	−6 ± 23[b]
OA alone	Nil	878	28 ± 9[b]
OA + CT	CT	939	19 ± 11[b]
Patients aged >50 years			
TAM alone	Nil	13,114	19 ± 3
TAM + CT	CT	8148	20 ± 4
CT alone	Nil	3745	14 ± 5
CT + TAM	TAM	3932	10 ± 7
	Total Patients	42,696	

Key: CT = polychemotherapy; TAM = tamoxifen; OA = ovarian ablation; SD = standard deviation.

[a]The annual odds of death is the probability of dying during the year divided by the probability of surviving the year. The ratio of the odds (called odds ratio) for the treatment group relative to the control group is a measure of whether the treatment reduces mortality. An odds ratio of 1.0 indicates equivalent outcomes for treatment and control groups, while an odds ratio of <1.0 indicates a reduction in the odds of death for the treatment group; 100 × (1.0 − estimated odds ratio) gives the percent reduction in annual odds of death.

[b]Estimated treatment effects that have an SD of 9 or greater are considered unstable (or insecure).

Source: The data are from the Early Breast Cancer Trialists' Collaborative Group in the *Lancet* 339:1 and 71, 1992. This table and analysis are adapted with permission from Gelber, R. D., et al. Adjuvant therapy for breast cancer: Understanding the overview. (International Breast Cancer Study Group) as published in *J. Clin. Oncol.* 11:580, 1993.

comparing various adjuvant treatment modalities for operable breast cancer. This analysis was a major, unique effort utilizing an "arithmetic construct" to increase statistical power that demonstrated the following:

a. Treated patients had a continuously increasing survival benefit for more than five years after adjuvant systemic therapy. Survival curves of patients treated with compared modalities continue to remain separated and to diverge further with additional follow-up. Comparable results were seen in the effect of treatments on disease-free survival.

b. Unequivocally, multiple agent cytotoxic chemotherapy improved survival in both premenopausal and postmenopausal women, although the magnitude of the benefit appeared to be greater in younger women.

c. Tamoxifen therapy showed not only a clear benefit in survival in ER-positive patients but also some benefit in ER-negative patients as well.

d. The combination of chemotherapy and endocrine therapy yielded additional benefit compared with either modality alone.

e. Ovarian ablation overwhelmingly improved both recurrence-free and overall survival for younger women but had no effect in women more than 50 years of age.

f. Single-agent chemotherapy was much less effective than polychemotherapy regimens, but the most powerful single agent (Adriamycin) was not studied.

g. This analysis could not determine the effect of tamoxifen treatment in younger women, the role of ovarian ablation in modern treatment programs for younger women, the effect of ER-status on the results of ovarian ablation, or the most effective combination chemotherapy regimen.

4. Adjuvant therapy: recommendations. Women at sufficiently high risk for such treatment include nearly all women with positive axillary lymph nodes and some with high-risk, node-negative disease as well. Precise recommendations for "adjuvant therapy" are beyond the scope of this section, but a summary of such treatment follows.

a. Premenopausal women with positive axillary nodes are offered either a six-month course of chemotherapy with CMF (cyclophosphamide, methotrexate, and 5-fluorouracil) or with an Adriamycin-containing regimen (FAC or CA) starting four weeks after surgery. Dosages for CMF, CA, and FAC are shown in Appendix A1.

b. Postmenopausal women with positive axillary lymph nodes and positive hormone receptors in the tumor are generally offered tamoxifen, 20 mg daily, for two or more years postoperatively. Because of the concern about the development of aggressive endometrial carcinomas in these patients, they should have an annual pelvic examination. Many clinicians also treat these patients with chemotherapy.

c. Postmenopausal women with positive axillary lymph nodes and negative hormone receptors are generally offered adjuvant chemotherapy, provided they have a life expectancy of at least 10 years.

d. Women with high-risk, node-negative disease who are offered systemic therapy include those with:

(1) Larger tumors (T2 or T3; offered chemotherapy or tamoxifen)

(2) Tumors larger than 1.0 cm and negative receptors for estrogen and progesterone (offered chemotherapy; see **4.a, c**)

(3) Tumors larger than 1.0 cm and positive hormone receptors (offered tamoxifen)

e. Women with 10 or more positive lymph nodes are offered dose-intense therapy in many centers, usually with autologous BMT (often as part of a clinical trial, but occasionally "off study").

f. Adjuvant systemic therapy is *not indicated* for:

(1) Women of any age with noninvasive, in situ carcinomas of any size

(2) Women of any age with very small primary tumors (≤ 1.0 cm) and negative axillary lymph nodes, irrespective of the status of hormone receptors in the primary tumor.

C. Advanced regional disease

1. Stage IIIA (operable). Firm guidelines for the management of stage III breast cancer do not exist. Surgical therapy is clearly of value in controlling local disease and is generally indicated. RT may be useful, but the bulk of tumor in such patients precludes a high chance of local control with RT alone. The biggest problem with these patients is early relapse and death from metastatic disease. Because of these considerations the first step in treatment for most patients is combination chemotherapy followed by total mastectomy with axillary lymph node dissection. Subsequent treatment is individualized.

2. Stage IIIB (inoperable) and inflammatory carcinoma. The management of this group of patients is also controversial. Increasingly, however, these patients are treated initially with three or four months of chemotherapy (either CMF, CA, or FAC) (see Appendix A1). RT is then given, followed in most cases by mastectomy. Systemic therapy is then resumed, with either CMF or FAC, or with tamoxifen (for hormone-positive tumors).

D. Systemic therapy for metastatic disease (stage IV). For most patients either chemotherapy or endocrine therapy is given as initial treatment. A flow diagram for the selection of systemic therapy is shown in Figure 10-1.

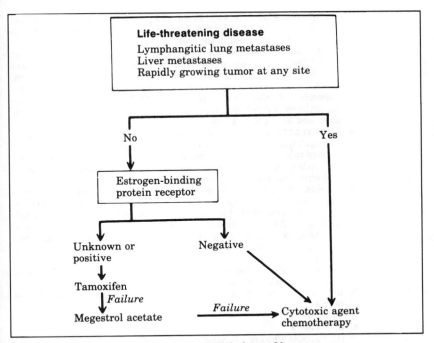

Fig. 10-1. Flow diagram for the management of advanced breast cancer.

1. **Endocrine therapy** is used for patients whose life is not in immediate danger from advancing cancer. Patients who develop recurrent disease within 1 year of primary treatment usually have rapidly growing tumors and have a poor response to endocrine treatments. Other factors that may influence the choice of endocrine therapy follow:

   a. **The hormone receptor status** of the tumor should be positive or unknown before embarking on endocrine manipulations. The response rate varies directly with the amount of ER and PgR present (Table 10-4). Patients with receptor-negative tumors should not be treated initially by endocrine manipulation because response is unlikely (<5%).

   b. **Tamoxifen** citrate (Nolvadex), 20 mg once daily, is an antiestrogen and the first endocrine therapy used in patients with ER-positive or ER-unknown tumors, regardless of the patient's age. Tamoxifen is given continuously until relapse occurs.

Table 10-4. Response rates of metastatic breast cancer to hormonal treatment are related to activities of estrogen receptor (ER) and progesterone receptor (PgR) in the tumor specimen

ER	PgR	Response rate
Negative	Negative	5%
Positive	Negative	25%
Negative	Positive	35%
Positive	Positive	70%
Unknown	Unknown	30%

c. **Megestrol acetate** (Megace), 40 mg q.i.d., is a progestin and an excellent second-line choice of endocrine therapy for eligible patients. It is the least toxic therapy used in the treatment of breast cancer.

d. **Aminoglutethimide,** 250 mg PO q.i.d., is used for patients who respond to and then subsequently fail endocrine treatment. The drug produces a medical adrenalectomy and is equivalent in effectiveness to surgical adrenalectomy. Hydrocortisone must also be given to prevent the pituitary-adrenal axis from overriding the effect of aminoglutethimide. Hydrocortisone is given orally, 10 mg in the morning, 10 mg in the afternoon, and 20 mg at bedtime.

e. **Other endocrine agents.** An estrogen (diethylstilbestrol, 5 mg t.i.d.) or androgen (fluoxymesterone, 10 mg q.i.d.) can be used in patients who respond to and then fail to respond to treatment with tamoxifen, megestrol acetate, or aminoglutethimide, but who show metastatic disease that still mandates endocrine therapy.

f. **Surgical castration** is still used by some practitioners to treat premenopausal women with relapsed breast cancer that is ER-positive. Sterilization can be accomplished by surgery or RT, although if the latter modality is used, lapse of time until response occurs is longer and response may be incomplete. Medical castration with leuprolide or a gonadotropin-releasing hormone (GnRH)-agonist (Zolodex) may also be considered in premenopausal women.

g. **Adrenalectomy or hypophysectomy** can cause difficult problems in medical management. Other therapeutic choices are preferable.

h. **BMT** is of uncertain benefit for patients with advanced metastatic breast cancer.

2. **Chemotherapy**
   a. **Indications**
      (1) Patients who are ER-negative
      (2) Patients who are ER-positive and who fail endocrine therapy
      (3) Patients with life-threatening disease: lymphangitic dissemination in the lungs, liver metastases, or rapidly advancing cancer in any site
   b. **Choice of cytotoxic agents.** Many cytotoxic agents used singly are effective in achieving partial (rarely complete) response in 20 to 35 percent of cases. Remission commonly lasts four to six months. The most effective single agent is Adriamycin.
      (1) **Combinations of cytotoxic agents** (see Appendix A1). The CMF regimen is a good choice for initial treatment, especially when combined with prednisone. Response rates of about 60 percent can be expected with a median duration of a year or more. Combinations of CA and FAC are also effective.
      (2) **Failure of combination chemotherapy.** After failing CMF or CA, sequential single agents can be tried. Drugs for end-stage disease are taxol, fluorouracil, methotrexate, vinblastine, vincristine, mitomycin C, and prednisone.

E. **Local therapy of metastatic disease.** Metastatic disease is generally treated systemically, but some local problems benefit from local RT.
   1. **Isolated painful bony metastases** usually respond well to local RT.
   2. **Massive axillary metastases** usually require local RT, either with or without surgical resection.
   3. **All cervical spine and femoral neck lesions** with or without symptoms should usually be treated with local RT. Femoral neck lesions may also require surgical fixation as well (see Chap. 33, sec. **I.E.4** and **I.E.5**).
   4. **Brain and orbital metastases.** A few patients survive several years after RT.
   5. **Chest wall recurrence.** These patients are generally treated first with systemic therapy. In some cases RT may be used, especially when the patient is otherwise without evidence of disease.

F. Carcinoma in situ (CIS). Improvements in mammographic technique and the increased utilization of screening have resulted in a dramatically increased incidence of noninvasive breast tumors in recent years, particularly ductal CIS.

1. **Ductal CIS** (75% of cases) is clearly a malignant disease and recurs in 30 to 40 percent of cases within 10 to 15 years if treated with excisional biopsy alone. The risk of recurrence is influenced by tumor grade, with low-grade lesions having a much better prognosis for local control than high-grade lesions. When axillary node dissection has been performed, metastases have been found in less than 3 percent of cases. When mastectomy has been performed, the disease is multicentric (additional CIS lesions more than 2 cm away from the main lesion) in 50 percent of cases. Cure rates are greater than 90 percent.

   a. Lumpectomy followed by RT appears to be as effective as mastectomy in treating patients who are motivated toward breast conservation and who have tumors that are small enough for total excision with clear margins and a residual breast that is cosmetically acceptable to the patient.

   b. Patients with small (<2.5 cm), well differentiated (low-grade, noncomedo) lesions detected as microcalcifications on screening mammograms and that are removed with generous margins may not require RT or mastectomy.

   c. Mastectomy is usually recommended for patients with tumors that are larger or that have margins involved by tumor.

   d. Axillary node dissection does not appear to be necessary.

2. **Lobular CIS** (25% of cases; also called "lobular neoplasia") is considered by many authorities to be a premalignant rather than a frankly malignant disease. It affects premenopausal women predominantly and tends to be multicentric. Treatment options include total mastectomy versus close follow-up with yearly mammograms and breast examinations by a physician every four months. This tumor is commonly bilateral (about 30%). The risk of developing cancer is 20 to 30 percent in the affected breast and 15 to 20 percent in the contralateral breast. High-risk patients may benefit from bilateral mastectomies.

G. Patient follow-up after primary therapy of local-regional breast cancer involves a repeat mammogram after RT (if it is used) and then once yearly thereafter. The goal of follow-up is to detect local-regional recurrent disease that is still amenable to curative therapy. Other laboratory studies should be chosen with the goal of cancer screening for unrelated, nonmammary malignant neoplasms (such as colon cancer and ovarian cancer, especially in patients with a strong family history of these disorders).

Patients should have a history and physical examination every six months for at least five years, with annual follow-up thereafter. Blood studies are rarely helpful in asymptomatic patients. Liver scans, bone scans, and other radiographic studies should not be done in the absence of abnormalities in symptoms or signs elicited on history and physical examination because treatment of advanced disease that is detected early has not been shown to improve survival compared to treatment when metastases become clinically evident.

Response to treatment in advanced disease is followed by monitoring previously abnormal tests. The blood CEA level may be a useful tumor marker for patients with disease limited to the skeleton.

VII. Special clinical problems

A. Postsurgical edema of the arm without pain was regularly associated with the traditional radical mastectomy but also occurs with less extensive surgery. The incidence is increased in patients who receive postoperative RT. The edema usually develops within a month after surgery. Therapy is not always helpful, but includes elevation of the arm, arm stockings, the Jobst pump, and exercise. The best treatment is prevention by good surgical technique and avoidance of postoperative irradiation of the axilla.

B. Postsurgical edema of the arm with pain or paresthesias occurring more than a month after surgery almost always reflects recurrent tumor. The cancer is often not clinically discernible because it resides high in the apex of the axilla or lung. Patients complain of tingling or pain in the hands and progressive weakness and atrophy of the hand and arm muscles (see Chap. 32, sec **IV.A**). If sufficient time passes, a tumor mass will become palpable in the axilla or supraclavicular fossa, but the patient is usually left with a paralyzed hand unresponsive to any therapy. These patients should receive RT to the axilla and supraclavicular fossa even if there is no evidence of tumor on physical examination or x-ray film. Such "blind" irradiation probably carries a more favorable risk-benefit ratio than exploration of the axilla and lung apex to confirm a tumor recurrence.

C. **Lymphangiosarcoma of the arm** is rare but develops as a complication of the chronically edematous arm five or more years after radical mastectomy. Typically, an area of ecchymosis resembling a bruise appears first. The edema worsens and the tumor ulcerates. Lymphangiosarcoma has a poor prognosis because of recurrence and metastatic spread after radical amputation. Although experience is limited, chemotherapy followed by RT may control this tumor.

D. **Chest wall radiation-induced ulcers** may occur as late as 25 years after treatment in women who had radical mastectomies followed by extensive RT. The ulcers occur in radiation ports involving thin skin stretched over bony prominences, are often progressive, and can penetrate through the chest wall. Management requires skilled surgical curettage to exclude the possibility of recurrent cancer. Therapy with hyperbaric oxygen is costly and requires several months but heals benign radiation-induced ulcers of less than 1-cm diameter in about 30 percent of cases. Generally, plastic surgery repair is necessary.

E. **Silicone-injected breasts** are potential sites for undetectable malignancies. Mammography does little for early detection, and palpable lumps cannot be clinically evaluated. Patients with silicone-injected breasts should be fully informed about the risks of undetectable cancer and referred to a plastic surgeon for implant removal and breast reconstruction, if necessary.

F. **Pregnancy** and considerations of fertility in patients with breast cancer are discussed in Chapter 26.

G. **Hypercalcemic crises or worsening bone pain following hormonal therapy** can occur. This "endocrine flair" is evidence of a hormonally responsive cancer. It is usually worthwhile to continue the treatment with hormones while treating the hypercalcemia. If hypercalcemia is refractory to treatment, the endocrine therapy should be discontinued and cytotoxic chemotherapy undertaken.

H. **A worsening bone scan in a clinically improving patient** may follow endocrine therapy of any type. The worsening probably reflects healing of diseased bone associated with increased or new uptake of isotopic tracers. This situation commonly indicates successful therapy, which should be continued.

Selected Reading

Blum, J. L., and Tomlinson, G. New insights on hereditary breast cancer. *Contemp. Oncol.* 4:23, 1994.

Dupont, W. D., and Page, D. L. Risk factors for breast cancer in women with proliferative breast disease. *N. Engl. J. Med.* 312:146, 1985.

Eddy, D. M. High-dose chemotherapy with autologous bone marrow transplantation for the treatment of metastatic breast cancer. *J. Clin. Oncol.* 10:657, 1992.

Gelber, R. D., Goldhirsch, A., and Coates, A. S. (for the International Breast Cancer Study Group). Adjuvant therapy for breast cancer: Understanding the overview. *J. Clin. Oncol.* 11:580, 1993.

Haskell, C. M., et al. Breast Cancer. In C. M. Haskell (ed.). *Cancer Treatment* (4th ed.) Philadelphia: W. B. Saunders, 1995.

Rosen, P. P., et al. Factors influencing prognosis in node-negative breast carcinoma: Analysis of 767 T1N0M0/T2N0M0 patients with long-term follow-up. *J. Clin. Oncol.* 11:2090, 1993.

Sacks, N. P. M., and Baum, M. Primary management of carcinoma of the breast. *Lancet* 342:1402, 1993.

Smith, T. J., and Hillner, B. E. The efficacy and cost-effectiveness of adjuvant therapy of early breast cancer in premenopausal women. *J. Clin. Oncol.* 11:771, 1993.

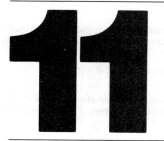

Gynecologic Cancers

Robin P. Farias-Eisner,
Donna L. Walker, and
Jonathan S. Berek

General Aspects

I. **Epidemiology.** Malignancies of the genital tract constitute approximately 20 percent of visceral cancers in women. The incidence and mortality according to primary site are shown in Table 11-1.

II. **Diagnostic studies**

  A. **Papanicolaou smears**

    1. **Frequency.** Early detection has greatly reduced the morbidity and mortality of cervical and endometrial cancer. The traditional annual Papanicolaou (Pap) smear has been questioned because it usually takes years for dysplasia to develop into invasive squamous cell carcinoma. However, some invasive lesions may develop de novo and bypass evolution through stages of dysplasia. In addition, the Pap smear may give a false-negative result, and the incidence of adenocarcinoma of the cervix is on the rise; the natural history of this malignancy and its precursors is less understood than squamous cell carcinomas. Thus, we recommend yearly Pap smears.

    2. **Technique.** The false-negative rate for Pap smears is 10 to 20 percent under optimal circumstances. The squamocolumnar junction, where cervical cancer arises, recedes upward and inward with advancing age. This process decreases the usefulness of cervical scraping alone to make the diagnosis. Sampling should be done by aspirating the cervical os with a glass pipette and scraping the exocervical circumference of the squamocolumnar junction with a divided wooden blade spatula. The specimens are smeared on clean glass slides and fixed immediately. Vaginal pool cytologies probably contribute little. The Pap smear is positive if class III or greater; a class II Pap smear requires treatment of infection and repeat smear.

  B. **Staging evaluation** is necessary regardless of the site of the primary lesion once cancer of the female genital tract is proved histologically. Potentially valuable studies include:

    1. Pelvic and rectal examinations (to determine whether the adnexae, vagina, or pelvic wall is involved).

    2. CBC, serum electrolytes, and liver and renal function tests.

    3. Chest x-ray film (for pulmonary metastases).

    4. Bone scan (if history, physical examination, or routine blood chemistries suggest an abnormality).

    5. Intravenous pyelogram (IVP) (to look for ureteral obstruction or deviation).

    6. Abdominal ultrasonography and CT scans (to delineate abnormal areas).

    7. Sigmoidoscopy with biopsy of abnormal areas and barium enema (for mucosal involvement or mass lesions).

    8. Cystoscopy with biopsy of abnormal areas (to look for bladder mucosal involvement) for cancers of the vulva, vagina, cervix, or endometrium.

    9. Cytologic evaluation of effusions.

III. **Managing treatment-related sexual dysfunction.** Patients treated for cancers of the female genital tract often have difficulty performing sexual intercourse.

  A. **Broaching the subject**

Table 11-1. Cancers of the female genital tract in the United States

Primary site	Proportion of female genital tract malignancies (%)	
	New cases	Deaths from cancer
Cervix (invasive carcinoma)	20	18
Endometrium	41	23
Ovary	32	55
Other sites	7	4
Total	100	100

Note: Cancers of the female genital tract accounted for approximately 75,300 new cancer cases and 25,200 cancer deaths in 1994.

1. Address changes in sexual function directly, preferably before therapy is undertaken; the patient's sexual partner should also be included.
2. Inquire about current sexual activities and about fears the patient or sexual partner might have about the cancer or therapy. Patients should be specifically reassured that the cancer is not contagious, that small amounts of bleeding following intercourse are not hazardous, and that a reasonably normal sex life is expected and desirable for most patients following therapy. See Chap. 26, for discussion of these issues.

B. Specific sexual problems

1. Following RT

   a. External beam radiation. Patients receiving external beam RT should be advised to continue their normal sexual activity; continued intercourse may help prevent vaginal stenosis. Should vaginal dryness develop, the patient should be advised to use petroleum jelly or other lubricants. Estrogen is also useful for treating vaginal dryness in patients with cervical cancer.

   b. Radiation implants. Patients with radiation implants should be advised against intercourse until 2 weeks after treatment. Implants are usually removed prior to discharge from the hospital. Manual foreplay to the point of orgasm is advised as a temporary substitute for intercourse.

   c. Vaginal stenosis secondary to RT may make penile penetration impossible. This complication is often preventable by using dilatation and lubrication during the course of irradiation. If penetration is impossible, some sensation of intercourse may be achieved by the woman's using tightly apposed and lubricated thighs. Manual foreplay, anogenital sex, and orogenital sex are alternatives. Surgical reconstruction by excision of scar tissue and placement of a split-thickness skin graft may yield excellent results.

2. Following hysterectomy the vaginal cuff may be foreshortened, resulting in dyspareunia. Vaginal reconstruction usually has excellent results. Alternatively, the woman can place her hips on a pillow to provide a better angle for penetration. The man can approach from the rear, which may be more comfortable. If these measures are unsatisfactory, lubricated hands placed at the base of the penis may give the sensation of a longer vagina.

3. Following vulvectomy, a major sensory modality for foreplay is removed. The patient should be apprised of this and the sexual partner instructed to stimulate other erogenous zones.

4. Following pelvic exenteration, the physician should emphasize the need to allow adequate time for healing of the wound and adjustment to the ostomies. Thereafter, sexual management is as recommended for the stenotic vagina (see sec. **1.c**). Patients can be advised that vaginal reconstruction can be accomplished during exenteration or 12 to 18 months postoperatively.

   5. Following vaginectomy. Reconstruction is often performed at the time of primary surgery. Both sexual and reproductive function can often be preserved after treatment for vaginal cancer. The gynecologist determines when intercourse can be resumed.

IV. Locally advanced cancer in the pelvis

   A. Pathogenesis. Massive pelvic metastases commonly develop in the course of gynecologic and urologic cancers, rectal carcinomas, and some sarcomas. Locally advanced cancers in the pelvis produce progressive pelvic and perineal pain, ureteral obstruction with uremia, and lymphatic and venous obstruction with pedal and genital edema. Invasion of the rectum or bladder can lead to erosion with bleeding, sloughing of tumor into the urine or bowel, and bladder or bowel outlet obstruction.

   B. Management

   1. Drug therapy is preferred initially because RT damages the pelvic bone marrow and prevents the subsequent administration of adequate chemotherapy dosages.

   2. RT frequently relieves symptoms and is useful when the tumor does not respond to chemotherapy.

   3. Surgery. A colostomy or suprapubic cystostomy may relieve bowel or urethral obstruction. Ureteral bypass can be accomplished by placement of ureteral stent catheters or by nephrostomy.

   4. No therapy. Patients with progressive pelvic disease unresponsive to irradiation or chemotherapy usually die of uremia. Uremia is usually the least painful death possible. Urinary stream bypass techniques are not recommended for patients with progressive, unresponsive pelvic pain syndromes or relentlessly eroding tumors.

V. Adverse effects of radiation to the pelvis

   A. Radiation cystitis

   1. Acute transient cystitis may occur during RT to the pelvis. The possibility of urinary tract infection should be investigated. Urinary tract analgesics and antispasmodics may be helpful for pain (see Chap. 5, sec. **V**).

   2. Late radiation cystitis occurs when high-dose, curative RT to the urinary bladder has been preceded by extensive fulgurations. The bladder becomes contracted, fibrotic, and subject to mucosal ulcerations and infections. Urinary frequency and episodes of pyelonephritis or cystitis (often hemorrhagic) are the clinical findings. If symptomatic management is not successful, cystectomy may be required.

   B. Radiation vulvitis of a moist and desquamative type usually begins at about 2500 cGy and may require temporary discontinuation of treatment for 1–2 weeks in up to 50 percent of patients.

   C. Radiation proctitis. See Chapter 30, sec. **VI.D.**

   D. Vaginal stenosis. See *General Aspects*, sec. **III.B.1.c.**

   E. Effects on gonads. See Chapter 26, sec. **III.**

Cancer of the Uterine Cervix

I. Epidemiology and etiology

   A. Incidence (see Table 11-1). The mortality of cervical cancer has declined by 50 percent over the past 40 years, probably as a result of early detection and treatment. One-third of all cases are invasive carcinoma and two-thirds are carcinoma in situ (CIS).

   B. Relationship to sexual history. The common denominator for increased risk of developing cervical cancer is early, frequent sexual intercourse. The incidence is highest in patients with a history of intercourse before the age of 16, early first pregnancy, multiple sexual partners, and venereal disease.

C. **Relationship to human papillomavirus (HPV).** A large body of evidence supports the relationship between HPV, cervical intraepithelial neoplasia (CIN or dysplasia), and invasive carcinoma. DNA transcripts of HPV have been identified by Southern blot analysis in more than 60 percent of cervical carcinomas. The viral DNA is typically integrated into the human genome rather than remaining in an intact viral capsid. Over 60 HPV subtypes have been identified. Types 6 and 11 are usually associated with benign condyloma acuminata, whereas types 16, 18, 31, and 33 are more likely to be associated with malignant transformation. Type 18 has been associated with poorly differentiated histology and a higher incidence of lymph node metastases. (See Chap. 36, sec. **V.D.2**).

II. **Pathology and natural history**
   A. **Histology.** Approximately 80 percent of cervical carcinomas are squamous cancers, 18 percent are adenocarcinomas, and 2 percent are sarcomas. The disease is believed to start at the squamocolumnar junction. A continuum from CIN to invasive squamous cell carcinoma is apparent. The average age of women with CIN is 15 years younger than that of women with invasive carcinoma, suggesting a potentially slow progression. The natural history of HPV infection is in part influenced by the host immune system; that all stages of CIN may regress spontaneously, remain unchanged, or progress to invasive carcinoma reflects this fact. A small percentage of lesions appear to bypass this progression and may evolve over a substantially shorter period of time.
   B. **Metastases.** Once invasive cancer is established, the tumor spreads primarily by local extension into other pelvic structures and sequentially along lymph node chains. Uncommonly, patients with locally advanced tumors may have evidence of blood-borne metastases, most often to the lung, liver, or bone.

III. **Diagnosis**
   A. **Symptoms and signs**
      1. **Symptoms** of early-stage invasive cervical cancer include vaginal discharge, bleeding, and particularly, postcoital spotting. More advanced stages often present with a malodorous vaginal discharge, weight loss, or obstructive uropathy.
      2. **Signs.** Findings on pelvic examination include the appearance of obvious masses on the cervix; gray, discolored areas; and bleeding or evidence of cervicitis. If a tumor is present, the extent should be noted; involvement of the vagina or parametria is an important prognostic factor.
   B. **Papanicolaou smears and biopsies.** Most patients with cervical cancer are asymptomatic, and cases are detected by routine Pap smear screening (see *General Aspects*, **II.A**). Biopsy specimens should be taken of all visibly abnormal areas, regardless of the findings on the Pap smear. Diagnostic conization may be required if the biopsy shows microinvasive carcinoma, if endocervical curettage shows high-grade dysplasia, or if adenocarcinoma in situ is suspected from cytology.
   C. **Patients with a positive Pap smear and no visible lesion** generally undergo **colposcopy,** which can detect 90 percent of dysplastic lesions. The colposcope is a magnifying instrument (10–20×) that usually detects class III to V lesions. Biopsy specimens are taken from areas that appear abnormal by colposcopy.
   D. **Endocervical curettage (ECC)** is required if colposcopy does not reveal a lesion; when the entire squamocolumnar junction cannot be visualized; when atypical endocervical cells are present on the Pap smear; or in women previously treated for CIN who have new abnormal findings on cytology. If the ECC reveals high-grade dysplasia, patients should undergo cervical conization.
   E. **Further diagnostic studies** in patients whose biopsy report shows cancer depend on the depth of invasion.
      1. For early CIS, other studies are not necessary.
      2. If blood or lymphatic vessels are invaded, or if the tumor penetrates more than 3 mm below the basement membrane, pretherapy staging studies are required (see *General Aspects*, sec. **II.B**).

IV. Staging system and prognostic factors
A. Staging system

Stage	Extent	Five-year survival (%)
0	Carcinoma in situ (no stromal invasion)	95–100
I	Strictly confined to cervix (disregard extension to the corpus)	80
Ia	Preclinical carcinoma (diagnosed only by microscopy)	
Ia1	Minimal microscopic stromal invasion	
Ia2	Microscopic stromal invasion that can be measured (≤5 mm from the originating epithelial base and 7 mm in horizontal spread)	
Ib	Lesions of greater dimensions than Ia2 whether seen clinically or not	
II	Cancer extends beyond the cervix but not to the pelvic sidewall	60
IIa	Lesion involves the proximal vagina (upper two-thirds)	
IIb	Obvious parametrial involvement	
III	Tumor extends to the pelvic sidewall, distal one-third of vagina, hydronephrosis, or nonfunctioning kidney	30
IV	Tumor extends beyond true pelvis, or biopsy-proven involvement of bladder or rectal mucosa	5

B. **Prognostic factors** in each stage include size of the primary tumor (tumor bulk), presence of lymph node metastases, and tumor grade; patients with poorly differentiated tumors do not do well.

V. Prevention and early detection (see *General Aspects,* sec. II.A).

VI. Management*

A. **Early disease.** The management of patients with positive cytologic findings or early carcinoma of the cervix is diagramed in Figure 11-1.

1. **CIN 1–3 (including CIS).** Treatment modalities include superficial ablative therapies, loop electrocoagulation diathermy excision procedure (LEEP), cone biopsy, and hysterectomy. CIN 1 lesions may be observed if the patient has good follow-up or may be treated with ablative therapy. Patients with high-grade (CIN 2–3) squamous lesions are suitable for ablative therapies, provided the entire transformation zone is visible on colposcopy, the histology of the biopsies is consistent with the Pap smear, the ECC is negative, and there is no suspicion of occult invasion. Ablative techniques include cryosurgery, carbon dioxide laser therapy, and electrocoagulation diathermy. LEEP, which involves the use of wire loop electrodes with radiofrequency alternating current to excise the transformation zone under local anesthesia, has become the preferred treatment for CIN which can be adequately assessed by colposcopy. Cone biopsy is preferred for lesions that cannot be assessed colposcopically or when adenocarcinoma in situ is suspected. If the patient has other gynecologic indications for hysterectomy, a vaginal or an extrafascial (type I) abdominal hysterectomy may be performed.

2. **Stage I disease** (see Table 11-2). Stage Ia1 and stage Ia2 with less than 3 mm invasion may be treated with excisional conization, provided the lesion has a diameter of less than 7 mm and no lymph-vascular space invasion. A vaginal or extrafascial hysterectomy is also appropriate if further childbearing is not desired. For patients with stage Ia2 disease and 3–5 mm of stromal invasion, the risk of nodal metastases is 5 to 10 percent. Bilateral pelvic

---

*"Point A" and "point B" are common terms used in the management of cervical cancer. Point A is 2-cm proximal and 2-cm lateral to the cervical os. Point B is 3-cm lateral to point A.

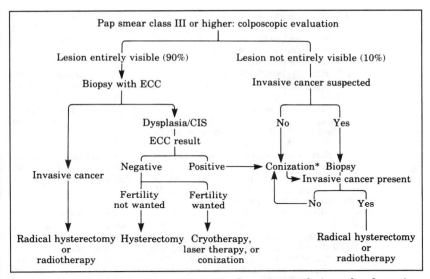

Fig. 11-1. Management of patients with positive Pap smear cytologies and early carcinoma of the uterine cervix. CIS = carcinoma in situ; ECC = endocervical curettage. (*) If invasion is not found on conization, patients are followed with Pap smears, biopsies, or repeat conization, depending on the patient and patient's age.

Table 11-2. Treatment of stage I cervical carcinoma

Stage	Typical treatment options
Ia1 and Ia2 with 1–3 mm invasion but without lymph-vascular space invasion	Therapeutic cone or type I hysterectomy
Ia2 with 1–3 mm invasion and with lymph-vascular space invasion	Type I or II hysterectomy with (?) pelvic lymph node dissection
Ia2 with 3–5 mm invasion	Type II hysterectomy and bilateral pelvic lymphadenectomy or RT for inoperable patients
Ib and IIa	Type III hysterectomy with bilateral pelvic lymphadenectomy with para-aortic lymph node evaluation or RT for inoperable patients

lymphadenectomy should be performed in conjunction with a modified (type II) radical hysterectomy. Stage Ib disease carries a 15 to 25 percent risk of positive pelvic lymph nodes and should be treated with a radical (type III) hysterectomy, bilateral pelvic lymphadenectomy, and para-aortic lymph node evaluation. In patients who are poor surgical candidates, or in whom the tumor is large (generally >5 cm), RT is preferred.

3. **Stage II disease.** Stage IIa disease is treated in the same manner as stage Ib disease. When the tumor extends to parametrium (IIb), patients should be treated with RT as discussed below.

4. Complications of therapy

    a. LEEP. Bleeding occurs in 1 to 8 percent of cases, cervical stenosis in 1 percent, and, very rarely, pelvic cellulitis or adnexal abscess.

    b. Conization. Hemorrhage, sepsis, infertility, stenosis, and cervical incompetence occur rarely.

    c. Radical hysterectomy. Acute complications include blood loss (average: 800 ml), urinary tract fistulae (1–3%), pulmonary embolus (1–2%), small bowel obstruction (1%), and febrile morbidity (25–50%). Subacute complications include transient bladder dysfunction (30%) and lymphocyst formation (<5%). Chronic complications include bladder hypotonia or atonia (3%) and rarely ureteral strictures.

    d. Pelvic irradiation. Radiation proctitis and enteritis with intractable diarrhea or obstruction, cystitis, sexual dysfunction because of vaginal stenosis and loss of secretions, loss of ovarian function, fistula formation, and 0.5 percent mortality either from intractable small bowel injury or pelvic sepsis (see *General Aspects,* sec. **V**).

B. Management of advanced disease

    1. Stage IIb and III disease. When the parametrium (IIb), the distal vagina (IIIa), or the pelvic sidewall (IIIb), are involved, clear surgical margins are not possible to achieve, and patients should be treated with maximum-dose (8500 cGy) RT delivered both externally and by brachytherapy. A variety of chemotherapeutic agents are being investigated for their ability to enhance the efficacy of RT. 5-FU and cisplatin have been shown to be radiation sensitizers and improve survival rates when compared to radiation alone.

    2. Stage IV disease

        a. RT. Radiation alone or with chemotherapeutic sensitizers rarely cures stage IV disease. External beam radiation is combined with intracavitary or interstitial radiation to a total dose of about 8500 cGy. The presence of tumor in the bladder may preclude cure with radiation, and removal of the bladder at the end of radiotherapy should be considered.

        b. Pelvic exenteration. A primary pelvic exenteration may be considered for disease with spread confined to the bladder or rectum. Cure rates are no better than for radiation, however, and exenteration carries a higher morbidity and mortality. Surgery should be abandoned if there is more extensive cancer than was clinically suspected (e.g., para-aortic or massive adherent pelvic lymph node involvement).

            (1) Indications. Central recurrent disease confined to the pelvis after the primary RT was completed.

            (2) Contraindications. Tumor fixation to the pelvic side wall, poor medical condition, or the unavailability of surgeons who are experienced in the technique and able to provide long-term postoperative management. Ureteral obstruction, leg edema, and sciatic pain usually suggest side wall disease.

            (3) Complications. Surgical mortality is less than 10 percent. The postoperative recuperative period may be as long as three months, and the massive fluid shifts and hemodynamic status that sometimes occur may require monitoring. Most postoperative morbidity and mortality result from sepsis, pulmonary embolism, wound dehiscence, and intestinal complications, including small bowel obstruction and fistula formation. A reduction in GI complications can be achieved by using unirradiated segments of bowel and closing pelvic floor defects with omentum. Five-year survival for patients undergoing total pelvic exenteration is 20 to 45 percent.

        c. Chemotherapy. Adjuvant chemotherapy is not curative for any stage. Distant metastases or incurable local disease should be treated as for any advanced malignancy. A number of chemotherapeutic regimens, such as a combination of cisplatin, bleomycin, and mitomycin C, produce short-term responses in 40 to 70 percent of patients.

3. **Lower vaginal recurrence** can occasionally be cured by radical RT or exenteration.
4. **Advanced cancer in the pelvis** is discussed in *General Aspects,* sec. **IV,** and obstructive uropathy is discussed in Chap. 31, sec. **II.**

VII. Special clinical problems
   A. **Chance finding of cancer at hysterectomy.** Cancer found in hysterectomy specimens removed for other reasons carries a poor prognosis unless treated with additional surgery or postoperative RT soon after surgery.
   B. **Uncertainty of recurrent cancer.** Recurrent cancer is usually manifested by pelvic pain, particularly in the sciatic nerve distribution, vaginal bleeding, malodorous discharge, or leg edema. Recurrence must be demonstrated by biopsy specimen because these symptoms and even physical findings are similar to radiation changes. If no tumor is found using noninvasive measures, a surgeon experienced in pelvic cancer should perform exploratory laparatomy.
   C. **Postirradiation dysplasia.** Abnormal Pap smears on follow-up examinations may represent postirradiation dysplastic changes or a new primary cancer. Suspected areas should be biopsied. If the biopsy findings show cancer, surgical removal is usually recommended.

Cancer of the Uterine Body

I. Epidemiology and etiology
   A. **Incidence** (Table 11-1). Endometrial cancer is the most common malignancy of the female genital tract in the United States. The peak incidence is in the sixth and seventh decades of life; 80 percent of patients are postmenopausal. Most premenopausal women with endometrial carcinoma have the Stein-Leventhal syndrome. Less than 5 percent of all cases are diagnosed before the age of 40.
   B. **Risk factors**
      1. Risk factors appear to be related to estrogen exposure that is unopposed by progestins. The risk of endometrial carcinoma from exogenous estrogen administration is increased 4- to 8-fold. Tamoxifen acts as a weak estrogen. Recent data suggest that the use of tamoxifen is associated with a 0.1 to 0.2 percent increased risk of endometrial cancer.
      2. **Medical conditions producing increased exposure to unopposed estrogens** and associated with increased risk of endometrial carcinoma are
         a. Polycystic ovarian disease (anovulatory menstrual cycles with or without hirsutism and other endocrine abnormalities)
         b. Anovulatory menstrual cycles
         c. Obesity
         d. Granulosa cell tumor of the ovary, or any other estrogen-secreting tumor
         e. Advanced liver disease
      3. **Other medical conditions** associated with increased risk for endometrial carcinoma
         a. Infertility, nulliparity, irregular menses
         b. Diabetes mellitus
         c. Hypertension
         d. History of multiple cancers in the family
         e. Patient history of breast or rectal cancer

II. Pathology and natural history
   A. **Histology.** Approximately 70 percent of uterine cancers are endometrial adenocarcinomas, 20 percent are adenocanthomas, and 10 percent are adenosquamous carcinomas. A small percentage are clear cell, small cell, or squamous carcinomas and sarcomas.
   B. **Role of estrogens.** Classically, unopposed estrogens cause a continuum of endometrial changes from mild hyperplasia to invasive carcinoma. More recent investigations, however, suggest that endometrial hyperplasia and endometrial

neoplasia are two biologically different diseases. Approximately 75 percent of women with endometrial hyperplasia that lacks cytologic atypia will respond to progestin therapy and are *not* at an increased risk of developing cancer. Endometrial hyperplasia with cytologic atypia should be considered endometrial intraepithelial neoplasia; 50 percent of these patients respond to progestins and approximately 25 percent go on to develop endometrial cancer.

C. Mode of spread. Tumors are confined to the body of the uterus (stage I) in 75 percent of cases. Endometrial cancer most commonly spreads by direct extension. Deep myometrial invasion and involvement of the uterine cervix are associated with a high risk of pelvic lymph node metastases. It is rare to find positive para-aortic nodes in the absence of positive pelvic nodes. The presence of cells in peritoneal washes suggests retrograde flow of exfoliated cells along the fallopian tubes. Hematogenous spread is an uncommon late finding in adenocarcinoma but occurs early in sarcoma. The lungs are the most frequent site of distant metastatic involvement.

III. Diagnosis
A. Symptoms and signs
1. **Abnormal vaginal bleeding** is the most common complaint (90%).
   a. **Premenopausal women** with prolonged menses, excessive menstrual bleeding, or intermenstrual bleeding must be evaluated for endometrial cancer, particularly if they have a history of irregular menses, diabetes mellitus, hypertension, obesity, or infertility.
   b. **All postmenopausal women** with vaginal bleeding more than 1 year after the last menstrual period are considered to have endometrial cancer unless proved otherwise. Even women who have been on estrogens to control postmenopausal symptoms must have histologic proof that withdrawal bleeding is not the result of an unrelated endometrial cancer.
2. **Asymptomatic patients** with abnormal Pap smears require evaluation for endometrial cancer if cervical cancer is not found; 10 percent of cases are detected in this manner. The findings of atypical histiocytes or normal endometrial cells in postmenopausal patients or in the second half of the menstrual cycle in premenopausal patients require histologic evaluation.
3. **Locally extensive tumors** may be palpable on pelvic examination.
4. **Advanced disease** is the original manifestation of cancer in 10 percent of cases. Presenting problems include ascites, jaundice, bowel obstruction, or respiratory distress from lung metastases.

B. Endocervical curettage and office endometrial biopsy should be performed in all patients suspected of having endometrial carcinoma. An endometrial smear and cell block should be made for optimal interpretation. The accuracy of endometrial sampling is about 90 percent. There is a false-negative rate of about 10 percent, and all symptomatic patients with a negative biopsy must undergo fractional curettage under anesthesia.

C. Fractional curettage is the diagnostic method of choice for endometrial cancer. The technique involves scraping the endocervical canal and then, in a set sequence, the walls of the uterus. If cancer is found by histologic evaluation, the fractional scrapings help to locate the tumor site. Often the gross appearance of the scrapings suggests cancerous tissue, which is gray, necrotic, and friable.

D. Jet-washout technique may be helpful in experienced hands as a screening procedure in high-risk patients. A stream of saline is forcibly injected onto the endometrial surface; cytologic examination of collections yields a 95 percent sensitivity.

E. Pap smears. Conventional Pap smears from endocervical aspiration or brushing have a much lower yield than fractional curettage or jet-washout. Pap smears alone should not be used to rule out suspected endometrial cancer. Only 50 percent of patients with endometrial cancer have abnormal cells on Pap smear.

F. Transvaginal ultrasound with or without color flow imaging is currently under investigation. Early data suggest a strong association between thickness of the

Table 11-3. Surgical staging system for cancer of the uterine body

Stage	Extent	Percent of cases	Five-year survival (%)
I	Cancer confined to the corpus	75	85
Ia	Tumor limited to endometrium		
Ib	Invasion to less than one-half the myometrium		
Ic	Invasion to more than one-half the myometrium		
	G1*: Well differentiated (≤5% of a nonsquamous or nonmorular solid growth pattern)		95
	G2*: Moderately differentiated (6–50%)		80
	G3*: Predominantly solid or undifferentiated		70
II	Cancer involves corpus and cervix but does not extend outside the uterus	11	60
IIa	Endocervical glandular involvement only		
IIb	Cervical stromal invasion		
III	Cancer extends outside the uterus but not outside the true pelvis	11	35
IIIa	Tumor invades serosa and/or adnexa or positive peritoneal cytology		
IIIb	Vaginal metastases		
IIIc	Positive pelvic and/or para-aortic nodes		
IV	Cancer extends outside true pelvis or invades bladder or rectal mucosa	3	10
IVa	Tumor invasion of bladder and/or bowel mucosa		
IVb	Distant metastases including intra-abdominal and/or inguinal lymph nodes		

*Adenocarcinomas with squamous differentiation are graded according to the nuclear grade of the glandular component. In serous adenocarcinomas, clear-cell adenocarcinomas, and squamous cell carcinomas, nuclear grading takes precedence. Notable nuclear atypia, inappropriate for the architectural grade, raises the grade of a grade 1 or 2 tumor by one.

endometrial strip and endometrial disease. Normal endometrium is usually less than 5 mm thick and false-positive results based on this criterion alone may be excessively high.

G. **Staging evaluation.** See *General Aspects,* sec. II.B.

IV. **Staging system and prognostic factors**

A. **Staging system** is shown in Table 11-3. If a patient is not a candidate for surgery, the 1971 FIGO clinical staging system is used. This system is based on endocervical curettage, hysteroscopy, cystoscopy, proctoscopy, and x-rays of the chest and bones.

B. **Prognostic factors**

1. **Histologic grade and myometrial invasion.** Increasing tumor grade and myometrial penetration are associated with increasing risk of pelvic and para-aortic lymph node metastases, positive peritoneal cytology, adnexal metastases, local vault recurrence, and hematogenous spread and thus have great prognostic value.

2. **Tumor histology.** Histologic types ranked from best to worst prognosis are adenocanthoma, adenocarcinomas, adenosquamous carcinomas, clear cell carcinomas, and small cell carcinomas.

3. **Vascular space invasion.** Vascular space invasion is an independent prognostic factor for recurrence and death from endometrial carcinoma of all histologic types.

4. **Hormone receptor status.** The average estrogen (ER) and progesterone receptor **(PgR)** levels are, in general, inversely proportional to the histologic grade. However, ER and PgR levels have also been shown to be independent prognostic indicators, with higher levels corresponding to longer survival.

5. **Nuclear grade.** Criteria for nuclear atypia vary, and intra- and interobserver reproducibility is poor. Despite these difficulties, a number of researchers have shown that nuclear grade is a more accurate prognosticator than histologic grade.

6. **Tumor size.** The larger the tumor, the larger the risk of lymph node metastases and, therefore, the worse the prognosis.

7. **DNA ploidy.** Aneuploid tumors comprise a fairly small percentage (25%) of endometrial carcinomas as compared to ovarian and cervical cancers. Aneuploidy is, however, associated with increased risk of early recurrence and death.

V. Prevention and early detection

A. **Prevention.** Unopposed exogenous estrogen administration should be avoided in postmenopausal women, and women who are anovulatory or who have endometrial hyperplasia should be treated with cyclic progestins.

B. **Early detection.** Patients in whom screening for endometrial carcinoma is justified include postmenopausal women on exogenous estrogens; obese postmenopausal women, particularly with a family history of endometrial, breast, bowel, or ovarian cancer; women who experienced menopause after age 52; and premenopausal women with anovulatory cycles (i.e., polycystic ovarian disease). Women in whom endometrial carcinoma must be ruled out include all postmenopausal women with bleeding, pyometra, or endometrial cells on Pap smear; perimenopausal women with intermenstrual or increasingly heavy periods; and premenopausal women with abnormal uterine bleeding, especially if anovulatory.

VI. Management

A. **Early disease**

1. **Surgery**

   a. **Total abdominal hysterectomy with bilateral salpingo-oophorectomy (TAH/BSO)** is the treatment of choice for patients with persistent hyperplasia after adequate progestin treatment and for all medically fit patients with stage I and stage II endometrial carcinoma with microscopic endocervical involvement and no expansion of the cervix. Removal of the vaginal cuff is not necessary. Any peritoneal fluid should be sent for cytology; if no fluid is found, a peritoneal wash with 50 ml normal saline should be performed. Any enlarged pelvic or para-aortic lymph nodes are resected. If the lymph nodes are not enlarged or are negative and the patient has stage Ia or Ib disease with grade 1 histology or grade 2 less than 2 cm, no further treatment is necessary. All other patients should have complete surgical staging, including pelvic lymphadenectomy.

   b. **Stage II disease** is treated with combined radiation and surgery or only hysterectomy, bilateral salpingo-oophorectomy, and bilateral pelvic lymphadenectomy. Patients with an expanded cervix may be treated with a type II (modified radical) hysterectomy; whereas those with microscopic involvement of the cervix may be treated with an extrafascial hysterectomy.

2. **RT**

   a. **RT alone** is used only for patients at high risk of surgical mortality because of concomitant medical conditions. The survival rate of patients with stage I or II disease treated with RT alone is significantly inferior to surgery alone or surgery combined with RT.

   b. **Postoperative RT.** In order to facilitate accurate surgical staging, many investigators have moved in favor of postoperative RT rather than preoperative.

   (1) Stage I patients who have undergone full surgical staging with negative lymph nodes should be treated with intracavitary vaginal vault radiation.

(2) External pelvic irradiation (approximately 5000 cGy) is indicated in all patients with grade 3 lesions, stage Ic, and stage II occult disease.

(3) Extended field radiation to the para-aortic nodes (4500 cGy) should be given to patients with biopsy-proven para-aortic nodal metastases, grossly positive or multiple positive pelvic nodes, grossly positive adnexal metastases, and Ic disease if grade 2 or 3.

(4) Whole abdominal radiation should be considered with positive peritoneal washings, adnexal involvement, peritoneal or omental metastases.

  c. Preoperative RT

(1) The use of preoperative brachytherapy is still sometimes advocated for patients with grade 3 stage 1 lesions.

(2) Clinical stage II disease (cervical enlargement) is often treated with preoperative external pelvic irradiation and intracavitary radiation followed in six weeks by TAH/BSO.

  3. Chemotherapy has no established role in the management of early endometrial cancers.

B. Advanced disease

  1. Stage III disease treatment should be individualized. It should aim to include TAH/BSO initially except in the presence of parametrial extension, when initial external and intracavitary radiation are more appropriate. Surgical removal of all macroscopic disease is of prime prognostic importance; all enlarged pelvic and para-aortic lymph nodes should be removed. Whole abdominal radiation should be considered for patients with positive peritoneal washings or micrometastases to the upper abdomen.

  2. Stage IV disease is rare and should also have individualized treatment. Treatment usually consists of a combination of surgery, RT, and progestins. If the tumor is removed it should be sent for ER and PgR levels. Pelvic exenteration may be considered for the occasional patient with disease extension limited to the bladder or rectum.

  3. Drug therapy. Patients with widespread metastases or with previously irradiated, recurrent local disease are treated with hormones and cytotoxic agents.

    a. Hormones. Response to progestins occurs in 20 to 40 percent of patients. The average duration of response is one year and expected survival in responding patients is twice that of nonresponders. A few patients survive in excess of 10 years. Hormone receptor studies are of predictive value. The drugs most frequently used are

(1) Repository form of medroxyprogesterone acetate (Depo-Provera), 1.0 g IM weekly for six weeks and monthly thereafter

(2) Megestrol acetate (Megace), 40 mg PO q.i.d. daily

(3) Tamoxifen, 10 mg PO b.i.d.

    b. Chemotherapy. Patients not responding to hormonal therapy can be treated with chemotherapy. Drug regimens containing Adriamycin are often effective; response may be produced in up to 40 percent of patients, which improves their expected survival by several months.

VII. Special clinical problems. Hormone replacement with Premarin (0.625 mg) and Provera (2.5 mg) daily for younger patients with stage I disease is important to protect against osteoporosis and cardiovascular disease. This treatment has not been associated with deleterious effects as previously feared. Other complications are discussed in *General Aspects.*

Vaginal Cancer

I. Epidemiology and etiology

  A. Incidence. Primary carcinoma of the vagina constitutes 1 to 2 percent of cancers of the female genital tract. Dysplastic changes of the vaginal mucosa appear to be precursors of CIS. The likelihood of vaginal carcinoma is increased in women with a history of cervical carcinoma. Eighty to ninety percent of cases of vaginal cancer are metastatic in origin and are treated according to the primary lesion.

B. HPV. HPV is associated with dysplastic changes of the vaginal mucosa referred to as vaginal intraepithelial neoplasia (VAIN). The exact potential of VAIN to progress to frankly invasive carcinoma is unknown but appears to be in the range of 3 to 5 percent when the dysplasia is treated with various methods.

C. Estrogens

1. The 2,000,000 daughters of women treated with diethylstilbestrol (DES) during the first 18 weeks of gestation are at risk for developing vaginal clear cell adenocarcinomas. As of February 1992, 580 cases of clear cell vaginal and cervical carcinomas have been reported by the Registry for Research on Hormonal Transplacental Carcinogenesis. DES exposure accounted for two-thirds of the reported cases. The actual risk of developing clear cell adenocarcinoma in DES-exposed women is estimated to be one in 1000, with the highest risk in women exposed before 12 weeks' gestation.

2. Vaginal adenosis is present in nearly 45 percent of women exposed to DES, and 25 percent have structural abnormalities of the uterus, cervix, or vagina. Almost all women with vaginal clear cell carcinoma also have vaginal adenosis.

II. Pathology and natural history

A. Histology. Approximately 85 percent of vaginal carcinomas are squamous carcinomas, and the remainder are adenocarcinomas, melanomas, and sarcomas.

B. Location. Primary vaginal cancers most commonly arise on the posterior wall of the upper one-third of the vagina. If the cervix is involved, the disease is defined as cervical rather than vaginal cancer. If the vulva is involved, the disease is defined as vulvar cancer.

C. Mode of spread

1. **Direct extension** to adjacent soft tissues and bony structures including paracolpos/parametria, bladder, urethra, rectum, and bony pelvis usually occurs when the tumor is quite large.

2. **Lymphatic dissemination** occurs to pelvic and then para-aortic nodes from the upper vagina while the posterior wall is drained by inferior gluteal, sacral, and deep pelvic nodes. The anterior wall drains into lymphatics of the lateral pelvic walls, and the distal one-third of the vagina drains into the inguinal and femoral nodes.

3. **Hematogenous spread** occurs late and is most often to lung, liver, bone, and supraclavicular lymph nodes.

III. Diagnosis

A. Symptoms and signs. The most frequent presenting complaints are vaginal discharge and bleeding. Vaginal adenosis is usually asymptomatic but may also produce a chronic watery discharge. Bladder pain and urinary frequency may occur early on. Advanced posterior tumors may cause tenesmus or constipation.

B. Diagnostic studies

1. Diagnosis of vaginal carcinomas is often missed on initial examination, especially when the tumor is located in the distal two-thirds of the vagina where the blades of the speculum may obscure the lesion. The speculum should always be rotated as it is withdrawn and the vaginal mucosa inspected carefully.

2. Vaginal Pap smears and biopsy of abnormal areas on pelvic examination are the mainstays of diagnosis. If no lesion is detected in with an abnormal Pap smear, application of Lugol's iodine and inspection with a colposcope may be helpful in identifying lesions.

3. Staging procedures are discussed in *General Aspects*, sec. **II.B.**

IV. Staging system and prognostic factors

A. Staging system. Several staging systems are used. Despite their clear influence on prognosis, however, tumor bulk and location of the primary lesion in the vagina are not included in any current system. Because expected survival depends on clinical stage, variable survival rates have been reported. A representative staging system and approximate survival are as follows:

		Five-year survival (%)
Stage	**Extent**	
0	Carcinoma in situ	100
I	Limited to vagina	70
II	Invasion of subvaginal tissues but not extending to pelvic wall	50
III	Extension to pelvic wall	20
IV	Extension beyond true pelvis or biopsy proof of bladder or rectal involvement	<10

   B. Prognostic factors. Generally, the greater the tumor size, the worse the prognosis. Cancers located in the upper vagina, however, have a better prognosis than those located in the lower vagina (upper posterior tumors can become quite large before invading the muscularis and changing the stage of disease).

V. Prevention and early detection

   A. Pap smears are the basis of screening the general population. Up to 30 percent of patients with vaginal cancer have a history of in situ or invasive cervical cancer; these patients should be screened with annual Pap smears.

   B. Females with a history of in utero exposure to DES should have a pelvic examination and Pap smear yearly from the time of menarche. Younger girls who have been exposed to DES should be examined at the first sign of bleeding or discharge, because clear cell carcinomas can occur in childhood. All suspected areas should be biopsied, and careful palpation of all mucosal surfaces is extremely important.

VI. Management

   A. Early disease

      1. Surgery. The close proximity of bladder, urethra, and rectum restricts the surgical margins that can be obtained without an exenterative procedure. In addition, attempts to maintain a functional vagina and the associated psychosocial issues play an important role in treatment planning.

         a. Vaginal mucosa stripping has been used for CIS.

         b. Stage I disease involving the upper posterior vagina may be managed with radical hysterectomy, partial vaginectomy, and bilateral pelvic lymphadenectomy. In a patient with prior hysterectomy, radical upper vaginectomy with bilateral pelvic lymphadenectomies can be used.

         c. Pretreatment exploratory laparotomy in patients requiring radiation allows for

            (1) More precise determination of disease involvement.

            (2) Resection of bulky involved lymph nodes.

            (3) Ovariopexy (ovarian transposition) to minimize the chance of radiation-induced infertility.

         d. Vaginal reconstruction may be performed using split-thickness skin grafts from the thighs or with myocutaneous flaps, usually with gracilis muscle.

      2. RT is an alternative treatment for patients with stage I disease; there are no controlled studies to prove that RT is as effective as surgery. Radiation is the treatment of choice for all higher stages, usually using combined external beam and intravaginal radiation.

      3. Chemotherapy. Topical fluorouracil, applied twice daily, has been used for CIS. Intense vaginal burning results, but it appears to consistently produce response. The long-range benefits of topical fluorouracil are not yet proved; this modality cannot be recommended as standard practice.

      4. Laser therapy is useful for stage 0.

   B. Advanced disease is managed as for cancer of the cervix (see *Cancer of the Uterine Cervix,* sec. **VI.B**). In otherwise healthy patients with stage IV disease or central recurrence after previous radiation, an exenterative procedure may be performed.

VII. Special clinical problems. Loss of genitalia and vaginal stenosis are discussed in *General Aspects,* sec. **III.**

Vulvar Cancer

I. Epidemiology and etiology

A. Incidence. Carcinomas of the vulva constitute 3 to 4 percent of malignant lesions of the female genital tract. The disease is most frequent in women over 50 years of age, with a mean age at diagnosis of 65 years.

B. Etiology

1. **Viruses** are suspected to play a role in the development of vulvar cancer. HPV has been isolated from vulvar condylomas, and about 5 percent of patients with vulvar cancer have genital condylomas. Herpes simplex virus (type II) nonstructural proteins have been demonstrated in invasive vulvar lesions, but no structural antigens have been demonstrated.

2. **Intraepithelial neoplasia** of the vulva (VIN), vagina (VAIN), and cervix (CIN) increase a woman's risk of developing carcinoma of the vulva.

3. **Medical history** associated with increased risk of vulvar cancer includes obesity, hypertension, diabetes mellitus, arteriosclerosis, menopause at an early age, and nulliparity.

II. Pathology and natural history

A. Histology. Malignant tumors of the vulva are squamous cell carcinoma in more than 90 percent of cases and melanoma in 5 to 10 percent. Adenocarcinoma, sarcoma, basal cell carcinoma, and other tumors constitute the remainder.

B. Location. The sites of tumor in order of decreasing frequency are labia majora, labia minora, clitoris, and perineum.

C. Natural history

1. **Squamous cell carcinomas** in the vulva have not been shown to develop as a continuum from VIN to CIS to invasive carcinoma. Most studies report that only about 2 to 4 percent of VIN lesions become invasive cancer. These cancers tend to grow locally, spread to superficial and deep groin lymph nodes, and then to pelvic and distant nodes. Hematogenous spread usually occurs after lymph node involvement, and death usually results from cachexia or respiratory failure secondary to pulmonary metastases.

2. **Malignant melanoma** of the vulva accounts for 5 percent of all melanoma cases, despite the comparatively small surface area involved and the paucity of nevi at this site (see Chap. 16, *Malignant Melanoma*). Therefore, all pigmented vulvar lesions should be removed.

3. **Paget's disease of the vulva** is a preinvasive lesion with thickened epithelium infiltrated with mucin-rich Paget's cells, which are derived from the stratum germinativum of the epidermis. Research shows that only 1 to 2 percent of patients with Paget's disease have an associated underlying adenocarcinoma of the vulva. Many older publications have reported a higher incidence of adenocarcinoma with Paget's disease, but this is probably a reflection of the underdiagnosis of the disorder. Paget's disease is associated with a synchronous primary cancer in another genital tract site in 25 percent of patients.

4. **Bartholin's gland adenocarcinoma** is extremely rare and is usually seen in older women. Inflammation of this gland is uncommon in women over 50 years old and is virtually nonexistent in postmenopausal women; gland swelling in women in these age groups should arouse suspicion for the presence of cancer.

5. **Basal cell carcinomas and sarcomas** of the vulva have natural histories similar to primary tumors located elsewhere.

III. Diagnosis

A. Signs and symptoms

1. Squamous cell carcinomas most often present with a vulvar lump or mass, often with a history of chronic vulvar pruritus. The tumors often ulcerate or become fungating. Bleeding, superinfection, and pain can develop with continued growth.

2. Paget's disease has a characteristic lesion that is velvety red with raised,

irregular margins. Lesions are pruritic with secondary excoriation and bleeding.
3. Basal cell carcinomas and melanomas are discussed in Chapter 16.
4. Lymph node enlargement may be palpable in the inguinal or femoral regions or in the pelvis.

B. Indications for wedge biopsy
1. Patches of skin that appear red, dark brown, or white
2. Areas that are firm to palpation
3. Pruritic or bleeding lesions
4. Any nevus in the genital region
5. Enlargement or thickening in the region of Bartholin's glands, particularly in patients 50 years of age or older

C. Staging evaluation (see *General Aspects*, sec. **II.B**).

IV. Staging system and prognostic factors for squamous cell carcinoma

A. Staging system.
The International Federation of Gynecology and Obstetrics (FIGO) has adopted a surgically based TMN staging system to avoid the problems associated with clinical assessment of lymph nodes.

FIGO stage	TMN	Clinical/pathologic findings
I	$T_1N_0M_0$	Tumor confined to the vulva or perineum, <2 cm in greatest dimension, lymph nodes negative
II	$T_2N_0M_0$	Tumor confined to the vulva and/or perineum, >2 cm in greatest dimension, lymph nodes negative
III	$T_3N_0M_0$ $T_{1,2,3} N_1M_0$	Tumor of any size with: adjacent spread to lower urethra or anus (T_3) or unilateral regional lymph node spread (N_1)
IVA	T_1 or T_2 or T_3, N_2M_0 T_4, Any N,M_0	Tumor invades upper urethra, bladder mucosa, rectal mucosa or pelvic bone (T4) or bilateral regional lymph node spread (N2)
IVB	Any T, Any N,M_1	Any distant metastasis, including pelvic lymph nodes

B. Prognostic factors and survival.
Survival is determined by stage, structures invaded, and tumor location.
1. **Lymph node involvement** is exceedingly important. Metastases to pelvic or periaortic nodes are rare in the absence of inguinal or femoral lymph node metastases.
2. The **five-year survival** in patients with negative or one microscopically positive lymph node is 95 percent. In contrast, five-year survival rates for two positive nodes is 80 percent, and for three or more positive nodes, 15 percent. Note that the risk of hematogenous spread with three or more positive nodes is 66 percent, in contrast to the risk with two or fewer nodes, which is only 4 percent.

V. Prevention and early detection.
The routine history and physical examination of all postmenopausal women should include specific questioning regarding vulvar soreness and pruritus followed by careful inspection and palpation of the vulva and palpation for firm or fixed groin nodes. All suspicious lesions should be biopsied.

VI. Management

A. Surgery is the treatment of choice for early-stage lesions.
1. **VIN.** Wide local excision for small lesions. Carbon dioxide laser of the warty variety is acceptable.
2. **Paget's disease.** This lesion usually extends well beyond the macroscopic lesion and requires a wide local excision. Underlying adenocarcinoma is usually apparent, but to avoid missing such a lesion, the underlying dermis should be removed for histologic evaluation.
3. **Invasive carcinoma with less than 1 mm invasion.** Radical local excision.
4. **Stage I with greater than 1 mm but less than 5 mm invasion.** Radical

local excision (modified radical vulvectomy) with ipsilateral groin lymph node dissection for lateralized lesions and bilateral node dissections for centralized lesions.

5. **Stage II** lesions may be treated with bilateral groin lymph node dissection and radical local excision, provided that at least 1 cm of clear margins in all directions can be achieved while preserving critical midline structures.

   a. **Complications** include wound breakdown, local infection, sepsis, thromboembolism, and chronic edema of the lower extremities. Using separate incisions for the groin node dissections reduces the incidence of wound breakdown and leg edema.

   b. **Pelvic lymphadenectomy** is reserved for patients with clinically suspicious groin nodes or three or more proven unilateral groin nodes.

B. RT

1. RT may be used to shrink stage III and IV tumors that involve the anus, rectum, rectovaginal septum, or proximal urethra preoperatively to improve resectability.

2. RT has been shown to improve survival and decrease groin recurrence when two or more groin nodes are positive.

3. Postoperative RT to the vulva may be used to reduce local recurrence when tumors exceed 4 cm or there are positive surgical margins.

4. External beam radiation to 5000 cGy with follow-up biopsy should be considered for small anterior tumors involving the clitoris, especially in young women to prevent the psychosocial issues involved with surgery.

5. Patients who have medical conditions precluding surgery may be treated with RT alone.

C. Chemotherapy

1. 5-FU or cisplatin chemotherapy is under investigation as a radiation sensitizer.

2. Systemic treatment with agents active against squamous cell carcinomas, such as cisplatin, methotrexate, cyclophosphamide, bleomycin, and mitomycin C, may be used for metastatic disease, but partial response rates are low (10–15%) and usually last only a few months.

Ovarian Cancer

I. Epidemiology and etiology

A. Incidence (see Table 11-1). Ovarian cancer is the fourth most frequent visceral malignancy in the United States and is the most lethal of all the gynecologic cancers. No major improvement of overall survival has been made during the last 30 years. The average age at diagnosis is 55 years.

B. Risk factors

1. The highest rates of ovarian cancer are recorded in industrialized countries. Physical, chemical, or dietary products may be etiologic. For example, Japanese women emigrating to the United States incur a higher risk than those who remain in Japan. No specific carcinogens have been determined.

2. Fewer than 5 percent of epithelial ovarian cancers have a familial or hereditary pattern. Patients at highest risk are those with two or more first-degree relatives with documented epithelial ovarian cancer. Women with a personal history of breast or endometrial cancer also have an increased risk for ovarian cancer.

3. Nulliparity with "incessant ovulation" is a risk factor.

II. Pathology and natural history

A. Histology. The World Health Organization's classification of neoplasms of the ovary is shown in Table 11-4.

B. Histologic grade. The percentage of undifferentiated cells present in tissue determines the grade of the tumors (as defined by Broder).

Table 11-4. Histology of ovarian neoplasms

A. Epithelial tumors (frequency) Serous cystadenocarcinoma (70%) Mucinous cystadenocarcinoma (20%) Clear cell (mesonephroma) (4%) Undifferentiated carcinoma (4%) Endometrioid carcinoma (2%) Brenner tumor Mixed epithelial tumor Unclassified	**B. Germ cell tumors** Dysgerminoma Endodermal sinus tumor Embryonal carcinoma Polyembryoma Choriocarcinoma Teratoma Mixed
C. Sex cord stromal tumors Sertoli-Leydig cell tumor Granulosa-stromal cell tumor Gynandroblastoma Androblastoma Unclassified	**D. Other tumors** Lipid cell tumors Gonadoblastoma Nonspecific soft tissue tumors Unclassified

Grade	Percentage of undifferentiated cells
G_1	0–25
G_2	25–50
G_3	>50

C. Biologic behavior

1. **Borderline tumors,** also called "tumors of low malignant potential," tend to occur in premenopausal women and remain confined to the ovary for long periods of time. Metastatic implants may occur and some may be progressive, leading to bowel obstruction and death.

2. **Other histologic subtypes** behave similarly when grade and stage are considered. Even in early stages, careful exploration frequently reveals subdiaphragmatic and omental implants. Organ invasion and distant metastases are less likely than spread over serosal surfaces. The lethal potential of ovarian cancer is most frequently related to encasement of intra-abdominal organs. Death usually results from intestinal obstruction and inanition.

D. Associated paraneoplastic syndromes

1. Neurologic syndromes are common. Peripheral neuropathies, organic dementia, amyotrophic lateral sclerosislike syndrome, and cerebellar ataxia are the most frequent occurrences.

2. Peculiar antibodies that cause difficulties in crossmatching blood can be corrected with prednisone.

3. Cushing's syndrome.

4. Hypercalcemia.

5. Thrombophlebitis.

III. Diagnosis

A. Symptoms and signs. Early ovarian carcinoma is typically asymptomatic. Symptoms, when they do occur, are often nonspecific and include irregular menses if premenopausal, urinary frequency, constipation, abnormal vaginal bleeding, abdominal discomfort, and distention. Physical findings include ascites and abdominal masses. Any pelvic mass in a woman who is over one year postmenopausal is suspicious for ovarian cancer.

B. Tissue diagnosis. Diagnosis requires biopsy of ovarian or other suspected abdominal masses.

1. **Adnexal masses**

   a. **Masses that are less than 8 cm** in premenopausal women are most commonly benign cysts. Patients should undergo **US** to confirm the cystic nature of the mass and receive suppression with oral contraceptives for two months. Benign lesions should regress.

    b. Surgical evaluation is necessary for masses that are
        (1) Less than 8 cm in diameter and cystic but still present after two months of observation in premenopausal women
        (2) Less than 8 cm in premenopausal women and solid on **US**
        (3) Greater than 8 cm in premenopausal women
        (4) Present in any postmenopausal patient
   2. Pap smears are not sensitive enough to detect ovarian cancer (25% yield).
  C. Serum tumor markers that are useful to monitor the response to therapy are CA 125 (see Chap. 1, sec. **III.D.5.d**) and CEA (see Chap. 1, sec. **III.D.2.b**). β-HCG (see Chap. 1, **III.D.3.a**) and α-FP (see Chap. 1, **III.D.2.a**) are useful in germ cell malignancies. None is useful for screening.
  D. Staging evaluation (see *General Aspects,* sec. **II.B**).
IV. Staging system and prognostic factors
  A. Staging system and five-year survival for epithelial tumors

Stage	Extent (proportion of cases)	Survival (%)
I	Cancer limited to ovaries (15%)	80
Ia	Limited to one ovary, no ascites	
Ib	Both ovaries involved, no ascites	
Ic	Ia or Ib with ascites or positive peritoneal washings	
II	Cancer of one or both ovaries with extension limited to pelvic tissue (15%)	60
IIa	Extension to uterus or tubes	
IIb	Extension to other pelvic tissues	
IIc	IIa or IIb with ascites or positive peritoneal washings	
III	Cancer involving one or both ovaries with peritoneal implants outside the pelvis and/or positive retroperitoneal or inguinal nodes. Tumor is limited to the true pelvis but with histologically proven extension to small bowel or omentum (65%).	30
IIIa	Tumor grossly limited to the true pelvis with negative nodes but with histologically confirmed microscopic seeding of abdominal peritoneal surfaces	(60)*
IIIb	Same as IIIa but abdominal peritoneal implants do not exceed 2 cm in diameter	(30)*
IIIc	Abdominal implants greater than 2 cm in diameter and/or positive retroperitoneal or inguinal lymph nodes	(5–10)*
IV	Distant metastases present (including cytology-positive pleural effusions and metastasis to liver parenchyma or peripheral superficial lymph nodes [5%])	5

  B. Prognostic factors. Extent, stage, and grade of disease are more important than specific histologic types. The extent to which the disease can be surgically debulked also affects prognosis.
V. Prevention and early detection. Women with strong family histories of epithelial ovarian cancer have a twofold increased risk for epithelial ovarian cancer, compared to other women, and women with family histories of breast or ovarian cancer or a personal history of breast cancer also have a twofold increased risk. The risk for women with Lynch II syndrome (see Table 9-2) is two to four times the general risk. All of the above mentioned groups should have proper genetic counseling and consider prophylactic oophorectomy when childbearing has been completed. Women should be advised that prophylactic oophorectomy does not offer absolute protection because peritoneal carcinomas occasionally occur after bilateral oophorectomy. The value of CA-125 for screening and transvaginal US in these women has not been clearly established.

*Estimates because this substaging is recent.

VI. Management of epithelial ovarian cancers (see *A* in Table 11-4)
   A. Surgical staging evaluation
   1. The ovarian tumor should be removed intact, if possible, and sent for frozen section. If the tumor is confined to the pelvis, a thorough surgical evaluation should be carried out.
   2. Any free fluid, especially in the pelvic cul-de-sac, should be sent for cytologic evaluation. If no free fluid is found, peritoneal washings should be obtained with 50–100 ml normal saline from the cul-de-sac, each paracolic gutter, and from beneath each hemidiaphragm.
   3. Systematic exploration of all peritoneal surfaces and viscera is performed. Any suspicious areas or adhesions of peritoneal surfaces should be biopsied.
   4. The diaphragm should be sampled by biopsy or by scraping and preparation of a cytologic smear.
   5. The omentum should be resected from the transverse colon (an infracolic omentectomy).
   6. The retroperitoneal surfaces are then explored to evaluate the pelvic and para-aortic lymph nodes. Any enlarged lymph nodes are submitted for frozen section. If frozen section is negative, a formal pelvic lymphadenectomy is performed.

   B. Borderline tumors. Treatment is surgical resection of the primary tumor. There is no evidence that subsequent chemotherapy or radiation improves survival.

   C. Stage Ia and Ib, Grade 1
   1. **Premenopausal** patients in this category may, after staging laparotomy is completed, undergo unilateral oophorectomy to preserve fertility. Follow-up should include regular pelvic examinations and determinations of CA-125 levels. Generally, the other ovary and uterus are removed when childbearing is completed.
   2. **Postmenopausal** patients and women in whom childbearing is not an issue should undergo TAH/BSO.

   D. Stage Ia and Ib, Grades 2 and 3, and stage Ic are treated with TAH/BSO followed by either chemotherapy or radiation.
   1. **Chemotherapy** with cisplatin or cisplatin plus cyclophosphamide (PC; see Appendix A1) for three to four cycles is recommended for young patients. It may be preferable to give older patients a course of melphalan (4–6 cycles).
   2. **Radiation** with intraperitoneal radioactive phosphorus (^{32}P) is an acceptable alternative for patients without significant adhesions.

   E. Stages II, III, and IV
   1. **Surgery** with exploration and removal of as much disease as possible should be carried out. Removal of the primary tumor and as much metastatic disease as possible is referred to as "cytoreductive surgery" or "debulking." Performance of a retroperitoneal lymph node dissection appears to improve survival.
   2. **Adjuvant therapy and results of debulking**
      a. **Optimal debulking with no macroscopic residual disease** warrants treatment with six cycles of chemotherapy or whole abdominal radiation.
      b. **Optimal debulking with macroscopic disease less than 2 cm** warrants treatment with six cycles of chemotherapy.
      c. **Nonoptimal debulking** should be followed by three cycles of chemotherapy and interval cytoreduction if there is a partial response to chemotherapy.
   3. **Second look laparotomy** should follow adjuvant therapy if there is no clinical evidence of disease. Serial CA-125 determinations should also be followed. CA-125 levels greater than 35 U/ml are nearly always associated with finding disease at second look operations. Negative CA-125, however, is not predictive of a negative second look. Laparoscopy has a 35 percent false-negative rate when used for second look assessments.
      a. If there is no pathologic evidence of disease at second look, patients may be observed or may be given consolidation chemotherapy.

  b. Microscopic or macroscopic disease less than 5 mm after second cytoreduction should be followed by intraperitoneal chemotherapy, possibly
radiation and further chemotherapy using a new agent, such as Taxol.
  c. Residual disease greater than 5 mm after second cytoreduction should
be treated with experimental protocols or palliative care.
4. Chemotherapy
  a. Single oral agent therapy with melphalan is reserved for patients who
cannot tolerate more toxic regimens or as a second line therapy.
  b. Cisplatin-based combination regimens have been the mainstay of treatment for advanced ovarian cancer (Appendix A1). Other drugs combined
with cisplatin include hexamethylmelamine, cyclophosphamide, Adriamycin, and Taxol. The roles of Adriamycin and hexamethylmelamine
remain controversial as they have considerable toxicities.
  c. Carboplatin has fewer gastrointestinal and renal side effects than cisplatin but more hematotoxicity. Carboplatin in combination with cyclophosphamide has a better therapeutic index than cisplatin plus cyclophosphamide (see Appendix A1). Studies investigating carboplatin and
Taxol show that this combination is as effective as cisplatin-based therapy.
  5. RT (whole abdominal radiation) appears to be useful in patients who have
optimal or microscopic disease after second look and is an alternative to
chemotherapy.
F. Patient follow-up after disease-free second look operations is clinical as there
are no reliable means of surveillance. CA-125 levels should be followed, but CT
and ultrasound have proven too insensitive to detect early recurrent disease.
CT may be used to follow known masses.
VII. Müllerian peritoneal tumors. The histology of peritoneal mesothelium is identical
to germinal epithelium. The peritoneum may transform into different forms of
benign and malignant müllerian epithelia that may mimic metastatic papillary
adenocarcinoma. Synonyms include papillary peritoneal neoplasia and benign
mesothelial proliferation with effusion.
A. Benign cystic mesothelioma is a benign cystic proliferation of peritoneal epithelia throughout the peritoneal cavity. Local recurrence after surgery is common but not fatal.
B. Malignant müllerian peritoneal tumors resemble advanced epithelial ovarian
carcinoma and present as implants throughout the peritoneal cavity (including
ovarian surfaces). Current management is the same as for stage III epithelial
ovarian carcinoma.
VIII. Germ cell tumors (see *B* in Table 11-4)
A. Epidemiology. Germ cell tumors make up 20 to 25 percent of all ovarian neoplasms, but only 3 percent of these tumors are malignant. These malignancies
constitute fewer than 5 percent of all ovarian cancers in Western countries and
up to 15 percent in Asian and African populations. Germ cell tumors make up
over 70 percent of ovarian neoplasms in the first two decades of life, and in this
age range, one-third are malignant.
B. Signs and symptoms. These tumors grow rapidly and often present with subacute pelvic pain and pressure and menstrual irregularity. Acute symptoms
related to torsion or adnexal rupture are often confused with acute appendicitis.
Adnexal masses greater than 2 cm in premenarchal girls and in premenopausal
women are suspicious; they usually require surgical investigation.
C. Diagnosis. Young patients should be tested for serum β-HCG and α-FP titers
along with other routine blood work. A karyotype should be obtained because
of the propensity of these tumors to arise from dysgenetic gonads. A chest x-ray
is essential, because germ cell tumors may metastasize to lungs or mediastinum.
D. Tumor types
  1. Dysgerminoma
    a. Natural history. Dysgerminomas are the most common germ cell malig-
nancy and represent up to 10 percent of ovarian cancers in patients
under 20 years of age. Seventy-five percent of dysgerminomas occur between the ages of 10 and 30 years. Approximately 5 percent are found

in dysgenic gonads. Three-quarters of cases are stage I, and 10 to 15 percent are bilateral. Unlike other ovarian malignancies, dysgerminomas often spread earlier via lymphatics than to peritoneal surfaces.

b. **Treatment** is primarily surgical; the minimal operation is unilateral oophorectomy and complete surgical staging. The chance of recurrence in the other ovary over the next two years is 5 to 10 percent, but these lesions are sensitive to chemotherapy. When fertility is an issue, the uterus and contralateral ovary should be preserved even in the presence of metastatic disease. If fertility is not an issue, a TAH/BSO should be performed. If a Y chromosome is found on karyotyping, both ovaries should be removed, but the uterus may be left in place. Chemotherapy is the adjuvant treatment of choice for metastatic disease. Most regimens use a combination of bleomycin, etoposide, and cisplatin (BEP; see Appendix A1). If fertility is not an issue metastatic disease may be treated with radiation as these tumors are very sensitive to it.

c. **Prognosis.** The five-year survival rate for patients with stage Ia disease is over 95 percent when the disease is treated with unilateral oophorectomy alone. Recurrence is most likely in patients with lesions larger than 10–15 cm in diameter, age under 20 years, and anaplastic histology. Patients with advanced disease that is treated with surgery followed by BEP chemotherapy have a five-year survival rate of 85 to 90 percent.

2. **Immature teratoma**

a. **Natural history.** Pure immature teratomas account for less than 1 percent of all ovarian cancers but are the second most common germ cell malignancy. They constitute 10 to 20 percent of ovarian malignancies in patients under the age of 20 years and account for 30 percent of ovarian cancer deaths in this group. Serum tumor markers (β-HCG, α-FP) are not found unless the tumor is of mixed type. The most common site of spread is the peritoneum; hematogenous spread is uncommon and occurs late.

b. **Treatment.** In premenopausal women in whom the lesion is confined to one ovary, a unilateral oophorectomy and surgical staging is warranted. In postmenopausal women, a TAH/BSO is performed. For patients with stage Ia, grade 1 tumors, no adjuvant therapy is required. For stage Ia, grade 2 or 3 or for higher stages with gross residual disease, adjuvant chemotherapy with BEP should be used. Chemotherapy is also indicated for patients with ascites, regardless of grade. RT is reserved for patients with localized disease after chemotherapy. Second look laparotomy is best reserved for patients at high risk of treatment failure (i.e., patients with macroscopic disease at the start of chemotherapy) because there are no reliable tumor markers for this disease.

c. **Prognosis.** The most important prognostic feature of immature teratomas is their histologic grade. The five-year survival rates are 82 percent, 62 percent, and 30 percent for patients with grades 1, 2, and 3, respectively. Patients whose lesions cannot be completely resected prior to chemotherapy have a five-year survival rate of only 50 percent as compared with 94 percent for completely resected disease.

3. **Endodermal sinus tumors** or yolk sac carcinomas are rare. The median age at diagnosis is 18 years. Pelvic or abdominal pain is the most common presenting symptom. Most of these lesions secrete α-FP and serum levels are useful in monitoring response to treatment. Treatment consists of surgical staging, unilateral oophorectomy, and frozen section for diagnosis. All patients are given adjuvant or therapeutic chemotherapy. A combination of cisplatin, vinblastine, and bleomycin (PVB; see Appendix A1, Testicular cancer) appears to be most effective. A seven-drug regimen has been developed for high-risk germ cell tumors of any histologic type and may be used in patients with massive metastatic disease or with liver or brain metastases.

4. **Embryonal carcinoma** is an extremely rare tumor that occurs in young females with a median age of 14 years. These tumors may secrete estrogens, producing symptoms of precocious pseudopuberty or irregular bleeding. Two-thirds are confined to one ovary at presentation, and they frequently secrete α-FP and β-HCG, which are useful to follow response to therapy. Treatment is unilateral or bilateral oophorectomy followed by chemotherapy with BEP.

5. **Choriocarcinoma of the ovary** is extremely rare; the majority of patients are under 20 years of age. β-HCG is often a useful tumor marker. Fifty percent of premenarchal patients present with isosexual precocity. The prognosis is usually poor, but complete responses have been reported with combination methotrexate, actinomycin D, and Cytoxan (MAC III; see Appendix A1).

6. **Mixed germ cell tumors** most commonly have a dysgerminoma or endodermal sinus component. Secretion of α-FP or β-HCG depends on component parts. Lesions should be managed with unilateral oophorectomy and chemotherapy with BEP. A second look laparotomy may be indicated when macroscopic disease is present at the start of chemotherapy to determine response to therapy in components that do not produce tumor markers.

IX. **Sex cord stromal tumors** (see *C* in Table 11-4) account for 5 to 8 percent of all ovarian cancers. Most tumors are a combination of cell types derived from the sex cords and ovarian stroma or mesenchyme.

A. **Granulosa-stromal cell tumors** include granulosa cell tumors, thecomas, and fibromas. Thecomas and fibromas are rarely malignant and are then called fibrosarcomas. Granulosa cell tumors are low-grade, estrogen-secreting malignancies that are seen in women of all ages. Endometrial cancer occurs with granulosa cell tumors in 5 percent of cases, and 25 to 50 percent are associated with endometrial hyperplasia. Inhibin, which may be secreted by some granulosa cell tumors, may be a useful tumor marker. Surgery alone is usually sufficient therapy with radiation and chemotherapy reserved for women with recurrent or metastatic disease. Granulosa cell tumors have a 10-year survival rate of about 90 percent. DNA ploidy correlates with survival.

B. **Sertoli-Leydig tumors** have a peak incidence between the third and fourth decades. These very rare lesions are usually low-grade malignancies. Most produce androgens, and virilization is seen in 70 to 85 percent of patients. Usual treatment is unilateral salpingo-oophorectomy with evaluation of the contralateral ovary. TAH/BSO is appropriate for older patients. The utility of radiation or chemotherapy is yet to be proven.

X. **Other tumors** (see *D* in Table 11-4)

A. **Lipoid cell tumors** are extremely rare with only slightly more than 100 cases reported. They are thought to arise from adrenal cortical rests near the ovary. Most are virilizing and are benign or low-grade malignancies. Treatment is surgical extirpation.

B. **Ovarian sarcomas** are also extremely rare and most occur in postmenopausal women. They are aggressive lesions with no effective treatment. Most patients die within two years.

C. **Lymphoma** can involve the ovaries, usually bilaterally, especially with Burkitt's lymphoma. A hematologist-oncologist should be consulted intraoperatively when lymphoma is found to determine the need for surgical staging. Treatment is as for lymphomas elsewhere in the body.

XI. **Special clinical problems**

A. **Pseudomyxoma peritonei** occurs in the setting of mucinous cystadenocarcinoma or "benign" mucinous adenomas. The peritoneum becomes filled with jellylike material that compresses bowel and produces painful abdominal distention. RT and chemotherapy may impede cellular production of the mucoid material but usually have little direct effect on the tumor. Periodic surgical debulking may be the only way to provide relief of abdominal symptoms. Occasionally the jelly can be liquefied by intraperitoneal instillation and aspiration of 5% dextrose in water.

B. **Obstructive complications.** Intestinal obstruction is discussed in Chapter 30, **II**. Rectal or urinary tract obstruction or dyspareunia in patients with advanced pelvic cancers may respond to either systemic chemotherapy or local irradiation (see *General Aspects,* sec. **IV**). We prefer to use chemotherapy first and retain the flexibility to use further cytotoxic agent treatment later in the course.

C. **Pregnancy with ovarian cancer** (see Chap. 26). Pregnancy is rarely complicated by the development of ovarian cancer. All pregnant patients have luteal cysts, which should be less than 5 to 6 cm in diameter. Masses that are larger or continue to enlarge over several weeks should be examined by laparoscopy at 16 weeks of gestation. Management of pregnant patients with ovarian cancer is the same as for nonpregnant patients who desire childbearing.

D. **Fallopian tube cancers** account for 0.3 percent of all cancers of the female genital tract. They are seen most frequently in the fifth and sixth decades. The classic triad of symptoms is a prominent watery vaginal discharge, pelvic pain, and pelvic mass. However, this triad is seen in fewer than 15 percent of patients. The histologic features, evaluation, and treatment are similar to those of ovarian cancer.

Gestational Trophoblastic Neoplasia

I. **Epidemiology and etiology.** Gestational choriocarcinoma accounts for less than 1 percent of malignancies in women. The etiology is unknown but certain risk factors and the relationship with hydatidiform mole are well recognized.

A. **Hydatidiform moles**

1. Hydatidiform mole develops in approximately 1:2000 pregnancies in North America and Europe. The incidence is 5 to 10 times greater in Asia, Latin America, and other countries.

2. Other factors that are associated with the occurrence of hydatidiform mole include:

   a. Patients who have had a prior molar pregnancy.

   b. Extremes of reproductive age.

   c. Presence of twin pregnancy.

B. **Malignant transformation.** Approximately 10 to 20 percent of molar pregnancies develop malignant trophoblastic neoplasia; two-thirds of the cases are locally invasive moles (chorioadenoma destruens) and one-third are choriocarcinoma. Thus, choriocarcinoma develops in 3 to 5 percent of moles. However, only 50 percent of choriocarcinoma cases have an antecedent hydatidiform mole; 25 percent follow pregnancies terminated by abortion, 20 percent follow delivery of a viable fetus, and 5 percent follow an ectopic pregnancy. The risk of choriocarcinoma is 5 times greater for an ectopic gestation than for an intrauterine gestation.

II. **Pathology and natural history**

A. **Pathology.** The fetal placenta is composed of mesenchymal tissue with blood vessels (the villus) and a covering epithelium (trophoblast). Hydatidiform mole results from an easily recognized grapelike hydropic degeneration of the villus (which may or may not be associated with changes in the trophoblast). Choriocarcinoma results from the malignant transformation of the trophoblast and is characterized by the absence of villi. A fine line separates benign from malignant disease. However, histology is not the critical feature of these disorders; the clinical course determines whether the growth is benign or malignant. Occasionally, malignant growth may not become clinically evident until years after the last gestation.

B. **Dissemination.** These tumors disseminate locally to the vagina and pelvic organs. Choriocarcinoma disseminates rapidly and widely via the bloodstream. The liver and lungs are the most common and important sites of distant metastases.

III. Diagnosis

A. Symptoms of molar pregnancy or malignant trophoblastic disease are

1. Vaginal bleeding during pregnancy (nearly all cases of molar pregnancy or malignant trophoblastic disease cause bleeding).
2. Hyperemesis gravidarum.
3. Passage of grapelike villi from the uterus.
4. Sweating, tachycardia, weight loss, and nervousness resulting from paraneoplastic hyperthyroidism (see sec. **VII.A**).
5. Pulmonary symptoms as a consequence of lung metastases.
6. Right upper quadrant pain or jaundice as a consequence of liver metastases.
7. Any neurologic abnormality resulting from brain metastases.
8. Abdominal (uterine) pain early in pregnancy.

B. Physical findings

1. The uterus is usually, but not always, larger than expected for the duration of pregnancy.
2. Fetal heart tones are absent (the coexistence of a viable fetus and a partial hydatidiform mole is uncommon).
3. The patient develops signs of toxemia of pregnancy (hypertension, retinal sheen, sudden weight gain, proteinuria, or peripheral edema). If signs occur in the first or second trimester, a molar pregnancy is strongly suspected.

C. Preliminary laboratory studies

1. CBC, platelet count, alkaline phosphatase level, LFTs.
2. β-HCG production is maximal in early pregnancy and decreases thereafter. Normal HCG values for pregnancy depend on the assay method used by the laboratory. HCG is elevated in all patients with choriocarcinoma; the serum concentration directly reflects the tumor volume. The serum half-life of HCG is 18 to 24 hours.

D. Special diagnostic studies

1. Ultrasonography of the uterus and Doppler examination reveal no evidence of fetal parts or heart beat in trophoblastic diseases. If these examinations show no fetus, plain x-ray films of the pelvic organs are obtained for confirmation.
2. A chest film should be obtained with molar pregnancies.
3. Radionuclide and CT scans are used to detect brain, liver, or other abdominal metastases. Scans and films of the abdomen and pelvis must be avoided until the absence of a fetus is proved.
4. Thyroid studies (serum T_4 concentration and T_3-resin uptake) are obtained in patients with clinical evidence of hyperthyroidism.

IV. Staging systems and prognostic factors. A staging system for choriocarcinoma is not yet established. A system in use at some centers divides patients into low- and high-risk groups.

A. Low-risk patients have a five-year survival expectancy of almost 100 percent. These patients have

1. Less than a four-month history suggestive of metastatic disease.
2. A serum HCG titer of less than 50 mIU/ml.
3. No evidence of liver or CNS metastases.

B. High-risk patients have a five-year survival expectancy of 50 percent. These patients have

1. More than a four-month history of metastatic disease, *or*
2. A serum HCG titer more than 50 mIU/ml, *or*
3. Liver or brain metastases, *or*
4. Disease following term pregnancy, *or*
5. Failure of chemotherapy.

V. Prevention and early detection. Early detection depends on careful attention to the signs and symptoms of trophoblastic disease in pregnant and postpartum patients.

VI. Management. All forms of gestational trophoblastic neoplasia, from hydatidiform mole to choriocarcinoma, are almost invariably lethal if not treated.

A. Early disease signifies a molar pregnancy without evidence of distant metastases by history, physical examination, LFTs, chest film, or scans.
  1. **Surgery.** Molar tissue is removed by suction curettage while oxytocin is being administered, and then by sharp curettement. Hysterectomy is recommended for women more than 40 years old. Disappearance of HCG is achieved within eight weeks in 80 percent of patients treated by surgery; virtually all of these patients are cured. The patient is followed by weekly blood assays for HCG.
  2. **RT** has no role in early disease.
  3. **Chemotherapy.** Following surgical treatment of a molar pregnancy with no suggestion of metastatic disease, weekly serum HCG titers are obtained. Chemotherapy is started for histologic diagnosis of choriocarcinoma, rising HCG titer (for two weeks), plateau of HCG titer (for three weeks), documentation of metastatic disease, or return of titers with no other explanation after achieving a zero titer. As long as titers continue to decrease, treatment is usually not started; in the past, treatment was started after a predetermined number of weeks.
      a. Methotrexate is the drug of choice in early gestational trophoblastic neoplasia. Methotrexate, 15 to 30 mg, is given IV daily for five days every two weeks. If there is significant toxicity, the drug is stopped. When the blood counts have become normal and other signs of toxicity have resolved, the drug is reinstituted at a dose reduced by 25 percent.
      b. Actinomycin D is used instead of methotrexate in patients with renal function impairment (creatinine clearance less than 60 ml/min). The dose is 8 to 13 µg/kg (usually 10 µg/kg) given in the same schedule as methotrexate.
B. Advanced disease
  1. **Surgery** is used to evacuate or excise the uterus for the same indications outlined in early disease (see sec. **A.1**).
  2. **RT** is clearly indicated for the primary management of patients with liver or brain metastases in combination with chemotherapy.
  3. **Chemotherapy** is the mainstay of management for metastatic trophoblastic disease. All patients undergo the restaging evaluation described in sections **III.C, III.D,** and **IV.**
      a. Low-risk patients are treated with methotrexate or actinomycin D as for early-disease patients. Patients not responding to one of these agents are switched to the alternative drug.
      b. High-risk patients are treated with combination chemotherapy regimens such as EMACO or MAC III (Appendix A1). RT is given if the liver or brain is involved by metastases.
      c. Duration of treatment. Chemotherapy should be continued until no HCG is demonstrable in the serum for three consecutive weekly assays. If the HCG titer rises or plateaus between any two measurements, the chemotherapy regimen must be changed.
C. Patient follow-up
  1. The HCG level is the single most important tumor marker in trophoblastic neoplasia. The assay should be repeated weekly during therapy. After therapy is completed, HCG titers are then obtained according to the following schedule: every two weeks for two months; every month for the next three months; every two months for the next six months; and every six months thereafter.
  2. Other studies that demonstrated disease at the start of therapy should be repeated monthly until complete remission is documented.
VII. Special clinical problems
  A. Thyrotoxicosis and even "thyroid storm" may result from the thyroid stimulating hormonelike effect of high concentrations of HCG. Clinical evidence of hyperthyroidism in choriocarcinoma occurs in the presence of widespread metastases and is associated with a poor prognosis. Laboratory confirmation requires a

serum T_4 concentration and T_3-resin uptake levels compatible with hyperthyroidism. If the symptoms are mild, propylthiouracil or methimazole can be used. In severe cases, patients must be given propranolol and Lugol's solution.

B. Development of choriocarcinoma long after the last pregnancy or even hysterectomy can occur. This development serves to emphasize that histologic diagnosis is necessary in metastatic cancer when the primary tumor is not evident. The diagnosis of choriocarcinoma can lead to life-saving therapy.

C. Subsequent pregnancies. Women with a history of trophoblastic disease can have normal pregnancies after successful treatment of the cancers.

Selected Reading

Cancer of the Uterine Cervix

Hatch, K. Cervical cancer. In Berek, J. S., and Hacker, N. F. (eds.). *Practical Gynecologic Oncology* (2nd ed.). Baltimore: Williams and Wilkins, 1994. Pp. 243–283.

Lawton, F. G., and Hacker, N. F. Surgery for invasive gynecologic cancer in the elderly female population. *Obstet. Gynecol.* 76:287, 1990.

Potter, M. E., et al. Early invasive cervical cancer with pelvic lymph node involvement: To complete or not to complete radical hysterectomy? *Gynecol. Oncol.* 37:78, 1990.

Soison, A. P., et al. Adjuvant radiotherapy following radical hysterectomy for patients with stage IB and IIA cervical cancer. *Gynecol. Oncol.* 37:390, 1990.

Stehman, F. B., et al. Carcinoma of the cervix treated with radiation therapy. I. A multivariate analysis of prognostic variables in the Gynecologic Oncology Group. *Cancer* 67:2776, 1991.

Vermorken, J. B. The role of chemotherapy in squamous cell carcinoma of the uterine cervix: A review. *Int. J. Gynecol. Cancer* 3:129, 1993.

Cancer of the Uterine Body

Farias-Eisner, R., Nieberg, R. K., and Berek, J. S. Synchronous primary neoplasms of the female reproductive tract. *Gynecol. Oncol.* 33:355, 1989.

Hacker, N. F. Uterine cancer. In Berek, J. S., and Hacker, N. F. (eds.). *Practical Gynecologic Oncology* (2nd ed.). Baltimore: Williams and Wilkins, 1994. Pp. 285–326.

Levenback, C., et al. Uterine papillary serous carcinoma (UPSC) treated with cisplatin, doxorubicin, and cyclophosphamide (PAC). *Gynecol. Oncol.* 46:217, 1992.

Lurain, J. R. The significance of positive peritoneal cytology in endometrial cancer. *Gynecol. Oncol.* 46:143, 1992.

Morrow, C. P., et al. Relationship between surgical-pathologic risk factors and outcome in clinical stage I and II carcinoma of the endometrium. *Gynecol. Oncol.* 40:55, 1991.

Parazzini, F., et al. The epidemiology of endometrial cancer. *Gynecol. Oncol.* 41:1, 1991.

Vaginal Cancer

Eddy, G. L., Singh, K. P., and Ganster, T. S. Superficially invasive carcinoma of the vagina following treatment for cervical cancer: A report of six cases. *Gynecol. Oncol.* 36:376, 1990.

Hacker, N. F. Vaginal cancer. In Berek, J. S., and Hacker, N. F. (eds.). *Practical Gynecologic Oncology* (2nd ed.). Baltimore: Williams and Wilkins, 1994. Pp. 441–453.

Reddy, S., et al. Radiation therapy in primary carcinoma of the vagina. *Gynecol. Oncol.* 26:19, 1987.

Vulvar Cancer

Berek, J. S., et al. Concurrent cisplatin and 5-fluorouracil chemotherapy and radiotherapy for advanced stage squamous carcinoma of the vulva. *Gynecol. Oncol.* 42: 197, 1991.

Farias-Eisner, R., et al. Conservative and individualized surgery for early squamous carcinoma of the vulva: The treatment of choice for stages I and II (T_{1-2}; N_{0-1}, M_0) disease. *Gynecol. Oncol.* 53:55, 1994.

Hacker, N. F. Vulvar cancer. In Berek, J. S., and Hacker, N. F. (ed.). *Practical Gynecologic Oncology* (2nd ed.). Baltimore: Williams and Wilkins, 1994. Pp. 403–439.

Podratz, K. C., et al. Melanoma of the vulva: An update. *Gynecol. Oncol.* 16:153, 1983.

Ovarian Cancer

Berek, J. S. Epithelial ovarian cancer. In Berek, J. S., Hacker, N. F. (eds.). *Practical Gynecologic Oncology* (2nd ed.). Baltimore: Williams and Wilkins, 1994. Pp. 327–375.

Bookman, M., and Berek, J. S. Biologic and immunologic therapy of ovarian cancer. *Hematol. Oncol. Clin. North. Am.* 6:941, 1992.

Einhorn, N., et al. A prospective evaluation of serum CA-125 levels for early detection of ovarian cancer. *Obstet. Gynecol.* 80:14, 1992.

Farias-Eisner, R., et al. The influence of tumor grade, distribution and extent of carcinomatosis in minimal residual epithelial ovarian cancer after optimal primary cytoreductive surgery. *Gynecol. Oncol.* 55:108, 1994.

Hoskins, W. J., et al. The influence of cytoreductive surgery on recurrence-free interval and survival in small volume state III epithelial ovarian cancer: a Gynecology Oncology Group Study. *Gynecol. Oncol.* 47:159, 1992.

Nguyen, H. N., et al. Ovarian carcinoma: A review of the significance of familial risk factors and the role of prophylactic oophorectomy in cancer prevention. *Cancer* 74:545, 1994.

Van der Burg, M. E. L., et al. Interval debulking surgery does improve survival in advanced epithelial ovarian cancer: An EROTC Gynecologic Cancer Cooperative Group Study. *Proc. Am. Soc. Clin. Oncol.* 29:818, 1993.

Gestational Trophoblastic Neoplasia

Berkowitz, R. S., and Goldstein, B. P. Gestational trophoblastic neoplasia. In Berek, J. S., and Hacker, N. F. (eds.). *Practical Gynecologic Oncology* (2nd ed.). Baltimore: Williams and Wilkins, 1994. Pp. 457–480.

Berkowitz, R. S., and Goldstein, B. P. The management of molar pregnancy and gestational trophoblastic tumors. In Knapp, R. C., and Berkowitz, R. S. (eds.). *Gynecologic Oncology* (2nd ed.). New York: MacMillan, 1993. Pp. 328–338.

Surwit, E. A., and Childers, J. M. High-risk metastatic gestational trophoblastic disease: A new dose-intensive multiagent chemotherapeutic regimen. *J. Reprod. Med.* 36:45, 1991.

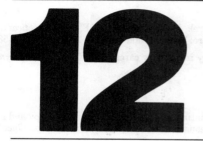

Testicular Cancer

Lawrence H. Einhorn and
Barry B. Lowitz

I. Epidemiology and etiology
A. Epidemiology
1. **Incidence.** Testicular cancer constitutes only 1 percent of all cancers in males but is the most common malignancy that develops in men between the ages of 20 to 40 years. Approximately 6000 new cases are diagnosed annually in the United States.
2. **Racial predilection.** The incidence of testicular cancer in African Americans is one-sixth that in whites. Asians also have a lower incidence than whites.
3. **Bilateral cancer** of the testis occurs in approximately 2 percent of cases.
B. Etiology
1. **Cryptorchidism.** Males with cryptorchidism are 10 to 40 times more likely to develop testicular carcinoma than are males with normally descended testes. The risk of developing cancer in a testis is 1:80 if retained in the inguinal canal, and 1:20 if retained in the abdomen. Surgical placement of an undescended testis into the scrotum before 6 years of age reduces the risk of cancer. However, 25 percent of cancers in patients with cryptorchidism occur in the *normal, descended testis.*
2. **Testicular feminization syndromes** increase the risk of cancer in the retained gonad by 40-fold. Tumors in these patients are often bilateral.
3. **Other risk factors.** The magnitude of other suggested risk factors, such as a history of orchitis, testicular trauma, or irradiation, is not known.
II. Pathology and natural history
A. Histology
1. Nearly all cancers of the testis in members of the younger age groups originate from germ cells (seminoma, embryonal cell, teratoma, and others). Other types, which account for less than 5 percent of cases, include rhabdomyosarcoma, lymphoma, and melanoma. Rarely, Sertoli cell tumor, interstitial cell tumor, or other mesodermal tumors develop.
2. In men more than 60 years old, 75 percent of neoplasms are not germinal cancers. Lymphomas are the most common testicular tumors in this age group.
3. Metastatic cancer to the testis is most often associated with prostatic carcinoma, lung cancer, melanoma, or leukemia.
B. Histogenesis. Each type of germinal cancer is thought to be a counterpart of normal embryonic development (Fig. 12-1). Seminoma is the neoplastic counterpart of the spermatocyte. The tissues of the early cleavage stage are the most undifferentiated and pluripotential and give rise to both the embryo and the placenta; the malignant counterpart is embryonal cell carcinoma. Teratomas are the neoplastic counterparts of the developing embryo. Choriocarcinoma is actually a more highly differentiated cancer; its aggressive biologic behavior reflects the capacity of its normal counterpart (the placenta) to invade blood vessels. The histologic similarity between germ cell cancer and normal embryology is illustrated by the following observations:
1. Pure choriocarcinomas metastasize only as choriocarcinomas.
2. Seminomas usually metastasize as seminomas; those that do not are be-

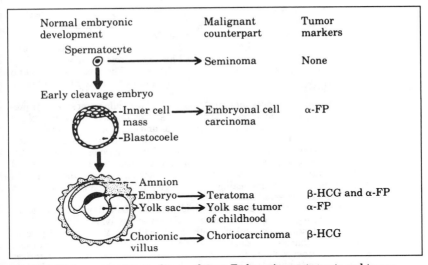

Fig. 12-1. Histogenesis of testicular neoplasms. Embryonic counterparts and tumor marker production are shown. β-HCG = β-subunit of human chorionic gonadotropin; α-FP = α-fetoprotein.

lieved to represent mixed tumors undetected on the original histologic examination.

3. Metastases from embryonal carcinomas may be found to consist of teratoma or choriocarcinoma elements.

4. In metastases from mixed tumors, chemotherapy destroys the rapidly growing, drug-sensitive embryonal cell elements. The more drug-resistant teratomatous elements may remain clinically evident but may become mature on histologic examination.

C. **Natural history.** The natural history of testis cancer varies with the histologic subtype. Both blood-borne and lymphatic metastases occur. Lymphatic drainage usually occurs in an orderly progression involving ileal and para-aortic lymphatic chains, as well as more lateral nodes near the kidneys (which are not assessed by pedal lymphangiography); inguinal and femoral nodes are normally not affected. Previous surgery, such as scrotal contamination with scrotal orchiectomy, disrupts normal lymphatic drainage patterns.

1. **Seminoma** (40–50% of testicular cancers) occurs in an older age group than other germ cell neoplasms, most commonly after the age of 30 years. Sixty percent of patients with cryptorchidism who develop testicular cancer have seminoma. Seminomas tend to be large, show little hemorrhage or necrosis on gross inspection, and metastasize in an orderly, sequential manner along draining lymph node chains. Approximately 25 percent of patients have lymphatic metastases, and 1 to 5 percent have visceral metastases at the time of diagnosis. Metastases to parenchymal organs (usually lung or bone) occur late. Seminoma is the type of testicular cancer most likely to produce osseous metastases. Three atypical forms of seminoma are the spermatocytic, poorly differentiated, and mixed subtypes.

   a. **Spermatocytic seminoma** (4% of seminomas) occurs mostly after the age of 50 years and is the most common germ cell tumor after age 70. It is more often bilateral (6% compared to 2%) and appears to have a much lower incidence of both lymphatic and parenchymal metastases (even to draining lymph nodes) when compared to typical seminoma.

   b. **Anaplastic seminoma** (10% of seminomas) is defined as a seminoma with three or more mitoses per high-power field. These tumors are clinically aggressive; however, stage for stage, their management and prognosis is identical to that of typical seminoma.

  c. **Mixed tumors** consist of seminoma together with embryonal or choriocarcinoma elements. Their natural history reflects the most aggressive histologic subtype of all cancers of the testis. The presence of visceral metastases in a patient whose primary tumor was apparently pure seminoma suggests the presence of another germ cell type.

2. **Embryonal carcinoma and teratoma** (50% of testicular cancers) occur predominantly in 20- to 30-year-old patients. Approximately two-thirds of these tumors are pure embryonal cell carcinomas and one-third have a preponderance of teratomatous features. The term **teratocarcinoma** refers to teratomas in combination with other elements. These subtypes are grouped together because teratomas appear to be dependent on the pluripotential embryonal cell line for their malignant potential. Any of the tissues in teratomas may become malignant (e.g., glandular structures may develop into adenocarcinoma).

     These tumors grow extremely rapidly, tend to be bulky and have areas of hemorrhage and necrosis, and spread by draining lymphatics and bloodborne metastases (particularly to the lung and liver). More than 65 percent of patients have evidence of metastatic disease at the time of presentation.

3. **Pure choriocarcinoma** (less than 0.5% of testicular cancers) metastasizes rapidly via the bloodstream to lungs, liver, brain, and other visceral sites.

4. **Yolk sac tumors** are common cancers in children and have a relatively unaggressive clinical course. Yolk sac elements in testicular cancer found in adult patients, on the other hand, portend a poor prognosis.

5. **Rare testicular tumors**
  a. **Gonadoblastomas** are found in patients with dysgenic gonads and chromosomal mosaicism. These tumors are mixtures of germ cell and stromal elements such as Sertoli cells. They vary in malignant potential but all can metastasize.
  b. **Polyembryomas** have a natural history similar to embryonal carcinoma.
  c. **Dermoid cysts** are fully mature teratomas and are exceptionally rare in the testis.
  d. **Rhabdomyosarcoma** of the testis occurs most often before the age of 20 years. Its clinical behavior is similar to that of embryonal carcinoma; metastases to draining lymph nodes and lung are common at the time it first appears.

III. Diagnosis
A. Symptoms and signs
  1. **Symptoms**
    a. **Mass and pain.** The most common symptom of testicular cancer is a painless enlargement usually noticed during bathing or after a minor trauma. Painful enlargement of the testis occurs in 30 to 50 percent of patients and may be the result of bleeding or infarction in the tumor. Acute pain in a patient with a cryptorchid testis suggests the possibility of torsion of a testicular cancer; rupture into the abdomen results in manifestations that may be indistinguishable from acute appendicitis and other causes of an acute abdomen.
    b. **Acute epididymitis.** Nearly 25 percent of patients with mixed teratoma and embryonal cell tumor present with findings indistinguishable from acute epididymitis. The testicular swelling from tumor may even decrease somewhat following antimicrobial therapy.
    c. **Gynecomastia** is the first sign of testicular cancer in about 10 percent of cases.
    d. **Infertility** is the primary symptom in about 3 percent of patients.
    e. **Back pain** from retroperitoneal node metastases is a presenting feature in 10 percent of patients.

f. **Other presenting symptoms.** Skin and retro-orbital metastases are unusual but occur most frequently with choriocarcinoma. Pyloric obstruction from epigastric lymph node metastases and bone pain from skeletal metastases are rare.

2. **Physical findings**

   a. **Scrotum.** A large testicular mass is nearly always present. The testis should be palpated using bimanual technique; the finding of irregularity, induration, or nodularity is indication for further evaluation.

   b. **Lymph nodes.** Patients must be carefully examined for lymphadenopathy, particularly in the supraclavicular region. Iliac nodes are especially liable to be affected in patients with spermatic cord or epididymal involvement. Herniorrhaphy alters the normal lymphatic drainage; as a result, the contralateral iliac and homolateral inguinal nodes become those likely to be involved.

   c. **Breasts.** Gynecomastia is associated with tumors that secrete high levels of HCG.

B. **Differential diagnosis**

   1. **Hydroceles** are usually benign but about 10 percent of testicular cancers are associated with coexisting hydroceles. The finding of a hydrocele in a young man should increase suspicion for an associated neoplasm.

      a. Benign hydroceles extend along the spermatic cord, often cause groin swelling, and can give the penis a foreshortened appearance. Hydroceles can be transilluminated.

      b. If the fluid prevents adequate palpation of the testis, a urologist should aspirate the fluid and reexamine the testis. Aspiration must avoid piercing a cancer (dissemination of tumor cells can result). Hydrocele fluid is clear and straw-colored; the presence of blood in the fluid mandates exploratory surgery.

   2. **Epididymitis** produces acute enlargement of the testis with severe pain, fever, dysuria, and pyuria. The same symptoms may be caused by an underlying testicular cancer.

      a. **Persistent pain or swelling** following treatment may result from a supervening testicular abscess or a coexisting tumor; surgical exploration is indicated.

      b. **Recurrent epididymitis** with a completely normal testis occasionally occurs. Surgical exploration should not be considered if physical examination between episodes is completely normal. Recurrent epididymitis per se does not necessarily indicate cancer.

   3. **Varicoceles** are swollen veins in the pampiniform plexus of the spermatic cord. The scrotum feels like it contains a "bag of worms." The veins collapse when the patient is in the Trendelenburg position.

   4. **Spermatoceles** are translucent masses that are located posterior and superior to the testis and feel cystic.

   5. **Inguinal hernias** generally are not a diagnostic problem.

   6. **Other masses** include gummatous and tuberculous orchitis, hematoma, and acute swelling from testicular torsion. None of these can be distinguished clinically from cancer, and all require exploratory surgery.

C. **Tumor markers** are the most critical and sensitive indicators of testicular cancer (see Fig. 12-1). HCG, particularly the β-subunit (β-HCG), and α-FP are the only markers of proven value. One or both of these serum markers are present in more than 90 percent of patients with nonseminomatous germ cell cancer of the testis. The incidences of these markers according to tumor histology are shown in Table 12-1.

   1. **HCG** is made by chorionic elements of the tumor. It is composed of two chains, α and β.

      a. **Whole two-component HCG** is a nonspecific tumor marker and may be found in patients with a variety of other tumors, including melanoma, lymphoma and sarcoma, or carcinoma of the lung, breast, ovary, or GI tract. Nonmalignant conditions associated with elevated HCG levels in-

Table 12-1. Incidence of tumor markers in testicular cancers

	Proportion of cases (%)	
Neoplasm	β-HCG[a]	α-Fetoprotein[b]
Seminoma	10	<1
Embryonal carcinomas with or without teratomas	65	>70
Choriocarcinoma	100	<1

[a] Normal levels of β-HCG = 0 ng/ml.
[b] Normal levels of α-fetoprotein = <40 μg/ml.

clude cirrhosis, peptic ulcer disease, and inflammatory bowel disease. The whole HCG molecule has a half-life in the blood of 24 hours.

    b. α-HCG is a component of several normal pituitary hormones and has been helpful in detecting certain occult neoplasms. α-HCG has a blood half-life of only 20 minutes.

    c. β-HCG is never found in normal men. Its presence always indicates a malignancy and has proved to be the most useful tumor marker to monitor response to therapy. In testicular cancer, the presence of β-HCG after orchiectomy constitutes proof that the patient has residual cancer and requires further treatment. The absence of β-HCG, however, does not exclude the presence of active cancer, particularly in previously treated patients. The blood half-life of β-HCG is 18 to 24 hours.

  2. α-FP is produced by yolk sac elements and is most commonly associated with embryonal carcinomas and yolk sac tumors. Elevated levels of α-FP are never found in patients with pure seminoma or pure choriocarcinoma. Elevated levels may also be explained by hepatocellular carcinoma, other cancers (occasionally), fetal hepatic production in pregnant women, infancy, and nonmalignant liver diseases (e.g., hepatitis, cirrhosis, necrosis). Elevated levels of α-FP following surgical therapy or cytotoxic agent therapy for testicular cancer indicate the presence of residual disease and the need for further therapy. The blood half-life of α-FP is five days.

  3. Placental alkaline phosphatase (PAP or Regan isoenzyme) is elevated in seminomas. It is especially sensitive when combined with LDH levels. Both studies are abnormal in 50 percent of stage I patients and 100 percent of stage II patients with seminoma. Combined PAP and LDH levels are useful both as an adjunct to diagnosis and in monitoring therapy and recurrence.

  4. CEA is elevated in 0 to 40 percent of patients with testicular cancer, is not correlated with disease extent or prognosis, and is not useful.

D. Laboratory evaluation

  1. Routine preoperative studies

    a. CBC, LFTs (especially LDH and alkaline phosphatase levels), renal function tests, and urinalysis

    b. Chest film including posteroanterior and lateral projections

    c. Blood levels of β-HCG and α-FP

  2. Routine postoperative studies are undertaken after the diagnosis of testicular cancer is proved. Studies performed in patients with all cell types include the following:

    a. Chest CT scan detects about 10 percent more metastatic lesions than do plain chest films.

    b. Abdominal CT scans assist assessment of retroperitoneal disease.

  3. Pedal lymphangiography is utilized only for patients with seminoma to complete staging evaluation and to plan RT fields. Its use in other cell types is restricted to certain controversial approaches to treatment (see sec. **VI.C.1**).

   4. Supraclavicular lymph nodes. Palpable lymph nodes should be biopsied for staging, if clinically appropriate.

IV. Staging system and prognostic factors

   A. Staging system and survival. The system presented is a pathologic staging system for nonseminomatous tumors for which lymphadenectomy is a standard practice. The system is also used for clinical staging of seminomas for which lymph node sampling is not part of management.

   The survival statistics for testicular tumors have been drastically altered by modern therapy. Five-year survival in patients with seminoma treated with RT alone is 95 to 99 percent for stage A and 70 percent for stage B; most patients with stage C are cured with chemotherapy. Five-year survival in patients with stage C nonseminomatous tumors is 70 percent.

Stage	Extent of disease
A	Disease confined to the testis
B	Metastases to the retroperitoneal lymph nodes are present
B_1	Five or fewer encapsulated lymph nodes positive for tumor
B_2	More than five lymph nodes positive for tumor
B_3	Massive retroperitoneal lymph node disease
C	Tumor involving supradiaphragmatic nodes, lungs, liver, bone, or brain

   B. Prognostic factors

   1. Elevated serum levels of α-FP or β-HCG following orchiectomy is prima facie evidence that the patient has residual cancer.

   2. Serum LDH levels correlate fairly well with tumor burden.

   3. The prognosis is worsened with

      a. Bulky abdominal disease that cannot be removed by surgery even after treatment with chemotherapy.

      b. Liver or brain metastases.

      c. Pure choriocarcinoma has a particularly poor prognosis in men because of the advanced disease present at the time of diagnosis.

V. Prevention and early detection. Cryptorchidism should be surgically corrected before puberty because the risk of developing malignancy is substantial. Prophylactic removal of undescended testes should be performed in postpubertal males; the complication rate is miniscule, the testes are functionless, and prostheses are available to fill the empty scrotum.

   The effectiveness of early detection by screening programs has not been tested. Most patients have symptoms or signs of a scrotal mass; few cases are detected by routine history and physical examination.

VI. Management

   A. Transinguinal orchiectomy is performed to make the diagnosis for all testicular cancers in all stages and is the treatment for stage A disease. A transinguinal approach is essential; the blood supply of the spermatic cord is immediately controlled. Transscrotal orchiectomy has been proved to result in tumor seeding to the skin and inguinal nodes. Likewise, transscrotal needle biopsy of a suspected testicular mass is *absolutely contraindicated.*

   The subsequent management of early-stage testicular tumors depends on whether the histopathology shows pure seminoma or nonseminomatous elements. Figure 12-2 diagrams an approach to the management of malignant testicular neoplasms.

   B. Management of seminomas: stages A and B

   1. Surgery. No further surgery is necessary after orchiectomy.

   2. RT. Bipedal lymphangiography is performed postoperatively in patients with seminoma. The retroperitoneal nodes are irradiated. Seminomas are exquisitely sensitive to RT.

   3. Chemotherapy is not necessary in most patients with stage A or B seminoma. Patients with bulky stage B (>5 cm disease) or stage C disease are treated the same as those with nonseminomatous germ cell cancer, and the results are similar (see sec. **D**).

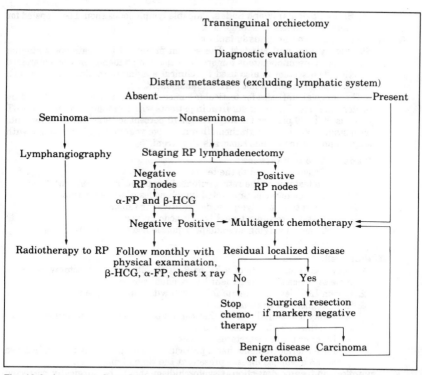

Fig. 12-2. An approach to the management of stage A, B_1, and B_2 testicular cancers. RP = retroperitoneal. β-HCG = β-subunit of human chorionic gonadotropin; α-FP = α-fetoprotein.

C. Management of nonseminomatous germ cell cancer: stages A and B

1. **Surgery.** Retroperitoneal lymphadenectomy is the current standard of practice at most centers in the United States in the following situations: when (1) staging evaluation does not reveal distant metastases and (2) there is no lymph node with a maximal tranverse diameter of 3 cm on abdominal CT. Lymphangiography is not routinely performed. If lymph node metastases are demonstrated at surgery, patients may be either treated with two courses of adjuvant chemotherapy or observed without treatment and achieve the same nearly 100 percent cure rate. Lymphadenectomy previously interrupted the sympathetic pathways and invariably resulted in sterility from failure of ejaculation, but not impotence (see Chap. 26, sec. **I.C.2**). However, modern nerve-sparing retroperitoneal lymph node dissections now routinely preserve fertility and allow antegrade ejaculation.

2. **Chemotherapy.** The agents used are discussed in **D**. Indications for chemotherapy are

   a. Elevated serum levels of β-HCG or α-FP after primary treatment.

   b. The presence of bulky retroperitoneal disease (>3 cm maximal transverse diameter of a node on abdominal CT) requires chemotherapy. If the abdominal CT scan becomes normal, retroperitoneal lymphadenectomy is not necessary. Otherwise, postchemotherapy retroperitoneal lymph node dissection is usually performed.

3. **RT.** Effective chemotherapy has made RT obsolete in the management of early-stage nonseminomatous tumors. RT compromises bone marrow re-

serves and may make administration of potentially curative doses of chemotherapy difficult.

D. Management of disseminated disease: stage C

1. Chemotherapy. Combination chemotherapy with BEP produces complete remission in 70 percent of patients. Complete remissions are obtained with all cell types and are long-lasting. Relapses may occur within one year of initiating therapy. Maintenance chemotherapy after achieving a complete remission is not necessary.

a. Etoposide is now used as first-line therapy instead of vinblastine because complete response rates are identical, and etoposide is associated with less bone marrow suppression, myalgias, paresthesias, and ileus than vinblastine.

b. BEP is administered every 3 weeks for three or four cycles. Dosages are as follows:

Bleomycin, 30 units IV weekly for nine to twelve weeks
Etoposide, 100 mg/m^2 IV daily for five days
Cisplatin, 20 mg/m^2 IV daily for five days

2. Resection of residual disease. After cytoreduction with chemotherapy, about one half of the patients without a complete remission (an additional 10–15% of all patients) can become candidates for surgical resection of the residual localized disease in the chest or retroperitoneum. Radiologic findings *cannot* distinguish benign from malignant processes in these patients.

a. The presence of elevated levels of tumor markers always signifies the continued presence of carcinoma and the need for further chemotherapy. The absence of tumor markers signifies that the residual disease in the thorax or retroperitoneum is either a benign process (fibrosis, inflammation), teratoma, or carcinoma.

b. Surgical resection of residual disease defines the subsequent treatment strategy in all of these patients and appears to be therapeutic in some. If surgical resection of residual disease reveals

(1) Fibrosis or teratoma, no further treatment is required.

(2) Carcinoma, two more cycles of cisplatin and etoposide therapy or salvage chemotherapy are given.

3. Salvage chemotherapy. Patients who do not achieve a complete remission with BEP are treated with cisplatin, vinblastine (0.11 mg/kg IV on days one and two of each cycle), and ifosfamide. In addition, high-dose chemotherapy with autologous BMT has been used.

VII. Special clinical problems

A. Gynecomastia and elevated blood β-HCG levels are occasionally found in patients with clinically normal testes and no other evidence of cancer. A number of other cancers can also produce β-HCG. Patients should be evaluated with ultrasonography of the testes and CT of the abdomen and chest. Thereafter, it is best to follow such patients clinically until there is demonstrable cancer or rising HCG levels. Blind or random biopsies in this setting are not likely to reveal a diagnosis, expose patients to unnecessary morbidity, and are contraindicated.

B. Extragonadal germ cell neoplasms, particularly seminomas, can occur in any anatomic site through which the normal germ cells migrate in the embryo. Such sites include the pineal gland, mediastinum, and presacral areas. Tumor markers (β-HCG and α-FP) should be measured. RT with or without chemotherapy, depending on the extent of disease, is used to treat seminomas. Intensive chemotherapy with BEP without RT should be used for nonseminomatous germ cell cancers. Results of treatment are less successful than for primary testicular cancer.

C. Solitary mediastinal masses with undifferentiated small cell histology may represent lymphoma, small cell carcinoma, melanoma, neuroblastoma, Ewing's sarcoma, or testicular cancer. Differentiation by histopathology may be impossible. If differentiation is impossible and the patient is in the correct age group

(20–30 years of age), a reasonable approach would be to treat the patient for disseminated nonseminomatous germ cell cancer. Mediastinal germ cell tumors are discussed in Chap. 19, sec. **I.B.3.**

Selected Reading

Bosl, G. J., et al. A randomized trial of etoposide plus cisplatin versus vinblastine, bleomycin, cisplatin, cyclophosphamide, and dactinomycin in patients with good prognosis germ cell tumors. *J. Clin. Oncol.* 6:1231, 1988.

Broun, E. R., et al. Long-term follow-up of salvage chemotherapy in relapsed and refractory germ cell tumors using high-dose carboplatin and etoposide with autologous bone marrow support. *Ann. Intern. Med.* 117:124, 1992.

Einhorn, L. H. Treatment of testicular cancer: A new and improved model. *J. Clin. Oncol.* 8:1777, 1990.

Einhorn, L. H., et al. Evaluation of optimal duration chemotherapy in favorable prognosis disseminated germ cell tumors: A Southeastern Cancer Study Group protocol. *J. Clin. Oncol.* 7:387, 1989.

Einhorn, L. H., et al. The role of maintenance therapy in disseminated testicular cancer. *N. Engl. J. Med.* 305:727, 1987.

Loehrer, P. J., et al. Salvage therapy with VP-16 or vinblastine plus ifosfamide plus cisplatin in recurrent germ cell cancer. *Ann. Intern. Med.* 109:540, 1988.

Saxman, S. B., et al. Mediastinal yolk sac tumors: The Indiana University experience, 1976–1987. *Thorac. Cardiovasc. Surg.* 102:913, 1990.

Thomas, G. M. Controversies in the management of testicular seminoma. *Cancer* 55:2296, 1985.

Williams, S. D., et al. Treatment of disseminated germ cell tumors with cisplatin, bleomycin, and either vinblastine and etoposide. *N. Engl. J. Med.* 316:1435, 1987.

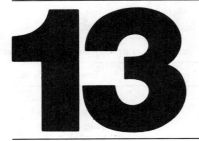

Urinary Tract Cancers

Robert A. Figlin and
Jean B. deKernion

The relative incidence and mortality of urinary tract malignancies according to primary site are shown in Table 13-1.

Renal Cancer

I. **Epidemiology and etiology**
   A. **Incidence** (see Table 13-1). Renal cancer constitutes 2 percent of all malignancies. The incidence has increased slowly in the past decade. Men are affected twice as often as women.
   B. **Etiology.** The cause of renal cancer is unknown.
      1. Factors that increase the risk of renal cancer include
         a. Smoking
         b. Urban living
         c. Family history of renal cancer
         d. Thorotrast exposure
         e. von Hippel-Lindau disease
      2. Unproven factors that may increase the risk of renal cancer include polycystic kidney disease, diabetes mellitus, and chronic dialysis.
II. **Pathology and natural history**
   A. **Adenocarcinomas** ("hypernephromas" or "Grawitz tumors") make up nearly all renal cancers in adults.
      1. The histologic variants include papillary, clear cell, granular cell, and spindle cell subtypes.
      2. These tumors originate in the kidney from proximal tubular cells, invade local structures, and metastasize by way of the lymphatics and bloodstream. The most common sites of distant metastases are the lungs, liver, bones, and brain. Adenocarcinomas may present with metastases to unusual sites such as the finger tips, eyelids, and nose. A primary renal cancer may be diagnosed based on the characteristic histology of a metastatic deposit.
      3. The natural history of hypernephroma is more unpredictable than most solid tumors. The primary tumor has variable growth patterns and may remain localized for many years. Metastatic foci may have long periods of indolent or apparently arrested growth or may develop many years after removal of the primary tumor.
   B. **Transitional cell carcinomas** are very uncommon tumors that arise in the renal pelvis and often affect multiple sites of urothelial mucosa, including the renal pelvis, ureters, and urinary bladder (see *Urinary Bladder Cancer*, sec. II). These tumors usually are low grade and discovered late in the course of the disease. Transitional cell carcinomas occasionally have a peculiar disposition to spread over the posterior retroperitoneum in a sheetlike fashion, encasing vessels and producing urinary tract obstruction. Hematogenous dissemination occurs, particularly to lung and bone.
   C. **Rare renal tumors**
      1. **Nephroblastomas** (Wilms' tumors) appear as large, bulky masses in children, but rarely occur in adults (see Chap. 18, *Wilms' Tumor*).

Table 13-1. Cancer of the urinary tract in the United States

	Proportion of urinary tract malignancies	
Primary site	New cases (%)	Deaths due to cancer (%)
Kidney	11	19
Bladder	21	18
Prostate	65	62
Testis	3	<1
Penis, urethra	<1	<1
Total	100	100

Note: Cancer of the urinary tract accounted for approximately 252,400 new cancer cases and 56,350 cancer deaths in 1993. Female genital tract malignancies are excluded.

    2. Lymphomas and sarcomas arising in the kidney have clinical courses similar to their counterparts elsewhere in the abdomen.

    3. Juxtaglomerular tumors (reninomas) are rare causes of hypertension and are usually benign.

    4. Hemangiopericytomas are associated with hypertension and are occasionally malignant (15% of cases).

    5. Benign renal adenomas. The existence of benign renal adenoma is controversial because it is not possible to determine malignant or benign biologic behavior only by histology on any lesion less than 3 cm in diameter.

  D. Paraneoplastic syndromes commonly occur with renal adenocarcinomas.

    1. Erythrocytosis. Renal adenocarcinomas are associated with erythrocytosis in approximately 3 percent of patients and account for 15 to 20 percent of cases of inappropriate secretion of erythropoietin. Elevated blood levels of erythropoietin are caused by ectopic erythropoietin production. A left flank mass of hypernephroma may be mistaken for an enlarged spleen resulting from polycythemia vera. The differential diagnosis of erythrocytosis is discussed in Chap. 34, *Increased Blood Cell Counts*, sec. I.

    2. Hypercalcemia, nearly always in association with widespread bony metastases, occurs in about 5 percent of patients.

    3. Fever caused by tumor occurs in 10 to 20 percent of patients.

    4. Hepatomegaly, with elevated serum levels of alkaline phosphatase and transaminase and without liver metastases, occurs in 15 percent of patients. These abnormalities are reversed after nephrectomy.

    5. Hypertension associated with renin production by the tumor occurs in up to 40 percent of patients and is alleviated by removal of the tumor.

    6. Hyperglobulinemia can result in elevated erythrocyte sedimentation rate.

    7. Amyloidosis occasionally occurs.

III. Diagnosis

  A. Symptoms and signs. Symptoms other than hematuria usually indicate large, advanced tumors. The classic triad of flank pain, a flank mass, and hematuria occurs in less than 10 percent of patients with hypernephroma. The combined picture of anemia, hematuria, and fever is rare but very suggestive of renal cancer.

    1. Symptoms

      a. Gross hematuria occurs in over 50 percent of patients.

      b. A steady, dull flank pain occurs in 50 percent of patients. Colicky pain may develop if blood clots are passed into the ureter.

      c. Weight loss is a presenting feature in 30 percent of patients.

      d. Left-sided varicocele that develops suddenly is a presenting feature in less than 3 percent of patients with adenocarcinoma of the left kidney.

      e. Leg edema is the result of locally advanced disease, which causes venous or lymphatic obstruction.

    f. Fever, plethora, or symptoms of hypercalcemia or anemia may be presenting features.

  2. Physical findings

    a. A flank mass is palpable in 50 percent of patients.

    b. Fever occurs in up to 20 percent of patients.

    c. Pallor from anemia occurs in about 40 percent of patients.

B. Diagnostic studies

  1. Urinalysis may reveal proteinuria and hematuria. One-third of patients have neither gross nor microscopic hematuria. *All patients* with macroscopic or microscopic hematuria of any degree must have a urologic evaluation.

  2. Routine studies

    a. CBC, liver and renal function studies.

    b. Hyperglobulinemia is frequently present in patients with hypernephroma because acute phase reactant proteins (α_1- and α_2-globulins) are elevated.

    c. Chest x-ray film may reveal multiple, large, round ("cannonball") metastatic deposits that are characteristic of metastatic genitourinary neoplasms.

  3. Scans should be performed in the following situations:

    a. Bone scan, if there is bone pain or elevated alkaline phosphatase levels

    b. CT scan of the brain, if there are signs or symptoms of CNS abnormalities

    c. Liver, CT scan, if there is hepatomegaly or abnormal LFTs

  4. Nephrotomography is the first diagnostic procedure to delineate mass lesions. Space-occupying lesions found by pyelography may represent cancers, cysts, or hamartomas (angiomyolipomas).

  5. Renal angiography is the most accurate study for distinguishing malignant from benign lesions prior to biopsy.

    a. Both renal cancers and hamartomas are vascular and both mandate surgical exploration. Renal cysts are hypovascular. The angiographic appearance of hamartomas may make preoperative diagnosis possible. Neovascularization and vascular parasitization are characteristic of cancer.

    b. Up to 25 percent of renal cancers, however, are hypovascular and resemble cysts on angiography. Epinephrine administered during angiography causes normal arterial smooth muscles to contract. Tumor vessels lack well-developed musculature and will produce a "tumor blush" after epinephrine is given; this may make previously obscure lesions more readily detectable.

  6. Ultrasonography of the kidney is relatively insensitive but may suggest the presence of a cyst; it may be used as an adjunct in the diagnosis of renal mass lesions but never as the final step.

  7. CT scans of the kidneys help to define cystic lesions and to determine the extent of tumor and adjacent organ involvement.

  8. MRI may be as accurate as CT and defines renal vein and caval extension more reliably in preparation for surgery.

  9. Inferior vena cavography is performed to locate tumor thrombi in all patients with large tumor masses, but has recently been replaced by MRI.

  10. Percutaneous thin-needle aspiration biopsy of a renal mass may result in tumor seeding in the needle track. This procedure should be restricted to patients with medical conditions that make angiography or surgery unduly hazardous, patients with metastatic disease where a tissue diagnosis is necessary, or patients who have findings strongly suggestive of a benign cyst.

  11. Exploratory surgery or nephrectomy may be necessary to define renal masses that cannot be accurately assessed by noninvasive methods, IVP, angiography, or aspiration.

C. Renal cysts. The following approach is recommended to evaluate potential renal cysts:

  1. A renal mass is demonstrated with nephrotomography. If the findings are not strongly suggestive of cancer, ultrasonography is performed to determine whether the mass is cystic.

2. Fluoroscopically directed, thin-needle aspiration is performed if the IVP and ultrasound examinations suggest a benign cyst and if expertise is available. If fluid is obtained, radiocontrast agent is injected in order to delineate the cyst walls. The cyst fluid is evaluated for cytology, glucose, LDH, and protein content and for histology of the cell block. The findings from nephrotomography and cyst fluid examination accurately predict a benign cyst in nearly 100 percent of cases.

3. Lesions that cannot be aspirated or are not suspected to be cystic are evaluated by renal angiography.

IV. Staging system and prognostic factors

   A. Staging system. The TNM system is commonly used to stage renal cancer. The following amended system is helpful in describing prognosis:

Stage	Extent of tumor	Five-year survival (%)
I	Tumor is confined to the renal parenchyma	50–60
II	Tumor extends into the perirenal fat but is confined to Gerota's fascia	50–60
	Tumor extends into renal vein or inferior vena cava	25–50
III	Tumor involves lymph nodes or other vascular structures	10–15
IV	Tumor invades adjacent organs or has distant metastases	<5

   B. Prognostic factors. The survival rate for untreated patients is less than 5 percent at three years and less than 2 percent at five years.

   1. **Histology.** Patients with clear cell carcinoma appear to have a better prognosis. Patients with undifferentiated and spindle cell cancers have five-year survival rates of less than 25 percent.

   2. **Venous extension.** Renal vein or vena cava involvement is not associated with a hopeless prognosis if managed properly; 25 to 50 percent of patients survive for five years.

   3. **Disease-free interval.** The length of time between nephrectomy and the development of metastases affects the survival of patients with metastatic disease.

      a. Nearly all patients who have metastases at the time of surgery or who develop metastases within one year of surgery die within two years if untreated.

      b. Patients who develop metastases more than two years after nephrectomy have a 20 percent five-year survival from the time metastases are recognized.

   4. **Spontaneous regression** of renal cancer following resection of the primary tumor is very rare and occurs in less than 1 percent of patients.

V. Prevention and early detection. The incidence of renal cancer might be reduced if tobacco smoking habits could be controlled. Early detection depends on prompt attention to hematuria and other symptoms suggestive of these cancers.

VI. Management

   A. Early disease

   1. **Surgery**

      a. **Nephrectomy** with removal of Gerota's fascia, the adrenal gland, and tumor in the renal vein or vena cava is the treatment of choice.

      b. **Partial nephrectomy** is sometimes adequate for small peripheral or polar lesions, even when the opposite kidney is normal. Patients with bilateral cancer and only one functional kidney may undergo partial nephrectomy. It is occasionally necessary to remove the kidney entirely, excise the tumor ("bench nephrectomy"), and then perform autotransplantation.

c. **Preoperative occlusion of the renal artery** using angiographic techniques has been advocated by some urologists but is seldom indicated. The hypervascular nature of renal cancer often results in hemorrhage during surgery, particularly with large, bulky tumors. Occlusion procedures make the operation technically easier but the patient may suffer considerable discomfort from pain, fever, and nausea.

d. **Contraindications to surgery** include high surgical risk due to unrelated medical diseases or evidence of distant metastases.

2. **RT** has no established role in the management of early renal cancers.

3. **Chemotherapy** has no established role in the management of early renal cancers.

B. **Advanced disease**

1. **Surgery**

a. **Nephrectomy.** The chance of a spontaneous regression of metastases following nephrectomy is well known but is far exceeded by the surgical morbidity and mortality. The hope for spontaneous regression is never an indication for surgery. Nephrectomy for the palliation of pain or hematuria can be considered in patients with metastatic disease if all of the following criteria are met:

(1) The performance status of the patient is at least 30 percent on the Karnofsky scale (see inside back cover) or is expected to improve substantially if hemorrhage was controlled.

(2) The only symptoms are in the area of the primary tumor. Sites of metastatic disease must be asymptomatic.

(3) The tumor should have a reasonable chance of being resectable as evaluated by the renal angiogram.

b. **Resection of metastases.** Metastases of hypernephroma can be considered for resection only if the following criteria are met:

(1) The interval from nephrectomy to the detection of metastases is at least two years.

(2) The metastasis is proved to be solitary by all of the following studies:

(a) Physical examination

(b) Normal LFTs (normal CT scan if LFTs are abnormal)

(c) Bone scan

(d) Chest CT scan

(e) CT scan of the brain if the patient has neurologic symptoms

2. **RT** is used to control bleeding and pain from the primary tumor and to palliate symptoms from metastases to the CNS and bone. Generally, renal tumors are relatively radioresistant.

3. **Drug therapy**

a. **IL-2** administered alone in high-dose regimens produces a response rate of 15 to 20 percent in good risk patients and durable remissions often lasting years. Significant morbidity and mortality have been associated with high-dose IL-2 therapy. IL-2 administered in lower dosages or in combination with IFN, however, produces comparable results with less morbidity and mortality. For example, 6 million IU/m^2 given daily by continuous intravenous infusion for four days weekly for four weeks out of six is a lower dose IL-2 regimen. IL-2 was approved by the FDA in 1992 for the treatment of metastatic kidney cancer.

b. **α-IFN** has been reported to have a response rate of 15 to 20 percent (particularly for intrathoracic metastases) but no effect on survival.

c. **Progestins** have been used to treat patients with metastatic adenocarcinomas. Medroxyprogesterone acetate (Depo-Provera), 500 mg IM weekly for four weeks and monthly thereafter, and megestrol acetate (Megace), 40 to 80 mg PO q.i.d., have been used. Tumor responses have been reported in less than 15 percent of patients with progestin therapy, and no improvement in survival has been reported.

d. **Cytotoxic agents** have produced negligible effects on metastatic hypernephroma and no improvement in survival. Agents reported to produce occasional responses (15–20% of patients) include the fluoropyrimidines and vinblastine.

  e. Transitional cell cancers of the renal pelvis and ureters may respond to cisplatin, Adriamycin, cyclophosphamide, or fluorouracil.
VII. Special clinical problems. Carcinomas of the ureter and pelvis and vermiform blood clots in association with hypernephroma can cause obstructive uropathy and death. If the cancer is otherwise not producing discomfort, the obstruction can sometimes be relieved by placement of a ureteral stent catheter.

Urinary Bladder Cancer

I. Epidemiology and etiology
  A. Incidence (see Table 13-1). Bladder cancers constitute 4 percent of visceral cancers in the United States. The disease is 2.5 times more frequent in men than women and is most frequent in industrial northeastern cities. The average age of onset is the sixth to seventh decade.
  B. Risk factors and carcinogens
    1. Industry. Aniline dye workers are 30 times more likely to develop bladder cancer than the general population. Aromatic amines that are chemical intermediates of anilines, rather than the aniline dyes themselves, have been shown to be etiologic. Leather, paint, and rubber industry workers also appear to have an increased risk of bladder cancer. Proven chemical carcinogens in these industries are 2-naphthylamine, benzidine, 4-amino-biphenyl, and 4-nitro-biphenyl.
    2. *Schistosoma haematobium* infection of the bladder is associated with bladder cancer, particularly with squamous cell histology, in endemic regions of Africa and the Middle East.
    3. Smoking increases the risk of bladder cancer twofold. Eighty-five percent of men who die of bladder cancer have a history of smoking.
    4. Pelvic irradiation increases the risk of bladder cancer by a factor of four.
    5. Drugs. Cyclophosphamide unequivocally increases the risk of bladder cancer. Other drugs that have been implicated in animal studies but not proved in human beings are phenacetin, sodium saccharin, and sodium cyclamate.
    6. Abnormal tryptophan metabolism has been found in up to 50 percent of patients with bladder cancer. Certain metabolites are carcinogenic in animals.
II. Pathology and natural history
  A. Pathology
    1. Histology. Ninety percent of bladder cancers are transitional cell (urothelial) and 8 percent are squamous cell types. Adenocarcinomas, sarcomas, lymphomas, and carcinoid tumors are rare.
    2. Sites of involvement. Bladder tumors often involve the posterior and lateral walls and involve the superior wall least often. Patients with bladder carcinoma also frequently have carcinomas in other urinary tract sites.
    3. Types of bladder cancer
      a. Single papillary cancers are the most common type and the least likely to show infiltration
      b. Diffuse papillary growths with minimal invasion
      c. Sessile cancers are often high grade and invasive
      d. CIS. Appearance is either the same as normal mucosa or a velvety red patch.
    4. The "field defect." Bladder cancer appears to be associated with premalignant changes throughout the urothelial mucosa. This co-called field defect is suggested by the folllowing observations:
      a. Up to 80 percent of patients treated for superficial tumors develop recurrences at different sites in the bladder.

    b. Multiple primary sites are present in 25 percent of all patients with bladder cancer.

    c. Random biopsies of apparently normal areas of mucosa in bladder cancer patients frequently show CIS.

    d. Depending on the reported series, patients with bladder CIS will also have ureteral CIS in 10 to 60 percent and urethral CIS in 30 percent of cases.

    e. Approximately 40 percent of patients presenting with carcinoma of the renal pelvis or ureter will develop tumors elsewhere in the urinary tract, usually in the bladder.

B. Natural history

  1. CIS of the bladder is multifocal and can affect the entire urothelium. Up to 80 percent of patients with untreated CIS develop invasive bladder cancer within 10 years after diagnosis; the disease is lethal for the majority of these patients.

  2. Low-grade superficial carcinomas have a better prognosis than CIS. Even though the recurrence rate is 80 percent, 80 percent of patients with these tumors survive five years. Invasive cancer develops in only 10 percent of patients with superficial tumors, often in association with CIS. More than 80 percent of patients with both superficial cancers and CIS develop invasive malignancies.

  3. High-grade or invasive tumors are associated with adjacent areas of CIS in 85 percent of cases. Squamous cell cancers are usually high grade and are the most aggressive carcinomas of the bladder.

  4. Mode of spread. Bladder cancers spread both by lymphatic channels and the bloodstream. High-grade lesions are more likely to metastasize. Thirty percent of patients with distant metastases do not have involvement of the draining lymph nodes. Distant sites of metastases include bone, liver, lung, and, less commonly, skin and other organs. Uremia from local extension into pelvic organs, inanition from advancing cancer, and liver failure are the usual causes of death.

  5. Role of instrumentation. Bladder cancer cells exfoliated by cystoscopy, brushing, transurethral biopsy, or resection may seed other areas of the bladder. Mucosal sites damaged by inflammation or instrumentation appear to be most receptive to such implants. Implanted tumors may become invasive.

  6. Associated paraneoplastic syndromes

    a. Systemic fibrinolysis

    b. Hypercalcemia

    c. Neuromuscular syndromes

III. Diagnosis

A. Symptoms and signs

  1. Symptoms

    a. Hematuria occurs as a presenting feature in 90 percent of patients.

    b. Bladder irritability occurs in 25 percent of patients. Hesitancy, urgency, frequency, dysuria, and postvoiding pelvic discomfort may mimic prostatitis or cystitis. These symptoms occur in patients with CIS, as well as with tumors that are large, extensive, or near the bladder neck.

    c. Pain in the pelvis or flank is associated with locally advanced disease.

    d. Edema of the lower extremities and genitalia develops from venous or lymphatic obstruction.

  2. Physical findings. The patient is carefully examined for metastatic sites. Bimanual examination is performed by the urologist through the rectum while the patient is under general anesthesia for cystoscopy.

B. Special diagnostic studies

  1. Routine studies

    a. CBC, renal and liver function tests

   b. Urinalysis
   c. Chest x-ray

2. Cystoscopy is the cornerstone for diagnosing bladder cancer. Grossly abnormal areas are biopsied. Biopsies of both suspected areas and normal areas at random are also taken to search for CIS. Cystoscopy is followed by bimanual pelvic examination under anesthesia in both men and women. Cystoscopy is indicated for patients with

   a. Hematuria and a normal IVP (except patients with a single episode of acute bacterial cystitis)
   b. Unexplained or chronic lower urinary tract symptoms
   c. Urine cytology positive for cancer
   d. A history of bladder cancer

3. Urography. An IVP is performed on all patients with unexplained hematuria or cystoscopic or cytologic evidence of tumor. To search for primary sites in the ureters or renal pelves, the IVP is performed before cystoscopy in patients with positive urine cytology.

4. Urine cytology, often accompanied by flow cytometry, detects about 70 percent of bladder cancers that are subsequently diagnosed by cystoscopy. Cytologic evaluation should not be the primary diagnostic method for patients suspected of having bladder cancer. Urine cytologies are useful for

   a. Following patients with a history of bladder cancer
   b. Screening asymptomatic patients who are exposed to environmental carcinogens
   c. Evaluating patients with chronic irritative bladder symptoms before cystoscopy is done

5. Scans. Abdominal CT and bone scans should be performed in patients with bone pain or elevated serum alkaline phosphatase or transaminase levels.

IV. Staging system and prognostic factors

   A. Staging system. The staging system for bladder cancer is based on clinical findings rather than on pathologic data obtained at surgery. The system most commonly used in the United States is being revised to incorporate tumor grade.

Stage	Extent of disease	Proportion of patients (%)	Five-year survival (%)
0	Papillary cancer confined to mucosa	55	80
A	Invasion of lamina propria		
B	Invasion of muscle	25	40
B_1	Superficial or minimal muscle invasion		60
B_2	Deep muscle invasion		20
C	Invasion into perivesical fat	10	20
D	Metastases in draining lymph nodes or distant metastatic sites	10	<10

   B. Prognostic factors. Untreated patients have a two-year survival of less than 15 percent and a median survival of 16 months.

   1. Histology. Squamous cancers and adenocarcinomas have poorer prognoses than transitional cell carcinoma.

   2. Invasion of muscle, lymphatic, or perivesical fat is associated with a poor prognosis. Invasive cancer is associated with a 50 percent mortality in the first 18 months after diagnosis.

   3. CIS progresses to invasive carcinoma in 80 percent of patients within 10 years of diagnosis.

   4. Tumor grade
      a. The close relationship of tumor grade and stage of disease is shown in Table 13-2.
      b. Tumor grade alone affects survival in patients with superficial tumors. The five-year survival is 85 percent with low-grade lesions and 30 per-

Table 13-2. Tumor grade and extent of disease in bladder cancer

Grade	Description	Affected patients (%)	Incidence of invasion (%)	Incidence of metastases (%)
G_1	Well differentiated	25	5	<10
G_2	Moderately well differentiated	50	50	30
G_3	Poorly differentiated	25	80	80

cent with high-grade lesions. Virtually all high-grade superficial tumors become invasive if left untreated.

- c. Chromosome number correlates with tumor grade. Tetraploid cells are more likely to be found in invasive tumors and diploid cells in low-grade, noninvasive tumors.

5. **Size** of the primary tumor does not correlate with the risk of dissemination. Large superficial lesions, however, are more likely to recur after therapy than small lesions.

V. Prevention and early detection

A. Prevention. Protecting factory workers in certain industries from continuous exposure to bladder carcinogens (e.g., with protective clothing) may be beneficial. The benefit gained by reducing the intake of coffee or artificial sweetener has not been determined. All persons should be discouraged from smoking.

B. Early detection depends on prompt evaluation of all patients with hematuria or chronic irritative bladder symptoms.

VI. Management

A. Early disease

1. **Overview**

   a. **Superficial low-grade tumors** not associated with CIS are managed by transurethral resection and intravesical chemotherapy (see **4.a**). Although the recurrence rate is 80 percent with this management, the prognosis is good. Fulguration is added if there are excessive numbers of small lesions.

   b. **CIS** is usually multifocal, persistent, and recurrent; it is highly likely to evolve into invasive cancer, which often involves the urethra and ureters. Choice of therapy may be based on the degree of urothelial atypia; however, the pathologic distinction between severe dysplasia and CIS is often difficult to make.

      (1) **Borderline cases.** Patients should have repeated urine cytologies; cystoscopy and biopsy are repeated every three to six months. Some patients have a very indolent course, and years pass before frank CIS is found.

      (2) **True CIS.** Opinion is divided on the optimal therapeutic approach for apparently localized CIS. Localized, unifocal areas of CIS may be fulgurated. CIS localized to the bladder, without ureteral or urethral involvement, may be initially treated by intravesical therapy (see sec. **4.a**), provided there is no history of invasive tumor. Multifocal CIS, particularly if high grade, diffuse, or symptomatic, is treated with radical cystectomy; urethrectomy and/or ureterectomy may also be necessary.

   c. **Invasive tumors or superficial tumors with CIS** are best treated by pelvic lymph node dissection and radical cystectomy in females and radical cystoprostatectomy in males. Segmental resections of the bladder may be used in highly selected cases (see section **VI.A.2.b**). Radiotherapy and chemotherapy may be appropriate in some cases (see sections **VI.A.3** and **4**).

2. **Surgery**
   a. **Transurethral resection** or fulguration is used for superficial low-grade carcinomas (stage A) and borderline urothelial atypia.
   b. **Segmental resection** is associated with a high risk of recurrence. Only about 5 percent of patients are candidates for this procedure. Segmental resection can be considered if the tumor
      (1) Is solitary, *and*
      (2) Is localized to the bladder dome, *and*
      (3) Is not associated with areas of CIS sought by multiple biopsies of urothelial mucosa, *and*
      (4) Can be removed with a 3-cm margin of healthy tissue
   c. **Radical cystectomy** includes excision of the bladder, pericystic fat, and attached peritoneum; ureters are diverted through a loop of ileum that functions as a bladder to an abdominal stoma (Bricker's procedure). In addition, males undergo removal of the entire prostate and seminal vesicles; females undergo en bloc removal of the uterus, adnexa, and cuff of the vagina. Alternative urinary drainage procedures include direct cutaneous implantation of the ureters and ureterosigmoidostomy. Continent urinary reservoirs, such as the Kock pouch or an ileal bladder anastomosed directly to the urethra, may be offered to selected patients. Lymphadenectomy is controversial; it does not improve survival, but adds little morbidity and provides information for staging.
      (1) **Indications**
         (a) Superficial low-grade (stage A) tumors that are diffuse, multiple, and frequently recurring
         (b) True, severe CIS
         (c) High-grade tumors
         (d) Invasive tumors
      (2) **Complications of cystectomy**
         (a) Mortality of 3 to 8 percent.
         (b) Impotence in men; potency can be preserved in some men by sparing the corporal nerves.
         (c) Ureterocutaneous fistulae, wound dehiscence or infection, or small bowel obstructions or fistulae occur in about 30 percent of patients. Small bowel fistulae are associated with a 50 percent mortality.
      (3) **Complications of urinary diversion**
         (a) Urinary tract infection.
         (b) Obstruction due to stenosis.
         (c) Urinary calculi occasionally occur after Bricker's procedure; calcium stones are most common.
         (d) Hyperchloremic acidosis from the rapid reabsorption of chloride by the sigmoid colon may become a problem after ureterosigmoidostomy.
3. **RT** does not appear to favorably alter the course of CIS.
   a. **Indications**
      (1) **Preoperative radiation** is seldom employed. RT does not appear to improve expected survival beyond that achieved by radical surgery alone, although local recurrence is reduced.
      (2) **Postoperative radiation** has no proven role in bladder cancer.
      (3) **RT alone** is an alternative to surgery in patients who desire to retain their bladder and potency and are willing to accept a 20 percent lower cure rate.
      (4) **RT combined** with cisplatin alone or M-VAC (see sec. **VI.B.3**) may spare the bladder in patients who are not candidates for cystectomy.
   b. **Complications** are discussed in Chapter 11, *General Aspects*, sec. **V.A** (Radiation cystitis) and Chapter 30, sec. **VI.D** (Radiation proctitis).

4. Chemotherapy

a. Topical therapy. Superficial low-grade bladder cancers may be treated with intravesical chemotherapy after sites of gross disease are resected transurethrally. The incidence of tumor recurrence is reduced with topical therapy, but how much topical therapy improves survival is not known. Thiotepa, mitomycin C, BCG, and Adriamycin are effective. Patients with CIS may benefit from BCG or mitomycin C.

Thiotepa is the most commonly used topical agent: 30 to 60 mg in 100 ml of sterile water or saline is instilled through a catheter into the previously emptied bladder and retained for two hours. Several different treatment schedules are employed. A widely used method is to repeat the instillation weekly for six months, then monthly for one year, and bimonthly for three years from the start of therapy. Repeat cystoscopic examinations with biopsy of questionable areas are performed every three months for the three-year period; evidence of progression or invasive carcinoma indicates the need for radical cystectomy.

b. Adjuvant therapy with systemic cytotoxic agents (cyclophosphamide, doxorubicin, cisplatin) for patients undergoing cystectomy has been associated with a delay in time to progression and improved survival time. Confirmatory studies are in progress.

c. Neoadjuvant therapy is an attempt to provide the earliest possible treatment of micrometastatic disease and to facilitate definitive local therapy. Multiple single institution trials of M-VAC (see section **B.3**) indicate high response rates (60%) and complete responses (20–25%) on surgical resection. This approach remains experimental pending confirmatory trials.

B. Advanced disease

1. Surgery

a. Large, bleeding tumors can occasionally be fulgurated.

b. Urinary diversion with a ureterocutaneous conduit is indicated in the patient with severe hemorrhage or voiding symptoms.

2. RT ameliorates hemorrhage in about 50 percent of patients and provides substantial local pain relief in areas of bone involvement. Tumor masses that threaten extension through the skin, particularly in the perineum, should be irradiated early. Bacterial cystitis should be treated effectively before the institution of RT if possible.

3. Chemotherapy. Combinations of methotrexate, vinblastine, Adriamycin, and cisplatin (M-VAC) have produced sustained complete responses in up to 40 percent of patients and represent the best current therapy for advanced bladder cancer. Alternative regimens are shown in Appendix A1. Arterial infusion of these agents is experimental. M-VAC is administered in 28-day cycles in the following dosages:

Methotrexate, 30 mg/m^2 IV on days 1, 15, and 22
Vinblastine, 3 mg/m^2 IV on days 2, 15, and 22
Adriamycin, 30 mg/m^2 IV on day 2
Cisplatin, 70 mg/m^2 IV on day 1

C. Patient follow-up

1. Patients with severe urothelial dysplasia should have urine cytology repeated every two to three months, and cystoscopy with random biopsies every three to six months.

2. Patients with superficial low-grade cancer treated with intravesical chemotherapy should have cystoscopy performed at three-month intervals.

3. Patients who have undergone cystectomy should be evaluated every three months for the first two years, every six months for the next three years, and yearly thereafter. Urinalysis and urine cytology should be performed at six-month intervals to search for the development of new primary cancers in the upper urinary tract. Hematuria or a positive cytology should be evaluated with intravenous urography.

VII. Special clinical problems

A. Hematuria may complicate the course of locally advanced bladder cancer. Transurethral fulguration may help. The bladder may be catheterized and filled with sterile water under pressure to attempt tamponade. Some physicians advocate instillation of 4% formaldehyde and 1% silver nitrate into the bladder under general anesthesia; the agent is retained for 15 minutes, then thoroughly rinsed out with 10% alcohol followed by normal saline. Irrigation of the bladder with dilute alum is very effective in controlling hemorrhage. RT is effective for bleeding from tumor in 50 percent of cases; side effects of bladder irritation or proctitis are treated symptomatically.

B. Obstructive uropathy from benign conditions. Uremia may develop in patients with ileal bladder or ureterocutaneous fistulae. Obstruction due to benign conditions, such as stones or stenosis, must be ruled out. The urine should be examined for malignant cells, crystals, and blood. If the ureteral orifice can be located, a retrograde pyelogram is performed. Otherwise, IVP or renal radionuclide scan may show obstruction. If these techniques are unrewarding, a CT scan may show hydronephrosis. Exploratory surgery should be undertaken in patients who otherwise are clinically free of cancer if a ureteral catheter cannot be passed.

C. Impotence complicates radical cystectomy in men. Penile prostheses are available, which permit penetration and, often, orgasm.

D. Management of urinary symptoms is discussed in Chap. 5, sec. **V**.

Prostate Cancer

I. Epidemiology and etiology

A. Incidence (see Table 13-1)

1. **Clinically evident cancer of the prostate.** The risk of clinically detectable prostate cancer increases with age from 0.02 percent at the age of 50 years to 0.8 percent at age 80. The risk of prostate cancer in black men increases at a faster rate than in whites.

2. **Subclinical (latent) cancer of the prostate** is a common incidental finding in autopsies. Latent cancer increases by 1 percent per year of age starting at the age of 50 years; the incidence is 10 percent at 50 years and 30 percent at 70 years.

B. Etiology. The cause of prostate cancer is unknown. Several factors are associated with an increased risk.

1. **Demography.** The risk of developing prostate cancer is highest in Sweden, intermediate in the United States and Europe (and Japanese men who migrated to the United States), and lowest in Taiwan and Japan. Jews of all age groups appear to be at low risk.

2. **Marital status.** The risk is lowest for single men and increases, in order of increasing risk, for married, widowed, and divorced men. The risk also appears to increase with the number of children parented.

3. **Occupation.** Higher rates of prostate cancer are reported in workers exposed to cadmium, loggers, chemists, farmers, textile workers, painters, and rubber tire workers.

4. **Hormones.** Altered estrogen and androgen metabolite levels have been detected in patients with prostate cancer or hyperplasia. The association of liver cirrhosis with increased risk of prostate cancer further suggests that an altered hormonal milieu plays a role in the etiology.

II. Pathology and natural history

A. Histology. Almost all prostate cancers are adenocarcinomas. Sarcomas and transitional, small, and squamous cell carcinomas are rare. The prostate may be the site of metastases from bladder, colon, or lung cancer or from the melanomas, lymphomas, or other malignancies.

B. Location. Prostate cancer tends to be multifocal and frequently involves the gland's capsule. Both of these characteristics make removal by transuretheral resection unfeasible.

C. **Mode of spread.** The biology of adenocarcinomas of the prostate is strongly influenced by tumor grade. Low-grade tumors may remain localized for long periods of time. The disease metastasizes along nerve sheaths, through lymphatic chains, and hematogenously. Distant metastases may occur without evidence of nodal involvement. Distant metastases are nearly always present when lymph nodes are involved.

D. **Metastatic sites.** Bone is the most common site of prostate cancer metastases, almost always producing dense osteoblastic metastases. Occasionally, patients demonstrate uncharacteristic osteolytic lesions. Liver involvement also occurs, but metastases to the brain, lung, and other soft tissues are rare.

E. **Associated paraneoplastic syndromes**
   1. Systemic fibrinolysis
   2. Neuromuscular abnormalities

III. **Diagnosis**

A. **Symptoms and signs**
   1. **Symptoms**
      a. Early prostatic cancer is usually asymptomatic and can only be detected by the routine rectal examination. The presence of symptoms indicates advanced disease. Symptoms include hesitancy, urgency, nocturia, poor urine stream, dribbling, and terminal hematuria.
      b. The sudden onset and rapid progression of symptoms of urinary tract obstruction in men of the appropriate age is most likely to be caused by prostate cancer.
      c. Pain in the back, pelvis, shoulders, or over multiple bony sites is the most common presenting complaint in patients with distant metastases.
      d. The sudden onset of paraplegia and incontinence resulting from extradural spinal metastases may be a presenting feature or may develop during the course of the disease.
   2. **Physical examination**
      a. Check for induration or nodularity of the prostate, which often represents prostatic cancer. Approximately two-thirds of patients with malignancy found on biopsy have palpable induration. Nodules of prostatic cancer are typically stony hard and not tender.
      b. Examine for normal lateral sulci and palpable (i.e., abnormal) seminal vesicles.
      c. Evaluate inguinal nodes for metastatic disease.
      d. Evaluate for distant metastases.

B. **Differential diagnosis of the enlarged prostate**
   1. **Acute prostatitis.** Bacterial infection causes dysuria, pain, and, often, fever. The prostate is tender and enlarged but not hard. Examination and culture of prostatic fluid obtained by prostate massage reveal the infectious agent.
   2. **Chronic and granulomatous prostatitis** caused by bacterial, tuberculous, fungal, or protozoan infection may produce a mass that cannot be clinically distinguished from cancer. Biopsy may be necessary to make the diagnosis.
   3. **Nodular hyperplasia** (benign prostatic hypertrophy) is found in men 30 years of age and over and in 80 percent of men by 80 years of age. Urinary obstructive symptoms are common. Palpable nodules that are indistinguishable from cancer necessitate biopsy.
   4. **Other possibilities.** Rarely, calculi, amyloidosis, benign adenomas, or infarction of a hyperplastic nodule may cause obstruction or a mass suggestive of cancer.

C. **Laboratory studies**
   1. **Routine studies.** Urinalysis; CBC, renal and liver function tests; alkaline phosphatase, calcium, and phorphorous levels; chest x-ray film.
   2. **Tumor markers**
      a. **Acid phosphatase (AP)** levels in the serum are increased in 70 to 80

percent of patients with disseminated disease. AP is not sensitive enough for screening of patients with localized disease. Blood levels should be assayed before digital rectal examination and prostate manipulation, which result in elevated serum concentrations.

  (1) AP is produced by several tissues, including the prostate, kidney, breast, granulocytes, and platelets. Elevated blood levels of the enzyme are found in 80 percent of prostate cancer cases with skeletal metastases, 60 percent of untreated cases, and 20 percent of cases apparently without extracapsular extension.

  (2) Elevated levels of serum AP are also found in patients with thrombocytosis, Gaucher's disease, osteitis deformans, breast cancer, and bony involvement from other tumors (particularly breast cancer and osteosarcoma).

  (3) The AP produced by the prostate, both normal and cancerous, is tartrate resistant. Radioimmunoassay of the enzyme has a high rate of false-positive results and is not yet recommended for routine screening or follow-up.

b. Prostatic-specific antigen (PSA) is a specific marker for prostate carcinoma and is more sensitive than AP.

  (1) Approximately 15 percent of patients with nodular hyperplasia have elevated PSA levels, but elevation usually indicates carcinoma. PSA values can also be increased with prostatic inflammation, surgery, or endoscopy, but not with rectal examination. PSA values have occasionally been elevated in patients with cancer that did not originate in the prostate.

  (2) PSA can detect primary or recurrent tumors of very low volume and is useful in diagnosis and follow-up. When PSA is combined with transrectal ultrasound and prostatic biopsies, cancer is detected in 20 percent of patients with PSA values between 4.0 ng/ml and 10 ng/ml and in 60 percent of patients with values exceeding 10 ng/ml. Although PSA is not sensitive enough to be the sole screening method for prostate cancer, it is useful when combined with digital rectal examination and transrectal ultrasound.

  (3) About 10 percent of patients with biopsy-proven prostate cancer have normal PSA levels. About 10 percent of patients with metastatic prostate cancer have elevated AP levels with normal PSA levels.

  (4) PSA values may show a progressive increase several years before metastatic disease becomes evident. Such a rise is an indication to look for local recurrence in previously treated patients using physical examination or transrectal ultrasound but not an indication to conduct a detailed, unbeneficial search for metastatic disease.

c. CEA is increased in too few patients with prostate carcinoma and in too many other conditions to be clinically useful.

3. Needle biopsy is the standard method to diagnose prostate cancer. Biopsy of nodules, suspect indurations, and multiple random areas detects cancer in only one-half of patients with induration of the prostate. Biopsy also helps determine whether the cancer is multifocal. Needle biopsy fails to detect cancers found by other surgical techniques in up to 30 percent of patients. The fine-needle aspiration biopsy is less painful and has less morbidity than the standard large needle and is the method of choice in many institutions with pathologists skilled in its interpretation.

4. Transurethral resection of the prostate for benign hyperplasia is the most common means of diagnosing patients with stage A prostate cancer.

5. Bone scans should be performed in all patients with a histologic diagnosis of prostate cancer even if the disease appears to be localized.

6. IVPs with cross-table lateral views are routinely obtained in all patients except those with stage A_1 lesions.

    7. CT scans and ultrasonography are used to demonstrate pelvic and abdominal lymph node enlargements in patients with scrotal and lower extremity edema.

IV. Staging and prognostic factors

    A. Staging system. A system based on clinical findings and commonly used in the United States is presented.

Stage	Extent of disease (proportion of patients)	Ten-year median survival (%)
A	Incidental histologic finding of cancer; prostate normal to palpation (10%)	60
A_1	Single focal area of well-differentiated tumor	
A_2	Multiple areas of cancer in the gland or cancer is poorly differentiated	
B	Tumor palpable but confined to prostate (10%)	40
B_1	Single nodule <2 cm in diameter	
B_2	Multiple nodules or single nodule >2 cm in diameter	
C	Tumor is localized to periprostatic area (45%)	30
C_1	No involvement of seminal vesicles and tumor <70 gm	
C_2	Involvement of seminal vesicles and tumor <70 gm	
D	Advanced disease (35%)	10–20
D_1	Pelvic node metastases or ureteral obstruction	
D_2	Distant metastases	

    B. Prognostic factors

      1. Tumor grade strongly affects prognosis. Higher tumor grades are more frequently associated with lymph node and distant metastases.

Grade	Five-year survival (%)
G_1	60
G_2	35
G_3	15
G_4	5

      2. Involvement of seminal vesicles is associated with a poor prognosis even in apparently early disease.

      3. The incidence of regional lymph node metastases is as follows:

Grade	Patients with lymph node metastases (%)
A_1	0
A_2	20
B_1	15
B_2	30
C	50
D	100

V. Prevention and early detection.
Early detection of prostate cancer necessitates careful examination of the prostate. Although screening for prostate cancer remains controversial the use of transrectal ultrasound, serum PSA, and biopsy with ultrasound-guided automatic gun hold promise and are the subjects of large clinical trials. Patients with any questionable induration or mass should be referred to a urologist for biopsy.

VI. Management.
The management of all stages of prostate cancer is highly controversial. This disease has a long natural history and substantial numbers of patients survive 15 or more years after the diagnosis. Investigators and clinicians vary widely in their use of surgery, RT, and hormonal manipulation for treating each stage of disease. Most clinicians agree, however, that treatment of early-stage disease with either surgery or radiation therapy results in comparable survival.

A. Early disease (stages A, B, and C)
   1. Surgery
      a. Stage A_1 prostate cancer is discovered by histologic evaluation of speci-
      mens taken from transurethral resection for prostatic hyperplasia. Once
      a focus of cancer is discovered, random needle biopsies are obtained to
      look for other areas of cancer. If none is found, no further therapy is
      necessary since patients with this stage of disease have the same sur-
      vival expectancy as normal age-matched controls. The extent of disease
      is followed with frequent digital examinations. Needle biopsies are per-
      formed for changes noted on rectal examination (some urologists perform
      a repeat transurethral resection three months after the first surgery). If
      the biopsy shows cancer, the patient is reclassified as stage A_2 and man-
      aged accordingly.
      b. Stages A_2, B_1, B_2, and C. These patients are offered either RT or radical
      prostatectomy. Urologists may recommend that patients with these clin-
      ical stages undergo pelvic lymphadenectomy for pathologic staging be-
      fore prostatectomy is done. The results of staging would then determine
      subsequent therapy.
      c. Complications of prostatectomy and lymphadenectomy
         (1) Prostatectomy causes incontinence in 4 percent and stress inconti-
         nence in up to 30 percent. Potency can be spared by a skilled surgeon
         in 60 to 80 percent of patients with small B_1, B_2, or with A_2 tumors.
         (2) Complications of staging lymphadenectomy occur in approximately
         20 percent of patients and include lymphocele, pulmonary embolus,
         wound infection, and lymphedema.
      d. Contraindications to prostatectomy and lymphadenectomy
         (1) Physiologic age over 75
         (2) High-grade cancers
         (3) Invasion of the seminal vesicles (stage C_2)
         (4) Metastases to pelvic nodes (stage D_1)
         (5) Disseminated cancer (stage D_2)
   2. RT
      a. Indications. RT is widely employed in the treatment of patients with
      stage A_2, B_1, B_2, and C_2 tumors. Therapy of patients with stage C disease
      is also controversial, but most authorities recommend RT. Other indica-
      tions for RT include
         (1) The patient's medical condition precludes surgery.
         (2) Node involvement is found at staging lymphadenectomy (radical
         prostatectomy is not performed).
         (3) Residual malignant pelvic disease after prostate surgery.
      b. Complications following approximately 7000 cGy given in seven to
      eight weeks and their approximate incidences in treated patients
         (1) Impotency: 50 percent.
         (2) Suprapubic or perineal edema or induration: 20 percent.
         (3) Radiation proctitis with diarrhea, blood-streaked stools, and rectal
         urgency: less than 5 percent (see Chap. 30, sec. **VI.D**).
         (4) Dysuria; urinary urgency and frequency: less than 5 percent (see
         Chap. 11, *General Aspects*, sec. **V.A**).
         (5) Perineal fistulae: less than 1 percent.
         (6) Fecal and urinary incontinence: uncertain incidence.
         (7) Hard induration of the prostate: 80 percent. This develops approxi-
         mately one year following RT and is the result of fibrosis. The gland
         may be "rock-hard" and be clinically indistinguishable from cancer
         recurrence.
         (8) Persistent tumor occurs in 10 to 30 percent of patients, depending
         on tumor stage.
   3. Systemic therapy. Neither hormonal manipulation nor chemotherapy
   clearly improves the survival of patients with early prostate cancer.

B. Advanced disease (stage D)
1. **Surgery.** Transurethral resection of the prostate may be used to relieve bladder outlet obstruction even in the presence of advanced disease; however, orchiectomy alone is usually effective.
2. **RT** is useful in treating the following problems commonly encountered in cancer of the prostate:
   a. Isolated, painful bony metastatic sites after endocrine therapy has ceased to be effective.
   b. Pelvic pain syndromes, urinary tract obstruction, and gross hematuria.
   c. Metastases to retroperitoneal lymph nodes, which produce back pain and scrotal and lower extremity edema.
   d. Spinal cord compression from vertebral and extradural metastases is a common and rapidly progressive complication of prostate cancer. Cord compression is an emergency; myelography and definitive therapy must be undertaken within a few hours after onset of symptoms (see Chap. 32, sec. **III**).
3. **Endocrine therapy** is the mainstay of treatment for *symptomatic* advanced prostate cancer. Asymptomatic patients with advanced disease do not appear to have improved survival with treatment when compared to untreated patients; treatment of asymptomatic patients with advanced disease is not essential. Orchiectomy, LHRH agonists, antiandrogen, or DES is the treatment of choice. Each produces symptomatic relief in 80 percent of patients. Improvement is often dramatic; many bedridden patients crippled with bone pain return to a more functional status in a few days.
   a. **DES** (3 mg/day PO). Testosterone is produced by the testes and is the only natural androgen that has a substantial stimulatory effect on the prostate. The 3-mg dose of DES reduces plasma testosterone levels to those produced by orchiectomy. Patients should be given a brief course of RT to the breasts *before* starting DES to prevent painful gynecomastia. Patients being treated with DES must be observed for the development of congestive heart failure and thrombophlebitis.
   b. **Orchiectomy** is preferred for treatment of patients with a history of cardiovascular disease (particularly congestive heart failure), stroke, or thromboembolic phenomena. These conditions are potentially aggravated by DES therapy.
   c. **LHRH agonists,** such as leuprolide, appear to be as effective as orchiectomy or DES and do not produce the cardiovascular, mammary, or GI side effects of DES. The cost of treatment with leuprolide is substantially greater than with either DES or orchiectomy.
   d. **Antiandrogens combined with LHRH agonists** are superior to LHRH agonists alone and result in a small but significant survival benefit for "total androgen blockade." Flutamide, an antiandrogen, is given at a dosage of 250 mg PO t.i.d. Leuprolide is given at a dose of 7.5 mg IM monthly.
   e. **Diethylstilbestrol diphosphate** (Stilphostrol) may be tried (50–200 mg PO t.i.d.) in patients failing orchiectomy or DES. This drug is a high-dose equivalent form of DES, which is presumably activated by acid phosphatase inside prostate cancer cells.
   f. **Other endocrine agents** that may be helpful
      (1) The long-acting estrogen, chlorotrianisene (TACE), 12 to 25 mg PO each day (same precautions as for short-acting estrogens).
      (2) Progestins such as megestrol acetate, 40 mg PO q.i.d.
      (3) Drugs that inhibit androgen synthesis (aminoglutethimide, ketoconazole) have also been shown to be effective.
4. **Chemotherapy** provides symptomatic relief in 20 to 30 percent of patients with prostate cancer. Effective agents include cyclophosphamide, fluorouracil, Adriamycin, and dacarbazine. Cyclophosphamide is at least as effective as any other single agent. Multiagent chemotherapy has not been

shown to be superior to single agents. Prednisone often provides symptomatic improvement in patients who no longer respond to other endocrine or cytotoxic therapies.

VII. Special clinical problems

A. Anemia in prostate cancer is usually part of the end-stage process caused by extensive involvement of the bone marrow by tumor or RT to major marrow-bearing sites. The anemia is typically normochromic and normocytic, frequently associated with other cytopenias, and sometimes a part of a leukoerythroblastic peripheral blood smear. Other causes of anemia must be ruled out.

B. Obstructive uropathy and uremia may be the fatal complication of prostate cancer. Orchiectomy or RT (followed by endocrine therapy or chemotherapy) may relieve the obstruction. Unlike uremic patients with other pelvic tumors, some patients with prostate cancer and ureteral obstruction may benefit from surgical intervention. Patients without pelvic pain syndromes and low-grade cancers should be considered for ureteral bypass by stent catheters, nephrostomy, or reimplantation of the ureters into the bladder. Patients with pelvic pain syndrome or high-grade cancer are likely to have progressive disease; surgical relief of ureteral obstruction would remove an important mechanism of palliation in end-stage disease and probably should not be considered.

C. Dense bone sclerosis on x-ray in an adult man of the appropriate age who has bone pain usually is diagnostic of prostate cancer. Bone containing prostate cancer is so densely sclerotic that attempts at marrow biopsy often result in "dry taps" and damaged biopsy needles. The radiologic appearance of Paget's disease is distinguished by the fluffy, cottonlike appearance of lesions, by thickening of the bone cortex, and by the dense sclerosis of the pelvic brim ("brim sign").

D. Extraosseous extension of prostate cancer is common. Extension of skull or vertebral lesions can produce neurologic deficits. Extension of rib lesions can produce subcutaneous or pleuropulmonary masses. Retro-orbital and cavernous sinus masses can result in proptosis and visual loss. Extraosseous extension of bony lesions necessitates RT.

E. Systemic fibrinolysis. Activators of the fibrinolytic enzyme, plasmin, abound in prostatic tissue. Prostatic disease, especially carcinoma of the prostate, is among the few medical conditions that can produce both significant systemic fibrinolysis and disseminated intravascular coagulation (see Chap. 34, *Coagulopathy*, sec. III, for diagnosis and management).

Urethral Cancer

I. Epidemiology and etiology. Urethral cancer is extremely rare; fewer than 1500 cases have been reported in the literature. Women are affected three times as often as men. The age of onset is usually more than 60 years. The etiology is not known, but urethral cancer may be associated with gonorrheal urethritis, strictures, or transitional cell carcinoma in the bladder.

II. Pathology and natural history

A. Histology. Eighty percent are squamous cell carcinomas, usually arising from the stratified squamous epithelium of the proximal (bulbous) urethra or distal (penile) urethra. Fifteen percent are transitional cell carcinomas arising in the prostatic urethra. Adenocarcinomas possibly arise from Cowper's glands.

B. Clinical course. Urethral cancer involves inguinal nodes early on and also spreads hematogenously to distant organs. Lesions of the anterior urethra are less likely to be associated with widespread metastases than posterior lesions.

III. Diagnosis. Patients have urinary hesitancy, hematuria, palpable mass, urethral discharge, perineal pain, or enlarged inguinal nodes. Transurethral biopsy establishes the diagnosis.

IV. Management. In females total urethrectomy and pelvic lymph node resection are required. In males penectomy is required if the tumor invades the corpora cavernosa. Ilioinguinal lymphadenectomy is performed in patients with clinical evidence of node metastases. Preoperative combination chemotherapy may reduce the size of large tumors.

Penile Cancer

I. **Epidemiology and etiology**
   A. **Incidence.** Penile cancer constitutes less than 1 percent of all cancers in males in the United States. The incidence is greatly increased in populations that do not uniformly practice circumcision. The average age of onset is about 60 years.
   B. **Etiology.** The etiology of penile cancer is not known. Venereal disease is not a causative factor. The following data suggest that circumcision is preventative.
      1. The disease is almost nonexistent in Jewish males, who are all circumcised shortly after birth.
      2. In Africa and other countries where circumcision is not performed, penile cancer constitutes 20 percent of all cancers.
      3. Moslems have an intermediate risk of penile cancer. Moslem boys are circumcised at puberty.

II. **Pathology and natural history**
   A. **Premalignant lesions**
      1. **Erythroplasia of Queyrat** occurs on the glans and prepuce of uncircumcised males. The lesions are flat and reddened or are velvety plaques. Cancer develops in 10 percent of patients with erythroplasia.
      2. **Bowen's disease** appears as a small eczematoid plaque anywhere on the penis. Squamous carcinoma in situ is demonstrated by histology. Bowen's disease of the penis, like squamous carcinoma in situ in other areas of the skin not exposed to sun, is associated with a high incidence of carcinoma of the gastrointestinal tract and lungs.
      3. **Leukoplakia.** Nonspecific plaques of leukoplakia on the glans are almost always associated with squamous carcinoma. Unlike leukoplakic lesions elsewhere, penile lesions are not white.
      4. **Giant penile condyloma** (Buschke-Löwenstein tumor) grossly resembles a cauliflowerlike squamous cell cancer and may have foci of cancer. Surgical excision is mandatory.
   B. **Histology.** Squamous carcinoma, usually well differentiated, constitutes nearly all penile cancers. Rare penile cancers include melanoma, sarcoma, and metastatic tumor. The squamous lesions may be an ulcer, nodule, or cauliflowerlike mass.
   C. **Clinical course**
      1. Squamous penile cancer usually starts on the glans or coronal sulcus. As the disease progresses, the corpora cavernosa are invaded. The urethra is usually spared until late in the course.
      2. The rich lymphatic drainage of this region results in metastases to the inguinal nodes (only one-third of palpable nodes are involved with tumor by histology). Lymphatic metastases are not common if the tumor is confined to the glans or prepuce.
      3. The tumor disseminates through the lymphatic system and the blood to distant organs, most often to the lungs, and less frequently to bone and other sites.
   D. **Paraneoplastic syndromes.** Hypercalcemia can develop.

III. **Diagnosis**
   A. **Symptoms and signs**
      1. The earliest lesion of penile carcinoma is described by patients as a nonhealing "sore." Frequently there is an associated foul-smelling discharge. Phimosis may mask penile cancer until erosion through the prepuce occurs. Many patients have a long history of a mass. Urinary tract symptoms, such as pain and hematuria, are signs of locally advanced disease.
      2. Physical examination usually reveals an exophytic mass. Infection of the tumor is usually present when the patient is examined for symptoms.

B. Laboratory studies

1. Routine blood tests, urinalysis, and chest x-ray film are obtained.
2. Biopsy or imprint slides should be done for all patients with a penile mass or with any finding compatible with a precancerous lesion.
3. Lymphangiograms have not been reliable and are not recommended for routine cases.
4. Liver and bone scans should be obtained only if abnormalities seen on physical examination or blood studies suggest liver or bone involvement.

IV. Staging system and prognostic factors

A. Staging system

Stage	Extent of disease	Five-year survival (%)
I	Tumor limited to the glans or prepuce	80
II	Tumor invasion of shaft or corpora	60
III	Stage I or II with regional lymph node metastases	25
IV	Inoperable lymph node or distant metastases	0

B. Prognostic factors. Poor prognostic features include endophytic and high-grade lesions, invasion of the shaft, and involvement of draining lymph nodes, especially at the iliac level or higher. Approximately 20 percent of patients with clinical stage I or II tumor have inguinal node involvement proved by surgery.

V. Prevention and early detection.
Prevention of penile cancer can be accomplished by routine early circumcision of male babies. Circumcision should be performed in patients with phimosis and penile discharge, inflammation, or induration. Early detection of penile cancer requires regular inspection of the prepuce and glans at physical examination and biopsy of suspected lesions.

VI. Management

A. Surgery is the principal modality of therapy for penile cancer in the United States. Partial penectomy is sufficient therapy if there is a 2-cm tumor-free margin.

1. Total penectomy is necessary for lesions that invade the body of the penis or are very large.
2. In younger patients with tumor confined to the prepuce, circumcision may be used if close follow-up can be assured; however, the recurrence rate is high.
3. Routine sampling of the superficial inguinal nodes of patients with stage I or II disease is recommended by some authorities; if the nodes contain tumor, a radical ilioinguinal lymphadenectomy is necessary. Radical lymphadenectomy is routinely performed in patients with stage III tumors.

B. RT. The primary role of RT is to avoid penectomy, especially in younger patients. This modality has been used for treating small primary stage I lesions (<3 cm diameter); the results for RT alone (along with salvage surgery for failures) appear to be the same as those obtained when partial amputation is used as primary therapy.

C. Chemotherapy

1. Premalignant lesions may respond to topical therapy with fluorouracil or to laser therapy in selected cases.
2. Penile cancer appears to be responsive to cisplatin, methotrexate, and bleomycin. Some authorities use these drugs as an adjunct to surgery for stage II and III tumors. Response rates of advanced cancer to these drugs are not known, but may be as high as 50 percent. The effect of chemotherapy on survival is not known.

Selected Reading

Renal Cancer

Belldegrun, A., et al. Immunotherapy for metastatic renal cell carcinoma. *World J. Urol.* 9:157, 1991.

Krown, S. E. Interferon treatment of renal cell carcinoma: Current status and future prospects. *Cancer* 59:647, 1987.

Rosenberg, S. A., et al. Observations of the systemic administration of autologous lymphokine-activated killer cells and recombinant interleukin-2 to patients with metastatic cancer. *N. Engl. J. Med.* 313:1485, 1985.

Stenzl, A., and DeKernion, J. B. Pathology, biology, and clinical staging of renal cell carcinoma. *Semin. Oncol.* 16(suppl 1):3, 1989.

Urothelial Cancers

Daniels, J. R., et al. The role of adjuvant chemotherapy following cystectomy for invasive bladder cancer: A prospective comparative trial. *Proc. Am. Soc. Clin. Oncol.* 9:31, 1990.

Herr, H. W. Conservative management of muscle-infiltrating bladder cancer: Prospective experience. *J. Urol.* 138:1162, 1987.

Maldazys, J. D., and DeKernion, J. B. Management of superficial bladder tumors and carcinoma in situ. In DeKernion, J. B., and Paulson, D. F. (eds.) *Genitourinary Cancer Management.* Philadelphia: Lea & Febiger, 1987. Pp. 51–52.

Scher, H., et al. Neoadjuvant chemotherapy for invasive bladder cancer: Experience with the M-VAC regimen. *Br. J. Urol.* 64:250, 1989.

Prostate Cancer

Garnick, M. B. Prostate cancer: Screening, diagnosis, and management. *Ann. Intern. Med.* 118:804, 1993.

Pienta, K. J., and Esper, P. S. Risk factors for prostate cancer. *Ann. Intern. Med.* 118:793, 1993.

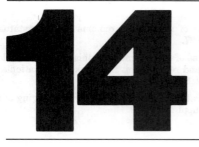

Neurologic Tumors

Ellen E. Mack

I. Epidemiology and etiology

A. Incidence. Primary brain cancers represent 1 percent (12,000 cases) of all cancers and 2.5 percent (10,000 cases) of cancer deaths annually in the United States (Table 14-1). They are more common in males than females by a ratio of 3:2. The incidence peaks at 5 to 10 years of age and again at 50 to 55 years. Brain cancers are the most common solid tumors in children; brain cancers occurring in childhood are discussed further in Chap. 18, *Brain Tumors*.

B. Etiology

1. **Environmental factors,** such as tobacco, alcohol, and diet, have not been associated with primary CNS tumors. Exposure to ionizing radiation, however, can induce the formation of meningiomas, nerve-sheath tumors, sarcomas, and less commonly astrocytomas. Occupational exposure to vinyl chlorides is a risk factor for astrocytomas; animal studies have shown that exposure to *N*-nitroso compounds, aromatic hydrocarbons, triazenes, and hydrazines increases the risk of astrocytoma formation.

2. **Hereditary causes**

   a. **Neurofibromatosis I** is a dominantly inherited condition of multiple neurofibromas that is also associated with optic gliomas, intracranial astrocytomas, schwannomas, neurofibrosarcomas, neural crest-derived tumors (glomus tumor, pheochromocytoma), embryonal tumors, and leukemia. The gene for this disorder is on chromosome 17 and its gene product, neurofibromin, has been identified.

   b. **Neurofibromatosis II** is a condition of multiple schwannomas, especially acoustic neuromas, that is also associated with ependymomas and meningiomas. The gene for this disorder is located on chromosome 22.

   c. **Tuberous sclerosis** (Bourneville's disease) is a dominantly transmitted disease associated with giant-cell astrocytomas.

   d. **von Hippel-Lindau disease** is a dominantly transmitted disorder characterized by hemangioblastomas of the retina, cerebellum, and less commonly the spinal cord. Other associated malignancies include renal carcinoma and pheochromocytoma. The gene for this disorder is located on chromosome 3.

   e. **Turcot syndrome** is a rare familial syndrome associated with colon cancer, glioblastoma, and medulloblastoma.

   f. **Nevoid basal-cell carcinoma syndrome** (Gorlin's syndrome) is a syndrome of multiple basal-cell carcinomas that may be associated with medulloblastoma, meningioma, craniopharyngioma, and some systemic tumors.

   g. **Li-Fraumeni syndrome** is a clinical syndrome of familial breast cancer, sarcomas, and primary brain tumors that is associated with germline p53 (chromosome 17) mutations.

3. **Immune suppression.** Transplant patients and patients with AIDS have a markedly increased risk of primary CNS lymphoma.

II. Diagnosis

A. Clinical presentation depends on the location of the tumor and its rate of growth. In general, slow-growing tumors cause little in the way of focal deficits because the nervous tissue is slowly compressed and compensatory mechanisms

Table 14-1. Features of common central nervous system tumors

Tumor type	Age	Common location	Clinical features	Survival	RT	Chemotherapy
Astrocytoma	Adult > child	Supratentorial	Slow-growing, may be present for years	5 yr (MS)	Yes	At recurrence
Anaplastic astrocytoma	Adult	Supratentorial	Rapidly growing	2 yr (MS)	Yes	Yes
Glioblastoma multiforme	Adult, elderly	Supratentorial	Rapidly growing, highly malignant	1 yr (MS)	Yes	At recurrence
Oligodendroglioma	Any	Supratentorial, often frontal	Seizures more common	5 yr (MS)	Yes	Yes
Brainstem glioma	Child > adult	Brainstem, especially pons	Marked morbidity from cranial nerve deficits	1 yr (MS)	Yes	Seldom
Pilocytic astrocytoma	Child > adult	Cerebellum and hypothalamus	Cure with total resection	80% 10 yr	Yes	Yes
Ependymoma	Child, adult	Fourth ventricle, cauda equina	Cure with total resection; can disseminate in CSF	70% 5 yr	Yes	Seldom
Medulloblastoma	Child > adult	Cerebellum	Likely to disseminate in CSF	55% 5 yr	Yes	Yes
Meningioma	Adult	Convexity, clival, thoracic	More common in women; cure with total resection	Long-term	Yes	Rare
Primary CNS lymphoma	Adult	Multifocal, periventricular	CSF/ocular dissemination common	2 yr (MS)	Yes	Yes
Germinoma	Second and third decades	Pineal and suprasellar	Highly sensitive to chemotherapy and RT	80% 5 yr	Yes	Yes
Nongerminoma germ cell tumor	Second and third decades	Pineal	Mixed histologies, often marker-positive	25% 5 yr	Yes	Yes

Key: MS = median survival; CSF = cerebrospinal fluid; CNS = central nervous system; RT = radiation therapy.

seem to occur. However, once they reach a certain size, CSF pathways may be obstructed, causing evidence of increased intracranial pressure (ICP). Fast-growing tumors tend to be associated with considerable surrounding cerebral edema; the edema, in addition to the tumor mass, is more likely to cause focal deficits. Usually, the deficits caused by edema are reversible, whereas those caused by a mass are much less so. Specific signs and symptoms associated with tumors of the CNS include:

1. **Headaches** are most likely to occur with fast-growing tumors and are typically deep, dull, and not intense or throbbing. They are characteristically worse on arising in the morning and are exacerbated by straining or lifting. Lateralization of headaches occasionally facilitates tumor localization.

2. **Seizures.** In 20 percent of patients over the age of 20 years, the onset of seizures is caused by a neoplasm. The seizures may be generalized or partial (focal). Simple partial seizures commonly consist of transient sensory or motor phenomena of a single limb or side. Complex partial seizures, often of temporal lobe origin, consist of changes in the level of consciousness or awareness of surroundings, frequently in conjunction with abnormal olfactory or gustatory phenomena. Speech arrest may also occur. Generalized seizures result in loss of consciousness, bowel and bladder incontinence, and bilateral tonic-clonic movements. In patients with brain tumors, generalized seizures are often partial or focal in onset, and evidence of focality may be found on postictal examination of the patient.

3. **Increased ICP** may result from a large mass or from obstructive hydrocephalus. Large masses cause progressive obtundation and can lead to transtentorial herniation, which classically presents with a third cranial nerve palsy and hemiparesis. Hydrocephalus causes gait ataxia, nausea, vomiting, headache, and eventually a decrease in level of consciousness. If left untreated, hydrocephalus can lead to central herniation, which is not heralded by a third nerve palsy. Papilledema is a sign of increased ICP. Unusual signs and symptoms of increased ICP include visual obscurations, dizziness, and the so-called falsely localizing signs. Of these unusual indications, the most classic is diplopia from sixth cranial nerve dysfunction due to stretching of the nerve from downward pressure caused by a large supratentorial mass.

4. **Supratentorial lobar** tumors usually present with focal signs and symptoms including hemiparesis (frontal lobe), aphasia (left frontal and posterior temporal lobes), hemi-neglect (parietal lobe), and hemianopsia (occipital lobe).

5. **Hypothalamic** tumors may be associated with disturbance of body temperature regulation, diabetes insipidus, hyperphagia, and, if the optic chiasm is involved, with visual field deficits.

6. **Brainstem** tumors, such as brainstem gliomas, present with multiple cranial nerve deficits and long-tract signs (weakness of the extremities).

7. **Nerve-sheath** tumors, such as acoustic neuromas, result in deficits of the involved cranial or spinal nerve. As the tumor enlarges, surrounding neural structures may also be compressed, leading to further symptoms.

8. **Cerebellar** tumors are associated with dysmetria, ataxia, vertigo, nystagmus, and vomiting.

9. **Spinal cord** tumors present with spastic paraparesis and sensory loss below the level of the tumor, as well as with disturbances of bowel and bladder function.

10. **Meningeal** involvement by primary nervous system tumors is less common than with metastatic tumors, and is seen mostly with medulloblastomas, pinealoblastomas, germinomas, primary lymphomas, and to a lesser degree ependymomas. The hallmark for meningeal disease is neurologic dysfunction at multiple levels of the neuraxis. Nonspecific features include seizures and changes in mentation.

B. **Evaluation.** Imaging studies must be performed to evaluate cases of suspected CNS mass lesions.

1. **CT and MRI** are the primary imaging modalities for evaluating presumed

CNS tumors. MRI is preferable because of its greater sensitivity, especially for mass lesions in the brainstem, posterior fossa, medial temporal lobes, and spinal cord. Contrast studies should always be performed because most, but not all, tumors show contrast enhancement.

2. **Lumbar puncture** is almost never a part of the initial evaluation of a suspected CNS tumor, and in fact is often contraindicated in this setting. It is used primarily to stage tumors known to disseminate along the neuraxis or to evaluate patients with clinical or radiographic evidence of meningeal dissemination (see sec. **II.A.10**).

3. **Angiography** is usually not required in the evaluation of suspected nervous system tumors. It is most useful in the preoperative evaluation of highly vascular tumors and tumors for which the blood supply may be shared with other neural structures. The need for angiography is determined by the neurosurgical consultant.

4. **Systemic evaluation.** Once a mass lesion is demonstrated on a CT or MRI scan, its specific etiology must be determined. The differential diagnosis includes primary tumors of the nervous system, metastatic tumors, stroke, and inflammatory or infectious processes (e.g., multiple sclerosis, cerebral abscess). Radiographic features can help differentiate between these diagnoses; combined with the patient's history and physical examination, they can lead to a presumptive diagnosis with reasonable certainty. However, basic screening tests are often performed to rule out an underlying systemic malignancy. A reasonable evaluation includes
   a. Posteroanterior and lateral chest x-rays.
   b. CBC, renal and liver function tests, electrolytes, calcium, magnesium, glucose, and thyroid function tests.
   c. Mammogram and pelvic examination, especially if they have not been performed recently or routinely.
   d. Stool guaiac for occult blood.

5. **Surgery** is required for definitive diagnosis in most cases of suspected primary nervous system tumors and usually is a cornerstone of treatment as well. Exceptions include tumors that can be diagnosed radiographically and do not require surgical extirpation (e.g., neurofibroma, optic nerve glioma). In addition, patients in whom non-neoplastic processes (e.g., stroke, multiple sclerosis) cannot be ruled out may elect to be managed by clinical and radiographic observation.

III. **Astrocytoma and glioblastoma multiforme**

A. **Pathology.** Astrocytomas are highly infiltrative tumors that are graded by their degree of anaplasia. Well-differentiated tumors are classified as astrocytoma, those with more evidence of atypia as anaplastic astrocytoma, and those with highly malignant features as glioblastoma multiforme (GBM). Glioblastomas with sarcomatous features are referred to as gliosarcomas. The incidence of astrocytomas increases with age, and as the age of the patient increases, the astrocytoma is more likely to be of a higher grade. Astrocytomas are most commonly supratentorial but may occur in the cerebellum, brainstem, and spinal cord.

B. **Radiology.** On CT or MRI scans, astrocytomas are usually solitary lesions, appearing as large translucent zones localized to the white matter. The mass is usually solid but may have cystic components. As the tumor grows, it tends to follow white-matter tracts. Most astrocytomas, especially high-grade lesions, enhance after administration of contrast material and are surrounded by focal edema. GBMs often have central necrosis and are described as "ring-enhancing" lesions.

C. **Treatment**

1. **Dexamethasone** reduces the cerebral edema associated with brain tumors by decreasing vascular permeability through its action on endothelial junctions. Neurologic dysfunction from brain tumors is often due to surrounding edema rather than to the tumor itself. Therefore treatment with steroids often results in considerable neurologic improvement. Dosing schedules

vary, but the typical starting dose is 4 mg PO or IV q6h. After treatment is initiated, patients should be monitored for hypertension and hyperglycemia. Doses should not be reduced until definitive treatment has been undertaken (usually postoperatively or during RT). Thereafter, the drug is gradually tapered off as tolerated.

2. **Surgical resection** should be performed whenever technically feasible. Not only is surgery necessary for adequate tissue sampling for pathologic diagnosis, but it can also lead to neurologic improvement from reduction of mass effect. The degree of surgical resection has been shown to correlate with survival, especially for higher grade lesions. The term "gross total resection" refers to removal of all or nearly all tumor visualized radiographically. Postoperative MRI scans should be performed within two days of surgery to determine the extent of surgical resection. However, based on the infiltrative nature of astrocytomas, residual tumor always remains.

3. **RT** substantially improves survival, and a dose-response relationship has been documented. Astrocytomas and anaplastic astrocytomas are usually treated with 54 Gy and 60 Gy, respectively, of focal radiation. Glioblastomas are treated with either 60 Gy to a focal field or with a lesser dose to the whole brain followed by a boost to deliver 60 Gy to the tumor and a surrounding margin. Radiation sensitizers have not been definitively shown to be beneficial in the treatment of astrocytomas.

4. **Chemotherapy** used on an adjuvant basis has been shown to provide a modest survival advantage to patients with anaplastic astrocytoma or GBM. The absolute increase in survival has been shown to be approximately 10 percent at one and two years. In general, the most effective agents are the nitrosoureas and procarbazine, often given in combination as the PCV regimen in 42-day cycles:

   CCNU, 110 mg/m^2 PO on day 1 of cycle
   Procarbazine, 60 mg/m^2 PO on days 8 through 21
   Vincristine, 1.4 mg/m^2 IV on days 8 and 29

   Treatment is usually continued until tumor progression is evident or a maximum of six or seven cycles have been administered. Monitoring pulmonary function tests may be necessary in selected patients.

5. **Treatment at recurrence.** Astrocytomas, including GBM, are responsive to treatment at recurrence and treatment strategies usually parallel those given at diagnosis. Low-grade astrocytomas are more likely to respond to continued sequential treatments than high-grade tumors. The decision to treat at recurrence therefore depends not only on patient characteristics, such as age and performance status, but also on tumor characteristics, such as histologic grade and surgical accessibility.

   For patients who elect further therapy, dexamethasone should be reinstituted for neurologic symptoms and further surgical debulking should be performed as much as possible. Postoperatively, either further irradiation using focused techniques, such as radiosurgery or interstitial brachytherapy, or chemotherapy should be employed. Agents other than the nitrosoureas and procarbazine that have activity against astrocytomas include carboplatin, etoposide, α-IFN, and melphalan.

6. **Patient follow-up.** Patients with astrocytomas require lifelong follow-up. Low-grade astrocytomas can recur, often as higher grade lesions, as long as 20 years after treatment. Tumor recurrence is usually at the primary site, but occasionally astrocytomas can become multifocal or recur at distal sites within the neuraxis. Metastasis to systemic tissues is exceedingly rare. Monitoring for tumor recurrence can best be achieved with serial neurologic examinations and neuroimaging. The rate of monitoring is individualized and depends on the grade of the tumor, the performance status of the patient, and the intention for further therapy.

D. Survival. Median survival is approximately five years for astrocytoma, 2.5 years for anaplastic astrocytoma, and one year for glioblastoma. Approximately 5 percent of patients with GBM survive for five years or more.

IV. Other glial neoplasms
A. Oligodendroglioma
1. **Pathology.** Oligodendrogliomas arise from the oligodendrocytes or myelin-producing cells of the CNS and may occur in conjunction with astrocytomas as a mixed tumor. Most are lower grade lesions, but highly anaplastic forms analogous to GBM also occur.
2. **Clinical features.** Compared with astrocytomas, oligodendrogliomas are more likely to result in seizures and have a higher tendency to hemorrhage and to disseminate to the meninges. Oligodendrogliomas often have a lobar location and are most common in the frontal lobes. Radiographically, they often contain calcifications.
3. **Treatment** is similar to that for astrocytomas and includes dexamethasone for control of symptoms, aggressive surgical resection, and postoperative RT. Oligodendrogliomas are usually more responsive to chemotherapy than astrocytomas, and PCV is often employed. Median survival is approximately five years.

B. Juvenile pilocytic astrocytoma (JPA)
1. **Pathology.** Pilocytic astrocytomas differ in histology and clinical behavior from the astrocytomas discussed in section **III**. They are less invasive, more circumscribed, and much less likely to progress to a more anaplastic state.
2. **Clinical features.** Pilocytic astrocytomas tend to occur in children and young adults and have a predilection for the cerebellum, hypothalamus, optic chiasm, and thalamus. Radiographically, they are well-demarcated masses that enhance densely and homogeneously and may have cystic components.
3. **Treatment.** Because JPAs tend not to be infiltrative or histologically progressive, and they can often be cured surgically, small residua of subtotally resected tumors may either be electively observed or treated with focal irradiation. Nonresectable tumors are usually treated with RT (54 Gy, focal fields) or, in very young patients, with chemotherapy. JPAs respond to nitrosoureas, procarbazine, cyclophosphamide, vincristine, platinum compounds, and etoposide.
4. **Survival** depends on tumor location and extent of resection. The overall median survival rate is 80 percent at 10 years and 70 percent at 20 years.

C. Ependymoma
1. **Pathology.** Ependymomas arise from ependymal cells. Therefore these tumors localize to the ventricular system and spinal canal, most often in the fourth ventricle and in the region of the cauda equina. They are more frequent in children but occur in adults as well. The majority are histologically benign, but some types, including anaplastic ependymoma, ependymoblastoma, and myxopapillary ependymoma, can disseminate to the spinal fluid.
2. **Treatment.** Ependymomas can be cured by total resection. Unfortunately, their location often makes them not completely resectable, and RT must often be administered postoperatively. Radiation is usually given to focal fields to a dose of 54 Gy. Anaplastic ependymomas and ependymoblastomas are often treated like medulloblastomas (see sec. **VI**). Chemotherapy plays less of a role in the treatment of ependymomas, but when used, platinum compounds are considered most effective.

D. Brainstem gliomas
D. Brainstem gliomas are astrocytomas that arise in the brainstem, usually the pons, and are more common in children than adults. Because their location has a major impact on the clinical course and survival of patients, brainstem gliomas are classified separately from astrocytomas. Multiple cranial nerve nuclei are usually involved, and therefore patients often have significant neurologic compromise and are at great risk for aspiration and sepsis. Surgical resection is also not possible due to tumor location and, since the radiographic and clinical findings are often characteristic, tissue confirmation by biopsy is often not pursued. Treatment consists of focal RT, usually to 60 Gy. Median survival for patients with diffuse brainstem gliomas is approximately one year. Patients with more localized, discrete tumors have a longer survival.

V. Primary CNS lymphoma (PCNSL) is discussed in Chap. 21, *Non-Hodgkin's Lymphoma,* sec. **VI.B** and Chap. 37, sec. **II.G.** Compared with gliomas, PCNSLs are more likely to cause subcortical dementia, cranial neuropathies, and visual loss, and are less likely to cause seizures. These clinical features reflect the tendency of PCNSLs to localize to deep, subcortical midline structures and to involve the meninges. PCNSLs are often elusive in their presentation and occasionally have a relapsing-remitting course similar to that of multiple sclerosis. Radiographically, these tumors tend to be multifocal and enhance homogeneously. They may involve midline structures such as the corpus callosum or basal ganglia. Radiographic evidence of leptomeningeal enhancement should always be sought. All patients require complete examination of the neuraxis, including the eyes.

VI. Medulloblastoma

   A. Pathology. Medulloblastomas are embryonal tumors arising from primitive germinal cells in the cerebellum; they most commonly localize to the vermis and fourth ventricle. They are more common in childhood but occur in young adults as well. Other small cell primary malignancies of the brain (e.g., neuroblastoma, pineoblastoma, ependymoblastoma) are similar histologically and clinically and are treated like medulloblastomas.

   B. Clinical features. Because of their close proximity to CSF pathways, medulloblastomas often cause obstructive hydrocephalus. Patients therefore often present with signs of hydrocephalus (e.g., gait ataxia, headache, nausea and vomiting) rather than with signs localizing to the site of their tumor.

   C. Staging and treatment. Patients require full staging of the neuraxis, i.e., contrast-enhanced MRI of the head and full spine and cytologic examination of CSF. Spinal imaging can often be performed preoperatively. CSF should be obtained intraoperatively or not until two weeks after surgery in order to avoid false-positive results.

   1. Surgery. The extent of surgical resection correlates with survival in patients with medulloblastoma, and gross total resection should be attempted. Patients with persistent hydrocephalus may require placement of a shunting device. Dexamethasone is used to control cerebral edema, especially in the perioperative period.

   2. RT consisting of craniospinal irradiation is the cornerstone of therapy, even for patients with negative staging studies. Doses range from 30–36 Gy to the whole brain and spine with an additional boost to the tumor to 60 Gy.

   3. Chemotherapy is administered to patients with evidence of tumor dissemination on staging studies. There is no established first-line chemotherapeutic regimen, but active agents include the nitrosoureas, procarbazine, cyclophosphamide, and cisplatin.

   D. Prognosis. Patients with medulloblastomas who have had a gross total resection and who show no evidence of tumor dissemination have a five-year survival rate of 60 to 75 percent. In cases of disseminated tumor, the addition of chemotherapy has increased the median survival to approximately five years.

VII. Germ cell tumors

   A. Pathology. Germ cell tumors arising in the nervous system are usually localized in the pineal and suprasellar regions. They are of two basic types, germinomas and nongerminomas. The former are highly sensitive to radiation and are analogous to systemic seminomas and dysgerminomas. The latter, including teratomas, choriocarcinomas, endodermal sinus tumors, and some tumors of mixed histology, are resistant to radiation. All germ cell tumors except mature teratomas are malignant. They are more common in males and in Japanese people, and they occur mostly in the first three decades of life.

   B. Evaluation. Since germ cell tumors can readily disseminate in the neuraxis, all patients require complete staging, including contrast MRI of the brain and full spine, CSF cytologic examination, and determination of serum and CSF α-FP and β-HCG levels.

   C. Treatment. Previously, patients with pineal tumors underwent a trial of RT; if the tumor responded rapidly, the diagnosis of germinoma was inferred. However, with improved surgical techniques and the advent of histology-directed therapy, surgical resection or biopsy should be performed first. Resection constitutes complete therapy for benign tumors (e.g., mature teratomas). Germinomas with no evidence of neuraxis dissemination and with negative tumor markers are subsequently treated with irradiation of the tumor and surrounding ventricular system. Nongerminoma, tumors with positive markers, and tumors with evidence of neuraxis dissemination are treated with craniospinal irradiation and chemotherapy. Regimens are similar to those used for systemic germ cell tumors. The prognosis for patients with germinomas is good, the five-year survival rate being greater than 60 percent, but nongerminomas are resistant to therapy, and the five-year survival is less than 25 percent.

VIII. Benign nervous system tumors

A. **Meningiomas** are tumors arising from arachnoidal cells. Their incidence increases with age and they are more common in females. The location of meningiomas may be over the convexities, parasagittal along the falx, along the sphenoid wing, retroclival, or along the thoracic spine. Although the great majority of these tumors are benign, some are histopathologically classified as aggressive or malignant. The tumors are recognized radiographically by their extra-axial location and their dense, homogeneous pattern of contrast enhancement. Treatment is by surgical resection, which is often curative. Recurrent or incompletely resected tumors may be treated with RT. These tumors have not been shown to respond to chemotherapy.

B. **Craniopharyngiomas** are congenital suprasellar tumors thought to arise from epithelial remnants of Rathke's pouch. They present clinically with dysfunction of the optic chiasm or hypothalamic-pituitary axis due to tumor compression. The tumor may contain calcifications and an oily, cellular debris that causes a severe chemical meningitis if introduced into the spinal fluid. The tumor is histologically benign and can be cured by total resection. Unfortunately, this is often not possible, and RT is eventually required for tumor control.

C. **Pituitary adenoma.** Adenomas of the pituitary gland can either be secreting or nonsecreting tumors. Secretory tumors can cause acromegaly, infertility, galactorrhea, amenorrhea, or Cushing's disease. These tumors, especially those secreting adrenocorticotropic hormone, are often very small and may be difficult to demonstrate radiographically, even with MRI. In such cases, venous sampling of the petrosal sinuses may be required to help localize the tumor. Nonsecretory tumors can result in bitemporal hemianopsia due to mass effect, pituitary apoplexy due to hemorrhage into the tumor, or hypopituitarism. Treatment usually consists of surgical resection, usually by the transsphenoidal route, except in the case of prolactinomas, which are initially treated with a trial of bromocriptine. Incompletely resected tumors may require RT as well.

D. **Schwannoma/acoustic neuroma.** Schwannomas, which are tumors arising from schwann cells in spinal nerve roots, are referred to as acoustic neuromas when present in the cerebellopontine angle, where they usually arise from the vestibular nerve. Acoustic neuromas lead to sensorineural hearing loss, tinnitus, and vertigo that can progress to involve adjacent neural structures, causing facial weakness, facial numbness, dysphagia, and ataxia. On contrast-enhanced MRI scans, these tumors are seen as homogeneously, densely enhancing mass that follow the eighth cranial nerve into the internal acoustic canal. Brainstem-evoked potentials are also useful for early diagnosis and monitoring. Management depends on the extent of hearing loss and whether bilateral tumors are present, but therapeutic options include surgical resection and focal irradiation with radiosurgery. Bilateral acoustic neuromas constitute the diagnosis of neurofibromatosis II. Spinal schwannomas cause a radiculomyelopathy and can be cured by total resection. Rarely, these tumors can have sarcomatous degeneration.

IX. Special clinical problems

A. **Seizures.** The prophylactic use of anticonvulsants is controversial in the setting of brain tumors. Because these drugs are often administered perioperatively, they are frequently continued, even in the absence of a history of seizures. Information regarding possible seizures, such as unexplained, transient neurologic events that could represent partial or focal seizures, should always be sought. Several anticonvulsants are available; the choice of a specific agent depends mostly on the side effect profile, the desired route of administration, and the urgency for treatment. If seizures have been multiple, prolonged, or generalized, a loading dose of anticonvulsants may be required. Otherwise, patients can be started on maintenance therapy and monitored until therapeutic levels are achieved. Commonly used agents include

1. **Phenytoin (Dilantin)**
   a. **Loading dose** is 18 mg/kg (usually 1 gm for adults). Maintenance doses are 5 mg/kg/day (usually 300 mg/day for adults). Phenytoin given orally is usually administered in a long-acting formulation such that once-a-day administration is adequate. For intravenous administration, the same doses are used, but are given every six to eight hours at a rate not exceeding 50 mg/min.
   b. **Therapeutic levels** are 10–20 μg/ml. Dose adjustments should be made gradually, because phenytoin has zero-order kinetics, and small increases in the dose can sometimes result in large increases in serum levels.
   c. **Side effects** of phenytoin include gingival hypertrophy, hirsutism, megaloblastic anemia, leukopenia, and hepatic dysfunction. Allergic reactions manifesting as eosinophilia and a rash are not uncommon and can proceed to a Stevens-Johnson reaction. Toxicity is progressively manifested by nystagmus, ataxia, and lethargy.

2. **Phenobarbital** is often the second-line agent in the emergent setting because an intravenous formulation is available. The loading dose is 20 mg/kg and may be administered up to a rate of 100 mg/min. Maintenance doses are 1–5 mg/kg/day, usually 90–120 mg/day in adults, and may be given before bedtime as a single dose. Therapeutic levels are 15–40 μg/ml. Sedation is the primary side effect.

3. **Carbamazepine** is often a first-line agent in the nonemergent treatment of seizures. It is available only in an oral form, and doses must be slowly increased to maintenance levels because rapid loading is not tolerated. Doses range from 7–15 mg/kg/day, divided into b.i.d. or t.i.d. fractions, typically 600–1000 mg/day for an adult. Therapeutic serum levels range from 6–12 μg/ml. Side effects include granulocytopenia, diplopia, nystagmus, fatigue, hepatic dysfunction, and allergic dermatitis. Monitoring of blood counts is required.

4. **Valproate** is administered orally at a dose of 15 mg/kg/day divided t.i.d. and elevated by 5 mg/kg/day as needed to control seizures; the therapeutic dose is 50–100 μg/ml. Side effects include hepatic and pancreatic toxicity, thrombocytopenia, nausea, tremor, and alopecia. Monitoring of LFTs is required.

B. **Hydrocephalus** can result from obstruction of CSF pathways, especially with intraventricular tumors or tumors in the upper brainstem. Patients with hydrocephalus present with headaches, nausea, vomiting, gait ataxia, urinary incontinence, and progressive lethargy. Large ventricles above the level of obstruction can be diagnosed with a noncontrast CT scan. Treatment consists of placement of a ventriculoperitoneal shunt.

C. **Radiation necrosis** can result from RT and is not uncommon after high-dose and interstitial irradiation. Clinically and radiographically, it is often indistinguishable from tumor recurrence. Position emission tomography (PET) is useful in distinguishing tumor recurrence from radiation necrosis. Radiation necrosis can be treated with dexamethasone, but surgical debulking is often required to relieve mass effect and to provide a definite tissue diagnosis.

D. **Deep venous thrombosis** occurs in approximately 20 percent of patients with high-grade gliomas. Ideal treatment consists of placement of an inferior vena cava filter. Although some physicians have expressed concern that anticoagulation poses increased risk of intracranial hemorrhage in patients with primary brain tumors, most studies have not substantiated this risk. Anticoagulation should therefore be used as therapy for patients with brain tumors and deep venous thrombosis or pulmonary embolism in whom a filter cannot be placed.

E. Herniation results from progressive mass effect in patients with large, edematous tumors. Herniation can be central in the case of midline tumors and hydrocephalus, uncal in the case of hemispheric lesions, or tonsillar in the case of posterior fossa tumors. Once recognized, herniation is an emergency that must be treated with methods to decrease intracranial pressure. These include

1. Elevation of the head of bed.
2. Hyperventilation to a P_{CO_2} of approximately 30 mm Hg.
3. Creation of an osmotic gradient by administration of mannitol at 1 gm/kg IV (usually 50–100 gm in adults).
4. Dexamethasone, up to 100 mg IV.

Selected Reading

Black, P. M. Brain tumors. *N. Engl. J. Med.* 324:1471, 1991.

DeAngelis, L. M., et al. Combined modality therapy for primary CNS lymphoma. *J. Clin. Oncol.* 10:635, 1992.

Fine, H. A., et al. Meta-analysis of radiation therapy with and without adjuvant chemotherapy for malignant gliomas in adults. *Cancer* 71:2585, 1993.

Kornblith, P. L., and Walker, M. W. Chemotherapy for malignant gliomas. *J. Neurosurg.* 68:1, 1988.

Leibel, S. A., and Sheline, G. E. Radiation therapy for neoplasms of the brain. *J. Neurosurg.* 66:1, 1987.

Shapiro, W. R. Brain tumors. *Semin. Oncol.* 13:1986.

Endocrine Neoplasms

Harold E. Carlson,
Barry B. Lowitz, and
Dennis A. Casciato

I. **General considerations.** Cancers of endocrine glands constitute less than 1 percent of all malignancies. Most malignant neoplasms derived from endocrine organs are not associated with clinical endocrinopathies, although several do produce unique syndromes and biochemical markers.

   A. **Steroid hormones** are never ectopic tumor products. They are always produced by the tissue that normally produces them, such as the adrenal cortex and gonads, whether that tissue is healthy or cancerous. The mechanism of action for most steroid hormones depends on specific receptors in the target cell cytoplasm.

   B. **Peptide hormones and catecholamines** appear to act at the cell surface where they attach to specific receptors and modify intracellular concentrations of cyclic nucleotides, calcium, and kinases.

      1. **Amine precursor uptake and decarboxylation (APUD) cells** are theoretically derived from embryonic neuroectoderm (melanocytes, thyroid C cells, adrenal medulla, paraspinal ganglia, argentaffin cells of the intestine). These cells produce hormone mediators such as serotonin, catecholamines, histamine, and kinins. Neoplasia of these tissues gives rise to carcinoid tumors, pheochromocytoma, and medullary thyroid cancer; these tumors may also produce peptide hormones (e.g., ACTH, vasoactive intestinal polypeptide [VIP]) in addition to their natural products. Other peptide-producing endocrine tissues (e.g., parathyroid, pancreatic islet) demonstrate some APUD characteristics, even though they may not be derived from neuroectoderm.

      2. **Peptide hormones,** such as ACTH, HCG, and calcitonin, are produced by a wide variety of neoplastic tissues that may or may not normally synthesize detectable amounts of these hormones. Many of these peptides are synthesized as a "prehormone." A segment of prehormone is enzymatically cleaved to form a storage molecule, a "prohormone." The prohormone is further cleaved into the active hormone, which is secreted into the blood.

      3. **Gastrointestinal hormones,** such as insulin, glucagon, somatostatin, VIP, and gastrin, are normally produced by gut endocrine cells and the pancreatic islets. Neoplasms of these tissues commonly produce one or more of these hormones; gut hormones are also normally produced in the brain and may be products of a wide variety of other neoplasms.

   C. **Multiple endocrine neoplasia (MEN)** are inherited Mendelian dominant endocrine tumor syndromes. Two categories of the syndrome are recognized.

      1. **MEN-I** (Wermer's syndrome; gene located at 11q13)

         a. **Pituitary tumors** (acromegaly, nonfunctioning adenoma, prolactinoma, or ACTH-producing adenoma)

         b. **Pancreatic islet cell tumors,** including gastrinoma, VIPoma, glucagonoma, and insulinoma

         c. **Parathyroid hyperplasia**

      2. **MEN-II.** Medullary carcinoma of the thyroid is present in all patients with this syndrome. Cushing's syndrome may develop as a consequence of ectopic ACTH production by medullary carcinoma or pheochromocytoma.

         a. **MEN-IIA** (Sipple's syndrome; *ret* oncogene located on chromosome 10)

> **(1)** Medullary carcinoma of the thyroid
> **(2)** Pheochromocytomas (bilateral)
> **(3)** Parathyroid hyperplasia
> **b. MEN-IIB** (also called MEN-III)
> > **(1)** Medullary carcinoma of the thyroid
> > **(2)** Pheochromocytoma (bilateral)
> > **(3)** Multiple mucosal ganglioneuromas (lips, tongue, eyelids)
> > **(4)** Marfanoid body habitus, high-arched palate, pes cavus, diverticulae, and sugar-loaf skull often accompany the endocrine abnormalities in MEN-IIB

II. Carcinoid tumors

A. Epidemiology and etiology. Carcinoid cancers represent less than 1 percent of visceral malignancies. The cause of these tumors is unknown, but they may be associated with MEN-I.

B. Pathology and natural history

1. **Primary tumor.** Carcinoid tumors belong to the APUD system of tumors (see sec. **I.B.1**). The primary tumors are usually small and most commonly arise in the small intestine. They also develop in the stomach, colorectum, lung, ovary, and, rarely, in other organs. Appendiceal carcinoids are common, but are usually of no clinical significance.

2. **Metastases** tend to develop primarily in the liver. Bone metastases, which are often osteoblastic, also occur. Carcinoid metastases are indolent or slowly progressive and evolve over many years. Carcinoid tumors tend to produce desmoplastic responses, which can result in mesenteric fibrosis and bowel obstruction ("parachute intestine"). Hormonally inactive tumors usually cause death by replacing hepatic tissue, which leads to liver failure.

3. **Tumor products.** Hormonally active tumors occur in 30 to 50 percent of patients and produce a variety of potentially lethal complications ("carcinoid syndrome").

   a. Small intestine carcinoids never produce the carcinoid syndrome in the absence of liver metastases; the responsible hormonal mediators are degraded in their first pass through the liver.

   b. Benign and malignant lung carcinoids occur with about equal frequency; those that produce the carcinoid syndrome are malignant. Lung carcinoids can potentially produce hormonal effects without metastasizing; active tumor products pass directly into the circulation without being filtered by the liver. However, most patients with endocrinologically active lung carcinoids also have liver metastases. Bronchial carcinoids that produce ACTH or growth hormone–releasing factor may be benign, and Cushing's syndrome or acromegaly may be the only endocrine manifestation.

   c. Symptomatic ovarian carcinoids are rarely associated with liver metastases.

   d. Humoral mediators of the carcinoid syndrome are serotonin, histamine, kinins, prostaglandins, and other hormonally active tumor products.

   (1) The major source of serotonin is dietary tryptophan, which normally is mostly metabolized to nicotinic acid. In carcinoid syndrome, tryptophan metabolism is directed to the production of serotonin (Fig. 15-1). Most patients with carcinoid syndrome develop chemical evidence of niacin deficiency, and some may develop clinically recognizable pellagra.

   (2) Other hormones and hormone metabolites that are found in some patients with carcinoid include: calcitonin, gastrin, growth hormone–releasing factor, and ACTH. These substances may or may not produce clinical syndromes, but they should be searched for in patients with serum calcium abnormalities, peptic ulcer, or Cushing's syndrome.

C. Diagnosis

1. **Symptoms: endocrinologically inactive carcinoids.** The majority of carci-

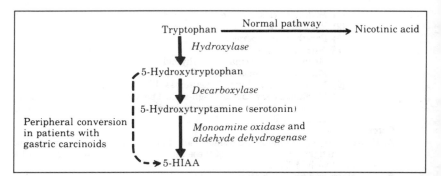

Fig. 15-1. Hepatic metabolism of tryptophan and serotonin in carcinoid syndrome. The normal pathway (*thin arrow*) of tryptophan metabolism is impaired in carcinoid syndrome, resulting in excessive production of serotonin. Monoamine oxidase inhibitors interfere with the metabolism of serotonin and are contraindicated in patients with carcinoid syndrome. 5-HIAA = 5-hydroxyindoleacetic acid.

noid tumors are endocrinologically inactive. Patients who have these tumors may have appendicitis, bowel obstruction, or a painful, enlarged liver that results from metastases.

2. **Symptoms: endocrinologically active carcinoids**
   a. **Humoral mediators** produce attacks of flushing, diarrhea, hypotension, light-headedness, and bronchospasm in various combinations. Attacks may be spontaneous or precipitated by emotional stress, alcohol ingestion, exercise, eating, or vigorous palpation of a liver that contains metastatic deposits.
   b. **Heart failure** from valvular lesions commonly occurs in patients with long-standing carcinoid symptoms. Ileal carcinoids produce tricuspid valve stenosis and insufficiency and pulmonary valve stenosis. Bronchial carcinoids with venous drainage into the left atrium can produce mitral valve disease.

3. **Physical findings**
   a. The characteristic flush differs somewhat according to the site of the primary tumor.
      (1) **Ileal carcinoid.** Purple flush involves the upper trunk and face and usually lasts less than 30 minutes.
      (2) **Bronchial carcinoid.** Deep, dusky purple flush over the entire body.
      (3) **Gastric carcinoid.** Generalized urticarialike, pruritic, and painful wheals, probably related to histamine production.
   b. Chronic skin changes involve repeated episodes of flushing, especially with bronchial carcinoids, which cause thickening of the facial features, telangiectasis, enlargement of the salivary glands, and leonine facies. A pellagrous skin rash characterized by photosensitivity, atrophy of the lingual mucosa, and thickened skin may develop.
   c. Right heart failure with evidence of tricuspid valve disease.
   d. Hepatomegaly.
   e. Cushing's syndrome and, occasionally, acromegaly.

4. **Laboratory studies in all patients**
   a. Routine blood tests, particularly LFTs.
   b. Liver sonogram or CT scan if hepatomegaly is present or if LFTs are abnormal.
   c. Chest x-ray film to search for bronchial carcinoids.
   d. Upper barium series.
   e. Nuclear scanning using a radiolabeled somatostatin analogue.
   f. A histologic diagnosis is essential for management. Biopsy the site that

is associated with the least morbidity and that has been determined by noninvasive tests to probably be affected.

5. **Laboratory studies in symptomatic patients** consist of 24-hour urine collections for 5-hydroxyindoleacetic acid (5-HIAA). Serotonin is a product of tryptophan metabolism and is metabolized to 5-HIAA (see Fig. 15-1). The normal value for 5-HIAA excretion is less than 9 mg/24 hr.

   a. **Causes of elevated 5-HIAA excretion include**

      (1) Carcinoid syndrome.

      (2) Other tumors that produce 5-HIAA include biliary, pancreatic islet, and medullary thyroid cancers.

      (3) Dietary intake of nuts, bananas, avocados, or pineapples within 48 hours of urine collection.

      (4) Medications that must be stopped one day before urine collection include mephenesin and guaifenesin.

      (5) Malabsorption syndromes (celiac disease, Whipple's disease, and tropical sprue) rarely increase 5-HIAA urine excretion above 20 mg/24 hr.

   b. **Causes of false low 5-HIAA excretion.** Phenothiazines interfere with the color reaction of the test and must be stopped two to three days before the collection of urine.

   c. **Interpretation.** A level of 5-HIAA greater than 9 mg/24 hr in patients without malabsorption or greater than 30 mg/24 hr in patients with malabsorption is pathognomonic for carcinoid unless interfering foods or drugs have been ingested. The magnitude of 5-HIAA excretion in the urine roughly corresponds to the tumor volume; 5-HIAA excretion can also be used to monitor therapy.

D. **Management.** The most important principle of management of metastatic carcinoid tumors is therapeutic restraint. These patients often survive for more than 10 years without antitumor treatment. Patients with endocrinologically active tumors have an especially high risk of developing complications from any procedure requiring anesthesia. Therapy should be focused on controlling the endocrine symptoms.

   1. **Surgery** is useful for patients with localized primary carcinoids or metastatic tumors that produce obstruction. For patients with incidental appendiceal carcinoids that are 2.0 cm or less in diameter (very rarely metastasize), appendectomy is adequate treatment.

      Partial hepatectomy has been recommended by some physicians, particularly if the metastases are confined to one lobe of the liver. However, the 20 percent mortality of hepatectomy and the long natural history of the disease often dissuades the physician from recommending the procedure.

   2. **Hepatic artery occlusion** performed surgically or by catheterization and embolization of hepatic metastases has been successfully used to palliate endocrine symptoms or pain. Objective regression of manifestations occurs in 60 percent of patients for a median of four months. Side effects of arterial occlusion include fever, nausea, and LFT abnormalities. Both the response rate and median duration of response appear to improve when occlusion is followed by sequenced chemotherapy (see **II.D.4**).

   3. **RT** is used to palliate liver pain caused by far-advanced metastatic disease unresponsive to other treatments. However, carcinoid tumors are relatively radioresistant.

   4. **Chemotherapy** is used late in the course of disease for treatment of symptomatic metastases and for patients with severe endocrine symptoms that do not respond satisfactorily to pharmacologic maneuvers (see sec. **5**). Chemotherapy with various combinations of fluorouracil, streptozocin, cyclophosphamide, Adriamycin, cisplatin, and α-IFN have been associated with response rates of about 50 percent with variable median durations of response; the responses to treatment with α-IFN have generally been the most transient. Endocrine symptoms may be palliated, but the effects of chemotherapy on survival are not known.

   a. Combination regimens. The largest experience in the treatment of metastatic carcinoid tumors has been gained with the combination of 5-FU and streptozocin administered every 42 days (see **4.b.** for dosages). Cisplatin (50 mg/m^2) in combination with Adriamycin (50 mg/m^2) every three to four weeks has been effective in a variety of apudomas. Cisplatin in combination with etoposide is useful for anaplastic neuroendocrine carcinomas.

   b. Sequenced chemotherapy following hepatic arterial occlusion is initiated about three weeks after the procedure, which is performed for symptomatic hepatic metastases from carcinoid tumors or islet cell carcinomas. Substantial or complete relief from the endocrine syndromes is achieved in about 80 percent of patients, with a median duration of 18 months.

   The following two regimens are alternated every four to five weeks until the patient has stabilized with maximum tumor regression (usually about six months).

   (1) Adriamycin (60 mg/m^2 IV on day 1) and dacarbazine (250 mg/m^2 IV daily for five days)

   (2) Streptozocin (500 mg/m^2) and 5-FU (400 mg/m^2), both given daily IV for five days.

5. Pharmacologic management. It is probably not possible to completely control the symptoms of carcinoid syndrome with aggressive dietary tryptophan restriction and high-dose antiserotonin drugs alone.

   a. Octreotide, a somatostatin analogue, inhibits the release of tumoral neurotransmitters and ameliorates symptoms in about 90 percent of patients. The dosage is usually 100–600 μg SQ daily in two to four divided doses.

   b. Hypotension, the most life-threatening complication of carcinoid syndrome, is mediated by kinins (and perhaps prostaglandins) and can be precipitated by catecholamines. β-Adrenergic drugs (e.g., dopamine, epinephrine) must be strictly avoided since they may aggravate hypotension. Pure α-adrenergic (methoxamine, norepinephrine) and vasoconstrictive (angiotensin) agents are preferred for treating hypotension in carcinoid syndrome.

   (1) Methoxamine (Vasoxyl) is given IM at a dose of 0.5 ml (10 mg) or IV, 0.25 ml (5 mg) over one to two minutes (using a tuberculin syringe). The dose is repeated as necessary to maintain the blood pressure.

   (2) Angiotensin amide (Hypertensin), rather than methoxamine, is recommended by some anesthesiologists.

   (3) Corticosteroids may prevent episodes of hypotension.

   c. Flushing is mediated by kinins and histamine and may respond to several agents.

   (1) Prochlorperazine (Compazine), 10 mg PO q.i.d., *or*

   (2) Phenoxybenzamine (Dibenzyline), 10 to 20 mg PO b.i.d., *or*

   (3) Cyproheptadine (Periactin), 4 to 6 mg PO q.i.d.

   (4) Prednisone, 20 to 40 mg PO daily, is useful for flushing due to bronchial carcinoids, and occasionally for patients with other kinds of carcinoids.

   (5) The combined use of histamine H$_1$- and H$_2$-receptor antagonists has been effective in patients with carcinoid flush and documented hypersecretion of histamine. Diphenhydramine hydrochloride (Benadryl), 50 mg PO q.i.d., *plus* cimetidine (Tagamet), 300 mg PO q.i.d., has been used with success in some patients.

   (6) Methyldopa (Aldomet) is useful in some patients.

   (7) Monoamine oxidase inhibitors are *contraindicated* in carcinoid syndrome because they block serotonin catabolism and can aggravate symptoms (see Fig. 15-1).

   d. Bronchospasm is mediated by histamine and managed with aminophylline. Adrenergic agents, such as isoproterenol, do not appear to worsen bronchospasm for carcinoid and also may be used.

e. Diarrhea is mediated by serotonin and is often difficult to control. A recommended sequence for treatment is

   (1) Belladonna alkaloids and phenobarbital combination (DonnagelPG), 15 ml q3h as needed. Patients are directed to take 15 ml q.i.d. if they have more than two or three diarrheal stools a day.

   (2) Diphenoxylate and atropine (Lomotil), two tablets q3h while awake.

   (3) Cyproheptadine (Periactin), 4 to 6 mg PO q.i.d.

   (4) Methysergide maleate (Sansert), started at 8 to 12 mg/day and gradually increased to 20 to 22 mg/day if needed.

f. Preparation for anesthesia. Patients with carcinoid syndrome are at high risk for the development of flushing and hypotensive episodes during surgery. Stimulation of adrenergic hormone release and use of drugs that induce hypotension (morphine, succinylcholine, and curare) must be minimized.

   (1) Preoperative period. Patients should be premedicated with cyproheptadine, 4 to 8 mg PO. Methotrimeprazine, 10 mg IM, is given one hour before surgery. Methotrimeprazine is a phenothiazine with amnesic, analgesic, antihistaminic, and catechol blocker properties. This drug permits the use of lower doses of anesthetics and allows the avoidance of morphine.

   (2) During surgery. Aminophylline can be used for bronchoconstriction, methotrimeprazine for flushing, and methoxamine for hypotension. Rapid, dramatic improvement has been reported following administration of intravenous somatostatin.

E. Special clinical problems associated with carcinoid syndrome

   1. Bowel obstruction may result from dense fibrosis of the mesentery. Surgical relief is impossible. Patients may improve with simple nagogastric decompression and fluid replacement.

   2. Right ventricular failure results from tricuspid and pulmonic valve lesions. These lesions develop with far-advanced carcinoid syndrome, which has a poor prognosis independent of the heart lesions. Because of the high surgical risk in these patients, valve replacement is usually not warranted. Heart failure should be medically managed with diuretics.

   3. Pellagrous skin lesions may be treated with daily oral vitamin preparations containing 1 to 2 mg of niacin.

III. Thyroid cancer

A. Epidemiology and etiology

   1. Incidence. Thyroid cancer accounts for less than 1 percent of visceral malignancies; there are 10,000 new cases and 1000 cancer deaths in the United States annually. The risk increases with age. Women are affected more than men in a ratio of 3:2.

   2. Radiation exposure. Radiation fallout and RT given over the neck region in intermediate doses (<2000 cGy) for benign conditions (such as acne in teenagers, or enlarged tonsils or thymus glands in children) increase the risk of thyroid cancer, particularly the papillary type.

   a. The lag time between radiation exposure and the onset of thyroid cancer averages 25 years, but ranges from 5 to 50 years. Most patients under 20 years of age with thyroid cancer have a history of neck irradiation.

   b. About 4 percent of patients with thyroid cancer have a history of radiation to the neck. Between 5 percent and 10 percent of patients who have a history of neck irradiation develop thyroid cancer; 25 percent have an abnormal thyroid by palpation.

   c. Thyroid cancers after neck irradiation are often multifocal but have an indolent course and a prognosis similar to spontaneous tumors.

   d. Neck irradiation also increases the risk of hyperparathyroidism and parotid gland tumors.

3. **Hereditary factors.** Medullary cancer of the thyroid may arise sporadically or as a dominantly inherited syndrome of MEN-II (see sec. **I.C.2**). Thyroid tumors (including papillary and follicular carcinomas), as well as breast neoplasms, also occur frequently in Cowden's multiple hamartoma syndrome. Several oncogenes and tumor suppressor genes have been implicated in the pathogenesis of thyroid neoplasms.

4. **TSH.** An increased risk for thyroid cancer may be present in patients with chronic TSH elevation, such as patients with congenital defects in thyroid hormone formation.

B. **Pathology and natural history.** The more aggressive histologic subtypes of thyroid cancer tend to affect older patients.

1. **Papillary cancers** (70% of thyroid cancers in adults) affect younger patients. Psammoma bodies are usually present in histologic sections. Regional lymph nodes that drain the thyroid are involved in 50 percent of patients. Mixed papillary-follicular cancers behave like pure papillary cancer. All combinations of papillary and follicular carcinoma have indolent courses. Distant metastases to lungs, bone, skin, and other organs occur late, if at all.

2. **Follicular cancers** (20% of thyroid cancers) have a peak incidence at 40 years of age. They tend to invade blood vessels and to metastasize hematogenously to visceral sites, particularly bone. Lymph node metastases are relatively rare, especially compared to papillary cancers.

3. **Anaplastic giant and spindle cell cancers** (5% of thyroid cancers) occur most often in patients over 60 years of age. Anaplastic thyroid cancers are aggressive cancers, which rapidly invade surrounding local tissues and metastasize to distant organs.

4. **Medullary thyroid cancers** (5–7% of thyroid cancers) secrete calcitonin. ACTH, histaminase, and an unidentified substance that produces diarrhea may also be secreted by these tumors. Large amounts of amyloid are evident by histologic examination. Metastases are mostly found in the neck and mediastinal lymph nodes and may calcify. Widespread visceral metastases occur late.

5. **Hürthle cell cancer** is an uncommon variant of follicular carcinoma and has a relatively aggressive metastatic course.

6. **Other tumors** found in the thyroid include Hodgkin's disease, lymphomas, a variety of soft tissue sarcomas, and metastatic cancers of lung, colon, and other primary sites. Small cell cancers of the thyroid are rare, histologically similar to lymphoma, and spread to both lymph nodes and distant sites.

C. **Diagnosis**

1. **Symptoms and signs**

   a. **Symptoms.** Some patients with thyroid cancer complain of an enlarging mass in the neck. Hoarseness may be the result of recurrent laryngeal nerve paralysis. Neck pain or dysphagia occasionally is a complaint. Asymptomatic patients may have thyroid cancer discovered at thyroidectomy done for other reasons.

   b. **Physical findings.** Thyroid cancer may be found on routine physical examination as a mass in the thyroid or in the midline up to the base of the tongue (thyroglossal duct remnant). Thyroid masses less than 1 cm in diameter often are not palpable. Most patients have a single palpable nodule; others have a normal, multinodular, or diffusely enlarged thyroid gland. Anaplastic cancer is often manifested by obvious masses infiltrating the skin of the neck or by respiratory distress. Cervical lymph nodes are frequently palpable.

2. **Laboratory studies**

   a. **Routine studies.** Chest x-ray film and serum alkaline phosphatase level should be obtained to look for evidence of metastatic disease in the lung, liver, or bone. Liver and bone scans and selected skeletal x-rays are indicated when the alkaline phosphatase level is elevated.

   b. **Thyroid scans** may be obtained in nonpregnant patients with palpable abnormalities of the thyroid. Nonfunctional "cold" nodules are found in 90 percent of patients with palpable nodules, both benign and malignant, but only about 10 percent of cold nodules prove to be cancer.

  c. **Thyroid ultrasonography** may be obtained in patients with palpable abnormalities of the thyroid, but may be unreliable for excluding cancer, depending on the experience of the ultrasonographer. Purely cystic lesions, found in about 10 percent of patients with palpable nodules, are reported to be malignant in less than 1 percent of cases. Benign and malignant lesions cannot be distinguished by ultrasonography if they are mixed with solid and cystic components or are entirely solid.

  d. **Diagnostic use of thyroxine.** Some clinicians treat cold nodules with thyroid hormones at physiologic doses for three months or longer to try to distinguish benign from malignant lesions. Although the majority of thyroid cancers remain unchanged or enlarge during this treatment, some cancers may temporarily partially regress.

  e. **Thyrocalcitonin assay.** Patients with a family history of medullary thyroid cancer should be given a pentagastrin or calcium infusion test for thyrocalcitonin. Patients with positive tests require neck exploration regardless of findings on physical examination or thyroid scan.

3. **Thyroid gland biopsy**

  a. **Needle aspiration biopsy** is invaluable for cytologic diagnosis of thyroid nodules and for preventing unnecessary thyroidectomies. Many authorities recommend needle biopsy as the first step in evaluation of any thyroid lump, even before thyroid scan is done, because 90 percent of all thyroid nodules are "cold." The accuracy of needle biopsy of the thyroid is over 90 percent for benign lesions; the false-negative rate is 5 to 10 percent. Only approximately 10 percent of cold nodules are cancerous. Roughly, if 100 patients with cold nodules underwent needle biopsy rather than thyroidectomy and if patients with benign histopathology were excluded from surgery, one cancer would be missed, nine cancers would be appropriately resected, and ten patients would have undergone unnecessary surgery. Therefore the needle biopsy saves 80 of 100 patients from unnecessary surgery at the expense of missing one cancer, which is usually indolent and can be detected later.

  b. **Open biopsy.** Nodules interpreted as suspicious on needle biopsy should undergo open biopsy. Solid nodules that grow during suppressive therapy should be excised despite negative cytology.

D. **Survival and prognostic factors**

  1. **Papillary and papillary-follicular adenocarcinomas.** Decreased survival is not noted when compared with age-matched populations until 12 years after the diagnosis. Only 3 to 12 percent of patients die as a result of thyroid cancer. Even with distant metastases, patients often survive many years without therapy. The raw 10-year survival is 95 percent for patients under 40 years of age and 75 percent for patients over 40 years of age.

  a. **Factors that have no adverse effect on prognosis**

    (1) Sex

    (2) Radiation-related neoplasms

    (3) Regional lymph node metastases (increased recurrences, but normal survival)

  b. **Factors that adversely affect prognosis** both increase the recurrence rate and decrease the survival rate and include

    (1) Age of more than 40 years

    (2) Size of nodule greater than 5 cm (compared with less than 2.5 cm)

    (3) Tumor extends through the thyroid capsule

    (4) Presence of symptoms, such as hoarseness or dysphagia

    (5) Distant metastases

    (6) Residual tumor fails to take up ^{131}I

    (7) Subtotal thyroidectomy (compared with "near-total" thyroidectomy) for tumors greater than 1.5 cm in diameter

(8) Probably, postoperative therapy with thyroid hormone alone (compared with thyroid hormone and ^{131}I)

2. **Follicular adenocarcinoma** without vascular invasion has essentially the same survival as papillary carcinoma for age-matched populations. With significant vascular invasion, the 10-year survival drops to 35 percent.

3. **Medullary carcinoma** without lymph node involvement is nearly always cured with surgery. With lymph node involvement, five-year survival decreases to 45 percent.

4. **Anaplastic carcinoma.** Nearly all patients die within six to eight months.

E. **Management.** No uniform opinion exists regarding the management of indolent varieties of thyroid cancer.

1. **Surgery.** Total or near-total thyroidectomy is the treatment of choice for all types of thyroid cancer. Subtotal thyroidectomy is associated with double the recurrence rate and a lower survival rate than total thyroidectomy for papillary and follicular cancers. Medullary cancer of the thyroid is often bilateral and total thyroidectomy is imperative.

   a. **Neck nodes** that are involved clinically should be removed. However, neck dissection does not improve the rate of survival or relapse, except in medullary carcinoma, and is responsible for increasing the rate of major complications.

   b. **Complications.** The major complications of thyroidectomy are hypoparathyroidism and vocal cord paralysis; death is rare. Combinations of these problems and other complications occur in 10 to 15 percent of patients subjected to total thyroidectomy; the incidence is doubled to tripled if neck dissection is added to the procedure.

2. **Thyroxine.** TSH suppression following thyroidectomy is essential because TSH stimulates most papillary and follicular tumors. Thyroxine is given in a dose sufficient to suppress serum TSH to subnormal levels. Patients must be monitored for signs of hyperthyroidism and the dose of thyroxine decreased to keep the patient clinically euthyroid. If ^{131}I is given, thyroxine is begun afterward.

3. **Radioactive iodine.** Fears of the leukemogenic potential of ^{131}I have abated since little increase in the incidence of acute leukemia has been found in many long-term studies. Iodine 131 given postoperatively (usually about 50–100 mCi) to ablate thyroid remnants may improve survival in patients with papillary, follicular, and mixed papillary-follicular tumors. Thyroid tumors that do not take up ^{131}I are not ablated by the isotope. See Chap. 2, sec. IV.A.

   a. **Indications for ^{131}I.** The true value of ^{131}I is not known and is difficult to determine since the isotope has been given to patients with thyroid cancer as part of standard practice for many years. Theoretically, radioactive iodine may not be necessary in all patients. Clear indications for postoperative ^{131}I in patients in whom the residual tumor demonstrates uptake include the presence of

      (1) Multiple tumors of the thyroid gland
      (2) Tumors larger than 2.5 cm
      (3) Locally invasive tumors
      (4) Remote metastases

   b. **Administration.** Iodine 131 may be given either when the patient demonstrates biochemical evidence of hypothyroidism or after treating the patient with TSH. Both methods are based on the principle that TSH stimulates ^{131}I uptake in both residual thyroid tissue and residual carcinoma, and that it permits ablation of both.

      (1) **Waiting for hypothyroidism** means postponing treatment for three to six weeks after thyroidectomy. Hypothyroidism is defined as serum TSH levels greater than 30 μU/ml by radioimmunoassay.

      (2) **Giving TSH.** The patient is treated with bovine TSH (10 units IM for three or four days) and then given ^{131}I in therapeutic doses. A thyroid and body scan is obtained 72 hours later to look for areas of

residual thyroid tissue or metastatic disease. Exogenous bovine TSH may be allergenic; recombinant human TSH is under evaluation.

4. **Patient follow-up.** Patients may need to be retreated with ^{131}I. Thyroxine therapy is discontinued for three to six weeks and the TSH level is checked weekly until it exceeds 30 μU/ml. The ^{131}I body scan is repeated, and ^{131}I therapy is given if needed. Thyroxine maintenance is then resumed. Withdrawal of thyroxine and ^{131}I scans are repeated every 6 to 12 months until a negative scan is obtained. In most patients with papillary and follicular cancers, serum levels of thyroglobulin correlate with residual thyroid tissue (either normal or neoplastic) and can be used as a tumor marker after all normal thyroid remnants have been ablated.

5. **Relapsing disease** develops in about 12 percent of patients who have no evidence of disease after primary therapy. Tumors that are not treatable by the combination of surgery, thyroxine therapy, and repeat doses of ^{131}I respond poorly to external beam RT and chemotherapy.

   a. **External beam RT** is probably indicated as adjuvant therapy following surgery for anaplastic thyroid cancer and for all patients with known residual cancers that do not take up ^{131}I.

   b. **Chemotherapy** for symptomatic, widespread metastatic thyroid cancer that is unresponsive to ^{131}I can occasionally produce short-range palliation. Adriamycin as a single agent produces up to a 30 percent tumor response rate. Adriamycin is the most active agent in anaplastic thyroid cancer as well. The effect of chemotherapy on survival is uncertain.

F. **Special clinical problems associated with thyroid cancer**

   1. **Hypoparathyroidism** complicates total thyroidectomy in 10 to 15 percent of patients; it is rare following ^{131}I therapy. Hypoparathyroidism is transient in 5 to 10 percent of cases; blood calcium levels normalize in one or two weeks.

      a. **Acute therapy.** Blood calcium levels and clinical evidence of hypocalcemia are checked daily. If the blood calcium is below 8 mg/dl, oral calcium lactate (2 gm q.i.d.) or calcium carbonate (2.5 gm/day) is given. If the patient manifests tetany or the blood calcium is 6 mg/dl or less, IV calcium gluconate or lactate is given (1 gm q4–6h), and calcium blood levels are monitored more frequently.

      b. **Chronic therapy.** Patients with persistent hypocalcemia one week after thyroidectomy usually require chronic calcium supplements. If hypocalcemia recurs after two more weeks of therapy that has been followed by weaning off supplements, vitamin D therapy is necessary as well. Dihydrotachysterol (DHT) is started at a dose of 0.4 mg/day PO; calcium lactate or carbonate are continued. Calcium level measurements are repeated weekly; if less than 8 mg/dl, the DHT is increased in 0.2-mg increments weekly until the calcium level has normalized. Despite stable calcium levels during many years of treatment, vitamin D intoxication can develop suddenly. Therefore, serum calcium should be evaluated every three to four months in the absence of symptoms and whenever any symptoms appear. Serum calcium should be maintained in the low-normal range (8.5–9.5 mg/dl) to avoid hypercalciuria.

   2. **History of neck irradiation.** Patients who have a history of neck radiation exposure and no palpable abnormalities should be followed by careful annual physical examination. Repeated radionuclide scans are potentially carcinogenic, especially in young adults. Radiation-induced thyroid cancer typically has a very indolent course and does not necessitate anxiety-provoking management.

IV. **Pheochromocytoma**

A. **Epidemiology and etiology.** Pheochromocytomas (PCCs) are very rare tumors; they belong to the APUD system and produce symptoms by elaborating catecholamines. Certain hereditary syndromes are associated with an increased risk for PCC.

   1. Dominantly inherited MEN-II (see section I.C)

2. Dominantly transmitted PCC
3. Neurofibromatosis (von Recklinghausen's disease)
4. von Hippel-Lindau disease of cerebellar hemangioblastoma with retinal angiomas and polycythemia

B. Pathology and natural history

1. PCC **originates** in the adrenal medulla (90% of patients) or in the paraganglia of the sympathetic nervous system. The paraganglia range from the organ of Zuckerkandl at the aortic bifurcation to the carotid bifurcation. Bilateral PCC frequently occurs in inherited syndromes and in 10 percent of noninherited cases.

2. **Metastases** to bone, liver, and lung occur in 10 percent of cases of PCC despite a histologically benign appearance. Metastases have an indolent growth pattern but are lethal because they often produce cardiovascular complications.

3. **Hyperglycemia** is very common in patients with PCC. Patients also have an increased incidence of gallstones.

4. **Paraneoplastic complications** of PCC include
   a. Polycythemia
   b. Hypercalcemia
   c. Cushing's syndrome

C. Diagnosis

1. **Symptoms and signs**
   a. **Symptoms.** The most common symptoms of PCC are episodes of various combinations of the following: headache, sweating, tachycardia, palpitations, pallor, nausea, and feeling of impending death. Episodes may be triggered by exercise, emotional upset, alcohol ingestion, physical examination in the area of the tumor, or micturition. Vague complaints of anxiety, tremulousness, fever, dyspnea, or angina are often mistaken for psychosomatic illness or thyrotoxicosis. Weight loss is common, but one-third of patients are overweight.
   b. **Hypertension** is present in 90 percent of patients. The hypertension is fixed (66% of patients) or paroxysmal (33%). Orthostatic hypotension occurs in 70 percent of patients.
   c. **Catechol cardiomyopathy.** Patients may have cardiovascular collapse after a vague history of arrhythmias and anxiety.

2. **Selection of patients for study.** Young patients without hypertension but with documented atrial arrhythmia, evidence of an unexplained hypermetabolic state, or cardiomyopathy should be screened for PCC and thyrotoxicosis. The presence of PCC should be sought in patients with hypertension and any of the following:
   a. Age less than 45 years (PCC is a remediable, though rare, cause of hypertension)
   b. A family history of a hereditary PCC syndrome
   c. Episodic attacks typical of the syndrome

3. **Chemical tests**
   a. **Catecholamine metabolites.** A 24-hour urine collection for vanillylmandelic acid (VMA) or total metanephrines (TMN) collected during a hypertensive episode is the best screening test for PCC (>90% sensitivity). Plasma assays and plasma catecholamine assays are also available. The upper limit of normal is 6.8 mg for VMA, and 0.9 mg for TMN per 24-hour urine specimen. Elevated levels suggest the presence of PCC and mandate further studies. A large number of drugs affect either the metabolism or assay of catecholamines. All drugs, except perhaps mild tranquilizers, sedatives, and analgesics, should be discontinued 72 hours prior to urine collection if possible.
      (1) **Misleading elevations in urinary catecholamine metabolites.** Phenothiazines and tricyclic antidepressants increase levels during acute therapy but may decrease catecholamine excretion during

chronic therapy. Increased excretion of metabolites is commonly found with drugs that are catecholamines (e.g., isoproterenol) or catecholamine releasers (e.g., ephedrine, amphetamines, methylxanthines). Other agents include L-dopa, nalidixic acid, or para-aminosalicylic acid (which affect the VMA level) and methyldopa and monoamine oxidase inhibitors (which affect the TMN level).

    (2) Misleading low values may be due to incomplete urine collections or the following drugs:

        (a) Alpha-methyl-paratyrosine, clonidine, reserpine, guanethidine, monoamine oxidase inhibitors, clofibrate, mandelamine (affect VMA level)

        (b) Alpha-methyl-paratyrosine, clonidine, reserpine, guanethidine (affect TMN level)

  b. Fasting hyperglycemia is almost always present in patients with PCC; its absence makes the diagnosis doubtful.

  c. Pharmacologic tests (e.g., production of a vasodepressor response with phentolamine) are hazardous, have a poor predictive value, and no longer have a role in the diagnosis of PCC. Failure to suppress plasma catecholamines by clonidine, however, may be useful in diagnosis.

4. Radiographic techniques are used for localization of tumor in patients with a chemical diagnosis of PCC.

  a. Chest x-ray may reveal a paraganglionic tumor.

  b. CT scan may identify PCC.

  c. Selective venography. During this procedure, blood catecholamines can be sampled from several areas of the venous system to help locate small tumors. Venography is useful

    (1) If less-invasive studies fail to show the tumor

    (2) To search for multiple primary sites, especially in patients with MEN syndromes

  d. Isotope scanning with ^{131}I-metaiodobenzyl guanidine may be useful in demonstrating PCC.

D. Management

1. Pharmacologic control of PCC is essential before invasive diagnostic tests or surgery is done.

  a. Phenoxybenzamine (Dibenzyline), 10 to 20 mg PO b.i.d., is a pure α-adrenergic blocker that controls both episodic and fixed hypertension.

  b. Propranolol (Inderal), 10 to 40 mg PO q.i.d., is a β-adrenergic blocker that is useful for treating sweating, hypermetabolism, and arrhythmias. Propranolol should be used only after adequate α-adrenergic blockade is established to avoid hypertension.

  c. Alpha-methyl-paratyrosine (Demser) blocks catecholamine synthesis in doses of 2 to 4 gm/day PO.

2. Surgery

  a. Before surgery

    (1) Long-acting α- and β-adrenergic blockers should be continued preoperatively and throughout surgery.

    (2) Close attention should be paid to maintaining fluid and electrolyte balance. Preoperative volume expansion may be useful.

    (3) Central venous and arterial catheters should be placed to closely monitor blood volume and pressure changes.

  b. During surgery

    (1) Close ECG monitoring is necessary to manage arrhythmias.

    (2) Hypertensive episodes, which may occur while the tumor is being manipulated, are managed with nitroprusside infusion or rapid IV boluses of phentolamine (Regitine, 1–2 mg IV).

    (3) Hypotensive episodes, which occur after the tumor's blood supply has been isolated, should be treated with IV fluids and norepinephrine.

    (4) Obvious tumors and paraspinal ganglia should be carefully inspected. All visible tumor is removed. In patients with metastatic PCC, as much tumor as possible is removed to reduce catecholamine secretion.

   c. After surgery

     (1) Hypertension may develop as a result of fluid overload during surgery and is treated with IV furosemide and fluid restriction until the blood pressure is controlled.

     (2) If hypertension persists for two or three days postoperatively, residual PCC must be suspected.

     (3) All patients should have 24-hour urine studies for VMA and TMN repeated about one week after surgery. Unsuspected residual tumors and tumor recurrences should be surgically removed.

  3. Metastatic disease

    a. RT is useful for palliating locally symptomatic metastases.

    b. The usefulness of **chemotherapy** for unresectable disease is not established, although the combination of cyclophosphamide, vincristine, and dacarbazine produces objective responses in the majority of patients. Symptoms of catecholamine excess are managed pharmacologically (see sec. **D.1**).

    c. Some patients may respond to therapeutic doses of ^{131}I-metaiodobenzyl guanidine.

V. Adrenal carcinoma

  A. Epidemiology. Adrenal cancer causes 0.2 percent of cancer deaths. The average age at diagnosis is 40 years, but the tumor occurs at all ages. Two-thirds of the patients are women.

  B. Pathology and natural history. Adrenal cancers are highly aggressive; they frequently metastasize to lungs, liver, and other organs and are large and bulky at the time of diagnosis. About 50 percent of these tumors produce functional corticosteroids, including cortisol, aldosterone, androgens, and estrogens.

  C. Diagnosis

    1. Symptoms and signs

      a. Hormonally inactive tumors are discovered as large abdominal masses in patients with abdominal pain, weight loss, or evidence of metastases.

      b. Hormonally active tumors present with the following:

        (1) Rapid virilization (hirsutism, clitoromegaly, oligomenorrhea, or amenorrhea) in women

        (2) Gynecomastia in men

        (3) Precocious puberty

        (4) Cushing's syndrome with hypertension and glucose intolerance

    2. Adrenal function tests. Patients with clinical or laboratory evidence (hypokalemic alkalosis) of hypercortisolism should have the dexamethasone suppression test and 24-hour urine collection for 17-ketosteroids performed. The differential diagnosis of causes of Cushing's syndrome is shown in Table 15-1.

      a. Dexamethasone suppression test. Before and after two days of treatment with dexamethasone, 0.5 mg PO every 6 hours, plasma cortisol and ACTH levels are obtained at 8 A.M. Dexamethasone dose is increased to 2.0 mg PO every 6 hours for 2 days, and 8 A.M. cortisol and ACTH levels are measured again. Both doses suppress the plasma cortisol to below 5 μg/dl in normal subjects; failure of the 8-mg/day dose to suppress cortisol blood levels suggests an adrenal source (adenoma or adenocarcinoma) of the hypercortisolism if ACTH levels are low. Nonadrenal tumors that produce ectopic ACTH also demonstrate failure of dexamethasone to suppress cortisol, but these patients have very high levels of ACTH in the plasma.

      b. 24-hour urine collection is obtained for urinary free cortisol (upper limit of normal is less than 100 μg/24 hr) and 17-ketosteroids (upper normal limit is less than 14–26 mg/24 hr, depending on the age and sex of the patient). The levels of both substances are elevated in Cushing's

Table 15-1. Differential diagnosis of causes of Cushing's syndrome

Etiology	Pituitary Cushing's syndrome	Ectopic ACTH secretion	Adrenal carcinoma	Adrenal adenoma
Serum potassium	N or ↓	↓ ↓	N or ↓	N or ↓
Urine 17-ketosteroids	↑	↑	↑ or ↑ ↑	↑ or ↑ ↑
Plasma ACTH	N or ↑	↑ ↑	↓	↓
Adrenal enlargement*	Bilateral	Bilateral	Unilateral	Unilateral
Suppression of plasma cortisol with dexamethasone	Yes	No	No	No

Key: ↓ = decreased; ↓ ↓ = markedly decreased; ↑ = increased; ↑ ↑ = markedly increased; N = normal.
*Adrenal gland enlargement is determined by CT scan.

syndrome, no matter what the cause. Levels of 17-ketosteroids in excess of 50 mg in 24 hours make the diagnosis of adrenal carcinoma likely; levels over 100 mg in 24 hours are diagnostic.

   3. Further studies
      a. Chest x-ray film to search for metastases.
      b. Abdominal CT scan to look for abdominal masses not clinically evident. Small (<6 cm) benign adrenal masses are common incidental findings on CT examination; laboratory findings and follow-up CT scans may help in the differential diagnosis.
      c. Biopsy
         (1) In patients with metastatic disease, the most readily accessible site is biopsied (e.g., superficial lymph nodes or liver with evidence of metastases).
         (2) If only intra-abdominal disease is evident, laparotomy is necessary for biopsy proof of the diagnosis.
   D. Management. The median survival for untreated patients is three months. Treated patients may survive up to five years, depending on the extent of disease.
      1. Surgery should be used to resect as much tumor as possible. The contralateral adrenal gland should be inspected and removed if there is evidence of tumor.
      2. RT is used to palliate symptoms from local metastatic sites.
      3. Chemotherapy may be useful for reducing tumor bulk and controlling endocrine symptoms. Mitotane (o,p′-DDD) produces objective tumor regression or improvement of endocrine symptoms in 30 percent of cases. The use of mitotane as an adjuvant to surgery in localized disease does not appear to improve results. Pharmacologic management of hypercortisolism is discussed in Chap. 27, sec. **VIII.C.**
VI. Islet cell tumors
   A. General aspects. Islet cell tumors of the endocrine pancreas are uncommon. In addition to the specific endocrine manifestations associated with each kind of tumor, some have been associated with ectopic production of ACTH (Cushing's syndrome). Many of these tumors are malignant and metastasize to the liver.
      1. Diagnosis. The diagnosis of islet cell tumor is usually suspected because of endocrine or biochemical abnormalities. Signs and symptoms of islet cell tumors are described according to the specific type. Once abnormal hormonal products are detected, the following studies are done in all patients to determine the tumor's location and extent.
         a. LFTs; liver imaging if there is hepatomegaly or abnormal liver function tests.

   b. Liver biopsy is the diagnostic method of choice if liver imaging suggests the presence of tumor.

   c. CT scan of the pancreas may reveal isolated tumors. Selective angiograms have less than a 50 percent yield. Somatostatin receptor scanning using radioiodinated octreotide frequently demonstrates primary and metastatic islet cell tumors. Endoscopic ultrasonography also appears to be useful in localizing tumors in the pancreas or duodenal wall.

   d. Exploratory laparotomy is indicated if there is clinical or laboratory evidence of an islet cell tumor, even if preoperative localization is unrevealing.

2. Management

   a. Surgery. Intra-operative pancreatic sonography is used to localize tumors. Benign tumors are excised. Debulking procedures for malignant tumors, such as partial hepatectomy in patients with metastases confined to one lobe of the liver, are hazardous and generally are not recommended. Hepatic artery occlusion, however, is frequently helpful (see sec. II.D.2).

   b. Chemotherapy has been useful in 50 percent of patients with metastatic disease, by both decreasing tumor mass and ameliorating otherwise refractory endocrine symptoms. The most studied regimen is the combination of fluorouracil and streptozocin, used either alone or sequenced with Adriamycin and dacarbazine following hepatic artery occlusion (see II.D.4). The combination regimens of cisplatin with either Adriamycin or etoposide (see II.D.4) and of dacarbazine with L-asparaginase have some reported therapeutic activity as well. Octreotide, a somatostatin analogue, inhibits hormone release and often relieves the symptoms of the associated clinical syndrome but usually has no effect on tumor mass.

B. Gastrinoma (Zollinger-Ellison syndrome). Approximately 60 percent of these tumors are malignant, 90 percent are multiple, and about 50 percent are associated with MEN syndromes.

   1. Diagnosis

      a. Symptoms include severe peptic ulcer disease refractory to medical management and, often, severe diarrhea.

      b. Laboratory studies

         (1) Upper GI contrast x-ray studies show severe ulceration and hypertrophic gastric folds.

         (2) Fasting serum gastrin level (normal value is less than 150 pg/ml) is usually elevated to more than 500 pg/ml. If gastrinoma is suspected but serum gastrin levels are not elevated, gastrin stimulation with calcium or secretin may be attempted. Calcium infusion (12 mg/kg of calcium gluconate over three hours) causes the gastrin level to more than double in patients with gastrinoma; the paradoxic increase in gastrin following secretin stimulation is used by some authorities to diagnose gastrinoma. Other causes of increased gastrin levels (atrophic gastritis, vagotomy, retained antrum after Billroth II gastrojejunostomy, and G-cell hyperplasia) must be differentiated from gastrinoma. Atrophic gastritis is differentiated by gastric acid studies.

         (3) Gastric secretory studies. After an overnight fast, a nasogastric tube is placed and four 15-minute aliquots are removed for analysis. Acid secretion of more than 10 mEq/hr along with a volume of more than 100 ml/hr suggest gastrinoma. These studies clearly distinguish gastrinoma from atrophic gastritis.

      c. Tumor location and extent. See sec. VI.A.1.

   2. Management

      a. Therapy with H_2-antihistamines, omeprazole, and liquid antacids controls symptoms in many patients.

      b. Surgery is necessary in cases refractory to medical therapy. Total gastrectomy is usually the procedure of choice to control peptic ulcer symptoms because of the multiplicity of tumors. Tumor excision may be possible in patients without hepatic metastases.

    c. Chemotherapy is used for metastatic disease (see sec. **VI.A.2.b**).

C. Insulinomas are most likely to occur between the ages of 40 and 60 years. Approximately 80 percent are benign, 10 percent are malignant, and 10 percent are multifocal; 80 percent are hormonally functional. Insulinomas are sometimes found in association with gastrinomas. A family history of diabetes mellitus is present in 25 percent of patients.

Insulinomas occur with equal frequency in the head, body, and tail of the pancreas; less than 1 percent develop outside the pancreas. Malignant tumors are more frequent in males. When malignant they metastasize to the liver primarily.

  1. Diagnosis. The differential diagnosis of hypoglycemia is discussed in Chap. 27, sec. **XII.A.**

    a. Symptoms. Fasting hypoglycemia, often alleviated by meals, is usually the presenting feature of insulinoma. Symptoms include diaphoresis, nervousness, palpitations, hunger pangs, anxiety, asthenia, confusion, weakness, seizures, and coma. Many patients have personality or other psychiatric changes noticed by the family. Weight gain is occasionally reported. Weight loss and liver failure may develop with metastases to the liver.

    b. Laboratory studies. Measurements of fasting blood glucose and insulin levels are the cornerstone for diagnosis of insulinoma.

      (1) Fasting hypoglycemia. An overnight fast is begun at 10:00 P.M. Blood glucose and insulin assays are obtained at 6:00 A.M., noon, 6:00 P.M., and midnight. An inappropriately elevated plasma insulin level (greater than 10 μU/ml) in the presence of hypoglycemia usually is diagnostic of insulinoma. A ratio of glucose (mg/dl) to insulin (μU/ml) of less than 2.5 is also strongly suggestive of insulinoma. If symptoms of hypoglycemia develop at any time, blood glucose and insulin levels should be measured; if the glucose concentration is less than 40 mg/dl, the test should be terminated by giving the patient food or a 50-ml IV bolus of 50% dextrose.

      (2) Other insulin assays. Proinsulin and C peptide are absent from commercial insulin preparations; their measurement by radioimmunoassay determines the role of exogenous insulin administration in the causation of hypoglycemia. In fasting patients, proinsulin levels are normally less than 20 percent of total insulin; a higher percentage of proinsulin is indicative of insulinoma.

    c. Tumor location and extent. See sec. **VI.A.1.**

  2. Management

    a. Surgery. Surgical removal of the tumor is the treatment of choice for insulinoma.

    b. RT as an adjuvant to surgery has not been shown to be helpful.

    c. Chemotherapy may be used for advanced disease (see sec. **VI.A.2.b**).

    d. Treatment of hypoglycemia

      (1) Diazoxide, 150 to 600 mg PO daily, is effective in managing hypoglycemic symptoms. The drug can induce hyperglycemia, hyperosmolar coma, or ketoacidosis; urine sugar and ketones should be monitored daily. A mild diuretic, such as hydrochlorothiazide, 50 mg b.i.d., should be given to counteract the sodium retention properties of diazoxide. Other complications of diazoxide therapy include cytopenias, lanugo hair growth, rashes, eosinophilia, and hyperuricemia.

      (2) Corticosteroids (prednisone, 40 mg/day, or hydrocortisone, 100 mg/day) may be given to patients who do not respond to diazoxide.

      (3) Patients with unresponsive hypoglycemia and unresectable insulinoma may be approached with several other, usually unsatisfactory alternatives, including: continuous IV infusion of 10% dextrose solutions through a Broviac or Hickman catheter, hepatic irradiation, or infusion of fluorouracil into the hepatic artery.

    (4) Subcutaneous injections of a long-acting somatostatin preparation (octreotide) can be used to inhibit insulin secretion and restore euglycemia.

D. Glucagonomas are usually malignant and usually will metastasize to the liver. The disease is suspected in patients who have diabetes mellitus that is moderately resistant to insulin and who have the following abnormalities:

  1. Diagnosis

    a. Symptoms and physical findings

      (1) Personality changes reported by family members

      (2) A peculiar erythematous migratory skin rash

      (3) Oral cavity ulcerations and sore tongue

      (4) Weight loss

    b. Laboratory studies

      (1) Anemia

      (2) Hyperglycemia

      (3) Hypercalcemia

      (4) Elevated fasting blood glucagon levels (normally less than 150 pg/ml)

    c. Tumor location and extent. See sec. **VI.A.1.**

  2. Management. See sec. **VI.A.2.**

E. Pancreatic cholera syndrome (VIPoma). These islet cell tumors are manifested by the release of VIP; 50 percent are malignant.

  1. Diagnosis

    a. Symptoms include severe watery diarrhea, muscle weakness due to hypokalemia, psychosis, and hypotension.

    b. Laboratory studies

      (1) Serum chemistries show hypokalemia and, often, hypercalcemia.

      (2) Gastric secretory studies show achlorhydria or hypochlorhydria.

      (3) Serum levels of VIP are elevated (normal is less than 70 pmol/ml).

    c. Tumor location and extent. See sec. **VI.A.1.**

  2. Management

    a. Surgery. Removal of solitary tumors controls manifestations of the pancreatic cholera syndrome, including hypercalcemia. Debulking of extensive tumor may palliate the diarrhea.

    b. Chemotherapy (see section **VI.A.2.b**) is useful for controlling symptoms in patients with metastatic tumor. Prednisone (80 mg/day PO) may reduce the diarrhea in some patients. Refractory diarrhea may respond to trifluoperazine (Stelazine), up to 38 mg/24 hr, or lithium carbonate, 300 mg PO q12h. A long-acting somatostatin preparation (octreotide) may lower VIP levels and reduce diarrhea.

F. Somatostatinoma. This exceptionally rare tumor produces diabetes mellitus, steatorrhea, diarrhea, gastric achlorhydria, and in many cases, gallstones. Liver metastases were present in two-thirds of reported cases. The disease is so uncommonly reported and has such obscure manifestations that no definite procedure for diagnosis has been established. Evaluation of diabetics for somatostatinoma is not worthwhile unless severe malabsorption is present. See sec. **VI.A** for diagnosis and treatment recommendations.

VII. Other endocrine cancers

A. Parathyroid carcinoma is extremely rare. Patients present with a neck mass and hypercalcemia. Tumor growth is slow and tends to involve the neck and upper mediastinum; widespread metastases are uncommon.

  1. Diagnosis

    a. Patients with parathyroid cancer usually have stigmata of hypercalcemia, including polyuria, polydipsia, constipation, mental status changes, bone disease, and hypercalciuria.

    b. High blood calcium levels are typical (15–16 mg/dl). Patients seem to tolerate these high levels relatively well, although hypercalcemic nephropathy and progressive bone disease ultimately complicate the course.

 c. The diagnosis is established by biopsy of obvious neck masses in patients with evidence of hyperparathyroidism.

 2. Management

  a. Surgery. Surgical extirpation of as much tumor as possible is necessary. Periodic repeated surgical debulking is warranted to try to control both the local effects of tumor and hypercalcemia.

  b. Hypercalcemia may be difficult to manage unless the tumor can be removed. Attempts should be made to normalize blood calcium levels; since this may be impossible, the alternative therapeutic goal is to reduce blood levels to the asymptomatic range. The management of patients with hypercalcemia is discussed in Chapter 27, sec. **I.** Chronic therapy with mithramycin (10–15 μg/kg every 4–5 days) may be necessary.

B. Pineal gland neoplasms are extremely rare and are usually found in boys and young men. Dysgerminoma is the most common tumor of the pineal gland, although gliomas, choriocarcinoma, and melanomas also occur. Most tumors are localized but spreading along the flow tract of CSF often occurs. See Chap. 14, sec. **VII** for diagnosis and management.

VIII. Metastases to endocrine organs

A. Adrenal gland metastases. The adrenal gland is frequently the site of metastatic tumors, particularly from lung cancer, breast cancer, and melanomas. Addison's disease, although rare, can develop with bilateral adrenal metastases.

 1. Diagnosis

  a. Symptoms and signs. Patients develop malaise, asthenia, weakness, decreased ability to taste salt, and salt craving. Hyperpigmentation of the skin and mucous membranes, particularly the gums, and orthostatic hypotension may occur.

  b. Laboratory findings include hyponatremia, hyperkalemia, and elevated blood urea nitrogen. Diagnosis is established by

   (1) Obtaining a baseline serum cortisol level that is low (<5 μg/dl), followed by:

   (2) Repeating the serum cortisol one hour after administering 0.25 mg of cosyntropin IV. Failure of the cortisol level to rise by at least 7 μg/dl to a peak value of at least 19–20 μg/dl is diagnostic of adrenal insufficiency.

 2. Management. Patients should be treated with hydrocortisone (30 mg daily) *and* fludrocortisone acetate (0.1 mg once or twice a day), *or* prednisone (5 mg daily) *and* fludrocortisone. The correct dose of fludrocortisone is determined by measuring orthostatic blood pressure changes and blood electrolyte levels. If the orthostatic drop in blood pressure is more than 10 mm Hg, the fludrocortisone is increased by 0.1-mg increments every few days until orthostasis is corrected. If the patient develops hypertension, hypokalemia, or alkalosis, the fludrocortisone dose is decreased.

B. Thyroid gland metastases. The thyroid gland is rarely involved with metastases and rarely the presenting site for metastatic tumors. Non-Hodgkin's lymphomas, Hodgkin's disease, and carcinomas of the breast, ovary, cervix, kidney, esophagus, colon, and lung have been reported to produce thyroid metastases. Diagnosis is established, if necessary, by needle biopsy of the thyroid masses. Therapy depends on the presence of local symptoms and the nature of the primary tumor.

C. Testicular metastases. Acute leukemia, melanoma, and carcinomas of the lung, prostate, bladder, and, occasionally, kidney can metastasize to the testes. A peritesticular mass, intratesticular mass, or a stony hard enlarged testis (particularly characteristic of leukemic infiltration) is found on physical examination. Biopsy is necessary to establish the diagnosis; a transinguinal approach is mandatory.

D. Ovarian metastases. Ovarian metastases may complicate melanomas and primary tumors of the breast, stomach, colon, lung, and, occasionally, other organs. Ovarian metastases are usually asymptomatic but occasionally are the presenting feature of the primary tumor. An ovarian mass is palpable on pelvic examination. Biopsy must be done to determine the diagnosis if no other sites of cancer are evident.

E. Pituitary metastases cannot be distinguished on clinical or biochemical grounds from pituitary adenomas. Patients with known cancers have approximately a 3 percent incidence of sellar or suprasellar metastases and a 1.5 percent incidence of pituitary adenomas. Radiologic discrimination is not possible. Primary cancers of the breast account for more than half of the cases; lung cancer accounts for 20 percent of cases; the remainder are caused by other carcinomas, melanomas, sarcomas, and leukemias. The triad of headache, extraocular nerve palsy, and diabetes insipidus is highly suggestive of sellar metastases whether or not the patient has a known cancer. Surgical exploration and decompression are essential unless precluded by progressive widespread metastases.

Selected Reading

Carcinoid and Islet Cell Tumors

Kvols, L. K., and Buck, M. Chemotherapy of endocrine malignancies: a review. *Semin. Oncol.* 14:343, 1987.

Kvols, L. K., et al. Evaluation of a radiolabeled somatostatin analog (I-123 octreotide) in the detection and localization of carcinoid and islet cell tumors. *Radiology* 187:129, 1993.

Moertel, C. G. An odyssey in the land of small tumors. *J. Clin. Oncol.* 5:1503, 1987.

Moertel, C. G., et al. The management of patients with advanced carcinoid tumors and islet cell carcinomas. *Ann. Intern. Med.* 120:302, 1994.

Rosch, T., et al. Localization of pancreatic endocrine tumors by endoscopic ultrasonography. *N. Engl. J. Med.* 326:1721, 1992.

Wynick, D., and Bloom, S. R. The use of the long-acting somatostatin analog octreotide in the treatment of gut neuroendocrine tumors. *J. Clin. Endocrinol. Metab.* 73:1, 1991.

Thyroid Cancer

Brennan, M. D., et al. Follicular thyroid cancer treated at the Mayo Clinic, 1946 through 1970: initial manifestations, pathologic findings, therapy and outcome. *Mayo Clin. Proc.* 66:11, 1991.

DeGroot, L. J., et al. Natural history, treatment, and course of papillary thyroid carcinoma. *J. Clin. Endocrinol. Metab.* 71:414, 1990.

Fagin, J. A. Molecular defects in thyroid gland neoplasia. *J. Clin. Endocrinol. Metab.* 75:1398, 1992.

Gagel, R. F., et al. Medullary thyroid carcinoma: recent progress. *J. Clin. Endocrinol. Metab.* 76:809, 1993.

Mazzaferri, E. L. Mananagement of a solitary thyroid nodule. *N. Engl. J. Med.* 328:553, 1993.

Nel, C. J. C., et al. Anaplastic carcinoma of the thyroid: a clinicopathologic study of 82 cases. *Mayo Clin. Proc.* 60:51, 1985.

Oertel, J. E., and Heffess, C. S. Lymphoma of the thyroid and related disorders. *Semin. Oncol.* 14:333, 1987.

Samaan, N. A., et al. Treatment modalities of well differentiated thyroid carcinoma. *J. Clin. Endocrinol. Metab.* 75:714, 1992.

Pheochromocytoma

Averbuch, S. D., et al. Malignant pheochromocytoma: effective treatment with a combination of cyclophosphamide, vincristine and dacarbazine. *Ann. Intern. Med.* 109:267, 1988.

Benowitz, N. L. Pheochromocytoma. *Adv. Intern. Med.* 35:195, 1990.

Hanson, M. W., et al. Iodine 131-labeled metaiodobenzylguanidine scintigraphy and biochemical analyses in suspected pheochromocytoma. *Arch. Intern. Med.* 151:1397, 1991.

Adrenal Carcinoma

Icard, P., et al. Adrenocortical carcinoma in surgically treated patients: a retrospective study on 156 cases by the French Association of Endocrine Surgery. *Surgery* 112:972, 1992.

Pommier, R. F., and Brennan, M. F. Management of adrenal neoplasms. *Curr. Probl. Surg.* 28:659, 1991.

Parathyroid Carcinoma

Wynne, A. G., et al. Parathyroid carcinoma: clinical and pathologic features in 43 patients. *Medicine* 71:197, 1992.

Pituitary Metastases

Branch, C. L., Jr., and Laws, E. R., Jr. Metastatic tumors of the sella turcica masquerading as primary pituitary tumors. *J. Clin. Endocrin. Metab.* 65:469, 1987.

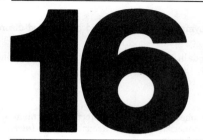

Skin Cancers

Richard F. Wagner, Jr., and
Dennis A. Casciato

Basal Cell and Squamous Cell Carcinomas

I. **Epidemiology and etiology**
   A. **Incidence.** At least 700,000 new cases of cutaneous basal cell carcinoma (BCC) or squamous cell carcinoma (SCC) are diagnosed annually in the United States. Men are more frequently affected than women. Although the most common of all malignancies, they account for less than 0.1 percent of patient deaths due to cancer.
   B. **Risk factors**
      1. **Actinic (sun) damage** appears to be a major carcinogenic factor. Ninety percent of these cancers develop in sun-exposed areas of the body. The incidence in white populations rises dramatically near the equator and is greater at higher altitudes than at sea level. Blue-eyed, fair-skinned, blond or red-haired persons, and those who are easily sunburned are at increased risk. The incidence in blacks is much lower than in whites.
      2. **Other carcinogens**
         a. **Arsenic.** Arsenical exposure predisposes to the development of Bowen's disease, multiple BCC, and SCC, and is also associated with a higher incidence of intestinal carcinoma. Hard, yellowish hyperkeratotic plaques on the palms and soles provide a clue that the individual was exposed to arsenic.
         b. **Irradiation** given for benign conditions (such as acne or hirsutism) or resulting from occupational exposure is associated with up to a 20 percent risk for skin cancer. The tumor develops many years after the initial exposure; latent periods may extend up to 50 years. About two-thirds of these cancers are BCC and one-third are SCC. Radiation-associated SCC tends to be aggressive and has a 10 percent mortality.
         c. **Coal tar and quinacrine exposures** appear to be risk factors for SCC.
         d. **Immunosuppression,** such as with renal transplantation, predisposes patients to an increased incidence of cutaneous SCC. Cyclosporin A is associated with cutaneous SCC and lymphoma.
      3. **Chronic inflammation and trauma**
         a. **Chronic draining osteomyelitis** predisposes to the development of SCC. The local tumor is usually evident but may first be manifested by metastases to a draining lymph node.
         b. **Fistulae, stasis dermatitis, and areas of irritative leukoplakia** can also give rise to skin cancers.
         c. **Thermal or electrical burns and chronic heat exposure** are associated with increased risk of high-grade, aggressive SCC. Certain ethnic groups are burned from hot coals used as bed or clothing warmers.
         d. **Atrophic skin lesions** of discoid lupus or epidermolysis bullosa give rise to SCC.
      4. **Hereditary factors**
         a. **Xeroderma pigmentosum** is an autosomal recessive disease with one

or more defects in DNA repair enzymes. Patients sunburn and freckle easily. Young children with xeroderma pigmentosum are at high risk for development of BCC, SCC, or malignant melanoma before their teenage years. Disturbances in speech, mentation, and convulsive disorders may also be present. A severe form (De Sanctis-Cacchione syndrome) comprises microcephaly, mental deficiency, dwarfism, and failure of gonadal development.

  b. Basal cell nevus syndrome appears to be inherited as autosomal dominant. Multiple BCC lesions appear over the face, arms, and trunk during the late teenage years. A large variety of associated lesions can occur and include: jaw cysts, palmar pits, bifid ribs, kyphoscoliosis, spina bifida, short metacarpals, and hyporesponsiveness to parathyroid hormone. Patients with this syndrome also appear to be at increased risk for medulloblastoma and ovarian fibroma.

5. **Infection**
  a. Epidermodysplasia verruciformis is primarily caused by human papillomaviruses (HPV) types 5 and 8 and results in in situ and invasive SCC synergistically with other carcinogens such as sunlight.
  b. SCCs of the genitals and anal regions are strongly associated with HPV types 16 and 18. Infection, usually through sexual transmission, increases the risk of regional SCC.
  c. Periungual SCC is associated with HPV type 16.
6. **Oncogene** (Ha-*ras*, Ki-*ras*, N-*ras*, c-*myc*) mutation and amplication, as well as anti-oncogene p53 mutations, have been reported for BCC and SCC.

II. Pathology and natural history
  A. SCC nearly always arises in skin that is visibly damaged. Lesions most commonly are ulcerative but may be exophytic.
  1. **Aggressive squamous cell cancers** are unlikely to arise from actinic keratosis or actinic skin damage. The lower extremities are frequently involved and may have to be amputated to effect cure. Aggressive SCC also develops from burn scars, radiation dermatitis, erythroplasia of Queyrat (see Chap. 13, *Penile Cancer*, sec. **II.A**), and Bowen's disease.
  2. **Bowen's disease** consists of small eczematoid plaques. By histology, the plaques demonstrate intraepithelial carcinoma in situ. Invasion may occur, so treatment is necessary. Although historically suspected, Bowen's disease is not associated with an increased risk of internal cancer.
  3. **Bowenoid papulosis** is characterized by multiple genital papules that are histologically indistinguishable from Bowen's disease. They are usually caused by HPV type 16 and when present on the female patient or her sexual partner may indicate increased risk for cervical carcinoma.
  4. **Metastases.** Tumors that metastasize are usually poorly differentiated. The incidence of metastasis is less than 3 percent for actinically induced SCC and 35 percent for nonactinically induced SCC. The draining lymph nodes are the most frequent sites of metastases, although distant organs are eventually involved.
  B. BCC is the most common type of skin cancer. It has several recognized subtypes.
  1. **Nodular-ulcerated BCC,** the most common type, usually appears on the face as a waxy papule with pearly or waxy borders. Some lesions are pigmented and clinically indistinguishable from melanoma. They spread both over the surface and deeply into the tissues to invade cartilage and bone. Ulceration is common ("rodent ulcer"). Inadequately treated BCC can result in severely deforming facial ulcerations and death through invasion of the vital structures of the head and neck. Distant metastases from BCC are extremely rare.
  2. **Superficial BCC** lesions usually arise on the trunk, are often multiple, and appear as red scaly patches with areas of brown or black pigmentation. They spread over the skin surface and may have areas of nodularity.
  3. **Sclerosing BCC** usually affects the face. The tumors closely resemble scars and may have an ivory-colored and ill-defined border. Histologically, the

cancer cells are surrounded by a dense bed of fibrosis ("morphealike"). Considering all types of BCC, they have the highest recurrence rate following treatment.

4. Cystic BCC is uncommon. The tumor undergoes central degeneration to form a cystic lesion.

III. Diagnosis. Skin biopsy is necessary to confirm the clinical suspicion of skin cancer. A shave or curette biopsy is usually adequate to diagnose BCC or SCC. If the first biopsy is negative and the tumor is still suspected, a deeper biopsy is necessary.

IV. Staging system and prognostic factors

A. The TNM system for classification of cutaneous carcinomas is shown in Table 16-1. The histopathologic grades for cutaneous carcinomas are as follows:

GX   Grade cannot be assessed
G1   Well differentiated
G2   Moderately differentiated
G3   Poorly differentiated
G4   Undifferentiated

B. BBC does not ordinarily require staging due to the rarity of metastases. However, the clinician should record the diameter and location of the lesion, and whether the tumor is primary or recurrent. The prognosis for BCC is worsened if the tumor is morpheaform, recurrent, greater than 2 cm in diameter, has poorly defined clinical borders, or is located in areas associated with high recurrence rates (see sec. **VI.B.2.a**).

C. Cutaneous SCC is clinically staged based on clinical examination of the lesion and regional lymph glands. No other metastatic workup is indicated. The prognosis for SCC is worsened if the tumor is recurrent, arises in a scar, occurs in immunocompromised patients, is greater than 4 mm thick or greater than 2 cm in diameter, is poorly differentiated, has perineural invasion, or appears in high recurrence areas (see sec. **VI.B.2.a**). Metastases to regional lymph nodes portend increased morbidity and mortality; visceral metastases are lethal.

V. Prevention. "Primary prevention" is largely achieved by encouraging patients and other responsible parties to minimize sunlight exposure and other reducible risk factors. Sunscreens (sun protective factor 15 or greater), and protective clothing,

Table 16-1. TNM classification of cutaneous carcinomas and melanomas

		Carcinomas[1]	Malignant melanomas[2]
Primary tumor			
TX		Primary tumor cannot be assessed	Primary tumor cannot be assessed
T0		No evidence of primary tumor	No evidence of primary tumor
Tis, pTis		Carcinoma in situ	Melanoma in situ (level I)
T1, pT1		≤2 cm in greatest dimension	≤0.75 mm thickness and level II
T2, pT2		2–5 cm	>0.75–1.5 mm thickness and/or level III
T3, pT3		>5 cm	>1.5–4.0 mm thickness and/or level IV
	pT3a	N/A	>1.5–3.0 mm thickness
	pT3b	N/A	>3.0–4.0 mm thickness
T4, pT4		Invades deep extradermal structures (i.e., cartilage, bone, skeletal muscle)	>4.0 mm thickness, level V, and/or satellite within 2 cm of primary tumor
	pT4a	N/A	>4.0 mm thickness and/or level V
	pT4b	N/A	Satellite within 2 cm of primary tumor

Table 16-1 (continued)

	Carcinomas[1]			Malignant melanomas[2]		
Regional lymph nodes						
NX	Regional lymph nodes cannot be assessed			Regional lymph nodes cannot be assessed		
N0	No regional lymph node metastasis			No regional lymph node metastasis		
N1	Regional lymph node metastasis			Metastasis ≤3 cm in greatest dimension in any regional node		
N2a	N/A			Metastasis >3 cm in any regional lymph node		
N2b	N/A			In-transit metastasis involving the skin or subcutaneous tissue more than 2 cm from the primary tumor but not beyond the regional lymph nodes		
N2c	N/A			Both N2a and N2b		
Distant metastasis						
MX	Presence of distant metastasis cannot be assessed			Presence of distant metastasis cannot be assessed		
M0	No distant metastasis			No distant metastasis		
M1	Distant metastasis present			Distant metastasis present		
M1a	N/A			Metastasis in skin or subcutaneous tissue or lymph nodes(s) beyond regional lymph nodes		
M1b	N/A			Visceral metastasis		
Stage grouping						
0	Tis	N0	M0	pTis	N0	M0
I	T1	N0	M0	pT1	N0	M0
				pT2	N0	M0
II	T2	N0	M0	pT3	N0	M0
	T3	N0	M0			
III	T4	N0	M0	pT4	N0	M0
	Any T	N1	M0	Any pT	N1	M0
				Any pT	N2	M0
IV	Any T	any N	M1	Any pT	any N	M1

[1]Excludes the eyelid, lip, vulva, and penis. In the case of multiple simultaneous tumors, the tumor with the highest T category is classified and the number of separate tumors indicated in parentheses, for example, T2(5).

[2]The extent of the primary tumor is classified after excision (pT classification). In case of discrepancy between tumor thickness and level, the pT category is based on the less favorable finding.

Key: N/A = not applicable.

Source: Adapted from Hermanek, P. and Sabin, L. H. (eds.). UICC: TNM Classification of Malignant Tumours, (4th ed., 2nd rev.). Berlin: Springer-Verlag, 1992.

including hats, are helpful. Skin erythema from solar exposure, even from ultraviolet light on cloudy days, represents skin damage that is cumulative over the years. The "healthy tan" represents the body's reaction to skin damage and freckling should be recognized as an early sign of skin injury. "Secondary prevention" is provided by lesional treatment.

VI. Management

A. Actinic keratoses may become SCC (1% risk). Lesions may be treated by liquid nitrogen or by curettage with electrical cautery of the base. The use of topical applications of fluorouracil or masoprocol can be successful in a highly motivated patient.

B. BCC and SCC are treated by several techniques, which have various cure rates.

1. **Traditional surgical resection** requires a surgical margin of 4 to 6 mm for primary tumors less than 2 cm in diameter (more margin for bigger primary tumors, tumors in high-risk areas, or recurrent tumors). Lack of complete visualization of tumor margins due to sampling error may result in tumor recurrence.

2. **Mohs' micrographic surgery** has the highest cure rates, maximally spares uninvolved tissue, and is less costly than RT or traditional excision surgery with frozen section control. With this method the tumor is microscopically mapped after it is excised. Mohs' surgery is indicated for

   a. **Primary BCC or SCC** with the following characteristics:

      (1) Located in regions at high risk for tumor recurrence (i.e., the periorbital area, nasolabial fold, nose-cheek angle, posterior ear sulcus, pinna, ear canal, nose, forehead, and scar tissue) *or*

      (2) Located in regions where tissue conservation is mandated *or*

      (3) Poorly defined clinical borders *or*

      (4) Diameter greater than 2 cm *or*

      (5) Perineural invasion *or*

      (6) Morpheaform, sclerotic, infiltrating, or basosquamous histopathologic features

   b. **Recurrent BCC or SCC.** Of all therapeutic modalities for recurrent tumors, Mohs' surgery has the greatest success rate (95%) and should ordinarily be considered the preferred treatment.

3. **Curettage** of the tumor with electrodesiccation of the apparently normal base to an additional depth of 3 or 4 mm is particularly useful for superficial BCC of the trunk or Bowen's disease.

4. **Cryosurgery** using liquid nitrogen to freeze the tumor to $-40°C$ should be considered for patients who refuse surgery or are poor surgical candidates. A probe to monitor freezing must be used for all tumors with the possible exception of superficial BCC. Cryosurgery is contraindicated for sclerosing BCC and cold-induced diseases.

5. **RT** has the same indications as cryosurgery. It is relatively contraindicated for patients with xeroderma pigmentosa, epidermodysplasia verruciformis, or the basal cell nevus syndrome because RT may induce more tumors in the treated field. RT may have adjuvant use for unusually aggressive SCC and is used with or without surgery, when metastasis involves regional lymph glands.

6. **Large, deeply eroding tumors** can partially or totally destroy the face. These far-advanced cancers often cannot be cured. CT or MRI scans are useful for determining the extent of disease due to local invasion. Often extensive reconstructive surgery is necessary following a surgical intervention. In the most severe cases, the patient may elect to wear a prosthesis.

7. **Chemotherapy.** Chemotherapy has no adjuvant use for BCC or SCC. Experience in treating metastatic skin cancers is extremely limited. Fluorouracil, cisplatin, methotrexate, bleomycin, retinoids, and cyclophosphamide given singly and in combination have produced temporary tumor regression. Excellent response rates have been reported for advanced cases of SCC and BCC treated with cisplatin in combination with either a five-day infusion of 5-FU (dosages similar to those used for head and neck cancers) or doxorubicin.

Malignant Melanoma

I. Epidemiology and etiology
A. Incidence
1. **Geography.** Approximately 32,000 new cases of melanoma are diagnosed in the United States annually and the incidence continues to rise.
2. **Sex.** The risk of developing melanoma is the same for men and women. Men are more likely to develop melanoma on the trunk, and women are more likely to develop lesions on the lower extremities.
3. **Age.** Melanoma is rare in young children. The incidence begins to rise with puberty, increases until the age of 65 to 70 years, and then decreases.
4. **Race.** The incidence of melanoma is low in people of color.
5. **Multiplicity.** About 5 percent of patients with a primary cutaneous melanoma have or will develop another primary melanoma or multiple primary melanomas.

B. Risk factors
1. **Sun exposure** appears to increase the risk of cutaneous and ocular melanoma.
2. **Hereditary factors.** Approximately 10 percent of melanomas occur in family clusters.
   a. **"Melanoma families"** appear to have a dominant mode of inheritance with incomplete penetrance. Ocular or cutaneous melanoma occurs in several members of these families. Members of melanoma families who get melanoma do so at a younger age and have a higher incidence of multiple primary tumors compared to sporadic melanomas.
   b. **Atypical mole syndrome (AMS) or dysplastic nevus syndrome (DNS)** is a recently described clinical syndrome of acquired atypical-appearing nevi that are associated with melanoma. Inheritance appears to be autosomal dominant with incomplete expression and penetrance.
3. **Nevi**
   a. Approximately 70 percent of patients with melanoma have had a preexisting nevus at the primary tumor site. Congenital nevi may engender increased risk for melanoma. Giant congenital nevi have an extremely high incidence of malignant transformation. Where feasible, removal is advised.
   b. White men have 20 to 40 moles by the third decade of life. Nevi continue to form throughout adult life. However, only one mole out of 500,000 becomes malignant.
4. **Other melanoma risk factors** include chemical exposure, physical agents (i.e., nonsolar ultraviolet radiation, ionizing radiation, trauma, burns), immunosuppression, and profession.
5. **Oncogene** mutations (N-*ras,* Ha-*ras,* Ki-*ras*) and amplications (N-*ras,* Ha-*ras*), as well as p53 anti-oncogene mutation, have been described.

II. Pathology and natural history
A. Melanocytes
are believed to migrate from the embryonic neural crest to the dermal-epidermal junction of the skin. The number of melanocytes per unit of skin surface appears to be the same for all races, even albinos. Pigmentary differences between races are dependent on how the melanin is "packaged" in each cell.

B. Histopathologic types of melanoma
1. **Superficial spreading melanoma,** or radial spreading melanoma (70% of melanomas), is more common in women and is most frequently located on the back. The lesion is a pigmented macule or a barely palpable plaque with variegated colors (black, tan, red, brown, or white). Irregularity of the margins, especially the presence of a notch, is a very suspicious feature. These tumors mostly manifest radial growth but eventually enter a vertical growth phase.
2. **Nodular melanoma** (15% of melanomas) occurs more frequently in men.

Most of these lesions are jet-black or dark-blue with a distinct border. Occasionally, no pigment is present and electron microscopy or special tissue stains are needed to determine the diagnosis. These tumors grow rapidly and vertically from the onset.

   3. Lentigo maligna melanoma (10–15% of melanomas) has no sexual predilection. The lesion appears as a large, flat, tan-to-black macule of up to 4 cm in diameter, developing in sun-exposed areas of older, light-skinned persons, most commonly on the face and neck. The in situ lentigo maligna lesion (or "Hutchinson's freckle") shows a horizontal growth phase for up to 20 years and eventually a vertical growth phase anywhere in the involved area. The vertical phase resembles superficial spreading melanoma rather than nodular melanoma.

   4. Acral lentiginous melanoma is melanoma involving the palms, fingers, soles, and toes.

   5. Unclassified and rare desmoplastic variants also exist.

C. Natural history

   1. Mode of spread. Most cutaneous melanomas are believed to arise near the basal lamina.

      a. Radial growth. The superficial spreading and lentigo maligna melanomas grow horizontally along the lamina (radial growth phase) before penetrating the deep skin structures (vertical growth phase). The radial phase may last as long as 20 years in lentigo maligna and five years in superficial spreading melanoma.

      b. Vertical growth. Nodular melanomas have a vertical growth phase from the outset. The vertical phase is associated with invasion of dermal blood and lymphatic vessels.

      c. Lymphatics. Local lymphatic spread results in satellite nodules of melanoma appearing near the site of the primary tumor ("satellitosis"). Draining lymph nodes are frequently involved once the vertical growth phase develops.

      d. Distant metastases. Metastatic melanomas can involve any organ in the body, including the placenta and fetus. Approximately 5 percent of patients with melanoma present with symptoms of distant metastases without an apparent primary site.

   2. Unusual primary sites of melanoma

      a. Melanomas can occur on the soles of feet and under fingernails, especially of the thumbs and large toes. These sites are more likely to be affected in people of color.

      b. Ocular melanoma can develop in the choroid, ciliary body, or uvea. Melanomas occurring in the eye itself have been divided into a variety of histologic subtypes, which have different prognoses. These tumors have a peculiar tendency of metastasizing to the liver, sometimes many years after diagnosis of the primary site, giving rise to the "syndrome" of hepatomegaly, unilateral scleral icterus, and a prosthetic glass eye.

      c. Melanomas may rarely arise in the palate or gingiva, usually in a site where increased pigmentation was previously noted.

      d. The anus and vulva are also potential sites for development of melanoma; 5 percent of melanomas in women occur on the vulva and 5 to 10 percent of vulvar cancers are melanomas, even though the vulva accounts for less than 2 percent of the body surface area.

      e. Internal sites with a melanocyte population, such as the foregut or CNS, may rarely be the site of a primary melanoma.

   3. Metastatic melanoma from unknown primary site accounts for 4 to 5 percent of all cases. To further complicate the problems of diagnosis and management, a melanotic melanoma may be mistaken for undifferentiated carcinoma. Patients usually have lymphatic metastases, but any organ may be involved. The occult primary site may have disappeared spontaneously or may have been excised or cauterized years before the appearance of the metastasis. The prognosis for these patients depends on the stage of disease and appears to be the same as for patients with clinically evident primary sites. This important clinical problem is discussed further in Chap. 20.

  4. Paraneoplastic syndromes associated with melanoma have a wide scope and include vitiligo, dermatomyositis, melanosis, gynecomastia, ectopic Cushing's syndrome, and neurologic abnormalities.

III. Diagnosis

A. Symptoms

1. **Change in a preexisting pigmented lesion** is the first sign of melanoma in 70 percent of patients. The lesion becomes lighter, darker, or variegated in color, increases in size, or may be associated with an itching sensation. Ulceration or bleeding usually represents advanced disease.

2. **De novo melanomas,** not associated with previously observed skin lesions, occur in about 30 percent of patients.

3. **Symptoms of distant metastases** depend on the anatomic site involved.

B. Physical examination.
Patients should be viewed completely for skin lesions. Special attention is given to areas not usually inspected, such as axillae, scalp, interdigital webs, mouth, genitals, and anal and oral regions. Paplation may reveal lymph node enlargement or organomegaly.

C. Differential diagnosis

1. **Pigmented skin lesions.** There are many pigmented skin lesions to consider in the differential diagnosis of melanoma. Common dark skin lesions include atypical mole, pigmented basal cell carcinomas, seborrheic keratoses, and sclerosing hemangiomas. It is often difficult to clinically distinguish early melanoma from a benign lesion.

2. **Signs that suggest melanoma** are variegated color and irregular borders. The presence of hair in the lesion does not assist in the differentiation of a benign lesion from melanoma. Specific findings that may indicate melanoma include:

   a. Changes in size, color, sensation, or surface characteristics of a preexisting nevus

   b. Lesions with variegated color (shades of brown, black, red, white, or blue)

   c. Lesions that contain bluish coloration even if not variegated

   d. Lesions with angular indentations or notches

   e. Other signs of possible malignancy are

      (1) Lesions that do not contain skin creases

      (2) Lesions that ulcerate or bleed

D. Laboratory studies

1. **Biopsy** of the lesions is the first diagnostic procedure to be undertaken. Suspected melanoma should not be observed for further signs. An excisional biopsy may be desirable based on size and location. An incisional biopsy may be performed when an excisional biopsy is not desired. There is no reliable evidence that incisional biopsies for melanoma result in increased morbidity or mortality.

2. **Patients with many small atypical nevi** (AMS, DNS). Several nevi should be excised and examined microscopically. Baseline total-body photographs are recommended. Significantly changed lesions should prompt excision. Monthly skin self-examination is recommended for the purpose of monitoring the atypical moles for malignant changes with interim physician examination as indicated. Lifetime physician follow-up is recommended for early melanoma diagnosis.

3. **S100 Protein** is a cytoplasmic protein that is present in malignant melanoma. The detection of this protein may help distinguish poorly differentiated amelanotic malignant melanoma from tumors of obscure histologic origin.

IV. Staging system and prognostic factors

A. Staging systems.
Several systems are in common use. The TNM classification, which integrates Clark's levels and the Breslow system, and stage groupings are shown in Table 16-1.

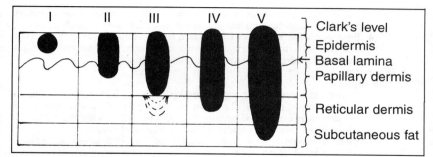

Fig. 16-1. Clark's levels of invasion for malignant melanoma.

1. **Clark's levels** by depth or invasion into the skin (Fig. 16-1).

Level	Tumor extent	Five-year survival (%)
I	Tumor is confined to epidermis (in situ)	100
II	Tumor extends beyond basal lamina into papillary dermis	85
III	Tumor extends into papillary dermis and abuts onto, but does not invade, the reticular dermis	65
IV	Tumor extends into reticular dermis	50
V	Tumor extends into subcutaneous fat	15

2. **Breslow system** by depth of tumor invasion from the basal lamina (measured with an ocular micrometer). Tumors with less than 0.85 mm of invasion have a very low metastatic potential.

Depth of tumor invasion	Five-year survival (%)
<0.5 mm	99
>3 mm	30

3. **Survival according to regional lymph node involvement**

Node involvement	Five-year survival (%)
Negative nodes	75
1–3 positive nodes	50
4 or more positive nodes	25

4. **Survival according to metastatic spread**

Stage	Extent	Five-year survival (%)
I	Primary cancer only	70
II	Local recurrence within 3 cm of primary site	30
III	Satellitosis and/or metastases to regional lymph nodes	<20
IV	Distant metastases	<10

B. **Recommended staging evaluation**
   1. Breslow or Clark's levels should be determined in all instances when a primary tumor is identified.
   2. Regional lymph nodes should be palpated and any suspicious finding should be biopsied. Lymph nodes containing melanoma require treatment.
   3. For melanomas thicker than 0.85 mm, LDH and chest x-ray films should be followed periodically. Radionuclide, CT, or MRI scans are performed if clinical or laboratory evidence suggests that specific organs are involved.

C. **Prognostic factors**
   1. Depth of invasion, presence of positive lymph nodes, or presence of distant metastases affects prognosis (see A).
   2. Women have a better prognosis than men when matched by age and stage of disease.

V. Prevention. "Primary prevention" of melanoma involves the avoidance of sun and other reducible risk factors. "Secondary prevention" depends on careful physical examination and biopsy of all suspicious skin lesions.

VI. Management

A. Surgery

   1. Management of the primary tumor

   a. Cutaneous melanoma. Local excision of early melanoma is the only proven method of curative therapy. The extent of tumor-free margins that is necessary remains controversial. However, in situ lesions are now treated with a 5-mm surgical margin, and thin melanomas (<.85 mm) only require a 1-cm surgical margin. Mohs' micrographic surgery should be considered for facial melanoma and other areas where tissue conservation is desired because of its equivalent cure rate. Tumor margin is often influenced by site. Large defects may require skin grafting or skin flaps.

   b. Historically, **choroidal melanomas of the eye** were treated by enucleation. Small tumors have been successfully treated with high-dose irradiation and local surgical measures; this treatment avoids removal of the eye.

   2. Management of lymph nodes. Prophylactic resection of clinically uninvolved draining lymph nodes for intermediate thickness stage I disease is controversial because it may not affect survival. Palpable nodes should be excised, however, because local growth of melanoma-involved nodes is disabling.

   3. Management of metastases. Highly selected patients may benefit from resection of metastases, particularly if they are solitary and completely excised.

   a. Solitary brain metastases. The brain is the third most frequent site for metastases. Operable solitary metastases may be excised, but prolonged survival is rare.

   b. Gastrointestinal problems. Melanoma has a tendency to metastasize to the gastrointestinal tract where it may cause bleeding, intussusception, or obstruction. Endoscopy should be an early study done on patients who have upper gastrointestinal tract bleeding. The characteristic "bull's eye" appearance on contrast studies of small bowel lesions is highly suggestive of melanoma. Patients with obstruction or uncontrolled bleeding from an apparently isolated intestinal lesion may temporarily benefit from resection of the tumor.

   c. Pulmonary metastases from melanoma are rarely beneficially resected, even if they appear to be solitary.

B. RT is occasionally useful as a primary or adjuvant modality for treating melanoma patients who are debilitated or who refuse surgery.

C. Systemic therapy. Caution must be used when interpreting responses of metastatic melanoma to systemic therapies of any kind, because melanoma is a capricious neoplasm that is associated with spontaneous regressions. Responses may be temporally but not causally related to treatment.

   1. Adjuvant therapy. The use of chemotherapy as an adjuvant to surgery has not been shown to improve survival.

   2. Limb perfusion. Patients with melanoma of the extremity and "in-transit" or "satellite" cutaneous metastases may be treated by limb perfusion with cytotoxic agents. The arterial and venous blood supplies of the involved extremity are isolated, and heated solutions of melphalan, dacarbazine, or other drugs are injected. Limb perfusion permits the administration of high doses of drugs while minimizing drug toxicity. Local tumor response rates are reported to be as high as 80 percent, but whether survival rate is affected is unclear.

   3. Cytotoxic agents. Patients with distant metastases can be treated with cytotoxic agents. Dacarbazine is the drug of choice. Response rates are 20 percent for skin and lymph node metastases but less than 5 percent for visceral metastases. The combination of a vinca alkaloid with either dacarbazine and cisplatin or procarbazine and lomustine appears to improve the response rate to 30 to 40 percent.

4. **Hormonal agents.** In women only, both response rate and survival are better for patients treated with tamoxifen and dacarbazine than with dacarbazine alone. Estrogen receptor activity on tumor cells may be a marker for a biologically more indolent form of melanoma.

5. **Immunotherapy.** The use of Bacillus Calmette-Guérin (BCG) or other immunotherapies does not affect survival of patients with malignant melanoma.

   a. **Satellite lesions** injected with BCG may regress in 40 percent of injected patients. This treatment can leave chronic, draining BCG infections or scabs on the skin, result in disseminated BCG infection (e.g., granulomatous hepatitis) that requires therapy with isoniazid, and produce a shocklike syndrome.

   b. **IL-2,** with or without lymphokine-activated killer cells, is associated with response rates of about 25 percent at the expense of high cost and considerable toxicity. Only a small proportion of patients achieve a durable remission.

   c. **α_2-IFN** therapy has response rates of less than 10 percent.

   d. **Tumor cell vaccines and gene therapies** are investigational.

VII. Special clinical problems associated with malignant melanoma

A. **Cardiac metastases** frequently occur with melanoma and can occasionally result in arrhythmia or cardiac rupture. Antemortem diagnosis is difficult in the absence of malignant pericardial effusion. Patients should be treated with appropriate antiarrhythmic agents. RT to the heart is probably of little benefit.

B. **Breast metastases.** Poorly differentiated or undifferentiated melanoma metastatic to breast can be confused with primary breast cancer.

C. **Slate-gray skin discoloration** (melanosis syndrome) results from widespread melanoma, which causes high blood and urinary melanogens. Affected patients often have urine that is dark or darkens on exposure to air.

D. **Black sputum,** similar to that seen in coal miners, may occur in patients who have pulmonary melanoma lesions that have eroded into the airways.

Kaposi's Sarcoma

I. **Epidemiology.** Historically Kaposi's sarcoma (KS) was a rare cutaneous tumor that mostly affects black southern African children and elderly whites. The occurrence of the malignancy in the United States has now been well described as part of the acquired immunodeficiency syndrome (AIDS) (see Chaps. 36 and 37).

A. **Older patients** with KS are usually over the age of 65 years and most have ancestry from the Mediterranean region. Lesions tend to be multifocal on the lower extremities and occasionally involve the hands, ears, and nose. The disease affects men 10 to 15 times more frequently than women and is relatively indolent.

B. **Black children** with KS in southern Africa tend to have tumors that involve the lymph nodes. This form of KS is generalized and aggressive.

C. **Patients with AIDS,** particularly homosexual men in the third or fourth decades of life, develop a widely disseminated, aggressive, and usually fatal form of the disease. Generalized cutaneous involvement, generalized lymphadenopathy, and visceral or gastrointestinal involvement are typical.

D. **Renal transplant recipients and Eskimos** also are more likely to have KS.

II. **Pathology and natural history.** This spindle cell tumor appears to originate in the dermis; the cell of origin is controversial. The tumor has vascular channels with variable fibrotic and lymphocytic components. The classic disease has a protracted indolent course, predominantly cutaneous manifestations, and expected survival of more than 15 years. Metastases may occur, but the rate of spread is variable. In African children and in AIDS patients the median survival appears to be less than five years.

III. **Diagnosis**
   A. **Signs.** KS typically presents as purplish blotches or nodules on the feet, which resemble venous stasis. However, because of the pleomorphic nature of this disease and of opportunistic infections in AIDS patients, any new skin lesion in this population should be investigated. Other skin sites, mucosa, or visceral organs may be involved. The lesions may be painful or pruritic. Tumor nodules may regress if thrombosis occurs. Edema is associated with involvement of the deep lymphatic system and veins.
   B. **Biopsy** of masses, or of what appear to be chronic, progressive venous stasis ulcers, reveals the diagnosis. Lymph node biopsy is necessary for evaluating the African form of the disease.
   C. **Staging.** No system is in widespread use, and no specific staging evaluation is universally accepted.
IV. **Management**
   A. **Surgery.** Surgical resection is used for localized nodular disease.
   B. **RT** is useful for local disease. KS is very radiosensitive.
   C. **Chemotherapy** is inconsistently effective. Vinblastine appears to be the most active agent. Responses are also reported for nitrosoureas, actinomycin D, and bleomycin. Response rates and effects on survival are unknown. The treatment of KS in AIDS is discussed in Chapter 36.

Selected Reading

Basal Cell and Squamous Cell Carcinomas

Kaspar, T. A., et al. Prognosis and treatment of advanced squamous cell carcinoma secondary to epidermodysplasia verruciformis: a worldwide analysis of 11 patients. *J. Dermatol. Surg. Oncol.* 17:237, 1991.

Miller, P. K., et al. Cutaneous micrographic surgery: Mohs' procedure. *Mayo Clin. Proc.* 67:971, 1992.

Rowe, D. E., Carroll, R. J., and Day, Jr., C. L. Long-term recurrence rates in previously untreated (primary) basal cell carcinoma. *J. Dermatol. Surg. Oncol.* 15:315, 1989.

Rowe, D. E., Carroll, R. J., and Day, Jr., C. L. Mohs' surgery is the treatment of choice for recurrent (previously treated) basal cell carcinoma. *J. Dermatol. Surg. Oncol.* 15:424, 1989.

Rowe, D. E., Carroll, R. J., and Day, Jr., C. L. Prognostic factors for local recurrence, metastasis, and survival rates in squamous cell carcinoma of the skin, ear, and lip. Implications for treatment modality selection. *J. Am. Acad. Dermatol.* 26:976, 1992.

Malignant Melanoma

National Institutes of Health Consensus Development on Early Melanoma. Diagnosis and treatment of early melanoma. *J.A.M.A.* 268:1314, 1992.

Roy, M. A., and Wagner, Jr., R. F. Prevention of primary cutaneous malignant melanoma: increasing cure rate in the 1990s. *Cutis* 50:365, 1992.

Shriner, D. L., Wagner, Jr., R. F., and Glowzwski, J. R. Photography for the early diagnosis of malignant melanoma in patients with atypical moles. *Cutis* 50:358, 1992.

Veronesi, U., et al. Inefficiency of immediate node dissection in stage I melanoma of the limbs. *N. Engl J. Med.* 297:627, 1977.

Kaposi's Sarcoma

Tappero, J. W., et al. Kaposi's sarcoma. *J. Am. Acad. Dermatol.* 28:371, 1993.

Sarcomas

Dennis A. Casciato and
Barry B. Lowitz

I. **Epidemiology and etiology.** Primary mesenchymal tumors localized outside the skeleton, parenchymatous organs, or hollow viscera are generally designated as soft tissue sarcomas (STSs). Kaposi's sarcoma is discussed in Chapters 16 and 37. Rhabdomyosarcoma and Ewing's sarcoma are discussed in Chapter 18. Sarcomas of the mediastinum, heart, and blood vessels are discussed in Chapter 19.

A. **Incidence.** Sarcomas constitute about 1 percent of all cancers and accounted for 8000 new cases in the United States in 1993. STS outnumber bone sarcomas by a ratio of 3:1. In children the majority of STS are rhabdomyosarcomas or undifferentiated tumors arising in the head and neck regions. In adults STSs occur most frequently on the extremities or retroperitoneum and least frequently in the head and neck region. Bone sarcomas occur mostly between the ages of 10 and 20 years (osteogenic sarcoma) or between 40 and 60 years (chondrosarcoma). Most sarcomas show no sexual predilection. Peak incidences occur in childhood and in the fifth decade.

B. **Etiology.** Certain kinds of sarcomas are associated with exposure to specific agents or with underlying medical conditions.

1. **Lymphangiosarcoma.** Prolonged postmastectomy arm edema (Stewart-Treves syndrome).

2. **Angiosarcoma and other STS.** Polyvinyl chloride, thorium dioxide, dioxin, arsenic, and androgens.

3. **Osteosarcoma.** Radium (watch dials) exposure; postmastectomy irradiation; Paget's disease of bone.

4. **Fibrosarcoma.** Postirradiation; Paget's disease of bone.

5. **Kaposi's sarcoma.** Cytomegalovirus and human immunodeficiency virus (HIV-1; discussed in Chap. 16, *Kaposi's Sarcoma,* and Chap. 37).

6. **Genetically transmitted diseases**

   a. **Li-Fraumeni syndrome.** Various sarcomas (especially rhabdomyosarcoma) and carcinomas of breast, lung, and adrenal cortex (p53 gene)

   b. **Beckwith-Wiedemann syndrome.** Wilms' tumor, genitourinary anomalies, aniridia, and hemihypertrophy

   c. **Neurofibromatosis.** Schwannoma (NF1 gene)

   d. **Familial retinoblastoma.** Osteosarcoma (RB1 gene)

7. **Chromosomal aberrations** are found in nearly all sarcomas. Characteristic translocations, particularly involving DNA transcription factors, are being defined.

II. **Pathology and natural history**

A. **Histology and nomenclature.** Sarcomas are given a bewildering variety of names that do not indicate biologic behavior and usually do not influence therapeutic approach. The multipotential capacities of the mesenchymal tissue and the appearance of several histologic elements in the same tumor often make clearcut histologic diagnosis difficult.

1. Sarcomas are named for the **tissue of origin** (osteosarcoma, chondrosarcoma, schwannoma, liposarcoma, etc.). These names may be combined to describe multicomponent tumors (e.g., fibrous histiocytoma).

2. Tumors are also named for **special histologic characteristics** or given a

nondescriptive name because the tissue of origin is unknown (alveolar soft parts tumor, Kaposi's sarcoma, Ewing's sarcoma).

3. **The degree of cellular differentiation (grade) and amount of necrosis** within the tumor are absolutely the most important factors in predicting tumor behavior and in determining treatment modalities for sarcomas. The other descriptive terms for the tumor are far less important. Expert pathologic evaluation is crucial.

4. **The presence of osteoid formation,** even in minimal amounts, assigns a tumor to a type of osteogenic sarcoma, which is biologically aggressive.

5. **Immunohistochemistry** may be helpful in confirming the diagnosis of rhabdomyosarcoma and synovial, clear cell, and epithelioid sarcomas. Electron microscopy is rarely helpful.

B. **Natural history.** Generally, sarcomas arise de novo and not from preexisting benign neoplasms. However, tumors occasionally "dedifferentiate" from benign to malignant forms or from a lower grade to a higher grade. Sarcomas spread without interruption along tissue planes; they invade local nerve fibers, muscle bundles, and blood vessels. Histologic sections usually show much greater local extension than is apparent on gross examination.

1. **Histologic grade.** The biologic behavior of sarcomas can usually be predicted by their histologic grade. Low-grade tumors tend to remain localized; high-grade tumors (especially those with a marked degree of necrosis) metastasize early. Virtually all osteogenic sarcomas, rhabdomyosarcomas, and synovial sarcomas are high-grade.

2. **Site of origin.** The site of origin of the sarcoma may suggest the cell type, as follows:

   a. **Head and neck**
      (1) Rhabdomyosarcoma (in a child)
      (2) Angiosarcoma (in an elderly person)
      (3) Osteogenic sarcoma (jaw)

   b. **Distal extremity**
      (1) Epithelioid sarcoma
      (2) Synovial sarcoma
      (3) Clear cell sarcoma
      (4) Osteogenic sarcoma (femur)

   c. **Proximal tibia or humerus.** Osteogenic sarcoma

   d. **Mesothelium.** Mesothelioma

   e. **Retroperitoneum and mesentery**
      (1) Leiomyosarcoma
      (2) Liposarcoma
      (3) Malignant fibrous histiocytoma

   f. **Genitourinary tract**
      (1) Rhabdomyosarcoma (in a child)
      (2) Leiomyosarcoma (in an adult)

   g. **Skin**
      (1) Angiosarcoma, lymphangiosarcoma
      (2) Kaposi's sarcoma
      (3) Epithelioid sarcoma
      (4) Dermatofibrosarcoma protuberans (on trunk)

3. **Metastases.** The lung is the major site of metastases for all sarcomas. Pulmonary metastases are almost always bilateral and multiple. Other structures, such as the liver, bone, and subcutaneous tissue, are affected by hematogenous dissemination much less frequently than are the lungs. Regional lymph node metastases are extremely uncommon in most types of sarcomas.

   a. **Sarcomas that metastasize to lymph nodes.**
      (1) Rhabdomyosarcoma
      (2) Synovial sarcoma
      (3) Epithelioid sarcoma

    b. Sarcomas that rarely metastasize and are associated with a favorable survival

      (1) Liposarcoma (myxoid and well-differentiated types)

      (2) Fibrosarcoma (infantile and well-differentiated types)

      (3) Malignant fibrous histiocytoma (superficial type)

      (4) Dermatofibrosarcoma protuberans

      (5) Parosteal sarcoma

      (6) Kaposi's sarcoma (not related to AIDS)

4. Paraneoplastic syndromes associated with sarcomas

    a. Hypoglycemia (particularly with retroperitoneal fibrosarcoma)

    b. Hypertrophic osteoarthropathy (sarcoma of pleura or mediastinum)

    c. Hypocalcemia

    d. Oncogenic osteomalacia

C. Clinical aspects of specific STS

1. Alveolar (septate) soft parts tumor

    a. Tissue of origin (incidence). Unknown (rare).

    b. Features. Unique histology with no benign counterpart; often indolent even with lung metastases, which are common. Commonly affects the thigh in adults and the head and neck in children. The five-year survival exceeds 60 percent.

2. Angiosarcoma (hemangiosarcoma, lymphangiosarcoma)

    a. Tissue of origin (incidence). Blood or lymph vessels (2–3%).

    b. Features of hemangiosarcoma. Affects the elderly; aggressive. Arises in many organs, notably the head and neck region, breast, and liver; especially affects the skin and superficial soft tissues (whereas most STS are deep). Dedifferentiation from a hemangioma is very rare. Five-year survival is less than 20 percent.

    c. Features of lymphangiosarcoma. Affects older adults; aggressive. Arises in areas with chronic lymphatic stasis (especially postmastectomy). The five-year survival is 10 percent.

3. Clear cell sarcoma

    a. Tissue of origin (incidence). Unknown (rare).

    b. Features. Affects adults under 40 years of age; painless, firm, spherical masses on tendon sheaths and aponeurotic structures of distal extremities. Very indolent. The five-year survival is 70 percent.

4. Epithelioid sarcoma

    a. Tissue of origin (incidence). Unknown (rare).

    b. Features. Affects young adults; aggressive; very typically appears on distal extremities. Differs from other STS by having a greater tendency to spread to noncontiguous areas of skin, subcutaneous tissue, fat, draining lymph nodes, and bone. The five-year survival is about 30 percent.

5. Fibrosarcoma

    a. Tissue of origin (incidence). Fibrous tissue (5–20%).

    b. Features. Affects all age groups; arises in many mesenchymal sites; usually involves the abdominal wall or extremities. Ninety percent are well-differentiated (desmoid). Dermatofibrosarcoma protuberans (rare) develops on the skin of the trunk and almost never metastasizes. Fibromyxosarcoma affects any soft tissue site but usually develops on the extremities. Ten percent are poorly differentiated (high-grade). Survival is directly related to tumor grade (see sec. **D.5**).

6. Malignant fibrous histiocytoma (MFH)

    a. Tissue of origin (incidence). Fibrous tissue and histiocytes (10–23%).

    b. Features. Age more than 40 years (<5% of affected individuals are less than 20 years old); histology is fibrosarcoma with infiltration of histiocytes. MFH has become a popular histologic diagnosis in recent years, often encompassing tumors that were previously classified as pleomorphic rhabdomyosarcoma or undifferentiated fibrosarcoma; it is the most common STS in some series. MFHs range from benign to atypical to frankly malignant. Develops in extremities (especially legs), trunk, and retroperitoneum. Superficial MFH develops close to the skin surface and is often low-grade; the five-year survival is 65 percent. Deep MFH usually is high-grade; the five-year survival is less than 15 percent (see sec. D.6).

7. **Hemangiopericytoma**
   a. **Tissue of origin (incidence).** Blood vessels (<1%).
   b. **Features.** Affects all ages. Develops under finger tips (glomus tumors), on lower extremities or pelvis, in the retroperitoneum, and elsewhere. Benign and malignant versions. The five-year survival is about 50 percent.

8. **Kaposi's sarcoma**
   a. **Tissue of origin (incidence).** Controversial (varied).
   b. **Features.** Classically affects older adults; extremely indolent lesions arise on lower extremities and rarely cause death. The epidemic and aggressive variety is associated with AIDS and Africans (see Chap. 16, *Kaposi's Sarcoma,* and Chap. 37, sec. **IV**).

9. **Leiomyosarcoma**
   a. **Tissue of origin (incidence).** Smooth muscle (7–11%).
   b. **Features.** Affects all age groups. Develops in gastrointestinal tract, uterus, retroperitoneum, and other soft tissues. Generally refractory to chemotherapy and radiotherapy. The five-year survival is 30 percent.
   c. **Leiomyoma peritonealis disseminata (LPD).** A condition in women, usually in reproductive years. Usually asymptomatic myriads of benign leiomyomas are scattered throughout the peritoneal cavity and range from 1 to 10 cm in size; they are stimulated by estrogen. LPD causes occasional mechanical problems with bowel or pain. Generally, no treatment is required; when symptomatic, treatment is with estrogens or antiestrogens.
   d. **Leiomyoma, benign metastasizing.** Histologically benign, these leiomyomas are typically discovered as persistent pulmonary nodules and possibly as a variant of LPD. Associated nodules in the pelvis are mostly in round ligaments of uterus and not as diffuse as in LPD. Treatment is surgical for symptomatic or progressive lesions.

10. **Liposarcoma**
    a. **Tissue of origin (incidence).** Fat tissue (15–18%).
    b. **Features.** Affects middle and older age groups, mostly men. Develops in thigh, groin, buttocks, shoulder girdle, and retroperitoneum. Does not arise from benign lipomas. The five-year survival is 80 percent for low-grade liposarcomas and 20 percent for high-grade liposarcomas.

11. **Mesenchymoma**
    a. **Tissue of origin (incidence).** Two or more distinct types of mesenchymal tissue (<1%).
    b. **Features.** Affects children. Tumors are composed of combinations of smooth or striated muscle, nerve sheath, vascular stroma, reticulum cells, osteoblasts, chondroblasts, or fat cells. Often low-grade with high survival rates; the five-year survival is greater than 80 percent.

12. **Mesothelioma**
    a. **Tissue of origin (incidence).** Mesothelium.
    b. **Features.** Age more than 50 years. Asbestos exposure is etiologic. Involves pleura and peritoneum; aggressively encases viscera. Highly lethal; the five-year survival is less than 10 percent. (See Chap. 8.)

13. **Myxoma**
    a. **Tissue of origin (incidence).** Mesenchymal tissues.
    b. **Features.** Usually found on extremities; has histologic appearance of umbilical cord. The five-year survival is about 80 percent.

14. **Neurofibrosarcoma (schwannoma, neurilemoma)**
    a. **Tissue of origin (incidence).** Nerve (5–7%).
    b. **Features.** Affects young and middle-aged adults and patients with von Recklinghausen's disease (about 10% develop sarcomatous changes dur-

ing lifetime). Histologically resembles fibrosarcoma. Presents with thickening of nerves and without anatomic predilection. Superficial variety is low-grade, spreads extensively along nerve sheaths without metastasizing, and has a five-year survival of over 90 percent. Penetrating variety is high-grade with nodular growth, vascular invasion, lung metastases and has a five-year survival of less than 20 percent.

15. Polyhistiocytoma (see **D.10**)

16. Rhabdomyosarcoma

   a. Tissue of origin (incidence). Striated muscle (5–19%).

   b. Features. By definition in the G-TNM staging system, all are grade 3. All types can occur in any age group, but the typical onset and distribution is noted below (see Chap. 18, *Rhabdomyosarcoma*).

   c. Features of embryonal rhabdomyosarcoma. Affects infants and children; sites are head and neck (70%) and genitalia (15–20%). Includes sarcoma botryoides. The five-year survival is about 50 percent.

   d. Features of alveolar rhabdomyosarcoma. Affects teenagers at any site; highly aggressive; histology resembles lung alveoli. The five-year survival is less than 10 percent.

   e. Features of pleomorphic rhabdomyosarcoma. Affects those over age 30; rare; develops in extremities. Often highly anaplastic; microscopically confused with MFH. The five-year survival is about 25 percent.

17. Synovial sarcoma

   a. Tissue of origin (incidence). Tenosynovial mesothelium (5–20%).

   b. Features. Affects young adults, but may occur from the second to fourth decade. Monophasic and biphasic subtypes microscopically; some authorities consider clear cell and epithelioid sarcomas as variants of synovial sarcoma. Presents with hard masses, often painful, near tendons in the vicinity of joints of the hands, knees, or feet. Often calcified with characteristic x-ray appearance. By definition in the G-TNM staging system, all are grade 3. Relatively high rates of local recurrence and lymph node metastases. The five-year survival is about 30 percent.

D. Clinical aspects of specific bone sarcomas

   1. Adamantinoma

      a. Tissue of origin (incidence). Unknown; nonosseous (<1%).

      b. Features. Osteolytic tumor; often develops on upper tibia; resembles ameloblastoma of mandible. Indolent behavior; the five-year survival is greater than 90 percent.

   2. Chondrosarcoma

      a. Tissue of origin (incidence). Cartilage (30%).

      b. Features. Age 40 to 60 years, fewer than 4 percent of patients are less than 20 years. Usually develops in shoulder girdle (15%), proximal femur (20%), or pelvis (30%). Chondrosarcomas are the most common malignant tumors of the sternum and scapula. Most tumors are grade 1 or 2; higher grade tumors metastasize frequently; however, tumor grade does not appear to affect prognosis. Refractory to both RT and chemotherapy; complete surgical removal is the main determinant of recurrence and survival. The five-year survival is about 50 percent.

      (1) Central chondrosarcomas (75%) arise within a bone; peripheral chondrosarcomas (25%) arise from the surface of a bone. Peripheral lesions can become quite large without causing pain; central lesions present with a dull pain but rarely with a mass. Pain means that the apparently "benign" cartilage tumor on x-ray is probably a central chondrosarcoma.

      (2) About 25 percent of chondrosarcomas represent malignant transformation of a preexisting endochondroma or osteocartilaginous exostosis. The presentation of multiple benign cartilaginous tumors has a higher rate of malignant transformation than the corresponding solitary lesions.

3. **Chordoma**
   a. **Tissue of origin (incidence).** Primitive notochord cells (5%).
   b. **Features.** Develops in the midline of the neural axis at base of skull or sacrococcygeal agea. The physaliferous cells are pathognomonic histologically. Indolent tumor with almost universal tendency for local recurrence. Low-grade but eventually fatal after many years due to complications associated with invasion into neural tissues. Treated with surgery and RT. The five-year survival is 50 percent.
4. **Ewing's sarcoma**
   a. **Tissue of origin (incidence).** Unknown; nonmesenchymal elements of bone marrow (15%).
   b. **Features.** Affects children 10 to 15 years of age; rare in blacks; highly aggressive; arises in many bones, but especially the femoral diaphysis (see Chap. 18, *Ewing's Sarcoma*).
5. **Fibrosarcoma of bone**
   a. **Tissue of origin (incidence).** Fibrous tissue (2%).
   b. **Features.** Affects middle-aged patients in major long bones; develops occasionally in conjunction with an underlying disease (bone infarcts, osteomyelitis, benign giant cell tumor, Paget's disease, following RT [see sec. **D.11**]). Resembles fibrosarcoma, but osteoid is detected in parts of the lesion. Often high-grade, which correlates with metastatic potential and survival (see **C.5**).
6. **Fibrous histiocytoma of bone**
   a. **Tissue of origin (incidence).** Fibrous and primitive mesenchymal tissue (5%).
   b. **Features.** Affects older patients; arises de novo or as a complication of Paget's disease. Most common sites are metaphyses of long bones, especially around the knee. In contrast to osteogenic sarcoma, serum alkaline phosphatase levels are normal. Pathologic fracture is often the first manifestation. Aggressive with high rate of regional lymph node and systemic dissemination (see **C.6**).
7. **Giant cell tumor of bone, malignant**
   a. **Tissue of origin (incidence).** Unknown (<1%).
   b. **Features.** Affects older patients, particularly females; develops predominantly in long bones, especially around the knee. Aggressive, locally recurrent tumor with low metastatic potential. Local recurrence is determined by the adequacy of surgical removal rather than the histologic grade. The entity is distinct from the tumor that arises from the transformation of a giant cell tumor that was thought to be benign; that transformation occurs in 10 to 20 percent of cases.
8. **Osteogenic sarcoma**
   a. **Tissue of origin (incidence).** Bone (40–50%).
   b. **Features of classic osteogenic sarcoma.** Affects any age but the onset is usually between 10 and 20 years; more common in males. Most tumors originate in the metaphysis of long bones, the region of highest growth velocity. Tender, boney masses in the distal femur, proximal tibia, and proximal humerus account for 85 percent of cases. Nearly always high-grade.
   c. **Features of low-grade osteogenic sarcoma.** Rare; resembles a desmoid tumor.
   d. **Features of osteogenic sarcoma of the jaw.** Affects individuals between the ages of 20 and 40 years; males are more commonly affected; frequently detected during dental examinations. High- and low-grade varieties are treated with hemimaxillectomy or hemimandibulectomy and reconstruction.
   e. **Features of telangiectatic osteogenic sarcoma.** Affects younger patients; a purely lytic tumor that can be confused with an aneurysmal bone cyst. Highly malignant; metastasizes early.

f. Features of multifocal sclerosing osteogenic sarcoma. Very rare; affects children under 10 years of age. Develops multiple simultaneous primary sites in metaphyses; rapidly metastasizes to lung and soft tissues.

g. Features of periosteal osteogenic sarcoma. Rare. Affects individuals between the ages of 15 and 25 years; arises on external bone surface growing into the overlying soft tissues as an enlarging painless mass with minimal involvement of medullary canal. Histologically confused with chondrosarcomas. More than 50 percent metastasize (see sec. **D.9**).

9. Parosteal (juxtacortical) sarcoma

    a. Tissue of origin (incidence). Bone surface (<2%).

    b. Features. A distinct clinical entity (see sec. **D.8.g**). Onset from 20 to 30 years of age. Characteristic exophytic lesion that is often on the posterior aspect of the distal femur or medial aspect of the proximal humerus. Presents as a fixed painless mass. Usually low-grade with a very indolent course; rarely involves medullary canal. Infrequently metastasizes; the five-year survival is 80 percent.

10. Polyhistiocytoma

    a. Tissue of origin (incidence). Mixed (<1%).

    b. Features. Typically affects patients in the first and second decades. Undifferentiated cells resembling Ewing's sarcoma are combined with differentiated mesenchymal elements. Any bone (e.g., ankle, skull) or soft tissue (e.g., orbit, meninges, heart valve) may be involved. Variable grade; the five-year survival about 50 percent.

11. Sarcomas of bone associated with other conditions

    a. Paget's disease of the bone. Affects individuals over the age of 60 years; the risk of sarcoma is 1000-fold greater than in the general population at this age. Sarcomatous transformation occurs in 0.7 percent of patients with Paget's disease and accounts for 5 to 14 percent of osteogenic sarcomas. The histologic form varies among reported series but is usually osteogenic sarcoma, MFH, or fibrosarcoma; chondrosarcoma, giant cell tumor, and other forms occur infrequently. Tends to affect the pelvis and proximal femur; frequently presents as pathologic fracture of the femur. Highly malignant.

    b. Following high-dose RT. Sarcoma develops within the irradiated field (bone or adjacent soft tissue structures) about 10 years after treatment. Highly malignant.

    c. Familial or bilateral retinoblastoma. A tumor suppressor gene (*RB*) has been identified on the 13q chromosome in some patients with retinoblastoma. Patients who have a 13q deletion are at increased risk for later development of osteogenic sarcoma, not only in the irradiated field but also in long bones distant from irradiated sites about 10 to 20 years later. Highly malignant.

III. Diagnosis

  A. Symptoms and signs are summarized in sec. **II.C** and **II.D**. Individuals with STS typically present with a painless, progressive swelling in an extremity; all such swellings are suspect for malignancy. Head and neck sarcomas manifest as proptosis, masses, or neurologic abnormalities. Retroperitoneal sarcomas present with back pain, lower extremity edema, and abdominal masses. Bone sarcomas usually result in visible enlargement of bone and pathologic fractures.

  B. Biopsy. *An accurate biopsy diagnosis is always essential.* An open-wedge biopsy that does not adversely affect subsequent resection has several advantages over needle biopsy (aspiration cytology is not sufficient); the advantages of wedge biopsy are

    1. The biopsy material obtained is adequate to determine tissue classification, which in turn affects management of the disease.

    2. A benign lesion, lymphoma, or metastatic lesion from an occult primary site of origin may be identified, thereby preventing excessive surgery at the first procedure.

C. X-ray studies

1. **Plain x-ray films** of soft tissues may demonstrate bone involvement. Stippled calcification may be present within the mass. Patients with painful or enlarged bones should have x-ray study of these areas. The following findings are helpful for making the diagnosis of osteogenic sarcoma:
   a. Mixed sclerotic or lytic areas.
   b. Periosteal reaction with elevated periosteum forming a ("Codman's") triangle with bone cortex. Any periosteal elevation in an apparent bone lesion is an indication for biopsy.
   c. Sunraylike spiculation of bones.
   d. Onionskin appearance (an uncommon finding in Ewing's sarcoma).
2. **CT scans** are most useful for evaluating retroperitoneal or head and neck regions. CT scanning of the extremities appears to be effective in delineating the extent of the tumor.
3. **MRI** is comparable to CT scans in defining the relation of the tumor to neurovascular and skeletal structures, but MRI might be better for predicting resectability.
4. **Arteriography** may be useful in certain cases to plan surgical resection.
5. **Bone scan** is performed in patients with STS to evaluate periosteal reaction, which may be helpful in planning resection.
6. **CT of the thorax** is necessary for all patients with sarcoma to detect lung metastases, which may be resected after the primary tumor is managed. An "old calcified granuloma" is an untenable radiologic diagnosis in a young person with sarcoma.
7. **Serum alkaline phosphatase** levels are elevated in 60 percent of patients with osteogenic sarcoma and rarely in other bone sarcomas. When elevated at the time of diagnosis, this result is an important tumor marker to evaluate response to therapy.

IV. Staging system and prognostic factors

A. Staging system. Tumor grade is the single most important prognostic factor in sarcomas and is incorporated into the G-TNM staging system.

1. **Grade (G).** All rhabdomyosarcomas and synovial sarcomas are grade 3 by definition.
   G1-Well differentiated
   G2-Moderately differentiated
   G3-Poorly differentiated
   G4-Undifferentiated
2. **Primary tumor (T)**
   a. **Bone sarcomas**
      T1: Tumor confined within the cortex
      T2: Tumor invades beyond the cortex
   b. **Soft tissue sarcomas (adults)**
      T1: Tumor ≤5 cm in greatest dimension
      T2: Tumor >5 cm in greatest dimension
3. **Regional lymph nodes (N)**
   N0: No regional lymph node metastases
   N1: Regional lymph node metastases present
4. **Distant metastases (M)**
   M0: No distant metastases
   M1: Distant metastases present

B. Prognostic factors

1. **Histologic grade** (the degree of differentiation, the amount of necrosis, and the number of mitoses per high-power microscopic field) is the single most important prognostic factor, especially for STS. The shortcoming of this system is the less than ideal reproducibility of grading among pathologists.
2. **Local recurrence** predisposes to further recurrences. Fibrosarcoma, neurofibrosarcoma, and synovial sarcoma seem to have the highest recurrence rates among patients with STS.
   The absence of clear surgical margins, with or without postoperative RT,

increases the rate of local recurrence in patients with STS but does not impact on survival. The development of distant metastases following local recurrence may be either directly related to the recurrence or only a reflection of the more aggressive tumor biology.

3. **Site of disease.** Fifty percent of deaths in patients with STS occur in the 8 percent of patients with retroperitoneal lesions.

4. **Tumor suppressor gene, p53,** is located on the short arm of chromosome 17. Nuclear accumulation of p53 protein appears to be a marker of tumor aggressiveness and may be a useful prognostic factor for STS.

C. **Stage groupings and survival for STS.** Note: Stage groups I through III can be further separated into substage A (for T1 lesions) and substage B (for T2 lesions).

Stage grouping	G-TNM stage			Two-year survival	Five-year survival
I	G1	T1-2 N0	M0	90%	80%
II	G2	T1-2 N0	M0	80%	70%
III	G3	T1-2 N0	M0	65%	45%
IV	G1-3 T1-2 N1		M0, *or*		
	G1-3 T1-2 N0-1 M1			25%	10%

D. **Cure.** Approximately 80 percent of all STS that recur will do so within two years. Patients with osteogenic sarcoma who survive three years without evidence of disease appear to be cured.

V. **Prevention and early detection.** The physician must suspect and biopsy all soft tissue masses, de novo bony abnormalities, and periosteal elevations with an apparent bone lesion.

VI. **Management**

A. **Treatment of STS.** Wide, adequate surgical resection with pathologically proven clear margins is the most effective therapeutic approach. Soft part resection can be accomplished without amputation in 50 to 60 percent of patients.

1. **Extent of resection.** Surgical exploration of the tumor demonstrates apparent encapsulation; this is actually a pseudocapsule. Local recurrences develop in 80 percent of patients treated only by enucleation of the pseudocapsule.

   The surgeon must remove the localized sarcoma *within a complete envelope of normal tissue:* normal structures must be sacrificed if necessary to encompass the tumor. The biopsy site, skin, and most of the subcutaneous tissue, fibrous tissue, and (often) the adjacent muscle group should be included in the resection. For muscle tumors, the entire group of muscles, from origin to insertion, must be removed.

2. **Regional lymph node dissection.** Only angiosarcomas and synovial sarcomas are commonly treated with regional node dissection because of the frequency of nodal metastasis with these tumors. Note dissection is usually not performed for other STS.

3. **RT** is administered to the tumor bed before or after surgery (depending on the treatment center) for high-grade or large STS to improve local control rates.

   a. **Microscopically positive surgical margins** increase the risk for local failure. The presence of microscopically positive surgical margins or the occurrence of local failure, however, does not affect overall survival. Adjuvant RT may be most important where achieving clear margins would require amputation or significant functional compromise of the extremity.

   b. Studies show that **for lesions distal to the elbow or knee,** postoperative RT raised the ability to perform limb salvage surgery to 95 percent and reduced the local recurrence rate to 10 percent. These results were the same as if radical amputation or muscle group excision were performed.

4. **Adjuvant chemotherapy** is standard practice in the management of rhabdo-

myosarcoma in children. Although adjuvant chemotherapy for STS in adults remains theoretically advantageous for patients with high-grade tumors, it is controversial and investigational. If the treatment is given preoperatively, no benefit has been proven. If given postoperatively, occasional marginal benefit has been reported.

5. **Treatment of STS for specific presentations**
   a. **Grade 1 and small grade 2 lesions** are treated with surgery alone; the relapse rate is less than 10% with surgery alone. Adjuvant RT is not required.
   b. **Grade 2 lesions that are proximal and large** are treated with surgery and postoperative RT.
   c. **Grade 3 or 4 lesions.** RT is advisable before or after surgery.
   d. **Head and neck STS.** Appropriate therapy is not defined. Wide surgical excision and RT before or after surgery is advisable.
   e. **Childhood rhabdomyosarcoma** is treated intensively with chemotherapy, RT, and surgery (see Chap. 18, *Rhabdomyosarcoma*).
   f. **Retroperitoneal STS** (mostly leiomyosarcomas and liposarcomas) must be radically extirpated. Complete resection is possible in about 65 percent of patients and strongly predicts outcome. Median survival with complete resection is 80 months for low-grade STS and 20 months for high-grade. Median survival with incomplete resection for all STS is only 24 months. The survival rate is not affected by tumor type or size.

B. **Treatment of osteogenic sarcomas** results in a 65 to 80 percent 10-year, disease-free survival. Relapse after three years of disease-free survival is unusual.

1. **Limb salvage surgery** is now the standard treatment for the vast majority of patients with osteogenic sarcomas of the extremities, where nearly 90 percent of these tumors originate. Only occasional patients require amputation. The widespread, successful use of limb salvage therapy has been made possible by
   a. Significant progress in the **development of modern prostheses** that are available immediately after surgery. For example, young children who would have had unacceptable leg-length discrepancy with limb salvage procedures can now be given a prosthesis that can be lengthened while the patient grows ("expandable prosthesis").
   b. Major advances in **orthopedic surgical techniques.** Furthermore, the historical fear of "skip metastases" (within the same bone of involvement) has proven to be excessive; the occurrence of "skip metastases" appears to be less than 10 percent.
   c. The use of **preoperative (neoadjuvant) chemotherapy,** which
      (1) Can result in enough tumor shrinkage to permit the use of prostheses and can allow time for fabrication of the prosthesis.
      (2) Provides an in vivo drug trial to determine the drug sensitivity of an individual tumor and to customize postoperative chemotherapy regimens. Patients who respond to preoperative chemotherapy are destined to do well and vice versa.
      (3) Provides a response rate of 60 to 85 percent with combination regimens, including high-dose methotrexate with leucovorin rescue (HDMTX).
   d. Whether gauging subsequent therapy based on the histologically evaluated response of the tumor (measured by assessing the amount of viable tumor within a mostly necrotic specimen) affects survival remains to be proved. Whether relapse-free survival is better with neoadjuvant chemotherapy than with adjuvant chemotherapy alone also needs to be confirmed.

2. **Amputation** provides definitive surgical treatment in patients in whom a limb-sparing resection is not a prudent option. The procedures include hip disarticulation, hemipelvectomy, and forequarter resection. Although these procedures were once utilized for technically difficult resections and proxi-

mal tumors, most sarcomas of the shoulder girdle or knee can now be resected rather than amputated with the extremity.

3. **Adjuvant RT** is usually not necessary for osteogenic sarcomas of the extremities. Tumors of the jaw, facial bones, and axial skeleton require combined RT and limited surgery.

4. **Adjuvant chemotherapy** is standard practice in the management of all patients with osteogenic sarcoma. Prospective, randomized, controlled studies demonstrated improvement in relapse-free survival for patients treated adjuvantly with chemotherapy compared with those treated with surgery alone (17% versus 65–85% at two years). A steep dose-response curve has been repeatedly observed for chemotherapy of sarcomas: the higher the dose, the higher the response rate.

   a. **HDMTX** with leucovorin rescue is clearly the most effective drug treatment for this disease; doses of 12 gm/m^2 are associated with a 50 percent response rate. Patients who responded to HDMTX have continued to do well.

   b. **Other single-agent chemotherapies** for osteogenic sarcoma have produced the following response rates: doxorubicin (90 mg/m^2), 30 percent; ifosfamide (6–10 gm/m^2 given over several days), 20 to 30 percent; and cisplatin (120 mg/m^2), 20 percent. Ifosfamide given in doses of 14 gm/m^2 (over several days) is reported to be associated with a 65 percent response rate.

   c. **Combination chemotherapy.** Doxorubicin, cisplatin, or etoposide is being given in escalating doses in combination with HDMTX and with hematopoietic growth factor support in an attempt to improve the already impressive cure rate.

C. **Treatment of other bone sarcomas**

   1. **Chondrosarcoma.** Complete surgical excision with limb-sparing procedures where applicable. Adjuvant RT or chemotherapy is not helpful.

   2. **MFH of bone.** Radical surgical resection. Because of the poor prognosis, adjuvant chemotherapy is justified but its efficacy has not been proved.

   3. **Fibrosarcoma of bone.** Surgery alone.

   4. **Chordoma.** The first surgical procedure has the best chance for cure. Inadequate surgery results in local recurrence and ultimate death. RT is also used adjuvantly with disappointing results. Heavy particle irradiation appears promising for improving local control.

   5. **Ewing's sarcoma** is discussed in Chap. 18, *Ewing's Sarcoma.*

   6. **Giant cell tumor of bone.** Surgical removal cures 90 percent of these tumors when benign. Amputation is reserved for massive recurrence or malignant transformation.

   7. **Cryosurgery,** using liquid nitrogen after curettage of a tumor cavity, can decrease local recurrence for aggressive benign bone tumors and low-grade sarcomas.

D. **Treatment of metastatic or advanced sarcomas**

   1. **Surgery**

      a. **Painful extremities.** Removal of a painful, functionless extremity that is the site of an eroding, necrotic tumor may be palliative, even in patients with metastatic disease. Surgery may be attempted after chemotherapy and RT have failed to control progressive disease.

      b. **Resection of pulmonary metastasis** is a reasonable measure in the selected patient with resectable pulmonary metastasis and no other evidence of disease (see Chap. 29, sec. II). The best results of this approach are observed in patients with sarcomas when compared to patients with carcinomas or melanomas.

   2. **RT**

      a. **Palliation.** The heterogeneity of sarcomas is reflected in their variable responses to RT. This group of tumors is only moderately sensitive to RT at doses that can be tolerated by most patients. Liposarcoma and the embryonal variety of rhabdomyosarcoma are the only STS in which an

objective response to RT is the rule. Objective tumor regression occurs in less than 50 percent of patients with other types of sarcomas.
  b. Inoperable disease. RT for patients who have inoperable lesions or who refuse surgery is of marginal value.
  c. Local hyperthermia used with chemotherapy or RT is an experimental modality that occasionally induces tumor responses.
3. **Chemotherapy**
  a. Effective agents. The combination of vincristine, actinomycin D, and cyclophosphamide in children with rhabdomyosarcoma produces a response rate of 90 percent even with disseminated disease. Responses to these agents in other sarcomas are usually minimal and brief.

  The response rates of STS to doxorubicin, ifosfamide, or dacarbazine used as single agents are 30 percent, 30 percent, and 15 percent, respectively. Dacarbazine is the only effective agent in the treatment of leiomyosarcoma, but that advantage is associated with minor improvement. Other drugs have minor activity ($\leq 15\%$ response rates) in the treatment of STS. See sec. **B.4** for the activity of single agents in osteogenic sarcoma.
  b. Combination chemotherapy regimens (e.g., CyVADIC [Appendix A1]) appears to provide no advantage over single agents for palliation or survival but is more toxic. Pulmonary and soft tissue metastases are more responsive than liver and bone metastases. Intra-arterial administration is not superior to IV administration.
  c. Dose intensity probably correlates with both response rates and survival in the treatment of sarcomas. High-dose combinations of ifosfamide (with mesna uroprotection), doxorubicin (Adriamycin), and dacarbazine (MAID regimen) results in a higher response rate (45%) than single agents but at the expense of substantial myelosuppression. Very high doses of ifosfamide ($14-18$ gm/m^2) given over several days with precautions for the development of renal tubular acidosis reportedly give much better responses to STS that were previously considered to be resistant to chemotherapy (e.g., synovial sarcoma). These dose-intensive regimens must be given with caution because of their substantial toxicity and the lack of corroborating evidence of efficacy.

Selected Reading

Antman, K. H., Eilber, F. R., and Shiu, M. H. Soft tissue sarcomas: current trends in diagnosis and management. *Curr. Probl. Cancer.* 13:339, 1989.

Casper, E. S., et al. Preoperative and postoperative adjuvant combination chemotherapy for adults with high grade soft tissue sarcoma. *Cancer* 73:1644, 1994.

Eilber, F. R., et al. A randomized prospective trial using postoperative adjuvant chemotherapy (Adriamycin) in high-grade extremity soft-tissue sarcoma. *Am. J. Clin. Oncol.* 11:39, 1988.

Elias, A., et al. Response to mesna, doxorubicin, ifosfamide, and dacarbazine in 108 patients with metastatic or unresectable sarcoma and no prior chemotherapy. *J. Clin. Oncol.* 7:1208, 1989.

Glasser, D. B., et al. Survival, prognosis, and therapeutic response in osteogenic sarcoma: the Memorial Hospital Experience. *Cancer* 69:698, 1992.

Hadjipavlou, A., et al. Malignant transformation in Paget disease of bone. *Cancer* 70:2802, 1992.

Jaques, D. P., et al. Management of primary and recurrent soft-tissue sarcoma of the retroperitoneum. *Ann. Surg.* 212:51, 1990.

Mark, R. J., et al. Postirradiation sarcomas. *Cancer* 73:2653, 1994.

Rosen, G., et al. Osteogenic sarcoma. Chap. 78 in Haskell, C. M. (ed.). *Cancer Treatment* (4th ed.). Philadelphia: W. B. Saunders, 1995.

Rosen, G., et al. Synovial sarcoma. Uniform response of metastases to high-dose ifosfamide. *Cancer* 73:2506, 1994.

Tanabe, K. K., et al. Influence of surgical margins on outcome in patients with preoperatively irradiated extremity soft tissue sarcomas. *Cancer* 73:1652, 1994.

Tran, L. M., et al. Sarcomas of the head and neck. *Cancer* 70:169, 1992.

Williard, W. C., Hajdu, S. I., and Casper, E. S. Comparison of amputation with limb-sparing operations for adult soft tissue sarcoma of the extremity. *Ann. Surg.* 215:269, 1992.

18

Cancers in Childhood

Carole G. H. Hurvitz

Incidence, Leukemia, and Lymphoma

I. **Incidence.** Although cancer is the second leading cause of death in children, it is still relatively uncommon. However, the incidence of cancer is increasing. Fortunately, with modern aggressive multidisciplinary therapy the majority of children with cancer survive.

Leukemia and lymphoma make up almost half the cases, followed by CNS tumors. The mortality rate of CNS cancers now exceeds that for acute lymphocytic leukemia. The incidence of malignant tumors in the United States in children is shown in Figure 18-1.

II. **Acute leukemia** (see Chap. 25)

    A. **Pathology.** Acute lymphoblastic leukemia (ALL) accounts for 80 to 85 percent of leukemia cases in childhood. Acute myelogenous leukemia (AML) accounts for 15 percent and chronic myelogenous leukemia for 5 percent of cases.

        In ALL, 25 percent of cases are T cell, 5 percent are B cell, and the remainder are pre-B cell. Of the pre-B leukemias, 70 percent possess the common acute lymphoblastic leukemia antigen (CALLA). They are usually also terminal deoxynucleotidyl transferase (tdt)-positive.

    B. **Treatment** of acute leukemias in childhood involves induction of remission, prophylaxis to the CNS, and maintenance therapy. Standard treatment for ALL leads to long-term remission in over 70 percent of cases. Induction therapy utilizes vincristine, prednisone, and L-asparaginase. Intensification therapy includes CNS prophylaxis. During maintenance therapy, oral mercaptopurine is given daily and methotrexate weekly for two to three years. Certain prognostic factors at diagnosis affect the outlook of children with ALL, and their treatment is modified accordingly. Children with poorer prognostic features require more intensive treatment than standard therapy.

        1. **Favorable prognostic factors** include initial WBC less than 10,000/μL, age 2 to 10 years, non-T/non-B leukemia, L1 morphology, hyperploidy, probable CALLA positivity, and lack of organomegaly.

        2. **Poor prognostic factors** include WBC greater than 50,000/μL, massive organomegaly, or lymphomalike features, CNS involvement at diagnosis, mediastinal mass, and certain chromosomal translocations. Average risk factors are those between favorable and poor.

        3. **BMT.** AML requires intensive therapy, often followed by allogeneic or autologous BMT. BMT is also often recommended for patients with ALL who relapse.

    C. **Survival.** In AML the five-year survival with the best available regimens is approximately 40 percent. The five-year survival is more than 80 percent in children with "good prognosis" ALL following standard therapy. Even children with poorer risk factors who receive intensive therapy have an overall long-term survival of at least 70 percent. Sites of relapse include the CNS, testes (in boys), and bone marrow. The risk of relapse after two years of therapy is very low.

III. **Malignant lymphoma** (see Chap. 21). In pediatrics, lymphomas can be considered to

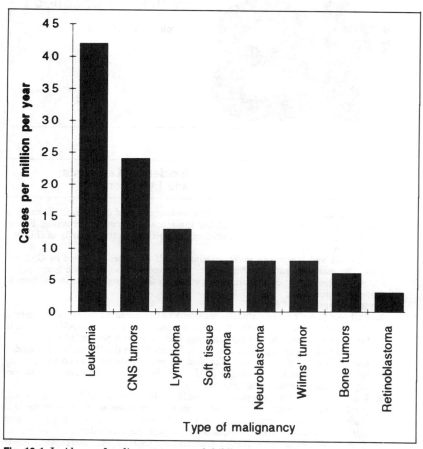

Fig. 18-1. Incidence of malignant tumors of childhood in the United States.

be lymphoblastic or nonlymphoblastic and localized or nonlocalized. Lymphoblastic lymphomas are usually T cell, and when nonlocalized may be the same entity as T cell leukemia; these illnesses are usually treated in the same way. Nonlymphoblastic lymphomas are usually B cell and are frequently Burkitt's (or Burkitt-like) lymphoma.

Different combination chemotherapeutic regimens are necessary for the subtypes of lymphoma. Localized lymphomas respond very well to chemotherapy even when very bulky and have a cure rate of greater than 90 percent. The prognosis for disseminated T cell lymphomas is the same as for T cell ALL. The outlook for disseminated nonlymphoblastic or B cell lymphoma is about 50 percent.

IV. **Hodgkin's disease** (see Chap. 21). There is no consensus on the treatment of Hodgkin's disease in children, with the exception of stage IV disease, which is primarily treated with chemotherapy. The role of staging laparotomy is still questionable, and splenectomy is contraindicated in young children because of fatal infectious complications. Chemotherapy rather than RT is generally preferred for all stages of disease. The alternation of MOPP and ABVD regimens is frequently recommended rather than either regimen alone. In children, local field rather than extended field radiation is also preferred.

Brain Tumors

The diagnosis and management of neurologic malignancies are discussed in Chap. 14.

I. **Epidemiology.** Brain tumors in children are associated with certain underlying diseases, including neurofibromatosis, tuberous sclerosis, and von Hippel-Lindau angiomatosis. Family clusters of CNS tumors have occasionally been reported.

II. **Pathology and natural history**

   A. **Pathology.** The vast majority of CNS neoplasms in children are primary tumors of the brain; the single exception is meningeal metastases, which are very common with leukemia and lymphoma. Astrocytomas are the most frequent type (30% of all cases). Medulloblastomas account for 25 percent of cases; ependymomas, 9 percent; and glioblastomas, 9 percent.

   B. **Sites of disease.** Brain tumors in children tend to occur along the central neural axis (i.e., near the third or fourth ventricle or along the brainstem). The majority of brain tumors that occur during the first year of life are supratentorial. Between 2 and 12 years of age, 85 percent are infratentorial. After the age of 12 years, the relative incidence of supratentorial tumors increases.

III. **Symptoms and signs**

   A. **Symptoms.** The most common symptoms include headaches, irritability, vomiting, and gait abnormalities. Morning headaches are most characteristic, but drowsiness and abnormal behavior are also quite common. Symptoms may be intermittent, particularly in very young children, who have open fontanelles.

   B. **Physical findings** include enlarged or bulging fontanelles in very young children, and cerebellar abnormalities, papilledema, and sixth cranial nerve abnormalities in older children.

IV. **Treatment and survival.** Survival rates for patients with low-grade astrocytomas are high if the tumor can be surgically removed (>90% at five years) and low if the tumor is high grade (<10% at five years). Survival for medulloblastoma depends on both local recurrence (<25% with RT and surgery) and spinal metastases (approximately 35% incidence without prophylactic spinal irradiation); this tumor is invariably recurrent when treated with surgery alone.

   Chemotherapy is now being used more frequently in children with brain tumors in an attempt to improve survival and to reduce the use of radiation, which has devastating effects in young children. RT is being deferred in children under three years of age.

Neuroblastoma

I. **Epidemiology and etiology.** Neuroblastoma is the most common congenital tumor and the most common tumor to occur during the first year of life. It rarely occurs in individuals more than 14 years of age. The incidence is 10 cases per million among children 0 to 4 years of age, and 4 per million among children 5 to 10 years of age. Rarely, family clusters are reported.

II. **Pathology and natural history.** Neuroblastoma has the highest incidence of spontaneous regression of any tumor in humans.

   A. **Histology.** Neuroblastoma closely resembles embryonic sympathetic ganglia. The tumors partially differentiate into rosettes or pseudorosettes, mature ganglion cells, or immature chromaffin cells. Though histologically similar to ganglioneuromas and pheochromocytomas, neuroblastomas are clearly distinctive. Electron microscopy shows typical dendritic processes that contain granules with dense bodies, probably representing cytoplasmic catecholamines. The most primitive histologic type of neuroblastoma is composed of small round cells with scant cytoplasm. The ganglioneuroma is composed of larger, more mature ganglion cells with more abundant cytoplasm.

   B. **Sites.** The most common primary site is the adrenal gland (40% of cases); a tumor of the adrenal gland produces an abdominal mass. Involvement of posterior sympathetic ganglion cells results in both intrathoracic and intra-abdominal masses, the so-called "dumb-bell tumor" that causes compression of the spinal cord.

C. Mode of spread. Most cases of neuroblastoma present with widespread metastatic disease. The most common metastatic sites include bone, bone marrow, liver, skin, and lymph nodes.

III. Diagnosis

A. Symptoms. Abdominal pain and distention, bone pain, anorexia, malaise, fever, and diarrhea.

B. Physical findings. Hepatomegaly, hypertension, orbital mass and ecchymosis, subcutaneous nodules (particularly in infancy), intra-abdominal mass, and Horner's syndrome.

C. Laboratory studies
1. CBC, serum chemistry panel
2. Urine for total catecholamines and metabolites, including vanillylmandelic acid (VMA) and homovanillic acid (HVA)
3. Chest x-ray and abdominal x-ray
4. Computerized tomography (CT) scan of the abdomen or thorax (possibly preceded by abdominal-renal ultrasound)
5. Bone scan
6. Bone marrow aspiration and biopsy to look for tumor cells
7. ^{131}I-MIBG, which is specific for neuroblastoma and pheochromocytoma. See Chap. 2, sec. II.E.
8. Examination of tumor for amplification of the N-*myc* gene

IV. Staging system and prognostic factors

A. Staging system

Stage	Extent of disease
I	Localized disease surgically removed in toto
II	Regional disease, unilateral
III	Tumor crossing the midline
IV	Metastatic disease
IVS	Stage I or II primary tumor with metastases to liver, skin, and/or bone marrow without radiographic evidence of bony involvement used in very young infants

B. Survival and prognostic factors. The prognosis for neuroblastoma is closely related to the age of the patient and stage of disease.

1. **Age.** Patients with congenital tumors have the most favorable prognosis even with widespread disease and also have the highest rate of spontaneous regression without treatment. Patients who are between one and five years of age do worse than patients less than one or more than five years of age.

2. **Stage.** Patients with advanced disease, except for stage IVS, have a poor survival rate. The overall two-year survival for neuroblastoma is greater than 80 percent for stages I and II and less than 30 percent for stage IV. Stage IVS has a 90 percent survival rate. Patients with stage III and IV disease who have amplification of the N-*myc* gene do worse.

3. The urinary VMA-HVA ratio is an indirect measure of dopamine hydroxylase. Absence of this enzyme may convey a poorer prognosis (i.e., if the VMA-HVA ratio is <1.5) and may cast doubt on the diagnosis of neuroblastoma.

V. Management

A. Surgery. Localized disease is managed primarily by surgical resection. For metastatic disease, biopsy or excision of the primary tumor is important for N-*myc* gene assessment. Complete resection is usually delayed until after chemotherapy is administered but may be done at the time of diagnosis.

B. RT is used for bulky tumor in combination with chemotherapy and as part of the conditioning regimen for BMT.

C. **Chemotherapy**
 1. **Residual localized or advanced disease.** Aggressive multimodal chemo-therapy with Adriamycin, cyclophosphamide, etoposide, and cisplatin combined with surgical resection and BMT has improved survival in stage III and IV disease.
 2. **Congenital disease.** In patients with congenital disease, specifically for stage IVS, chemotherapy is not used unless the tumor causes significant symptoms.
D. **BMT** (usually autologous) following intensive radiation and chemotherapy appears to improve the outlook for patients with advanced disease.

Wilms' Tumor
(Nephroblastoma)

I. **Epidemiology and etiology**
 A. **Incidence.** Wilms' tumor most frequently affects children between one and five years of age, and rarely those more than eight years of age. The incidence is about seven per million in the childhood age group. Familial clusters have been described, particularly in patients with bilateral Wilms' tumors.
 B. **Associated abnormalities.** Wilms' tumor has been associated with certain congenital anomalies including genitourinary anomalies, aniridia (absence of an iris), and hemihypertrophy (Beckwith-Wiedemann syndrome). Deletion of the short arm of chromosome 11 has been associated with a syndrome of Wilms' tumor, mental retardation, microcephaly, bilateral aniridia, and ambiguous genitalia.
II. **Pathology and natural history**
 A. **Histopathologic classification** most accurately predicts the prognosis.
  1. **Wilms' tumor.** Tumors that display mature elements and few anaplastic cells have the most favorable prognosis and are termed "favorable" histology. "Unfavorable" histology concerns tumors that have focal or diffuse anaplasia, rhabdoid sarcoma, or clear cell sarcoma. Unfavorable histology accounts for 12 percent of Wilms' tumors but almost 90 percent of deaths.
  2. **Congenital mesoblastic nephroma** is a rare benign tumor that is common in infancy (the most common renal neoplasm during the first month of life) and can be histologically confused with Wilms' tumor. This tumor consists of spindle-shaped, immature connective tissue cells that have a distinctive fibroblastic appearance with only minimal nuclear pleomorphism and mitoses.
 B. **Sites.** Approximately 7 percent of Wilms' tumors are bilateral at the time of diagnosis.
 C. **Mode of spread.** The lungs are the principal sites of metastases; liver and lymph nodes are the next most common sites. Bone marrow metastases are extremely rare and tend to be associated with clear cell subtypes of sarcomatous Wilms' tumor. CNS metastases are extremely rare.
 D. **Paraneoplastic syndromes.** Wilms' tumors have been rarely associated with increased erythropoietin (erythrocytosis) and with increased renin (hypertension).
III. **Diagnosis**
 A. **Symptoms.** The most common symptoms include enlarged abdomen, abdominal pain, and painless hematuria.
 B. **Physical findings.** A palpable abdominal mass is the most common finding. Hypertension is sometimes present.
 C. **Laboratory studies**
  1. CBC, serum chemistries, urinalysis, chest x-ray
  2. Plane x-ray films of the abdomen
  3. CT or MRI (preferably) scan of abdomen

IV. Staging and prognostic factors
A. Staging system

Stage	Extent of disease
I	Well-encapsulated tumor that is surgically removed in its entirety
II	Extension of tumor beyond renal capsule by local infiltration with extension along the renal vein, involvement of para-aortic nodes, and no residual macroscopic disease
III	Macroscopic residual disease or peritoneal metastases or contamination during nephrectomy
IV	Distant metastases, particularly to lung
V	Bilateral disease

B. Survival and prognostic factors.
The most important prognostic factors are the histopathologic classification and the clinical and surgical staging. Age at diagnosis is of minor importance, though younger patients seem to have a slightly better outcome. The overall two-year survival is greater than 95 percent for stages I, II, and III, with favorable histology, and about 50 percent for stage IV.

V. Management
A. Surgery.
All patients must have surgery for both staging and removal of as much tumor as possible. A transabdominal incision is mandatory to examine the vessels of the renal pedicle and the noninvolved kidney. The tumor bed and any residual tumor should be outlined with metallic clips at the time of surgery.

B. RT
is useful for treating stage III disease and metastatic disease to bone, liver, or lung.

C. Chemotherapy.
Multiple courses of combination chemotherapy are the preferred treatment. The major active chemotherapeutic agents are actinomycin D, vincristine, and Adriamycin. Cyclophosphamide is an effective second-line drug. Cisplatin is active against Wilms' tumor and is currently being used in investigational protocols. The National Wilms' Tumor Study is ongoing and several chemotherapeutic regimens are under study. The youngest patients are particularly susceptible to serious toxic effects from chemotherapy, particularly hematologic, and drug dosages should be reduced 50 percent for patients under 15 months of age.

D. Treatment according to stage of disease.
Surgery and chemotherapy are used for all stages of disease.
1. **Stage I.** RT is not necessary.
2. **Stages II and III.** RT is not needed for stage II favorable histology but is used for unfavorable histology and stage III.
3. **Stage IV or recurrent disease.** If possible, surgery can be used. Chemotherapeutic agents can be restarted if they were discontinued, or changed if relapse occurred during treatment. RT is useful for metastatic disease. Intensive chemotherapy with BMT is being evaluated.
4. **Stage V.** Bilateral Wilms' tumor necessitates a special approach. The most commonly used approaches are (1) nephrectomy of the most involved side with contralateral partial nephrectomy; or (2) bilateral total nephrectomy, with either renal allotransplantation or ectopic reimplantation of any remaining autologous renal parenchyma. Chemotherapy and irradiation to the tumor bed are given after surgery.

Rhabdomyosarcoma

I. Epidemiology and etiology.
Rhabdomyosarcoma is the most common soft tissue sarcoma in the pediatric age group; there are approximately eight cases per million

population. Suggestive evidence of C particle viruses in these tumors has been observed with electron microscopy but the viruses have not been isolated.

II. Pathology and natural history

A. Histology. Four major histologic categories of this striated muscle neoplasm have been described: embryonal (including sarcoma botryoides), alveolar, pleomorphic, and mixed. Z bands can be seen with electron microscopy. Rhabdomyoblasts have acidophilic cytoplasm, which is often PAS-positive.

B. Sites. The head and neck are involved in 35 percent of cases, the trunk and extremities in 35 percent, and the genitourinary tract in 30 percent.

C. Mode of spread. These tumors have a great tendency to recur locally and to metastasize early via the venous and lymphatic systems. Any organ may be involved with metastases.

III. Diagnosis

A. Symptoms. The most common presenting symptom is a painless, enlarging mass. Hematuria and urinary tract obstruction is seen with primary tumors of the genitourinary tract. The painless swelling is often noticed after minor trauma that calls attention to the enlarging mass.

B. Physical findings include mass lesions, urinary tract obstruction, and a "cluster of grapes" protruding through the vaginal canal (sarcoma botryoides). Exophthalmos or proptosis occurs with head and neck primaries.

C. Laboratory studies
1. CBC, LFTs
2. Plain x-ray films and MRI CT scans of involved areas
3. Bone marrow aspiration and biopsy
4. Gallium (and perhaps thallium) scans

IV. Staging system and prognostic factors

A. Intergroup Rhabdomyosarcoma Study Staging System

Stage	Extent of disease
I	Localized disease, completely resected
II	Localized disease, microscopic residual tumor
IIA	Grossly resected disease with microscopic residual tumor and negative lymph nodes
IIB	Regional disease, completely resected, with no microscopic residual disease
IIC	Regional disease with positive lymph nodes, grossly resected
III	Incomplete resection or biopsy with residual gross disease
IV	Distant metastases

B. Survival and prognostic factors. Survival is closely correlated with stage. The five-year survival with the standard VAC chemotherapy regimen is almost 100 percent for stages I and II, greater than 60 percent for stage III, and about 40 percent for stage IV. The overall survival rate is 70 percent.

V. Management.
The treatment of rhabdomyosarcoma should be aggressive, even with localized disease. Surgery, RT, and chemotherapy should be used for all cases with any residual disease.

A. Surgery should include total excision, if possible, but very radical surgery is unnecessary and unwarranted. Lymph node dissection is useful for staging in extremity or genitourinary tract tumors.

B. RT usually consists of 5000 to 6000 cGy in five to six weeks to the primary tumor site with wide ports so as to include margins of all dissected tumors.

C. Chemotherapy. A regimen that includes vincristine, actinomycin D, and cyclophosphamide (VAC) is most commonly given. Current studies are comparing Adriamycin, etoposide, and ifosfamide to VAC for advanced disease. Chemotherapy is necessary for patients:
1. Adjuvantly with stage I disease
2. With RT for stage II disease, *and*
3. To shrink the primary tumor either before or after surgery for stage III and IV disease and continued as adjunctive therapy

Ewing's Sarcoma

I. **Epidemiology and etiology.** The incidence of Ewing's sarcoma is approximately 1.5 cases per million population. The disease is very rare among black children. Seventy percent of patients are less than 20 years of age. The peak incidence is at 11 to 12 years of age for girls, and 15 to 16 years of age for boys. Males predominate at a ratio of 2:1.

II. **Pathology and natural history**
   A. **Histology.** Ewing's sarcoma is a small cell tumor of bone characterized by islands of anaplastic small round cells.
   B. **Sites of disease.** These tumors occur predominantly in the midshaft of the humerus, femur, tibia, or fibula, but also occur in the ribs, scapula, or pelvis. It also occurs as an extraosseous tumor (these behave more like rhabdomyosarcoma).
   C. **Mode of spread.** At the time of diagnosis, 20 to 30 percent of these tumors have metastasized. The majority of metastases are to the lung. Metastases to other bones or lymph nodes rarely develop. CNS metastases, particularly meningeal, have been reported but are very rare.

III. **Diagnosis**
   A. **Symptom.** Pain that is followed by localized swelling is the most frequent manifestation.
   B. **Physical findings** include tenderness and a palpable mass over the tumor site.
   C. **Preliminary laboratory studies** may show an elevated erythrocyte sedimentation rate and lytic bone lesions on x-ray film (frequently the lesions have an "onionskin" appearance). A chest x-ray film should be obtained in all patients.
   D. **Special diagnostic studies**
      1. Lung CT scan
      2. Bone scan
      3. MRI or CT scans of involved sites
      4. Gallium scan

IV. **Staging and prognostic factors**
   A. **Staging.** The two major stages for Ewing's sarcoma are
      1. Localized disease
      2. Metastatic disease
   B. **Survival and prognostic factors.** The prognosis for patients with metastatic disease at time of diagnosis remains grave; bone metastases have the worst prognosis. Patients with primary tumor of the pelvis have a higher incidence of local recurrence and a generally poorer prognosis than do patients with tumors in other primary sites. The diffuse histologic type that has uniform sheets of cells of moderate size, and stippled nuclei may have the fewest relapses and the best survival. The five-year survival of patients treated with surgery and RT alone is less than 20 percent.

V. **Management**
   A. **Treatment according to stage of disease**
      1. **Localized disease.** All patients with localized disease should receive intensive chemotherapy followed by complete surgical resection if possible. If resection is not feasible or complete, RT is given.
      2. **Metastatic disease** is treated with intensive chemotherapy followed by surgical resection, if possible, or RT. Ewing's sarcoma of bone rarely involves regional lymph nodes.
   B. **RT** is aimed at eradicating all disease while preserving limb function. The optimal volume of bone to be irradiated has not been determined.
      1. **Nonbulky lesions.** RT (6000–7000 cGy) with shrinking fields is given to the entire bone when leg-length discrepancies will not be excessive.
      2. **Leg-length discrepancies.** When the probabilities for leg-length discrepancies are excessive (e.g., for younger children with lesions near the knee),

patients should have primary amputation plus chemotherapy. This regimen usually results in better extremity function than limbs treated with ortho-voltage irradiation. Limb salvage procedures with chemotherapy are also frequently performed when appropriate.

    3. Pelvic primaries. Moderate doses of RT (4000 cGy) with limited surgery are used for pelvic primary tumors because an excessive morbidity is associ-ated with large doses of radiation delivered to bowel and bladder. Chemo-therapy is preferred for pelvic primaries.

C. Chemotherapy involves multiple drugs given in multiple cycles. The most ac-tive agents include vincristine, actinomycin D, high-dose cyclophosphamide, and Adriamycin. Ifosfamide and etoposide in combination have been shown to be very effective. Carmustine, methotrexate, and bleomycin also have activity against this disease and are useful in combination with the more active agents. The optimal combination of agents is controversial.

D. Surgery. The role of surgical resection is controversial. Surgery is helpful in selected patients with localized disease and in patients with bulky metastatic disease. The total removal of tumor is not necessary in instances where severe disabilities could result. Concerted efforts at limb preservation should be made.

Retinoblastoma

I. Epidemiology and etiology

    A. Incidence. Retinoblastoma occurs approximately once in 25,000 newborn in-fants. The average age of patients is 18 months, and more than 90 percent are less than five years old. The incidence in Asians is four times that in whites. Patients have a high risk for other neoplasms, particularly radiation-induced osteosarcomas that arise in treatment portals.

    B. Familial retinoblastoma. Bilateral disease occurs in 33 percent of affected pa-tients, and the majority of these cases are familial. Siblings have a 10 to 20 percent chance of developing retinoblastoma if the affected child has bilateral disease and about 1 percent if unilateral. The offspring of a patient who survived bilateral retinoblastoma have approximately a 50 percent chance of developing the disease.

II. Pathology and natural history

    A. Histology. Retinoblastoma appears histologically as undifferentiated small cells with deeply stained nuclei and scant cytoplasm. Large cells are sometimes seen forming pseudorosettes, particularly in bone marrow aspirates.

    B. Mode of spread. Multiple foci of tumor in the retina are typical at the outset. Most patients die of CNS extension through the optic nerve or widespread hema-togenous metastases.

III. Diagnosis

    A. Symptoms. The disease typically presents with a "cat's eye" (white pupil or leukokoria). A squint or strabismus is occasionally noted. Orbital inflammation or proptosis rarely occurs.

    B. Physical findings are usually limited to the eye, but patients must have a complete neurologic examination. Ophthalmologic examination under anesthe-sia is essential for infants and small children, for both those with symptoms and those at high risk for developing the disease. Two pathognomonic features are

        1. The typical pattern of fluffy calcifications in the retinas

        2. The presence of vitreous seeding by tumor cells

    C. Preliminary laboratory studies

        1. CBC, LFTs

        2. MRI or CT scans of head and orbit (both scans performed with contrast)

    D. Special diagnostic studies

        1. Lumbar puncture with CSF by cytocentrifuge.

        2. Bone marrow aspiration and biopsy.

3. Serum levels of CEA and α-FP, which are frequently elevated in this disease.

4. Urinary catecholamines, which are very infrequently elevated.

IV. **Staging system and prognostic factors**

A. **Staging system.** The Reese-Ellsworth classification is most frequently used.

Group	Extent of disease
I	Solitary lesion or multiple tumors less than 4 disc diameters in size at or behind the midplane of the eye
II	Solitary lesions or multiple tumors 4–10 disc diameters at or behind the midplane of the eye
III	Any lesions anterior to the midplane, or solitary lesions larger than 10 disc diameters and behind the equator
IV	Multiple tumors, some larger than 10 disc diameters, or any lesion extending anteriorly to the ora serrata (junction of the retina and ciliary body)
V	Massive tumor that involves more than half the retina, or presence of vitreous seeding or optic nerve involvement

B. **Survival and prognostic factors.** The prognosis is related to both stage and the interval between discovery of clinical signs and the initiation of treatment. Survival with preservation of useful vision is greater than 90 percent for groups I and II, greater than 65 percent for groups III and IV, and greater than 60 percent for group V. In recently reported studies, survival with preservation of useful vision has been as high as 100 percent for groups I and II and greater than 75 percent for groups III, IV, and V.

V. **Management**

A. **Surgery** is the primary modality of treatment. Prompt enucleation in unilateral disease and enucleation of the most extensively involved eye in bilateral disease are most commonly employed. Another approach has been to enucleate only those eyes with optic nerve involvement and to treat the remaining disease with RT. When enucleation is performed, as long a segment of the optic nerve as possible should be removed.

B. **RT** is given, in most cases, to either the tumor bed or to the nonremoved involved eye. Usually the dose given is approximately 3500 cGy in nine fractions over a three-week period to the posterior retina. This technique, particularly when using megavoltage irradiation, is used to attempt to spare the anterior chamber and avoid cataract formation; it is unsuitable for tumors at or beyond the midpoint of the eye.

1. **Radiocobalt applicators** have been used for single lesions or discrete groups of small lesions.

2. **RT without surgery** is usually reserved for patients with advanced disease in both eyes, residual tumor after surgery, or for tumors involving the optic nerve. Most patients should not have RT without surgery.

3. **Light coagulation** and **cryotherapy** have been used for discrete lesions, particularly for small recurrences.

C. **Chemotherapy** is useful for metastatic disease. Adjuvant therapy for localized disease has not been shown to increase longevity. Many chemotherapeutic agents are active (vincristine, actinomycin D, cyclophosphamide, and Adriamycin).

Selected Reading

Albright, A. L. Pediatric brain tumors. *CA* 43:272, 1993.

American Cancer Society. Workshop on children with cancer. *Cancer* 71:(10 suppl.), 1993.

Bleyer, W. A., et al. Monthly pulses of vincristine and prednisone prevent bone marrow and testicular relapse in low-risk childhood acute lymphoblastic leukemia: A report of the CCG-161 Study by the Childrens Cancer Study Group. *J. Clin. Oncol.* 9:1012, 1991.

Brugieres, L., et al. Screening for germ line p53 mutations in children with malignant tumors and a family history of cancer. *Cancer Res.* 53:452, 1993.

Israel, M. A. Pediatric oncology: model tumors of unparalleled import. *J. Natl. Cancer Inst.* 81:404, 1989.

Nathan, D. G., and Oski, F. A. *Hematology of Infancy and Childhood,* vol. 2 (4th ed.). Philadelphia: W. B. Saunders, 1993.

Neglia, J. P., et al. Second neoplasms after acute lymphoblastic leukemia in childhood. *N. Engl. J. Med.* 325:1330, 1991.

Smith, M. B., et al. Forty-year experience with second malignancies after treatment of childhood cancer: analysis of outcome following the development of the second malignancy. *J. Pediatr. Surg.* 28:1342, 1993.

Woods, W. G., et al. Intensively timed induction therapy followed by autologous or allogeneic bone marrow transplantation for children with acute myeloid leukemia or myelodysplastic syndrome: a Childrens Cancer Group pilot study. *J. Clin. Oncol.* 11:1448, 1993.

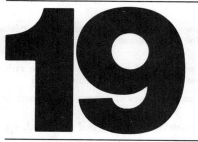

Miscellaneous Neoplasms

Dennis A. Casciato and
Barry B. Lowitz

I. Primary tumors of the mediastinum
A. General features
1. **Anatomy.** The mediastinum is bounded by the sternum anteriorly, the thoracic vertebral bodies posteriorly, the diaphragm inferiorly, and the first thoracic vertebrae superiorly. Its lateral boundaries are the parietal and pleural surfaces of the lungs. The mediastinum is arbitrarily divided into anterior and posterior segments by the heart.
2. **Incidence.** The annual incidence of mediastinal tumors is two per million population. Seventy-five percent of mediastinal tumors are benign. Most mediastinal malignancies represent metastases from other sites or lymphomas.
3. **Age and sex.** Most of the tumors show no sexual predilection. Mediastinal teratomas usually arise after the age of 30 years. Benign thymomas may occur in any age group. Thymic carcinomas are more common in elderly men, thymic sarcomas in young men. Tumors of nerve tissue origin may occur at any age but are more common in children.
4. **Symptoms and signs.** Presenting symptoms depend on the tumor location, type, and rate of growth. Symptoms are more likely to be present with rapidly growing, malignant tumors. Hypertrophic osteoarthropathy can occur with any primary mediastinal tumor, particularly sarcomas.
   a. **Anterior mediastinal tumors** present with retrosternal pain, dyspnea, upper airway obstruction, and development of collateral venous circulation over the chest. Dullness to percussion may be observed over the upper sternum.
   b. **Posterior mediastinal tumors** cause tracheal compression (cough and dyspnea), phrenic nerve compression (hiccoughs or diaphragm paralysis), involvement of left recurrent laryngeal nerve (hoarseness), esophageal compression (dysphagia), vena cava obstruction, Horner's syndrome or pain, or palsies in the brachial or intercostal nerve distribution.
5. **Evaluation**
   a. **Chest x-ray films** with posteroanterior and lateral views are obtained in patients with symptoms or signs suggestive of a mediastinal mass.
   b. **Sputum cytologies** are obtained if lung cancer is a possible diagnosis, especially if the patient has vena cava obstruction.
   c. **CT scans** of the chest are taken to determine the extent of the tumor in patients with unexplained symptoms or radiologic evidence of a mediastinal mass.
   d. **Angiography** is performed for large masses when hypervascularity of the tumor or involvement of the heart or large blood vessels is possible.
   e. **Exploratory thoracotomy** is performed for tissue diagnosis and resection of as much tumor as possible in patients considered to have primary mediastinal tumors.
B. Tumors of the anterior mediastinum
1. **Thymomas** represent 20 percent of all mediastinal tumors and are the most common cause of anterior mediastinal masses. They are composed of cells

of both lymphocytic and epithelial origin. Seventy percent of thymomas are benign and 30 percent are locally invasive. Invasive thymomas involve the pericardium, myocardium, lung, sternum, and large mediastinal vessels. Metastases are uncommon but can involve multiple organs, including liver, bone, and brain. Histologic details have little bearing on prognosis or evaluation of malignant potential; invasiveness of a thymoma at surgery is the best index of its malignancy.

   a. Paraneoplastic syndromes associated with both benign and malignant thymomas do not affect prognosis. These syndromes include:

     (1) Myasthenia gravis, which occurs in more than half of patients with thymoma; manifestations are improved in about 70 percent of patients who undergo thymectomy. Twenty percent of patients with myasthenia gravis have thymomas.

     (2) Pure red cell aplasia.

     (3) Ectopic Cushing's syndrome.

     (4) Acquired hypogammaglobulinemia.

     (5) Polymyositis, dermatomyositis, granulomatous myocarditis.

     (6) Systemic lupus erythematosus.

     (7) Hypertropic osteoarthropathy.

   b. Therapy

     (1) Surgical extirpation results in a cure rate that exceeds 95 percent for encapsulated, noninvasive thymomas. Surgery alone appears to be insufficient therapy for invasive thymomas. RT (3500 to 5000 cGY) given postoperatively for invasive thymoma (with or without complete resection) reduces the local recurrence rate from 30 percent to 5 percent.

     (2) Combination chemotherapy regimens for locally advanced or metastatic disease, which involve cisplatin, Adriamycin, and cyclophosphamide (with or without vincristine), result in 70 to 80 percent response rates, about half of which are complete responses. Corticosteroid therapy is also beneficial. The five-year survival rate for these patients is about 50 to 70 percent. The median duration of complete responses in widespread disease is about 12 months.

2. Thymic carcinomas are obviously malignant histologically and are usually not associated with paraneoplastic syndromes. Neoplasms that are well-circumscribed, are low-grade, and have a lobular growth pattern have a relatively favorable prognosis for survival. Therapeutic recommendations are not defined.

3. Germ cell tumors (see Chap. 12). Teratomas or dermoid tumors represent 10 percent of mediastinal cancers. Approximately 10 percent of these are malignant, usually with a predominant epithelioid component, but occasionally with sarcomatous or endodermal elements. Malignant germ cell tumors of the mediastinum are usually large and solid.

   a. Benign teratoma accounts for approximately 8 percent of all mediastinal tumors. They appear as a round, dense mass (often with a calcified capsular shell and teeth). The serum of a patient with benign teratoma contains no α-FP or β-HCG. These characteristics differentiate benign teratoma from germ cell malignancy. Benign tumors are also suggested by their small size and the presence of multilocular cysts. Approximately two-thirds of patients are symptomatic. Surgical excision is the treatment of choice.

   b. Seminoma is the most common malignant germ cell neoplasm of the mediastinum and occurs most frequently in 20- to 30-year-old men. Treatment of mediastinal seminoma is surgical excision followed by irradiation of the mediastinum and the supraclavicular nodes. The five-year survival for these patients is approximately 80 percent.

   c. Choriocarcinoma in the mediastinum presents with gynecomastia and testicular atrophy in 50 percent of patients. This aggressive cancer has widespread metastases at the time of diagnosis. Surgical resection is not justifiable after biopsy. Chemotherapy, similar to that used to treat testicular carcinoma, is undertaken, but the prognosis is dismal.

   d. Embryonal or yolk sac tumors of the mediastinum are highly aggressive cancers that are large and bulky at the time of diagnosis. They produce α-FP, which is useful in monitoring treatment response. Therapy consists of surgical debulking, followed by aggressive chemotherapy (as outlined for testicular cancer, see Chap. 12, sec. **VI.D**). Mediastinal irradiation delays the initiation of chemotherapy, compromises bone marrow reserve (thus limiting the chemotherapy doses), and probably should not be used.

  4. Other anterior mediastinal masses
    a. Goiter and thyroid cysts
    b. Parathyroid adenoma (20 percent of parathyroid tumors are mediastinal)
    c. Bronchogenic and thymic cysts
    d. Aortic aneurysm
    e. Soft tissue sarcomas and their benign counterparts
    f. Lymphoma and Hodgkin's disease
    g. Plasmacytoma
    h. Lymphangioma

C. Tumors of the posterior mediastinum
  1. Neurogenic tumors are the most common neoplasms in the posterior mediastinum; 15 percent are malignant. Surgical resection alone is curative for neurofibromas, schwannomas, paragangliomas, and pheochromocytomas. Some paragangliomas produce a syndrome identical to pheochromocytoma, and some malignant schwannomas are associated with noninsulin-producing paraneoplastic hypoglycemia.

  2. Mesenchymal tumors, including lipomas, fibromas, myxomas, mesotheliomas, and their sarcomatous counterparts, are very rare mediastinal tumors; more than 50 percent are malignant. Therapy necessitates surgical debulking. RT and/or chemotherapy is used as a surgical adjuvant for treating sarcomas.

  3. Other posterior mediastinal masses
    a. Goiter and thyroid cysts
    b. Pericardial and gastroenteric cysts
    c. Lymphoma and Hodgkin's disease

II. Retroperitoneal tumors

A. Etiology. Excluding renal tumors, 85 percent of primary retroperitoneal neoplasms are malignant. Approximately one-sixth of cases are Hodgkin's disease and one-sixth are non-Hodgkin's lymphoma. Sarcomas often appear in the retroperitoneum, particularly rhabdomyosarcoma (in children), leiomyosarcoma, and liposarcoma. Germ cell tumors, adenocarcinomas, and rare neuroblastomas account for most of the remainder of cases. Carcinomas of the breast, lung, and gastrointestinal tract can metastasize to retroperitoneal structures by way of the bloodstream or the spinal venous plexus.

B. Evaluation

  1. Symptoms. Back pain, upper urinary tract obstruction, and leg edema due to lymphatic or vena cava obstruction frequently are manifestations of retroperitoneal malignancies; arterial insufficiency does not appear to occur. Some patients develop fever or hypoglycemia as paraneoplastic syndromes.

  2. Laboratory studies. History, physical examination, chest x-ray film, and routine blood studies are performed. Uremia may result from entrapment of the ureters. IVP, barium contrast study of the colon, and abdominal CT scanning are performed to evaluate the extent of tumor.

C. Management. Exploratory surgery is necessary to establish the tissue diagnosis and to attempt resection of the tumor for potential cure, particularly for sarcomas. RT is used to treat residual disease. Chemotherapy is used for patients with lymphoreticular neoplasms or with tumors that are not responsive to RT. The specific chemotherapy selected depends on the tumor type.

III. Cardiovascular tumors. Primary cardiac tumors are exceedingly rare; cardiac metastases are more common (see Chap. 29, sec. **V**). Tumors of blood vessels are mostly sarcomas, which are discussed in Chapter 17. Some special types are discussed here.

A. Malignant heart tumors include fibrosarcoma, angiosarcoma, rhabdomyosarcoma, and endothelial sarcoma. Tumors usually arise in the right auricle and extend into the heart substance and valves. Their aggressive course is characterized by heart failure, angina, life-threatening arrhythmias, or cardiac rupture. The prognosis is hopeless.

B. Benign heart tumors

1. Fibroma, myxoma, lipoma, and hemangioma typically arise in the atria. Presenting features include intermittent valvular obstruction with syncope or episodes of dyspnea and cyanosis.

2. Atrial myxoma may cause a syndrome resembling microbial endocarditis with heart murmur, fever, joint pain, and systemic emboli. Patients with these findings and sterile blood cultures should have an echocardiogram, which is highly accurate for diagnosing myxoma of the heart. Occasionally the diagnosis is established by the finding of myxomatous tissue in arterial embolectomy specimens.

C. Hemangiopericytomas are tumors of the capillaries, which look like very cellular fibrosarcomas but are rarely malignant. Histologic appearance and grade do not closely correlate with the metastatic potential; metastases occur in cases with apparently benign tumors. These highly vascular tumors are treated by resection after embolic therapy (an absorbable gelatin sponge [Gelfoam] soaked in thrombin and injected into a vessel feeding the tumor). Postoperative RT may reduce local recurrence. Metastatic tumors respond to Adriamycin.

D. Primary intravascular sarcomas are rare tumors that present with signs of focal vascular obstruction. Venous sarcomas, particularly leiomyosarcomas, are the most common intravenous sarcomas. Vena cava tumors may produce the Budd-Chiari syndrome, renal failure, or pedal edema; patients may present with poorly defined back or abdominal pain. CT scan or venography suggests the diagnosis. Treatment is surgical resection, when technically feasible.

IV. Mastocytosis

A. Pathogenesis. Malignant mastocytosis is an uncommon disease; it is most frequently reported in Israelis and light-skinned whites. Mast cells infiltrate any organ that contains mesenchymal tissue (particularly the lymph nodes, liver, spleen, and bone marrow) and produce local destructive or fibrotic changes. Organ infiltration often indicates acceleration of the disease.

B. Clinical features

1. **Skin changes.** Urticaria pigmentosa is the most common early manifestation of systemic disease. Brownish skin nodules diffusely infiltrated with mast cells may be localized or diffuse, flat or raised, bullous or erythematous. Mild skin trauma may produce urticaria or dermographia.

2. **Organ infiltration** may develop years after skin lesions have appeared and is manifested by
   a. Hepatosplenomegaly
   b. Lymphadenopathy
   c. Bone pain (osteosclerotic lesions on x-ray films are common)
   d. Bone marrow fibrosis (common)
   e. Mast cell leukemia (occasional)
   f. Peptic ulcer and malabsorption (hyperchlorhydria occasionally occurs)

3. **Hyperhistaminemia symptoms** may be precipitated by exposure to cold, alcohol, narcotics, fever, or hot baths, and include
   a. Erythematous flushing, urticaria, edema, pruritus
   b. Abdominal pain, nausea, vomiting (occasionally diarrhea), flatulence, steatorrhea
   c. Sudden hypotension

C. Therapy. Results of various treatments have been unsatisfactory. Histamine antagonism by H_1 and H_2 blockade may help flushing, itching, and gastric distress. Cyclooxygenase inhibition may prevent prostaglandin D_2-induced hypotension when indicated. Oral chromalyn may prevent gastrointestinal symptoms and bone pain. Cytotoxic agents (especially alkylating agents) occasionally help.

V. Carcinosarcomas. Carcinosarcomas are rare tumors, which have a histologic appearance of combined sarcomatous and epithelial elements. Typically, they arise in the myometrium, prostate, or lung. Surgical resection is the treatment of choice. The role of postoperative irradiation is not clear.

VI. Adenoid cystic carcinoma ("cylindroma"). Adenoid cystic carcinomas are rare tumors, which most often arise in salivary glands or the large airways but also can develop in the skin, breast, and other sites. Local recurrence after surgery is common. Pulmonary metastases are radiologically dramatic but often have an indolent course over several years. Primary tumors are treated surgically. Local recurrences may respond to RT. Asymptomatic patients with lung metastases do not need specific treatment. Patients with symptomatic disease may respond to fluorouracil or Adriamycin.

VII. Dental tumors

A. Ameloblastomas appear to originate in dentigerous cysts. Eighty percent occur in the mandible (70% in the molar areas). The remaining 20 percent of histologically similar tumors arise in other bones and, occasionally, soft tissues. Ameloblastomas are locally invasive and have a high risk of local recurrence after surgery. Distant metastases do not occur. Therapy is by surgical resection. Some surgeons use intraoperative cauterization or cryotherapy for better local control. RT has no role in managing the tumor or recurrences.

B. Cementoma is probably an area or calcified fibrous dysplasia and not a neoplasm.

C. Other dental tumors. Ameloblastic adenomatoid tumors, calcifying epithelial odontoma, ameloblastic fibroma, dentinoma, ameloblastic odontoma, and complex odontoma are all benign tumors of the embryologic precursors of teeth. Surgical removal is the therapy of choice.

VIII. Olfactory esthesioneuroblastoma. Olfactory esthesioneuroblastoma is a tumor of the sensory epithelium of the nasal cavity close to the cribriform plate. This malignancy is considered in the differential diagnosis of poorly differentiated, round cell neuroectodermal neoplasms. Its aggressive biologic behavior is characterized by inapparent submucosal spread, local recurrence, atypical distant metastases, and poor long-term prognosis. Presenting features are unilateral nasal obstruction, epistaxis, rhinorrhea, sinus pain, or proptosis. Metastases to neck nodes develop in about 30 percent of patients. Surgical resection followed by RT appears to be the treatment of choice. Metastases are often sensitive to combination chemotherapeutic regimens.

IX. Urachal cancer. Urachal cancer arises in the primitive embryonic connection between the apex of the bladder and the umbilicus. Most of these tumors arise near the dome of the urinary bladder. The most common histologic type is adenocarcinoma. Adenocarcinomas evolve slowly and are asymptomatic until late in the course of disease. Presenting symptoms are painless hematuria, suprapubic mass, or passage of mucus in the urine. The presence of stippled calcification of a lower midline abdominal wall mass is almost pathognomonic for urachal carcinoma. Surgical resection is the therapy of choice.

X. Merkel cell carcinoma (MCC) is a rare cutaneous tumor that predominantly affects the skin in the head and neck region of older patients. These cells, first discovered by Merkel in the snout skin of voles in 1875, are thought to originate from the neural crest and to act as mechanoreceptors. MCC is a highly aggressive neoplasm with a marked propensity for local and distant metastases. Systemic disease is preceded by the appearance of nodal metastases and is uniformly fatal regardless of subsequent therapy. The five-year survival is 65 percent, especially in the absence of lymphadenopathy at the time of presentation.

The treatment of choice for MCC is wide excision of the primary tumor and early or elective regional lymph node dissection. RT may be palliative but has no proven role as an adjuvant. Chemotherapy produces a high rate of short-lived responses.

XI. Paragangliomas have also been called chemodectomas, receptomas, glomus tumors, carotid body tumors, and tympanic body tumors. These neoplasms originate in the neural crest and develop from paraganglia tissues, which are themselves chemoreceptor organs that are distributed throughout the body in association with the sympathetic chain. Nearly half originate in the head and neck region (particularly at the carotid bifurcation and in the temporal bone) and the remainder develop in the mediastinum, retroperitoneum, abdomen, and pelvis.

A. Occurrence. These uncommon neoplasms are either familial (predominantly men) or nonfamilial (predominantly women). They are multiple at several locations in 25 to 50 percent of the familial type and in 10 percent of the nonfamilial type.

B. Natural history. Paragangliomas, which are usually considered to be benign, are characterized by slow and inexorable growth from the site of origin. Manifestations depend on the cellular characteristics and tumor location. Approximately 5 percent of tumors are functional, manifest excessive secretion of neuropeptides and catecholamines, and produce a syndrome identical to pheochromocytoma. Metastases, which are the exception rather than the rule, develop in organs that do not contain paraganglia tissue (lungs, lymph nodes, liver, spleen, and bone marrow).

C. Evaluation. Paragangliomas must always be considered as potentially multiple, especially in those with a family history of such tumors. Patients should be screened for signs and laboratory evidence of excessive catecholamine secretion.

CT or MRI is useful in delineating the tumor(s). Arteriography may be useful for tumor embolization done just before surgery or for evaluating contralateral crossover blood supply. Radionuclide scintigraphy using MIBG may be helpful in localizing both paragangliomas and pheochromocytomas. These tumors have a rich blood supply; caution must be exerted not to cause hemorrhage during biopsy. Fine-needle aspiration cytology is often useful if performed carefully.

D. Treatment. Surgical extirpation is the treatment of choice, particularly for small head and neck lesions, but technical expertise in vascular surgery is mandatory. RT is effective in local control and is probably the treatment of choice for lesions that are large or erode bone, particularly in older patients. Chemotherapy is generally ineffective for metastatic disease. To do nothing is an acceptable option in some patients because these lesions are often well tolerated for long periods.

Selected Reading

Mediastinum

Adkins, R. B., Jr., Maples, M. D., and Hainsworth, J. D. Primary malignant mediastinal tumors. *Ann. Thorac. Surg.* 38:648, 1984.

Burke, A. P., Cowan, D., and Virmani, R. Primary sarcomas of the heart. *Cancer* 69:387, 1992.

Fornasiero, A., et al. Chemotherapy for invasive thymoma. A 13-year experience. *Cancer* 68:30, 1991.

Suster, S., and Rosai, J. Thymic carcinoma. A clinicopathologic study of 60 cases. *Cancer* 67:1025, 1991.

Miscellaneous Tumors

Batsakis, J. G., Hicks, M. J., and Flaitz, C. M. Peripheral epithelial odontogenic tumors. *Ann. Otol. Rhinol. Laryngol.* 102:322, 1993.

Davis, R. E., and Weissler, M. C. Esthesioneuroblastoma and neck metastasis. *Head Neck* 14:477, 1992.

Eden, B. V., et al. Esthesioneuroblastoma. Long term outcome and patterns of failure—the University of Virginia experience. *Cancer* 73:2556, 1994.

Harrison, L. B., Gutierrez, E., and Fischer, J. J. Retroperitoneal sarcomas: the Yale experience and a review of the literature. *J. Surg. Oncol.* 32:159, 1986.

Marney, S. R., Jr. Mast cell disease. *Allergy Proc.* 13:303, 1992.

Schild, S. E., et al. Results of radiotherapy for chemodectomas. *Mayo Clin. Proc.* 67:537, 1992.

Sclafani, L. M., Woodruff, J. M., and Brennan, M. F. Extraadrenal retroperitoneal paragangliomas: natural history and response to treatment. *Surgery* 108:1124, 1990.

Verniers, D. A., et al. Radiation therapy, an important mode of treatment for head and neck chemodectomas. *Eur. J. Cancer* 28A:1028, 1992.

Williams, C. J., et al (eds.). *Textbook of Uncommon Cancer*. Chichester: John Wiley and Sons, 1988.

Yiengpruksawan, A., et al. Merkel cell carcinoma. Prognosis and management. *Arch. Surg.* 126:1514, 1991.

Metastases of Unknown Origin

Dennis A. Casciato

Metastases of unknown origin (MUO) are defined as metastatic solid tumors for which the site of origin is not suggested by thorough history, physical examination, chest x-ray, routine blood and urine studies, and histologic evaluation.

There are two basic categories of MUO: (1) metastases that appear in the lymph nodes only (potentially curable with aggressive treatment), and (2) metastases to all other sites (usually carrying a dismal prognosis with any treatment).

I. Epidemiology

A. Incidence. About 4 percent of patients with cancer present with MUO. MUO is the seventh most frequent malignancy, ranking below only cancers of the lung, prostate, breast, cervix, colon, and stomach. Tumors that are responsive to treatment constitute only 25 percent of cases of MUO.

B. Age. The average age at onset is 58 years. Patients who present with a midline distribution of poorly differentiated carcinoma (10% of all MUO patients) have a median age of 39 years.

II. Histopathology

A. Establishing a histologic diagnosis should be the first order of business. Remarkably, physicians commonly engage in a diagnostic pursuit of the primary tumor for more than one week before proving the type of cancer causing the problem.

1. **Patients with metastases to neck lymph nodes only.** Suspicious cervical nodes should not undergo excisional biopsy until a complete diagnostic evaluation of the head and neck has been performed (see sec. **V.B.1**). Approximately 30 to 40 percent of these patients have potentially curable cancers of the aerodigestive tract. This is not the case for patients with supraclavicular lymph nodes, which may be directly excised for histologic examination.

2. **Other patients who have suspected metastatic cancer**

    a. **Biopsy of the most accessible site** should be performed **before** specialized blood or radiologic studies are done; the histologic findings provide an invaluable guide for a rational diagnostic workup. Biopsy proof of metastatic cancer is necessary *at only one site*. If several areas of tumor involvement are suggested by the findings from the screening evaluation, the preferred biopsy site is that associated with the least morbidity (e.g., peripheral lymph nodes when palpable, bone marrow when a leukoerythroblastic blood picture is present, cytology of sampled effusions, or suspect skin lesions). The biopsy specimen should be placed in a fixative that allows immunoperoxidase analysis (e.g., B5-fixative) and perhaps electron microscopy (e.g., Karnofsky fixative) to be done well.

    b. **Frozen sections of the biopsy material** should be obtained in female patients. If a frozen section shows adenocarcinoma, tissue should be submitted for ER determination. Although many tumors have ER, levels of more than 20 fmol/mg protein are strongly suggestive of breast cancer in women.

    c. **Poorly differentiated, undifferentiated, or anaplastic carcinomas** should be further evaluated with immunoperoxidase stains and, if possible, electron microscopy (see Appendices C1 and C2 for potentially helpful findings and markers).

        (1) Immunoperoxidase stains for cytokeratin, vimentin, leukocyte common antigen (for lymphoma), S100 protein (or other marker for melanoma), and PSA appear to be the most useful in the evaluation of patients with the MUO syndrome.

        (2) Immunoperoxidase stains for β-HCG and α-FP are frequently performed for the possibility of a germ cell neoplasm, but have not been found to be useful in these patients.

        (3) Electron microscopy for undifferentiated small cell and large cell neoplasms is used to evaluate for possible secretory granules, oat cell carcinoma, melanoma, and lymphoma (see Appendix C1).

B. Role of the pathologist. Close communication between the clinician and the pathologist is especially important in cases of MUO. Morphologic clues may make certain anatomic sites more likely and direct the sequence of investigation. Histologic problems include

    1. Poorly differentiated tumors, including adenocarcinomas, epidermoid carcinomas, and small cell neoplasms, may be indistinguishable by light microscopy.

    2. Squamous metaplasia overlying adenocarcinoma may be misread as squamous cell cancer.

    3. Extensive fibrosis, a common sequela of squamous cell carcinoma and breast adenocarcinoma, may mask the underlying tumor.

    4. Limitations of pathology. Pathologists are able to identify the primary site based on review of the biopsy alone in approximately 20 percent of cases of MUO. If they are given clinical information (especially the site of metastasis), the accuracy doubles. However, the histologic appearance of these tumors usually defies categorization for the origin of the tumor.

C. Histologic types of metastases

    1. Adenocarcinomas and undifferentiated carcinomas account for more than 75 percent of cases of MUO. The natural history, prognosis, and poor responsiveness to therapy are similar for both these histopathologies.

        a. Histologic clues for origin of adenocarcinomas are discussed in Appendix C1.

        b. Undifferentiated and poorly differentiated large cell neoplasms may represent carcinoma, extragonadal germ cell tumors, or large cell lymphoma. Lymphomas rarely are mistaken for adenocarcinomas, but the chance of confusion is increased if the tissue obtained is small or of poor quality. For example, gastric lymphoma and Ki-1 lymphoma (a T cell malignancy characterized by long survival times and spontaneous remissions) are frequently misdiagnosed as carcinoma. These lymphomas, in particular, require special study with immunoperoxidase or electron microscopy techniques.

        c. The primary site is determined antemortem in only 15 percent of cases, even with exhaustive diagnostic efforts. When a primary site is determined, the sites of origin and relative frequencies are as follows:

            (1) Pancreas (25%)

            (2) Lung (20%)

            (3) Stomach, colorectum, hepatobiliary tract (8–12% each)

            (4) Kidney (5%)

            (5) Breast, ovary, prostate (2–3% each)

            (6) Other sites (<1% each)

    2. SCCs account for 10 to 15 percent of all MUO cases and less than 5 percent if patients with metastases to cervical lymph nodes alone are excluded. Most squamous cancers that appear as MUO originate in the head and neck or lung. Other SCC primary sites include the uterine cervix, penis, anus, rectum, esophagus, and, occasionally, urinary bladder. Acanthocarcinomas (squamoid tumors) may develop in the GI tract, notably in the pancreas and stomach. Squamous skin cancer that arises in a chronic osteomyelitis fistula may not be apparent until regional draining lymph nodes become involved.

    3. Undifferentiated small cell neoplasms develop in the entire alimentary

Table 20-1. Histology of neck node metastases from unknown primary site

Lymph nodes	Histopathology: relative frequencies (%)			
	Squamous cell carcinoma	Undifferentiated carcinoma	Adenocarcinoma	Other*
Upper to middle cervical	60	25	10	5
Lower cervical	45	40	5	10
Supraclavicular	20	45	35	

*Malignant melanoma accounts for the majority of cases with other histologies.

canal, upper aerodigestive tract, thymus, uterine cervix and endometrium, breast, prostate, urinary bladder, and skin, as well as the lung; approximately 2.5 percent of small cell carcinomas originate in extrapulmonary sites. Although this subtype is only a small percentage of the patients who present with MUO, it represents one of the treatable varieties.

Very poorly differentiated small cell neoplasms may also represent a number of cancers that can be recalled with the mnemonic *MR. MOLTEN* (*M*yeloma, *R*habdomyoblastoma, *M*elanoma [amelanotic], *O*at cell carcinoma, *L*ymphoma, *T*esticular carcinoma [anaplastic seminoma], *E*wing's sarcoma, *N*euroblastoma).

4. **Melanoma** constitutes 2 to 5 percent of all cases of MUO. Approximately 4 percent of malignant melanoma cases present as MUO. It is important to distinguish melanoma from other histologies because metastases frequently involve lymph nodes alone, and these patients may be cured with appropriate therapy (see sec. **V.D**).

   a. Amelanotic melanoma may be mistaken as undifferentiated carcinoma. Malignant melanoma may be distinguished from tumors having obscure histology by use of electron microscopy, immunohistochemical techniques, and perhaps by measuring in serum or urine S100 protein (a cytoplasmic protein that is specific for nervous system tissue and is also present on human melanoma cell lines).

   b. Explanations of how melanoma can present as MUO
      (1) The primary lesion may have been destroyed (e.g., by prior excision or cautery), *or*
      (2) The primary lesion may have regressed spontaneously, *or*
      (3) The tumor may have arisen de novo within a lymph node.

III. **Sites of metastases, natural history, and survival**
   A. **Manifestations.** Symptoms of metastasis, which are present in nearly all patients with the MUO syndrome, are multiple in 30 percent of patients. The most frequent presenting features are
      1. Pain (60%)
      2. Liver mass or other abdominal manifestations (40%)
      3. Lymphadenopathy (20%)
      4. Bone pain or pathologic fracture (15%)
      5. Respiratory symptoms (15%)
      6. CNS abnormalities (5%)
      7. Weight loss (5%)
      8. Skin nodules (2%)
   B. **Sites of metastatic tumors**
      1. **Neck lymph nodes.** Neck masses in adults, other than thyroid nodules, are malignant in 80 percent of cases. After 50 years of age, 90 percent of neck masses are malignant. The histologic type of metastases to neck nodes varies in incidence according to anatomic location (Table 20-1); the probability for squamous carcinoma rises the higher the node is on the chain. Involved

nodes are single in 75 percent of patients, multiple but ipsilateral in 15 percent, and bilateral in 10 percent. Multiplicity is often associated with adenocarcinoma.

   a. Cervical nodes (70% of cases). The primary site of most squamous tumors that present as MUO in the upper half of the neck is the upper respiratory passages. With skillful endoscopic evaluation and modern CT scanning technology, a primary site can be determined in at least 30 percent of cases. Approximately 35 percent of these patients can potentially be cured.

   (1) Carcinomas of the nasopharynx, hypopharynx, base of the tongue, and tonsil present with cervical node MUO as the first manifestation of disease in 30 to 50 percent of cases. Studies have shown that these sites or the larynx harbored the primary tumor 95 percent of the time when the primary site was found to be head and neck cancer that initially manifested as MUO.

   (2) About two-thirds of metastases to the low cervical nodes originate in sites below the clavicle, most commonly in the lung.

   b. Supraclavicular nodes (30% of cases). Involvement of this group of lymph nodes with malignancy nearly always indicates disease that is far advanced. The primary site is detected in only about 15 percent of cases presenting as metastases to supraclavicular lymph nodes.

2. Axillary lymph nodes. Axillary lymphadenopathy that is excised for diagnosis is found to have benign disease in 75 percent of cases, lymphoma in 15 percent, and solid tumors (particularly adenocarcinoma) in 10 percent.

   a. The most likely sites of origin of a solid tumor metastasizing to the axilla are the breast, lung, arm, and regional trunk. In patients with isolated malignant axillary lymphadenopathy, the primary site is detected in only one-half of cases.

   b. Breast cancer. Breast cancer accounts for 70 percent of cases of MUO involving axillary lymph nodes in women when the primary site is eventually diagnosed. About 0.5 percent of all breast cancer patients present with masses palpable in the axilla and not in the breast.

3. Groin lymph nodes. The primary tumor is detectable in 99 percent of patients having malignant groin lymphadenopathy. Metastases are most likely to arise from the skin (especially the lower extremities and lower half of the trunk), genital and reproductive organs, rectum, anus, or urinary bladder. If a primary tumor is not evident, a lymphoproliferative disease is most frequently the cause.

4. Other sites of metastases. The incidence of clinically significant metastases to specific organs in patients with known primary tumor sites is shown in Table 1-2. The most likely primary tumor sites according to the histology and site of metastases are shown in Table 20-2. These correlations may have limited usefulness in patients with MUO, however, because of the frequent occurrence of atypical metastatic patterns (see sec. **III.C**). Special considerations for each site are

   a. Bone and bone marrow metastases

   (1) Bone cortex. When a primary site is found, carcinoma of the lung accounts for the great majority of patients with MUO who have bone metastases. When presenting as a MUO, pancreatic carcinoma frequently involves the skeleton. The median survival of patients presenting with MUO and predominantly bone metastases is three months.

   (2) Bone marrow is shown to be involved (by aspiration or biopsy techniques) in 10 to 15 percent of MUO cases during life, particularly in patients who prove to have lung, breast, or prostate cancer. Leukoerythroblastotic peripheral blood smears are the most accurate barometers of bone marrow involvement in patients with solid tumors (see Chap. 34, *Cytopenia*, sec. **I.A**). The median survival of patients

Table 20-2. Probability of primary site according to site of presentation

Presentation	Probable site of origin
Lymph nodes	
Upper and middle cervical	Head and neck tissues
Lower cervical and supraclavicular	
Right side	Lung, breast
Left side	GI, lung (upper lobe), breast
Axillary	Breast, upper extremity, stomach (very rarely)
Inguinal	Lower extremity, vulva, anus/rectum, bladder, prostate
Skin	Lung, breast, kidney, ovary, melanoma
Lower extremity	Kidney
Abdomen and upper extremity	Colon, bladder
Umbilicus	Stomach, pancreas, colon
Brain	Lung, breast, melanoma
Lung	Lung, breast, GI, GU
Pleura	Lung, breast, stomach, pancreas, liver
Pericardium	Lung, breast, lymphoma, melanoma
Liver	Pancreas, stomach, colon, lung, breast
Ascites	Ovary, pancreas, stomach, colon
Bone marrow	Breast, lung (small cell), prostate, thyroid
Bone	
Osteolytic lesions	Myeloma, breast, lung (non-small cell), thyroid
Osteoblastic lesions	Prostate, sarcoma, carcinoid, Hodgkin's disease, lung (small cell)
Mixed lesions	Breast
Spinal cord compression	Lung, breast, prostate, kidney, GI, sarcoma, lymphoma, myeloma
High thoracic	Breast, lung
Lumbar	Lymphoma, prostate
Migratory thrombophlebitis	Pancreas, lung, GI

Key: GI = gastrointestinal tract; GU = genitourinary tract.

presenting with MUO and marrow metastases is less than one month.

b. Intrathoracic metastases

(1) Pulmonary metastases may be solitary, and primary lung cancer lesions may be multiple. MUO presenting as a solitary pulmonary nodule is quite rare; when it does occur, it is most frequently associated with colorectal carcinoma or sarcoma. The median survival of patients presenting with MUO and predominantly intrathoracic metastases is variable.

(2) Effusions. Pleural effusions, when caused by malignant disease, are associated with an unknown primary tumor in 20 percent of cases. Pericardial effusions rarely occur as the predominant manifestation of MUO.

c. Intra-abdominal metastases most frequently involve the liver and originate in the GI tract, but the primary site is determined during life in only about 30 percent of cases.

(1) Liver metastases. Differentiating between primary hepatocellular carcinoma and metastatic carcinoma of unknown origin in the liver may be difficult. Carcinomas of the prostate or ovary metastasize to the liver more frequently when they present as MUO than when they occur as known primaries. The median survival of patients presenting with MUO and predominantly liver metastases is less than four months.

(2) Ascites, when caused by malignant disease, is associated with MUO in 10 percent of cases. The median survival of patients presenting with MUO and predominantly malignant ascites is less than one month except for women with peritoneal carcinomatosis that is considered to be a variant of ovarian carcinoma (see sec. **V.F**).

d. CNS metastases

(1) Brain metastases are most frequently associated with bronchogenic carcinoma and second most frequently with the MUO syndrome. The primary site eventually becomes evident during life in 40 percent of cases, and 90 percent of these are lung carcinoma. Excision of single metastatic brain lesions does not improve survival beyond that experienced by other patients with the MUO syndrome. The median survival of patients presenting with MUO and single brain metastasis that is resected is three to six months.

(2) Spinal cord compression is occasionally a manifestation of MUO syndrome. In these cases, laminectomy has been traditionally recommended as the first step to establish the histopathologic diagnosis. However, the median survival of patients presenting with MUO and epidural metastasis is less than two months, and such an aggressive approach is often not justified.

e. Cutaneous metastases are associated with carcinomas of the breast and lung in the vast majority of cases. When skin metastases represent the initial manifestation of cancer, renal adenocarcinoma or bronchogenic carcinoma is the most likely possibility. The region of the skin near the primary tumor is most often involved. **Umbilical nodules** ("Sister Joseph's nodules") represent intra-abdominal carcinomatosis. The median survival of patients presenting with MUO and predominantly skin metastases is seven months if the primary site does not prove to be the lung.

C. Aberrant natural history of tumors in the MUO syndrome compromises the ability to predict the primary site of disease.

1. Origin. Carcinomas that occur commonly in the general population (namely carcinoma of the breast, prostate, and bowel) make up only a small percentage of the patients with MUO. Approximately 75 percent of tumors in the MUO syndrome originate below the diaphragm.

2. Patterns of dissemination by tumors do not follow typical pathways in the MUO syndrome. Examples are

Metastatic site involved (% of cases)

Type of carcinoma	Site	With primary site known	With MUO
Lung	Bone	30–50	5
Pancreas	Bone	5–10	30
Prostate	Liver or lung	15	>50

D. Survival. *The prognosis in patients with the MUO syndrome is unaffected by whether the primary lesion is ever found.*

1. Five-year survivals according to sites of involvement are as follows:

a. Upper or middle cervical nodes alone (30–50%)

b. Axillary nodes alone (25%)

c. Groin nodes alone (50%) (perhaps)

d. Midline distribution with poorly differentiated adenocarcinoma, particularly in young men (30%)

e. Any other metastatic site (<5%)

2. Patients with metastases to sites other than peripheral lymph nodes

alone. The median survival for all patients ranges between less than one month and five months. Survival depends on the sites of metastases, extent of disease, and the patient's performance status. More than 75 percent of patients die within one year of diagnosis. Subcutaneous metastases have a more favorable prognosis if the primary site is not the lung; bone marrow and epidural metastases have the worst prognosis (median survival less than one month). Patients who are less than 57 years old and who have a good performance status have a relatively better prognosis.

IV. **Searching for the primary tumor site.** When the primary site of metastases is evident, the biopsy is performed one week earlier than when patients present with MUO, and the number of diagnostic tests ordered is significantly fewer than when patients present with MUO. Unfortunately, the usual behavior of physicians is to delay biopsy while in pursuit of a primary site via a prolonged investigative pathway with a bewildering scope of expensive, time-consuming, and potentially dangerous tests.

Even if all patients undergo exhaustive evaluation with barium enema, upper GI series, IVP, skeletal survey, lung tomography, mammography (women), abdominal and pelvic CT scans, endoscopy, and a variety of radionuclide scans, *less than 15 percent* of patients with the MUO syndrome (excluding those who have disease only in cervical nodes) have the primary site established before death. Part of the 15 percent includes patients in whom the primary tumor becomes clinically evident on follow-up. The primary tumor site remains undiagnosed in 30 percent of patients even after postmortem examination.

Searching for the primary tumor site should be guided by the following questions:

A. **What are the clinical clues?**
1. **Histology** (see sec. II). The finding of squamous carcinoma obviates the need to investigate organs in which adenocarcinomas develop. If the pathologist is not certain of the diagnosis because of the morphology or quality of the specimen, special studies (see sec. II.A.2) or another biopsy may be in order.
2. **Presentation.** The history, physical examination, and screening studies should be reviewed with awareness of the natural histories of the potentially causal malignancies. The atypical behavior patterns of certain malignancies when presenting as MUO should also be remembered (see sec. III.C).

B. **Which advanced malignancies are treatable?**
1. **Metastases to unilateral lymph nodes alone**
   a. Melanoma to peripheral lymph nodes in a single region
   b. Squamous cell or undifferentiated carcinoma in the upper two-thirds of the cervical chain
   c. Adenocarcinoma in the axillary chain
   d. Carcinoma in groin nodes
2. **Metastases that are exquisitely sensitive to chemotherapy**
   a. Small cell carcinomas
   b. Peritoneal carcinomatosis in women
   c. Poorly differentiated carcinoma metastatic to retroperitoneum, mediastinum, or peripheral lymph nodes, particularly in men
   d. Adenocarcinomas that are treatable in advanced stages (breast, ovary, prostate, and thyroid) constitute less than 15 percent of cases of MUO. These tumors should be considered in patients with appropriate constellations of findings.
   e. Lymphomas should be considered in any patient with a poorly differentiated or undifferentiated neoplasm (see sec. II.C.1.b).

C. **What are the limitations of diagnostic studies?** Despite subjection to an alarming battery of tests, more than 85 percent of patients with MUO do not have the primary site determined while they are alive. Furthermore, many of the diagnostic tests are *just as frequently misleading as they are helpful.*
1. **Pathology.** Review of the initial biopsy does not contribute to the origin of the malignant neoplasm in 80 percent of cases of MUO. Histopathologic classification of tumors can vary by more than 50 percent among different reviewers of the same specimen.

2. **Chest x-ray films.** No chest x-ray pattern, including the number of lesions, can distinguish a metastasis from a primary lung cancer.

3. **Upper GI series, barium enema (BE), and IVP.** Fewer than 5 percent of patients with MUO who undergo these studies have abnormal results in the absence of abdominal symptoms, occult blood in the stools, or hematuria. Abnormal results usually consist of findings that provide no useful information (e.g., organ displacement by tumor) in the presence of these manifestations. Upper GI series, BE, and IVP each suggest a primary malignant lesion in 5 to 10 percent of cases of MUO; the numbers of true-positive, false-positive, and the minimum number of false-negative results are about equal, however.

4. **CT scans** have not improved the frequency of detecting occult primary sites except in the head and neck.

5. **Radionuclide scans.** *Staging disease in asymptomatic sites is a dubious practice for patients with disease that is already considered lethal.*

   a. **Thyroid scans** are associated with equal frequencies of true-positive, false-positive, and false-negative results. Thus these scans are virtually useless in MUO.

   b. **Liver scans** are rarely abnormal in patients with no more than one abnormality on LFTs and a normal-sized liver on physical examination. The scans are abnormal in more than 70 percent of patients with MUO and either two or more abnormal LFTs (especially alkaline phosphatase) or palpable livers.

   c. **Bone scans** may be abnormal in the absence of symptoms related to the skeleton and may be useful for determining the extent of disease if that information is believed to be helpful.

   d. **Gallium scans** are useless in MUO.

6. **Ultrasonograms** have a high rate of false-positivity in the evaluation of MUO, giving particularly erroneous results in retroperitoneal areas.

7. **Arteriography and screening endoscopy,** including bronchoscopy, upper GI endoscopy, sigmoidoscopy, and colonoscopy, are overly invasive and of no value in the MUO syndrome.

V. **Management.** The author's recommendations for the treatment of patients with the MUO syndrome are diagramed in Figure 20-1.

A. **Malignant melanoma involving peripheral lymph nodes only**

1. **Evaluation**

   a. Inquire about skin lesions that may have been removed previously.

   b. Search the skin carefully for a possible primary lesion; biopsy any suspect lesion.

   c. Exclude visceral disease with history and physical examination (especially ophthalmoscopy), chest x-ray films, LFTs, and CT scans of the liver and brain.

2. **Recommended treatment** for malignant melanoma involving lymph nodes alone is *radical lymphadenectomy* of the affected nodal region. The procedure is repeated if the tumor recurs and the patient has no other evidence of disease.

3. **Results of treatment.** Both the five- and 10-year survivals using radical lymphadenectomy are 30 to 45 percent. The prognosis with lymphatic metastasis is affected neither by knowing the primary site nor by having a history of a preexisting lesion. The prognosis is best if the metastasis involves only one node, and not the cervical chain, and if surgical intervention is prompt and aggressive.

B. **Metastatic disease in neck lymph nodes only**

1. **Evaluation.** The recommended sequence of evaluation of cases of potentially cancerous cervical nodes is as follows:

   a. **Initial evaluation.** Carefully inspect and palpate all accessible areas of the mouth and nose. Then perform a complete evaluation of the upper airways, especially the nasopharynx, with mirrors or a Hopkin's laryngoscope.

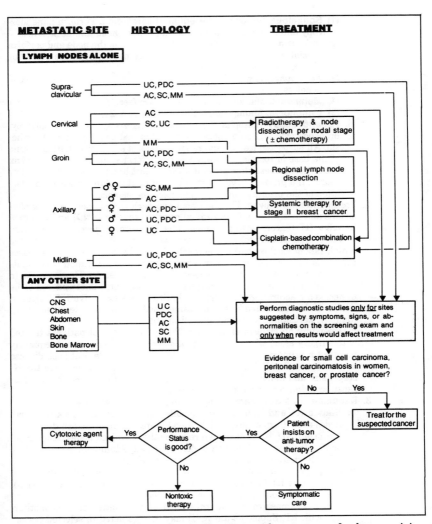

Fig. 20-1. An approach to the treatment of patients with metastases of unknown origin. AC = adenocarcinoma; PDC = poorly differentiated carcinoma; SC = squamous cell carcinoma; UC = undifferentiated carcinoma; MM = malignant melanoma; CNS = central nervous system.

    b. Imaging. Obtain a CT or MRI scan of the neck and paranasal sinuses to search for a primary tumor. [18F]-2-fluorodeoxyglucose imaging with position emission tomography (PET) appears to be a promising new method to detect the primary site for squamous cell carcinoma MUO of the head and neck.

    c. Biopsy. If these efforts fail to demonstrate any hint of a primary cancer and if pathologic expertise is available, fine-needle aspiration biopsy is performed. The results of cytologic evaluation direct further evaluation as follows:

(1) **Squamous cell or undifferentiated carcinoma.** Perform panendoscopy and manage the patient for a primary head and neck cancer.

(2) **Indeterminate or equivocal histology.** Excise the node and perform special studies on the tissue such as immunoperoxidase stains or electron microscopy as necessary.

(3) **Adenocarcinoma.** Manage as for MUO to viscera. The outlook is hopeless.

(4) **Melanoma.** Manage as discussed above (sec. **V.A**).

(5) **Lymphoma.** Manage accordingly (see Chap. 21).

d. **Panendoscopy** (nasopharyngoscopy, laryngoscopy with tracheoscopy, bronchoscopy, and esophagoscopy) is performed under general anesthesia. All suspected lesions and random areas of apparently normal tissue of the base of tongue, tonsillar fossa, pyriform sinus, and nasopharynx are biopsied; these sites are statistically most likely to harbor a primary source. If a primary tumor is found, treatment is planned with consideration of the primary and presumed neck metastasis.

2. **Treatment alternatives.** The treatment approach varies greatly among physicians and institutions. Both **radical neck dissection (RND)** and **comprehensive RT** (encompassing the nasopharynx, oropharynx, hypopharynx, and both sides of the neck), particularly when used in combination, achieve a high rate of local control in the involved neck. In theory, RT encompasses the undiscovered primary tumor. The complications associated with treatment are discussed in Chap. 7, *General Principles,* sec. **VI.** However, RT to encompass all potential nasopharyngeal drainage sites is considered to be unnecessary according to several authorities; less extensive RT has been shown to be associated with the same good results and less morbidity (namely, xerostomia and other complications).

Depending on criteria of selection, 20 to 50 percent of patients treated with surgery alone will develop contralateral neck disease or subsequently manifest a primary tumor site. The incidence of contralateral neck disease is much less after RT. The major factors influencing prognosis are the N-stage (size and multiplicity of nodes) and the presence or absence of extracapsular extension into connective tissue.

3. **Recommended treatment** (many centers use RT for all cases)

a. **Stages N1 and N2a** (solitary, mobile, upper or middle neck node; N1 nodes are 3.0 cm or less and N2a nodes are 6.0 cm or less in diameter). Perform RND. If the specimen reveals other involved nodes (stage N2b) or if extracapsular invasion is demonstrated, administer postoperative RT. Alternatively, treat patients with RT alone.

b. **Stage N2b** (multiple, larger [less than 6 cm] upper and middle neck nodes). Use RT followed by RND in three to six weeks (or vice versa). Adjuvant chemotherapy can be considered.

c. **Stage N3** (massive or bilateral nodes). Use cisplatin-based chemotherapy with RT. Supplemental RND may be considered in selected cases.

d. **Squamous cell carcinoma of low cervical or supraclavicular nodes or adenocarcinomas.** Administer RT alone (survival rates are poor no matter what is done; the goal of treatment is control of local disease).

4. **Results of treatment**

a. **Patients with upper neck nodes.** The five-year survival for all patients is 30 percent if the primary tumor is eventually found and 60 percent if it is not found.

(1) Stage N1 or N2a. The five- and 10-year survival is 80 percent.

(2) Stage N2b. The reported survival rates are variable.

(3) Stage N3. The five-year survival is 20 percent.

b. **Patients with low cervical or supraclavicular node metastases.** The five-year survival is 5 percent (median survival is seven months).

C. **Metastatic disease in unilateral axillary lymph nodes only.** The major treatable malignancies presenting as MUO in axillary lymph nodes are occult breast carcinoma, amelanotic melanoma mistaken as undifferentiated carcinoma, and malignant lymphoma mistaken as carcinomas. Axillary metastases from breast cancer without an evident breast mass are most likely to emanate from the upper outer quadrant of the ipsilateral breast.

1. **Evaluation**
   a. Search for a primary site in the breasts, lungs, and regional skin.
   b. If no primary lesion is found, perform an excisional biopsy.
   c. In women with adenocarcinoma or poorly differentiated carcinoma, mammography (although the diagnostic yield is poor) and ER assessment on the frozen section should be performed.

2. **Occult breast cancer** (axillary nodal metastasis without a clinically detectable primary tumor in the breast) accounts for 0.5 percent of all breast cancer patients. Ultimately, 30 to 50 percent of patients develop evidence for a primary breast cancer. The primary tumor becomes evident in less than 20 percent of these patients if the breast is treated with RT. Approximately 55 percent of these tumors are ER-negative.

3. **Recommended treatment**
   a. **Lymphoma.** See Chap. 21.
   b. **Malignant melanoma.** See sec. **D.**
   c. **Women with adenocarcinoma or poorly differentiated carcinoma.** Treat for stage II breast cancer. Mastectomy had been traditionally performed, but is not justifiable in these patients.
   d. **Other patients.** Axillary node dissection attempting to achieve local control and long-term survival.
   e. **RT** to the axilla is frequently given, but is not recommended because there is no evidence to indicate that survival is improved over that achieved with resection of the involved nodes alone.

4. **Results of treatment.** Patients who have MUO and prove to have breast cancer can be expected to have the same survival as patients with stage II disease. The five-year and 10-year survival rates are identical with and without mastectomy and with and without the primary tumor ever becoming manifest. All other patients who are treated with excision of clinically involved nodes or axillary dissection have a 20 to 25 percent long-term survival (2–10 years).

D. **Metastatic disease in unilateral groin lymph nodes only**
   1. **Evaluation**
      a. Search for a primary site on the skin, anus, rectum, pelvis, and lower urinary tract.
      b. If no primary lesion is found, perform an excisional biopsy.
   2. **Recommended treatment**
      a. **Lymphoma.** See Chap. 21.
      b. **Melanoma.** See sec. **V.A.**
      c. **Carcinoma.** Perform a superficial groin node dissection (affords local control with less morbidity than radical dissection). Simple excision of the involved node may be sufficient treatment, however.
      d. **RT** does not appear to be necessary.
   3. **Results of treatment.** Half of patients treated with excisional biopsy or superficial groin dissection alone appear to survive more than two years. A proportion of these patients had unclassifiable carcinomas that may have been amelanotic melanoma.

E. **Poorly differentiated carcinoma with a midline distribution** (especially in men)
   1. **Evaluation**
      a. Perform CT scans of the chest, abdomen, and pelvis.
      b. Measure serum levels of β-HCG and α-FP, but the results do not affect the probability of response to treatment.
   2. **Recommended treatment.** Administer four cycles of cisplatin-based combination chemotherapy using regimens recommended for testicular cancer.
   3. **Results of treatment.** The response rate with disease confined to the mediastinum, retroperitoneum, or peripheral lymph nodes is 75 percent, with complete remissions observed in 45 percent of patients and long-term sur-

vival in 70 percent of those achieving a complete remission. The five-year survival is 35 percent for patients with disease confined to the retroperitoneum and peripheral lymph nodes and 15 percent for those with disease affecting predominantly the mediastinum. For patients with metastases to other sites, the response rate is 20 percent and five-year survival rate is 7 percent.

F. Peritoneal carcinomatosis in women
  1. Evaluation
    a. Perform paracentesis with cytologic and biochemical analysis of the ascitic fluid.
    b. Rule out other causes of malignant ascites clinically.
    c. Perform CT scans of the abdomen and pelvis.
  2. Recommended treatment. If no extraovarian primary site is evident, perform exploratory laparotomy. If peritoneal carcinomatosis is confirmed without an extraovarian primary site, treat the patient as if she had ovarian carcinoma by performing total abdominal hysterectomy, bilateral salpingo-oophorectomy, omentectomy, and cytoreductive debulking of metastases. Thereafter, treat with a platin-based combination chemotherapy regimen for six to eight months. Second look laparotomy is not a consideration in these patients.
  3. Results of treatment. The median survival rates are 1.5 to 2.0 years for all patients, 2.5 years for patients with limited residual disease after surgery, and 1.0 year for patients with extensive residual disease after surgery. Ten to 25 percent of patients survive three years.

G. Small cell carcinoma MUO
  1. Evaluation
    a. Perform CT scans of the chest and abdomen.
    b. Perform bone marrow biopsy if the patient has a leukoerythroblastic anemia or increased serum alkaline phosphatase.
    c. Evaluate the biopsy with panneuroendocrine markers (e.g., chromogranin, synaptophysin, neuron-specific enolase).
  2. Recommended treatment. Use cisplatin-based combination chemotherapy. If a complete remission is obtained, consider administering RT to the known previous sites of disease. For patients with small cell carcinoma MUO to cervical lymph nodes alone, some authorities recommend treatment with RND or RT alone.
  3. Results of treatment. The response rate to chemotherapy is about 70 percent. Long-term survival is seen in patients who achieve a CR after treatment for limited disease. Prolonged survival also occurs in patients presenting with cervical node metastases from occult primary small cell tumors in the minor salivary glands or paranasal sinuses after treatment with RND or RT alone.

H. All other patients with the MUO syndrome
  1. Evaluation. Because of the very low frequency of detecting the primary site in patients with MUO and the frequently misleading results of radiologic studies, x-ray or radionuclide studies are justified only in the presence of either specific abnormalities in the screening evaluation or possibilities suggested by review of histopathology. When the initial database does not suggest a primary organ site, further evaluation is usually fruitless and is not indicated. Even when the primary site can be determined, therapy is not likely to be affected. It is important to recognize that these patients have *incurable* cancer that is usually *refractory to treatment.* With the exception of treatable malignancies, documenting a site is more important to the patient (or physician) psychologically than therapeutically.

  All patients should receive a complete history and physical examination (including the rectum and pelvis), chest x-ray film, urinalysis, CBC, and serum liver and renal function tests. In patients with **adenocarcinoma or undifferentiated carcinoma,** perform the following:

a. **Women.** Mammograms, careful pelvic examination, and ER assessment of the biopsy specimen.
b. **Men.** Careful examination of the testes and prostate gland, possibly in conjunction with random needle biopsies of the prostate (if there is an elevated serum acid phosphatase level, unexplained lower extremity edema, or pelvic bone metastases. Obtain the following:
   (1) Serum PSA
   (2) β-HCG and α-FP in men with findings consistent with a germ cell neoplasm (see sec. **V.E.1.b**)
2. **Recommended treatment** for patients who may have specific neoplasms is as follows for findings consistent with
   a. **Breast carcinoma** in women (e.g., bone or upper torso soft tissue metastases, even with negative mammography results)
      (1) **ER-positive tumors,** even with negative mammography results: tamoxifen
      (2) **ER-negative tumors:** CMF combination chemotherapy (see Appendix A1)
   b. **Prostate carcinoma** (e.g., men with metastases mostly to pelvic bones, particularly if the serum acid phosphatase level is elevated): diethylstilbestrol or leuprolide with flutamide.
3. **Recommended treatment for other patients.** Nearly 90 percent of patients who have MUO have metastases from cancers of the pancreas, GI tract, lung, and other or never-to-be-known sites that are usually refractory to chemotherapy. Only about 20 percent of patients with adenocarcinomatous MUO who have been treated with 5-FU (alone or in combination with other agents) experience partial tumor regression. Partial responses are associated with only a minimal (if any) improvement in survival. Combination chemotherapy regimens have response rates of less than 30 percent. Median survival is reported to be improved by four to six months in patients who respond to therapy compared with those who do not; this form of reporting data, however, is largely discredited.

   For most patients with MUO, particularly those with low performance status, we do not recommend chemotherapy. Our recommendations are as follows for patients who request therapy and who have
   a. **Good performance status.** Combination chemotherapy (see Appendix A1)
   b. **Poor performance status.** Fluorouracil alone, nontoxic drugs, or nontoxic drug dosages

---

Selected Reading

Abbruzzese, J. L., et al. The biology of unknown primary tumors. *Semin. Oncol.* 20:238, 1993.

Casciato, D. A. Chapter 103, Metastases of unknown origin. In Haskell, C. M. (ed.). *Cancer Treatment* (4th ed.) Philadelphia: W. B. Saunders, 1994.

Coster, J. R., et al. Cervical nodal metastasis of squamous cell carcinoma of unknown origin: indications for withholding radiation therapy. *Int. J. Radiat. Oncol. Biol. Phys.* 23:743, 1992.

Farag, S. S., et al. Delay by internists in obtaining diagnostic biopsies in patients with suspected cancer. *Ann. Intern. Med.* 116:473, 1992.

Hainsworth, J. D., Johnson, D. H., and Greco, F. A. Cisplatin-based combination chemotherapy in the treatment of poorly differentiated carcinoma and poorly differentiated adenocarcinoma of unknown primary site: results of a 12-year experience. *J. Clin. Oncol.* 10:912, 1992.

Kemeny, M. M. Mastectomy: is it necessary for occult breast cancer? *N. Y. State J. Med.* 92:516, 1992.

Le Chevalier, T., et al. Early metastatic cancer of unknown primary presentation. A clinical study of 302 consecutive autopsied patients. *Arch. Intern. Med.* 148:2035, 1988.

Remick, S. C., and Ruckdeschel, J. C. Extrapulmonary and pulmonary small-cell carcinoma: tumor biology, therapy and outcome. *Med. Pediatr. Oncol.* 20:89, 1992.

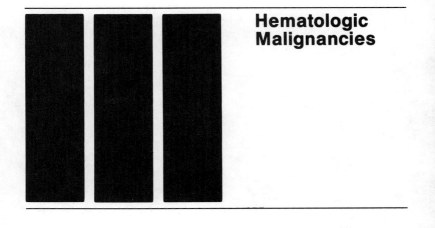

Hematologic Malignancies

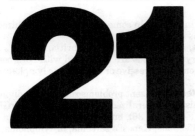

Hodgkin's Disease and Malignant Lymphoma

Peter J. Rosen

Evaluation of Suspected Lymphoma

I. Symptoms and signs
A. History
1. **Painless lymphadenopathy** involving any of the superficial lymph nodes is the most common chief complaint of patients with Hodgkin's disease (HD) and non-Hodgkin's lymphoma (NHL).
2. **Systemic symptoms.** Fevers, night sweats, and weight loss are characteristic in advanced presentations of HD and aggressive NHL but may be encountered in all stages and pathologic types of lymphoma. Marked fatigue and general weakness may also be reported.
   a. **Pruritus,** often intense, may be the presenting symptom in HD, particularly the nodular sclerosis subtype, and may antedate diagnosis by months or years.
   b. **Pel-Ebstein fever** is periodic, uncommon, but characteristic of HD.
3. **Pain**
   a. **Alcohol-induced pain** in areas of involvement is infrequent but is pathognomonic of HD.
   b. **Bone pain** may reflect localized areas of bone destruction or diffuse marrow infiltration.
   c. **Neurogenic pain** is caused by spinal cord compression, plexopathies, nerve root infiltration, meningeal involvement, and complicating varicella zoster.
   d. **Back pain** suggests massive retroperitoneal nodal involvement.
B. Physical examination should evaluate for hepatosplenomegaly, the presence of effusions, evidence of neuropathy, and signs of obstruction (e.g., extremity edema, superior vena cava syndrome, spinal cord compression, hollow viscera dysfunction). **Lymph node chains** must be carefully examined including the submental, supraclavicular, infraclavicular, epitrochlear, iliac, femoral, and popliteal nodes.
1. The lymph nodes are examined for size, multiplicity, consistency, and tenderness. Lymphomatous involvement typically imparts a rubbery consistency, not the rock-hard quality of carcinoma.
2. **The tonsils and oropharynx** are thoroughly examined. Waldeyer's ring involvement mandates complete evaluation of the naso-, oro-, and hypopharynx by endoscopy.
II. Differential diagnosis
A. Lymphadenopathy
1. **Infections.** Individuals, particularly young children with apparent viral or other infections, may develop striking lymphadenopathy. Such patients should be evaluated for infectious processes and observed for clear-cut resolution. Infectious diseases associated with lymphadenopathy include infectious mononucleosis, cytomegalovirus infection, toxoplasmosis, HIV infection, secondary syphilis, tuberculosis, atypical mycobacterial infection,

brucellosis, and some fungal infections. In some cases biopsy is required for diagnosis of specific infectious diseases.

2. **Systemic immune disorders,** such as rheumatoid arthritis, Sjögren's syndrome, and systemic lupus erythematosus are associated with both benign lymphadenopathy and lymphoma. Progressive or asymmetric lymphadenopathy mandate biopsy.

3. **Individuals at risk for HIV infection** present problems requiring individualization in management. Persistent generalized lymphadenopathy (PGL) is a part of the AIDS spectrum (see Chap. 36), but lymphadenopathy can also be caused by opportunistic infections, Kaposi's sarcoma, or lymphoma.

4. **Lymph nodes that are usually benign**
   a. **Occipital.** Consider scalp infection.
   b. **Posterior auricular.** Usually viral or scalp infection.
   c. **Shotty inguinal nodes.** Suggest lower extremity infection.

5. **Cervical nodes.** Patients with isolated enlargement of high or middle cervical lymph nodes often harbor occult primary carcinoma of the head and neck. The special approach required for these patients is discussed in Chap. 20, sections **III.B.** and **V.A.**

B. **Midline masses**

1. **Retroperitoneal masses** (see Chap. 19, sec. II)

2. **Mediastinal masses** may occur in a variety of non-neoplastic and neoplastic (both primary and metastatic) conditions (see Chap. 19, sec. I).

3. **Hilar masses.** Isolated symmetrical bilateral hilar lymphadenopathy (without mediastinal mass) is strongly suggestive of sarcoidosis, and many experts believe that observation alone could suffice in this clinical setting. Unilateral hilar masses are frequently secondary to lung cancer; metastatic disease must also be considered. Coccidioidomycosis and histoplasmosis enter the differential diagnosis in the appropriate clinical and geographic milieu.

C. **Splenomegaly.** The diagnosis can usually be made with careful history-taking and physical examination, laboratory evaluation, CT scans of abdomen, bone marrow biopsy or aspiration, and occasionally liver biopsy. When a diagnosis cannot be established by these means, careful follow-up of the patient is warranted. **Splenectomy** should be considered for diagnosis only in patients with massive or progressive isolated splenomegaly.

1. **Normal.** A palpable spleen is occasionally seen in otherwise healthy young adults of thin body habitus.

2. **Infections** include bacterial endocarditis, granulomatous infections, brucellosis, syphilis, infectious mononucleosis, cytomegalovirus infection, toxoplasmosis, and HIV.

3. **Secondary to portal hypertension** (congestive splenomegaly). Patients with chronic liver disease or portal or splenic vein thrombosis may have no other findings to direct the diagnostic search. Liver-spleen scanning reveals redistribution of the nuclide to the spleen and increased marrow uptake, strongly suggesting the diagnosis of portal hypertension.

4. **Storage diseases,** particularly Gaucher's disease, may produce prominent splenomegaly; characteristic cells are seen in the bone marrow in most cases.

5. **Tumors** are predominantly hematologic, including lymphomas and leukemias. Metastases particularly from melanoma and breast cancer and primary splenic sarcomas may also occur.

6. **Myeloproliferative disorders** such as polycythemia vera, myelofibrosis with myeloid metaplasia, essential thrombocythemia, and chronic myelogenous leukemia may cause marked splenomegaly.

7. **Autoimmune disorders.** Rheumatoid arthritis (Felty's syndrome), systemic lupus erythematosus, and autoimmune hemolytic anemia may produce splenomegaly (not isolated autoimmune thrombocytopenia) and can usually be diagnosed by history and associated laboratory findings.

Table 21-1. Comparison of Hodgkin's disease and non-Hodgkin's lymphomas

Characteristic	In Hodgkin's disease	In non-Hodgkin's lymphomas	
		Low-grade	Others
Site(s) of origin	Nodal	Extranodal ($\sim$10%)	Extranodal ($\sim$35%)
Nodal distribution	Centripetal (axial)	Centrifugal	Centrifugal
Nodal spread	Contiguous	Noncontiguous	Noncontiguous
CNS involvement	Rare (<1%)	Rare (<1%)	Uncommon (<10%)
Hepatic involvement	Uncommon	Common (>50%)	Uncommon
Bone marrow involvement	Uncommon (<10%)	Common (>50%)	Uncommon (<20%)
Marrow involvement adversely affects prognosis	Yes	No	Yes
Curable by chemotherapy	Yes	No	Yes

8. **Miscellaneous.** Splenic cysts, thyrotoxicosis, sarcoid, and amyloidosis are unusual causes of splenomegaly.
   D. **Comparison of HD and NHL** is shown in Table 21-1.
III. **Biopsy procedures**
   A. **Sites and methods of diagnostic biopsy.** Tissues or organs that are suspected of involvement are subjected to generous open biopsy for primary diagnosis wherever possible. Fine-needle aspiration cytology is mainly used for staging evaluation or for proving recurrence but may sometimes allow cytologic diagnosis *if expertise in interpretation is available.*
      1. **Peripheral node biopsy.** One of the largest accessible lymph nodes is biopsied whenever peripheral lymphadenopathy is present. Small lymph nodes may be more readily removed but may be uninvolved.
      2. **Inguinal lymph nodes** are frequently enlarged because of chronic inflammatory processes in the lower extremities. These nodes should only be biopsied when other sites are not suspect or when pathologic involvement is clearly anticipated.
      3. **Bone marrow biopsy** combined with aspiration is used for staging and may lead to diagnosis, particularly in the presence of abnormal circulating cells or cytopenias.
      4. **Mediastinoscopy or limited thoracotomy** (e.g., Chamberlain procedure) for definitive diagnosis is required for a substantial proportion of patients with mediastinal masses. These procedures are generally well tolerated and can be performed safely by experienced surgeons.
      5. **Laparotomy** is utilized to diagnose some cases of lymphoma restricted to the abdomen and should include biopsies of the liver and random lymph nodes as well as the primary area in question. If HD is suspected, splenectomy may be performed as part of a staging procedure. Staging laparotomy is performed infrequently in NHL.
      6. **Peritoneoscopy** assesses the liver and peritoneum and allows extensive biopsy, obviating the need for staging laparotomy in some patients.
      7. **Endoscopic biopsy** of gastric lymphoma may raise the possibility of carcinoma or reveal only reactive tissue. Repeated attempts with deeper biopsies

and immunoperoxidase staining for leukocyte common antigen and keratin intermediate filaments may be helpful in the differential diagnosis between lymphoma and carcinoma. Small bowel involvement beyond the duodenum usually requires open biopsy, although capsule biopsies may be suggestive of lymphoma in some cases.

8. **Retroperitoneal and mesenteric masses** may be evaluated by Trucut biopsy or fine-needle aspiration with immunologic analysis of the specimens, perhaps obviating the need for laparotomy. Such techniques are most useful for NHL and less so for HD.

B. **Handling the biopsy material.** The procured biopsy specimen is submitted to the pathologist directly and *not placed in a fixative* by the operating surgeon to ensure the best use of the available tissue. Pathology tissue processing includes

1. Performing **touch preparations** (imprints), which provide cytologic detail and material for immunologic phenotyping.

2. **Immunologic phenotyping** with monoclonal antibodies, which requires unfixed cells or tissue for indirect immunoperoxidase labeling or flow cytometry.

3. **Special handling of tissues** for procedures that may occasionally be utilized in difficult diagnostic problems or research such as electron microscopy, cytogenetics, and molecular genetic analysis.

4. Submission of material for **microbial culture** when the clinical picture or tissue suggests infection.

IV. **Clinical evaluation.** The extent of the staging evaluation is determined by the individual case presentation, the histopathologic diagnosis, and the impact of the stage on treatment planning.

A. **Evaluation of blood tests**

1. **Hematologic manifestations** are discussed in Chap. 34.

2. **Diagnostically abnormal circulating lymphoid cells** or lymphocytosis are seen in some patients with NHL, particularly the indolent forms. Lymphoid cells are characterized immunologically using flow cytometry and monoclonality may be established by kappa-lambda ratios (B cell) or gene rearrangement technology (T and B cell); these techniques are capable of detecting minute clones of circulating lymphoma cells not detectable by inspection of the blood smears.

3. **Evaluation of the erythrocyte sedimentation rate** (or other acute phase reactants such as serum copper, fibrinogen, and haptoglobin levels) may parallel disease activity especially in HD.

4. **LFTs** are unreliable in predicting lymphomatous involvement of the liver. Marked elevation of alkaline phosphatase and occasionally frank cholestatic jaundice may complicate HD as a paraneoplastic event without direct liver involvement. Extrahepatic biliary obstruction may also occur with lymphoma caused by enlarged nodes in the porta hepatis.

5. **Renal function tests.** Elevated creatinine and BUN suggest ureteral obstruction and, less commonly, direct renal involvement. Uric acid nephropathy or hypercalcemia may contribute to renal insufficiency. Frank nephrotic syndrome as a paraneoplastic phenomenon may complicate HD and other lymphomas (see Chap. 31).

6. **Serum uric acid.** Hyperuricemia is a common manifestation of high turnover rate (aggressive) NHL and may also be seen with extensive lower grade lymphomas. Treatment of high-grade NHL may provoke brisk tumor lysis leading to further elevation of uric acid and renal shutdown (see Chap. 27, sec. XIII.) Hypouricemia may be seen in HD.

7. **Hypercalcemia** has been noted in some cases of lymphoma and may be secondary to production of osteoclast activating factors such as lymphotoxin or activation of vitamin D by lymphoma tissue.

8. **Serum LDH** may reflect tumor bulk and turnover, particularly in the aggressive NHL.

9. **Serum immunoglobulins.** Diffuse (broad-based) hypergammaglobulinemia is commonly seen in HD and NHL. Hypogammaglobulinemia is particularly

common in the small lymphocytic lymphomas and late in the disease. Monoclonal spikes are seen occasionally in NHL patients.

B. Evaluation of the chest

1. **Chest x-ray** may demonstrate mediastinal and hilar lymphadenopathy, pleural effusions, and parenchymal lesions. A cavitating lesion is more typical of infection than lymphomas.

2. **CT scans** can demonstrate parenchymal and mediastinal abnormalities. Whole lung tomography may have a slight advantage in assessing the hilar regions.

3. **Thoracentesis and pleural biopsy** may demonstrate direct lymphomatous involvement of the pleura. Obstruction of mediastinal lymphatic-venous drainage may result in cytologically negative or chylous effusions.

C. Evaluation of the abdomen and retroperitoneum

1. **CT scans** are useful in delineating abnormal enlargement of nodes in retroperitoneal, mesenteric, portal, and other lymph node sites. The CT scan also detects splenomegaly and with constant enhancement may define space-occupying lesions in the liver, spleen, and kidneys.

2. **Bipedal lymphangiography (LAG)** visualizes the periaortic and iliac lymph nodes, not the mesenteric, celiac, and portal nodes. Enlargement or a foamy appearance of the nodes is characteristic of lymphomatous involvement. Experienced evaluators can achieve false-negative and false-positive rates for lymphomas that are less than 15 percent.

   a. **Advantages.** The LAG can guide the surgeon at laparotomy to verify that abnormal nodes are removed by checking intraoperative x-rays. The LAG dye persists for many months or years; abnormal nodes can be followed by abdominal flat-plate examinations. The LAG may also guide the radiotherapist in treatment planning.

   b. **Reactions.** Patients with prior pulmonary disease or extensive mediastinal or retroperitoneal involvement may develop respiratory insufficiency from the procedure because LAG dye is oil-based and results in lipid pulmonary emboli. Fever commonly complicates the procedure.

   c. **Contraindications to LAG** include iodine allergy, respiratory disease, prior pulmonary irradiation, extensive mediastinal or retroperitoneal involvement, right-left cardiac shunts, and insufficient radiologic expertise.

3. **Abdominal ultrasonography** is too insensitive to be useful in routinely assessing abdominal lymphadenopathy. It is occasionally helpful in distinguishing hepatic or splenic lesions (cystic versus solid) and in excluding an obstructive basis for renal insufficiency and jaundice.

D. Evaluation of the gastrointestinal tract. Direct involvement of the GI tract is uncommon in HD but is common in NHL. Patients with Waldeyer's ring lymphoma, suggestive GI symptoms, extensive abdominal, mesenteric nodal involvement or GI bleeding are evaluated with upper GI series and complete small bowel follow through. Barium enema may be necessary. Endoscopic examination and biopsy of accessible abnormalities are performed.

E. Evaluation of the central nervous system. Spinal fluid examination is routinely used to exclude occult lymphomatous involvement of the meninges in patients with Burkitt's lymphoma or lymphoblastic lymphoma, and is often performed in patients with intermediate- and high-grade lymphoma involving bone marrow, testes, or paranasal sinuses. Patients with AIDS-related lymphoma require CT scans of the brain and spinal fluid analysis. Symptoms suggestive of intracranial, spinal cord, or peripheral nerve involvement require immediate diagnostic evaluation.

F. Nuclear scans

1. **Gallium 67 (^{67}Ga)** scans are primarily used in assessing residual radiographic mediastinal and, less often, retroperitoneal abnormalities following therapy. Persistent ^{67}Ga uptake in these areas strongly suggests residual tumor instead of fibrosis or necrosis. To be useful in such follow-up, a ^{67}Ga body scan is recommended prior to therapy. ^{67}Ga scans are unreliable below

the diaphragm because of competing uptake in the GI tract, liver, and spleen (see Chap. 2, sec. II.B).

2. **The technetium diphosphonate (^{99}Tc) bone scan** is a sensitive technique in discovering early bone lesions and is performed whenever bone pain, alkaline phosphatase or calcium elevation, or equivocal radiographs are encountered. The ^{99}Tc bone scan is often insensitive to purely osteolytic bone lesions. HD is associated with predominantly osteoblastic bone lesions and the bone scan is hence very reliable.

Hodgkin's Disease

HD is a remarkable disorder of unknown cellular origin. The clinical spectrum varies from indolent to fulminant disease. Current therapy cures over 70 percent of patients.

I. **Epidemiology and etiology**
  A. **Incidence.** HD accounts for about 1 percent of new cancer cases annually in the United States, or 7000 to 8000 cases per year.
    1. **Age.** HD demonstrates a biomodal age-incidence curve in the United States and some industrialized European nations. The first peak, constituting predominantly the nodular sclerosis (NS) subtype, occurs in the twenties and the second peak after age 50. In third world countries, the first peak is absent, but there is a significant incidence of mixed cellularity (MC) and lymphocyte-depleted (LD) HD in male children.
    2. **Sex.** Approximately 85 percent of children with HD are male. In adults, the NS subtype of HD shows a slight female predominance, whereas the other histologic subtypes are more common in males.
  B. **Risk factors.** In Western countries the first peak of HD is associated with a higher social class, advanced education and small family size; a delayed exposure to a common infectious or other environmental agent has been suggested. Certain human leukocyte antigen (HLA) genotypes may be associated with increased susceptibility to HD; several examples of multiple sibling occurrences have been reported. Although an increased incidence of HD has not been demonstrated with HIV infection, HIV-associated HD often presents with constitutional symptoms, advanced stage (III, IV), and unusual sites of involvement (e.g., marrow, skin, leptomeninges).

II. **Pathology and natural history**
  A. **Histology**
    1. **Reed-Sternberg (R-S) cells** are giant cells that have more than one nucleus and large, eosinophilic, inclusion-like nuclei. The lineage of these cells is unknown. R-S cells and the accompanying mononuclear "Hodgkin's cells" are the putative neoplastic cells in HD.
      a. **The "lacunar cell,"** a variant of the R-S cell, characterizes NS and is often far more plentiful than classic R-S cells in that subtype.
      b. **R-S cells** in the lymphocyte-predominant (LP) subtype of HD, particularly the so-called nodular variant of LP HD, manifest B cell markers and leukocyte-common antigen (LCA). In the other types of HD, R-S cells are usually LCA-negative and express LeuM-1 (CD15) and Ki-1 (CD30), an antigen also observed in occasional NHLs (particularly the Ki-1 anaplastic large cell lymphomas).
      c. **R-S–like cells** are found in a variety of infectious, inflammatory, and neoplastic disorders, including infectious mononucleosis, lymphoid hyperplasia associated with phenytoin therapy, and immunoblastic lymphomas.
    2. **The pathologic diagnosis** of HD depends on the presence of R-S cells and their variants in an **appropriate pathologic milieu.** The bulk of lymphatic tissue involved by HD is **not** composed of neoplastic cells but rather a variety of normal-appearing lymphocytes, plasma cells, eosinophils, neutrophils, and histiocytes existing in different proportions in the four histologic

subtypes. Broad sheets of mature collagen bands subdivide the lymph nodes in NS.

3. **The Rye Classification** relates the histopathologic subtypes of HD to clinical behavior and prognosis as shown in Table 21-2.

B. **Mode of spread.** HD almost always originates in a lymph node (see Table 21-1). Whenever a primary diagnosis of HD is made in an extranodal site without contiguous nodal involvement, the diagnosis should be highly suspect. For much of its natural history, HD appears to spread in an orderly fashion via the lymphatic system by contiguity. Histologic types other than NS, however, often skip the mediastinum and disease appears in the neck and upper abdomen. Hematogenous dissemination occurs late in the course of disease and is characteristic of the LD subtype.

C. **Sites of involvement.** The axial lymphatic system is almost always affected in HD, whereas distal sites (e.g., epitrochlear and popliteal) are rarely involved.

1. **Peripheral lymph nodes.** Cervical or supraclavicular lymphadenopathy occurs in more than 70 percent of cases. Axillary and inguinal lymph nodes are less frequently involved. Generalized lymphadenopathy is atypical of HD. Left supraclavicular lymphadenopathy is more strongly associated with abdominal involvement than right-sided disease. Cervical or mediastinal involvement comprise the supradiaphragmatic presentation seen in more than 80 percent of cases.

2. **Thorax**
   a. The anterior mediastinum is a prime location for NS HD.
   b. Mediastinal precedes hilar lymph node involvement. Lung involvement may occur by direct contiguity with hilar involvement in HD as well as by hematogenous dissemination.
   c. Pulmonary involvement by HD may produce discrete nodules, irregular or interstitial, or even lobar infiltrates.
   d. Pleural effusion may occur secondary to mediastinal compression of vascular-lymphatic drainage and by direct pleural involvement. Chylous effusions occasionally occur.
   e. Pericardial involvement may be found on CT scans, but overt cardiac tamponade is uncommon.
   f. Superior vena cava syndrome may occur in HD but is more frequent in NHL.

3. **Spleen, liver, and upper abdomen**
   a. The spleen, splenic hilar nodes, and celiac nodes are the earliest abdominal sites of involvement in supradiaphragmatic HD. Mesenteric lymph nodes are rarely involved by HD.
   b. At least 25 percent of spleens not clinically enlarged harbor occult HD at laparotomy, and as many as one-half of spleens believed to be enlarged on physical examination or radiologic assessment are histologically normal. The spleen is frequently involved by HD in the absence of abnormalities on abdominal CT scan and LAG.
   c. Liver involvement is uncommon at diagnosis and is almost always associated with infiltration of the spleen.

4. **Retroperitoneal lymph node** involvement tends to occur relatively late in the course of supradiaphragmatic HD and after spleen, splenic hilar, and celiac nodal involvement. Periaortic involvement without splenic involvement is uncommon. The retroperitoneal nodes are, however, affected early in the course of inguinal presentations of HD.

5. **The bone marrow** is rarely involved at the time of diagnosis of HD. Patients with advanced stage, systemic symptoms, and MC or LD histologies have a higher risk of having bone marrow involvement. Biopsy is mandatory to evaluate the bone marrow since HD is difficult to diagnose on marrow aspirates.

6. **Bone.** Osseous involvement of HD usually produces an osteoblastic reaction mimicking prostatic carcinoma. Extradural masses may result in spinal cord compression. Sternal erosion by mediastinal NS HD may occur.

Table 21-2. Pathologic and clinical features of Hodgkin's disease subtypes

Histologic subtype	Frequency (%)	Pathology	Age (years)	Characteristics	Common stages
Lymphocyte predominant (LP)*	5	R-S cells rare; difficult pathologic diagnosis. Large polyploid cells. B cell lymphoma (nodular form)	20–40	Males; often localized disease. Late relapse; transformation to high-grade B-NHL	I–IIA
Nodular sclerosis (NS)	65–80	"Lacunar cells." Birefringent bands of collagen	15–40	Females; mediastinal, supraclavicular lymphadenopathy	I–IIIA or B
Mixed cellularity (MC)	20–35	R-S cells more frequent; necrosis; partial nodal involvement. Heterogeneous cellularity	30–50	Frequently retroperitoneal; often symptomatic	II–IVA or B
Lymphocyte depletion (LD)*	<5	Very rare. Most are probably peripheral T cell or Ki-1 lymphomas. Diffuse fibrosis and "reticular" forms	40–80	Febrile, wasting syndrome. Liver, bone marrow involvement	III–IVB

* Evolving data are consistent with the hypothesis that HD is composed of several disease entities. LP HD is almost certainly of B cell lineage. Clinically, patients with LP HD exhibit an unusual pattern of late recurrences and a high incidence of transformation to aggressive B cell NHL. Many cases previously diagnosed as LD HD are now believed to represent NHL, usually peripheral T cell lymphomas or Ki-1 anaplastic large cell lymphomas, when specialized studies are performed on fresh tissue.

7. **Other extranodal sites** are rarely involved in HD. Skin involvement is rare and usually a late manifestation of disease. CNS involvement is uncommon with the exception of spinal cord compression. Clinical involvement of meninges, brain, Waldeyer's ring, GI tract, kidney, and other extranodal sites is so rare as to suggest an alternative diagnosis.

D. **Immune abnormalities and infections.** Progressive loss of cell-mediated immunity with the development of cutaneous anergy, lymphocytopenia, and increased susceptibility to a variety of organisms is associated with advancing HD, even in the absence of therapy. Treatment with chemotherapy, corticosteroids, and radiation therapy accentuates these abnormalities. Late in the course of HD hypogammaglobulinemia may also develop.

1. **Infections associated with depressed cell-mediated immunity and therapy** (particularly corticosteroids) include *Listeria, Toxoplasma, Mycobacteria,* fungi, and slow viral infections (such as progressive multifocal leukoencephalopathy). Patients treated with corticosteroids are at a particularly increased risk for infections with *Pneumocystis carinii* and CMV.

2. **Herpes zoster** appears in over 25 percent of patients, particularly in irradiated dermatomes and in patients undergoing splenectomy. Generalized cutaneous involvement is not uncommon, but visceral involvement is rare.

3. **Splenectomy-related infections** involve encapsulated microorganisms, particularly pneumococci and less commonly *Haemophilus influenzae* and *Salmonella*. Pneumococcal infection in an asplenic host can be rapidly fatal. Vaccination with polyvalent pneumococcal vaccine is recommended prior to splenectomy, although its effectiveness in this population is not certain. Early aggressive treatment with antibodies of all febrile patients after splenectomy is mandatory.

III. **Staging system and prognostic factors**

A. **Staging** is the most critical determinant of prognosis and treatment in HD. The Ann Arbor staging system had previously been universally used but has been recently modified to take into account important prognostic factors particularly mediastinal bulk. The modified system is called "The Cotswolds Staging Classification of HD."

1. **Cotswolds staging classification of HD**

Classification	Description
Stage I	Involvement of a single lymph node region or lymphoid structure
Stage II	Involvement of two or more lymph node regions on the same side of the diaphragm (the mediastinum is considered as a single site, whereas hilar lymph nodes are lateralized). The number of anatomical sites should be indicated by a subscript (e.g., II_3)
Stage III	Involvement of lymph node regions or structures on both sides of the diaphragm
III_1	With involvement of splenic hilar, celiac, or portal nodes
III_2	With involvement of paraaortic, iliac, and mesenteric nodes
Stage IV	Involvement of one or more extranodal sites in addition to a site for which the designation "E" has been used

2. **Designations** applicable to any disease stage

A	No symptoms
B	Fever (temperature, >38°C), drenching night sweats, unexplained loss of >10% of body weight within the preceding six months
X	Bulky disease (a mediastinal mass exceeding one-third the maximum transverse diameter of the chest or the presence of a nodal mass with a maximal dimension greater than 10 cm)
E	Involvement of a single extranodal site that is contiguous or proximal to a known nodal site
CS	Clinical stage
PS	Pathologic state (as determined by laparotomy, or biopsy)

B. Prognostic factors

1. **Stage** is clearly the single most important prognostic factor in HD. Within each stage the presence of B symptoms confers a poorer prognosis. Approximately 60 percent of patients with HD in the United States are stages I or II at the time of diagnosis. The percentage of patients with stages III or IV is generally higher in third world countries or in lower socioeconomic enclaves.

2. **Histopathology** was formerly closely related to prognosis. With advances in therapy, the value of histopathologic subtype as an independent prognostic variable (apart from stage) is less clearly defined.

3. Age greater than 60, male sex, bone marrow involvement, bulk of disease, and poor Karnofsky performance status are so closely correlated with stage, systemic symptoms, and histopathology that it is difficult to prove independent prognostic importance.

IV. Diagnosis

A. Clinical evaluation.
See *Evaluation of Suspected Lymphoma*, sec. **I. Symptoms and signs, II. Differential diagnosis, III. Biopsy procedures,** and **IV. Clinical evaluation.**

B. Staging evaluation

1. Adequate surgical biopsy reviewed by experienced hematologist.
2. Thorough history and physical examination.
3. Laboratory tests: CBC, differential, platelet count, SMA-12 equivalent, protein electrophoresis, sedimentation rate, urinalysis.
4. Chest x-ray: PA and lateral.
5. CT scan of chest (include neck), abdomen, and pelvis with contrast.
6. LAG if CT scan is normal or equivocal (unless clearly stage IV) and in cases to be subjected to laparotomy or potential radiation therapy.
7. Bone marrow aspiration and biopsy (bilateral iliac crest) unless CS IA/IIA with no anemia or other blood count depression.
8. Bone scan in presence of bone pain, or elevated serum alkaline phosphatase or calcium.
9. ^{67}Ga scans, particularly high-dose SPECT scans, are optional but are useful in follow-up of residual masses on chest x-ray or CT scan after therapy.
10. Bone x-rays to corroborate findings on bone scan or in presence of bone pain.
11. Peritoneoscopic examination with directed liver biopsies is performed in some institutions to avoid staging laparotomy when there is a high index of suspicion of liver involvement on clinical evaluation. Staging laparotomy is discussed below.

C. Staging laparotomy

1. **Background.** Systematic evaluation by staging laparotomy revealed that at least 25 percent of patients with supradiaphragmatic presentations and negative clinical subdiaphragmatic evaluations had occult HD discovered at laparotomy (predominantly in the spleen, splenic hilar nodes, or celiac lymph nodes). Liver involvement was extremely uncommon in the absence of extensive splenic involvement.

   a. Therapeutic interventions can be substantially changed by findings at laparotomy, depending on the treatment philosophy of the institution or physician.

   b. Significant controversy regarding the employment of **routine** staging laparotomy in the evaluation of HD continues to the present day. **Laparotomy should be avoided unless the surgical findings will alter the treatment plan.**

   c. Many centers are now using chemotherapy alone for any disease discovered below the diaphragm. A number of centers are exploring the utility of nonleukemogenic chemotherapy plus local radiation to involved sites or extended field radiation in nonsurgically staged cases of HD as a method of reducing short- and long-term morbidity while maintaining excellent disease control.

2. **Possible indications for staging laparotomy** include patients with
   a. **Limited supradiaphragmatic** (CS IA/B and IIA) or **equivocal stage IIIA** (e.g., equivocal LAG) disease.
   b. **CS IIB** disease, which would also be considered for laparotomy if the treatment policy of the physician did not include full course chemotherapy.
3. **Patients who do not require staging laparotomy**
   a. Patients with clear-cut **CS IIIB or IV disease** (e.g., positive LAG) are treated with chemotherapy.
   b. Patients with **bulky mediastinal masses** involving more than one-third of the transverse diameter of the chest tolerate laparotomy poorly and require combined radiation and chemotherapy.
   c. Patients with **isolated** high cervical or axillary involvement by LP HD or patients with isolated and not massive mediastinal NS HD have a very low likelihood of harboring disseminated disease.
   d. Other groups with an **extremely low incidence** of positive laparotomies include females with CS I disease and females less than 26 years of age with three or fewer supradiaphragmatic sites of involvement.
   e. **CS IIIA** is successfully treated with chemotherapy alone; these patients will not benefit from laparotomy unless the radiographic findings are equivocal and the patient may actually be PS IIA.
4. **Possible benefits** of staging laparotomy (in addition to the more precise knowledge regarding stage) include:
   a. Elimination of the need to radiate the spleen; a portion of the left lower lobe of the lung and left upper pole of the kidney are thus spared from irradiation.
   b. Possible enhanced hematologic tolerance to therapy following splenectomy (never proved).
   These benefits alone do not justify "routine" staging laparotomy.
5. **Definition of an adequate staging laparotomy**
   a. Careful abdominal exploration.
   b. Wedge and needle biopsies of both lobes of the liver.
   c. Splenectomy with removal of splenic hilar lymph nodes.
   d. Biopsy of equivocal or abnormal nodes on LAG with intraoperative x-rays to prove that suspicious and abnormal nodes were removed.
   e. Selected random biopsies of celiac, iliac, portal, and mesenteric nodes.
   f. Biopsy of any node that is enlarged or feels abnormal.
   g. Open iliac crest bone marrow biopsy (if bone marrow biopsy was not performed prior to laparotomy).
   h. Oophoropexy, which moves the ovaries out of the direct radiation field, was formerly offered to young women undergoing staging laparotomy, but the declining use of pelvic radiation has almost eliminated this indication.
   i. The use of radiopaque clips is useful in delineating sites of biopsies, splenectomy, and large masses for treatment planning.
6. **Potential complications of staging laparotomy.** The operative mortality should be under 0.5 percent and the significant morbidity under 5 percent to justify this procedure. Older individuals (>50 years) and patients with significant respiratory, cardiac, or other serious illnesses should probably not undergo laparotomy. The most common anticipated complications include pneumonitis, pulmonary embolism, pancreatitis, and subdiaphragmatic abscess.

   Overwhelming pneumococcal sepsis is also a potential complication, but "radiation splenectomy" may produce similar complications. Patients who have undergone splenectomy should carry penicillin and must report any incident of fever or chills to a physician immediately.

V. **Management: Primary therapy**
   A. **Treatment philosophy.** More than one treatment approach may be utilized in

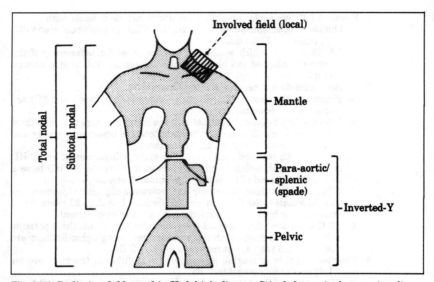

Fig. 21-1. Radiation fields used in Hodgkin's disease. Stippled area is the area irradiated. See text for descriptions.

the management of cases of HD. The current challenge is to determine a course of therapy that preserves cure while minimizing long-term neoplastic and non-neoplastic complications.

B. Surgery is limited to diagnosis, staging laparotomy, splenectomy for the very rare patient with hypersplenism, and laminectomy for spinal cord compression.

C. RT alone is used in the United States to treat many patients with stages IA and IIA disease. A few institutions also use RT alone to treat stages IIB and IIIA disease.

    1. Radiation dose. HD may be locally sterilized in almost all cases with 3500 to 4500 cGy given at a rate of approximately 1000 cGy/week.

    2. Radiation fields (Fig. 21-1)

        a. Mantle field encompasses the cervical, supraclavicular, infraclavicular, axillary, hilar, and mediastinal lymph nodes to the level of the diaphragm. Preauricular fields are added for patients with high cervical lymphadenopathy. The lungs and much of the heart are shielded by lead blocks, although many radiotherapists administer some radiation (≤1500 cGy) to the lung on the involved side, if hilar lymph nodes are enlarged. The whole heart may be treated if the pericardium is involved. A small gap must be left between the inferior border of the mantle field and the superior border of the periaortic field to obviate potential severe spinal cord injury caused by overlap.

        b. Inverted-Y field includes the spleen or splenic pedicle, celiac, periaortic, iliac, inguinal, and femoral lymph nodes. The kidneys, much of the pelvic marrow, and testes are shielded.

        c. Spade and pelvic fields. The inverted Y may be divided into a "spade field" encompassing the splenic pedicle (or spleen) and periaortic nodes, and a pelvic field including the iliac, inguinal, and femoral lymph nodes.

        d. Subtotal nodal or subtotal lymphoid irradiation consists of mantle and spade fields and is generally used for stages IA and IIA and sometimes PS IIB.

Table 21-3. Combination chemotherapy regimens for Hodgkin's disease

Drug (route)	Drug doses[a] in mg/m^2		
	MOPP	ABVD	MOPP/ABV
Mechloreth-amine	6 (1 + 8)		6 (1)
Vincristine (Oncovin) (IV)	1.4 (1 + 8)		1.4[b] (1)
Procarbazine (PO)	100 (1 → 14)		100 (1 → 7)
Prednisone (PO)	40 (1 → 14)[c]		40 (1 → 14)
Adriamycin (IV)		25 (1 + 15)	35 (8)
Bleomycin (IV)		10 (1 + 15)	10 (8)
Vinblastine (IV)		6 (1 + 15)	6 (8)
Dacarbazine (DTIC) (IV)		375 (1 + 15)	

[a] Days are given in 28-day cycles.
[b] Maximum dose is 2.0 mg.
[c] Cycles 1 and 4 only; omit if mediastinal radiation was previously administered.

    e. Total nodal or total lymphoid irradiation is now uncommonly used and consists of mantle and inverted-Y fields and is usually considered for stages IIB and IIIA.
    f. Involved field irradiation consists of sites of known disease only and is used with curative intent only in combination with chemotherapy.
D. Combination chemotherapy is used for stages IIIB and IV HD. It is being increasingly used either alone or with RT for stages IIB and IIIA. Chemotherapy is effective in treatment of early stage (IA/IIA) HD, but is currently **not** often utilized because of poorer patient tolerance compared with that of RT and the possible increased risk of long-term complications. However, many centers and cooperative groups are now exploring the role of nonleukemogenic chemotherapy (ABVD or variants) plus involved field or extended field radiation for patients with early *clinically staged* HD (CS I–IIA), thus hoping to eliminate the role of laparotomy and/or to reduce radiation fields.
    1. Useful chemotherapy regimens for HD are shown in Table 21-3. These regimens must be strictly followed since delays in therapy or reduction in dosages not indicated by the protocol can clearly compromise results. The total dose and dose rate (dose intensity) are important in achieving cure.
    2. MOPP (mechlorethamine, Oncovin, procarbazine, and prednisone). The NCI recommends that vincristine should not be limited to a 2-mg maximum dosage in this regimen but most clinicians sustain the 2-mg limit.
        a. MOPP therapy is administered in 28-day cycles for two additional cycles beyond the attainment of a restaged CR and a minimum of six cycles (months). Almost all patients who obtain CR require eight months or less of treatment.
        b. The CR rate using MOPP is between 70 and 80 percent for stages III and IV HD.
        c. Approximately 60 to 70 percent of CR cases are **durable** with relapses rare after 42 months. Fifty percent of patients are cured with some deaths caused by treatment-related or unrelated disease.
        d. Over 80 percent of patients with stage IIIA or IVA survive 10 years disease-free.

  e. Maintenance therapy beyond the initial complete course is unnecessary and not recommended.
  f. Histologic subtype appears to have little effect on results with MOPP.
  g. MOPP is associated with significant toxicities including hematosuppression, nausea, neuropathy, leukemogenesis, and infertility.

3. ABVD (Adriamycin, bleomycin, vinblastine, and dacarbazine) is an alternative regimen that appears to be as effective as MOPP but has much less reported leukemogenesis and infertility. Potential cardiac toxicity caused by Adriamycin and potential pulmonary toxicity caused by bleomycin have been infrequent problems using this schedule but are of concern, especially when combined with RT.

4. MOPP and ABVD in alternating cycles for 12 months have been found by Italian investigators as superior to MOPP alone with respect to CR rate and relapse-free survival for patients with stage IV disease. The duration of treatment is longer than most investigators have reported in U.S. studies.

5. MOPP/ABV hybrid. Canadian investigators have combined the two effective combinations (minus dacarbazine) into a single hybridized regimen administered for a minimum of eight months with excellent results.

6. Compared effectiveness. A large, randomized trial conducted by a cooperative group showed that ABVD alone may be as effective as MOPP plus ABVD and more effective than MOPP alone in the management of most patients with advanced HD. ABVD is increasingly being considered the treatment of choice for two reasons: (1) MOPP produces infertility in almost all male patients and in most females over 26 years old and (2) MOPP has been associated with the development of acute myeloid leukemia. It is possible that certain subsets such as stage IVB or older patients may benefit from MOPP-containing combinations (e.g., MOPP/ABV), but this is still uncertain.

7. Combined modality management (RT plus chemotherapy) is frequently employed in many stages of HD, but current data do not support this position except in bulky mediastinal HD (see sec. **E.3**). The use of RT as an adjunct in the management of stage III–IV HD has been studied in randomized trials; as yet, no conclusive evidence supports its use. The possible use of minimal radiation ports in conjunction with nonleukemogenic chemotherapy in early stage HD is under study.

E. Treatment controversies, results, and recommendations

1. Stages IA and IIA. Supradiaphragmatic presentations should be treated by subtotal nodal RT alone. Disease-free survivals exceeding 75 percent are anticipated in this population, and approximately 60 percent of relapsing patients are salvaged by chemotherapy.

  The role of the staging laparotomy for this group is controversial. Infradiaphragmatic presentations are frequently given the inverted-Y field for limited inguinal-femoral presentations and total nodal irradiation or chemotherapy for periaortic involvement. Research protocols are exploring the use of nonleukemogenic chemotherapy and lesser fields of radiation in supradiaphragmatic disease.

2. Stage IB and stage IIB management is very controversial. Either subtotal or total nodal irradiation produces 75 percent relapse-free seven-year survival in *pathologically staged* patients. Patients with fever *and* weight loss have only 48 percent freedom from relapse at seven years. Thus, subtotal nodal radiation may be considered for laparotomy-staged patients with *either* fever or weight loss. However, patients with stage IB or IIB disease are being increasingly managed with chemotherapy without laparotomy. Infradiaphragmatic presentations should receive chemotherapy. The role of adjunctive RT in stage I–IIB disease managed with chemotherapy is unclear.

3. Bulky mediastinal presentations. Approximately 60 percent of patients with large (> one-third of the transverse diameter of the chest) mediastinal masses (stage IA-IIB) fail treatment with RT alone; relapses occur predominantly in the mediastinum and lungs. Full course combination chemotherapy and involved field, mantle, or subtotal nodal lymphoid irradiation are recommended for these patients. Patients with bulky mediastinal and more advanced stages (IIIA-IVB) should also receive mediastinal RT. Using both modalities, results approaching the cure rate for patients without large mediastinal masses may be attained. Some centers administer all chemotherapy first, whereas others use a sequence such as chemotherapy-radiation-chemotherapy. These patients are high anesthetic risks and should not undergo laparotomy because they receive chemotherapy. No reliable data are available using chemotherapy alone.

4. **Stage IIIA.** Eighty percent of patients obtain 10-year disease-free survival using chemotherapy alone. Such results probably cannot be improved by combined modality therapy and RT alone is inferior. Patients with "early" stage IIIA (PS IIIA$_1$) who are discovered at staging laparotomy to have stage III disease only because of minimal splenic involvement (four nodules or fewer) or celiac and splenic hilar disease can be considered for subtotal or total nodal RT, reserving chemotherapy for relapse.

5. **Stage IIIB/IV.** ABVD is probably adequate management for most patients, although it remains possible that some subsets may benefit from MOPP plus ABVD or MOPP-ABV hybrid.

6. **E presentations.** Those patients with contiguous limited extranodal disease (such as a single bone involved adjacent to an involved lymph node) can sometimes be managed by radiation alone. Multiple E lesions or extensive E disease (such as a large pulmonary lesion) are best managed with chemotherapy or a combined approach.

7. **Extensive splenic involvement** (defined as more than four splenic nodules) has been associated with a high incidence of hepatic recurrence in some series. Chemotherapy is generally advised for these patients.

8. **Pediatric HD.** Because of the retarding effects radiation has on growing bone, combined modality therapy is frequently and effectively used.

VI. Management after primary therapy
A. Restaging
1. All CR resulting from either irradiation or chemotherapy must be verified by a restaging evaluation that consists of the repetition of all examinations, except laparotomy, that were initially abnormal.
2. The initial restaging occurs one to two months after completion of radiation and traditionally after three or four cycles of chemotherapy, providing that all palpable and radiographic disease has disappeared.
3. Restaging mandates **rebiopsy** of previously involved and accessible stage IV sites such as liver or bone marrow.
4. Contrast dye remaining from previous LAG may remain for many months and is useful in determining nodal size changes (architectural abnormalities may remain indefinitely).
5. **Persistent and stable abnormalities** on chest x-ray or CT scan in the mediastinum are not uncommon (particularly in patients treated for NS). Occasionally persistent stable abdominal masses or palpable nodal masses may also occur. These abnormalities demand close follow-up. However, in most cases these findings represent only fibrosis and do not require biopsy. ^{67}Ga uptake becomes negative in instances in which there is no longer viable disease. PET scanning (see Chap. 2, sec. **I.C.4**) may also be useful in distinguishing viable HD from fibrosis.

B. Follow-up
1. Most relapses following therapy occur within the first three to four years, although later recurrences have been observed.
2. Follow-up should occur every 2 months the first 2 years, every 3 months for the next 2 years and then every 6 to 12 months.
3. Follow-up examinations
   a. History and physical examination.
   b. CBC with sedimentation rate and chemistry panel.

      c. Chest x-ray; KUB (if dye remains).

      d. T_4 and TSH levels—at least annually (see sec. **VII.A.1**).

C. Salvage therapies

1. RT failures are generally treated with combination chemotherapy with results at least as successful as with de novo chemotherapy.

2. Chemotherapy failures

    a. Failure to achieve a CR with effective combination chemotherapy is a very poor sign. Although alternate combinations (i.e., ABVD when MOPP fails) may be temporarily useful, long-term disease control is very unlikely. Such patients may be candidates for autologous (or allogeneic) BMT.

    b. Relapses after chemotherapy-achieved CR. The initial combination can be used again if the unmaintained CR lasts more than one year, but it should not be used again if the CT lasts less than one year. No known available regimen is capable of producing long-term disease-free survival in more than 10 to 20 percent of chemotherapy relapsed cases; autologous (or allogeneic) BMT should be considered.

    c. Patients who are resistant to MOPP and ABVD may experience brief (although occasionally long) responses to alternate chemotherapy (single-agent therapy with a nitrosourea, or etoposide or combinations of these and other agents). Chemotherapy failures with predominantly nodal relapses may benefit from extended field irradiation with some long-term disease-free survivors.

3. Intensive chemo(radio)therapy with autologous stem cell rescue has undergone extensive study in the last decade. High doses of chemotherapy (potentially myeloablative), often combined with total body radiation, are administered ("conditioning regimen"), and either autologous bone marrow or peripheral stem cells (mobilized by growth factors) are used to rescue the patient from prolonged myelosuppression. This procedure is currently performed in most centers with a mortality rate of less than 5 percent; the hospital stay averages three to four weeks. Candidates include patients who have either relapsed following CR or who have never achieved CR with adequate combination chemotherapy. The precise indications for the procedure and comparison with other salvage chemotherapy programs remain subjects for further studies. Perhaps 40 percent of chemosensitive candidates may achieve prolonged disease-free survival and some may be cured.

D. Other therapies

1. Radioisotope-tagged ferritin antibody appears capable of producing responses in some refractory HD, but its eventual place in the therapeutic armamentarium is uncertain.

2. Biologics. Interferons as single agents have proved disappointing though some studies report minor activity in HD. Interleukin-2 with and without interferons may have limited applicability in the treatment of HD.

VII. Special clinical problems in HD

A. Sequelae and complications of therapy

1. Hypothyroidism. Overt hypothyroidism can be expected in 10 to 20 percent and elevation of serum TSH in up to 50 percent of patients treated with mantle field RT. Replacement therapy obviously corrects the problem.

2. Sterility. RT poses problems for female patients who receive pelvic irradiation. The testes are shielded during radiation. MOPP therapy produces near-universal sterility in males and can be anticipated to produce sterility in women in their late twenties or older. Sperm banking is encouraged in males about to receive MOPP, although many patients have oligospermia prior to therapy.

3. Radiation pneumonitis. Mantle radiation routinely produces a paramediastinal fibrosis that is usually not clinically significant. When very large ports are necessitated by large mediastinal-hilar masses, the potential for more severe reaction exists. In addition, patients given MOPP with a prior history of mantle irradiation may experience an abrupt episode of pneumonitis presumably secondary to steroid withdrawal. Therefore, prednisone is omitted from MOPP after mantle radiation even if the radiation was administered years earlier.

4. **Cardiac damage.** The risk of radiation pericarditis is relatively small when modern anterior-posterior weighted radiation ports are used and when large portions of the heart are not radiated. However, radiation pericarditis with or without pericardial effusion or tamponade can develop. The effusion occasionally requires surgical drainage. Constrictive pericarditis is a rare complication of radiation. In addition, accelerated atherosclerosis and the interaction between Adriamycin and mantle radiation are causes of concern.

5. **Aseptic necrosis of the femoral heads** has been reported and is probably secondary to prednisone therapy in MOPP.

6. **Depressed cellular immunity** has been discussed above (see sec. **II.D**).

7. **Secondary neoplasms**
   a. **Acute myelogenous leukemia** often preceded by a prodrome of **myelodysplastic syndrome** develops in 2 to 10 percent of patients treated with MOPP or combination modality therapy. The problem appears greatest in patients over 40 and may be increased in patients undergoing splenectomy. The leukemia generally occurs between 3 and 10 years after treatment, is often associated with total or partial deletion of chromosomes 5 and 7, and has an extremely poor prognosis. Acute leukemia is extremely uncommon in patients treated with radiation alone and seems rare in patients treated with ABVD.
   b. **NHL** may occur during the course of HD and may represent an evolution of the natural history of disease rather than a treatment complication. Most reported cases are high-grade B cell tumors with a particularly high incidence in cases of LP HD (especially the nodular variant). As previously noted, LP HD may be a B cell lymphoma (see footnote, Table 21-2). High-grade peripheral T cell lymphomas have also complicated HD, particularly the NS type.
   c. **Epithelial tumors and sarcomas** are being increasingly reported as complications of radiation and possibly of combined modality therapy and actuarial statistics suggest a rate of second neoplasms approaching 20 percent with prolonged follow-up. Tumors may include breast cancer, sarcoma, melanoma, lung cancer, and other solid tumors.

8. **Neurologic complications**
   a. **Lhermitte's sign,** which follows thoracic radiation for HD, is an innocuous but worrisome finding for the patient. It consists of shocklike sensations down the back and legs often precipitated by flexing the neck and gradually disappears.
   b. **Transverse myelopathy** is a rare but serious complication of RT that is usually caused by failure to leave an appropriate gap between the mantle and abdominal ports.

9. **Retroperitoneal fibrosis** has been described as a complication of HD treatment.

B. **Synchronous neoplasms.** HD is said to be associated with an increased risk of simultaneous Kaposi's sarcoma, leukemia, NHL, and myeloma.

C. **Nephrotic syndrome,** as a remote effect of malignancy, occurs most often in patients with HD. Lipoid nephrosis is typical (see Chap. 31, sec. **IV**).

D. **Pregnancy in HD.** See Chap. 26.

E. **Ichthyosis.** Adult onset ichthyosis is associated with HD in 75 percent of cases (see Chap. 28, sec. **II.H**).

Non-Hodgkin's Lymphoma

NHLs are a group of lymphoproliferative disorders with wide variations in growth rate, progression, and response to therapy.

I. **Epidemiology and etiology**
   A. **Incidence.** NHL occurs roughly four to five times as frequently as HD, with

approximately 40,000 new cases annually in the United States. The incidence is rising dramatically and this increased incidence cannot be totally explained by the AIDS epidemic.

B. Age and sex. Small lymphocytic lymphomas occur in the elderly. Lymphoblastic lymphoma has a predilection for male adolescents and young adults. Follicular lymphomas occur mainly in midadult life. Burkitt's lymphoma occurs in children and young adults.

C. Etiology. Viral etiology and abnormal immune regulation have been implicated in the development of lymphomas. The two mechanisms may be interrelated.

    1. Viruses

        a. RNA viruses. HTLV-I is associated with adult T cell leukemia-lymphoma (ATLL). HIV produces AIDS and the resultant immune deficiency is associated with high-grade B-cell lymphomas.

        b. DNA viruses. EBV has been found in the genome of African Burkitt's lymphoma cells. This virus has also been associated with lymphomas in patients with the x-linked lymphoproliferative syndrome, organ transplantation, and, in many instances, HIV-associated lymphoma. More recently, EBV sequences have been reported in some T cell lymphomas as well. The precise role of EBV in lymphomagenesis remains unsettled.

    2. Immunodeficiency states associated with development of lymphomas

        a. AIDS

        b. Organ transplant recipients

        c. Congenital immunodeficiency syndromes (e.g., agammagobulinemia, ataxia-telangiectasia, Wiskott-Aldrich)

        d. Autoimmune disorders (e.g., Sjögren's syndrome, rheumatoid disease, lupus erythematosus, Hashimoto's thyroiditis)

    3. Treatment-related. The potential role of chemotherapy or RT in the development of NHL following HD and myeloproliferative disorders remains uncertain.

II. Pathology and natural history

A. The Working Formulation (Table 21-4) for the classification of NHL is currently the most commonly used system. This scheme was developed as the result of a consensus panel made up of distinguished hematopathologists, each espousing his or her own classification. The Working Formulation fails to incorporate currently accepted information regarding B or T cell origin of lymphomas, however, and does not recognize a large variety of newly described clinical-pathologic entities.

    1. Basis. The Working Formulation was developed based on the following observations:

        a. Small, resting lymphocytes are capable of "transformation" by mitogens or antigens into large, activated, highly proliferative cells with a neoplastic appearance. This phenomenon explains the common observation of "mixed" lymphomas that are composed of small "resting" and large "activated" cells (formerly called histiocytes).

        b. Lymphomas are the neoplastic counterparts of normal B and T cell lymphocyte biology. Approximately 80 percent of NHLs in the United States are of B cell origin. T cell lymphomas make up a higher proportion in Asian societies.

        c. Follicular (nodular) lymphomas are tumors of the germinal center (or follicular center) of lymph nodes. The cells making up the follicles are called follicular center cells and are of B lineage.

    2. Grades. The Working Formulation divides NHLs into low, intermediate, and high grades that reflect their biologic aggressiveness. The dividing line between these categories is arbitrary. In general, low-grade NHLs are characterized by small cell size, round or cleaved nuclei, and a low mitotic rate. The intermediate/high-grade NHLs usually manifest larger cell size, prominent nucleoli, and a higher mitotic rate.

        a. Clinically, it is useful to consider low-grade NHLs as **indolent** or **nonaggressive,** whereas the intermediate and high-grade NHLs are **aggres-**

Table 21-4. Classification of non-Hodgkin's lymphomas: The Working Formulation* based on a study of 1014 patients

Grade	Malignant lymphoma type	Frequency (%)	Median age (years)	Stage III/IV (%)	Bone marrow involvement (%)	Survival Median (yrs)	Five-year (%)
Low-grade	A. Small lymphocytic	3.6	60	89	71	5.0	59
	CLL-type						
	Plasmacytoid						
	B. Follicular, small cleaved cell	22.5	54	82	51	7.2	70
	C. Follicular, mixed (small cleaved and large cell)	7.7	56	73	30	5.1	50
Intermediate-grade	D. Follicular, large cell	3.8	55	73	34	3.0	45
	E. Diffuse, small cleaved cell	6.9	58	72	32	3.4	33
	F. Diffuse, mixed (small and large cell)	6.7	58	55	14	2.7	38
	G. Diffuse, large cell	19.7	57	54	10	1.5	35
High-grade	H. Immunoblastic (large cell)	7.9	51	49	12	1.3	32
	I. Lymphoblastic	4.2	17	73	50	2.0	26
	J. Small, non-cleaved	5.0	30	66	14	0.7	23
	Burkitt's						
	Non-Burkitt's						
	Total = 88.0%*						

* The Working Formulation does not include cutaneous T cell lymphomas, adult T cell leukemia-lymphoma, diffuse-intermediately differentiated lymphocytic lymphoma, and malignant histiocytosis, which constitute 12% of cases.

Source: Rosenberg, S. A., et al. National Cancer Institute-sponsored study of classifications of non-Hodgkin's lymphomas. *Cancer* 49:2112, 1982.

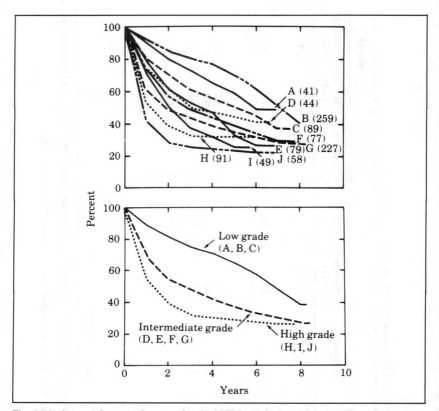

Fig. 21-2. Actuarial survival curves for the NCI formulation subtypes of lymphomas. The upper panel shows the curves for individual subtypes (A through J with the numbers of patients in parentheses). The lower panel shows the curves for the three major prognostic categories (grades); each curve is significantly different from the other (p < 0.0001). Table 21-4 defines the subtypes A through J and the grades. (Reprinted with permission from S. A. Rosenberg, et al. *Cancer* 49:2112, 1982.)

    sive diseases with a short, untreated natural history. Many clinicians approach immunoblastic lymphomas in a similar fashion to the intermediate-grade NHLs and consider lymphoblastic lymphomas and the small, noncleaved NHLs, particularly the Burkitt variant, as high-grade NHLs requiring specialized clinical management.

    b. Survival curves for the Working Formulation are shown in Figure 21-2.

    3. An updated "clinical" classification system that incorporates T or B cell derivation and recognizes newly established clinical-pathologic entities is presented in Table 21-5. This scheme represents the author's current distillation of information regarding the large spectrum of lymphoma types and is not yet all-inclusive.

B. Natural history. NHL exhibits a remarkable range of natural histories, with doubling times varying between days (e.g., Burkitt's lymphoma) to years (some low-grade NHLs). Treatment tends to have a much more dramatic effect on intermediate/high-grade NHLs than on low-grade NHLs. NHLs, particularly the low-grade types, are characterized by early bone marrow involvement and

Table 21-5. Clinical classification of non-Hodgkin's lymphomas (NHLs)

B Cell NHLs	T Cell NHLs
Low-grade:	**Prethymic:**
Small lymphocytic lymphoma	Lymphoblastic lymphoma
Plasmacytoid lymphocytic lymphoma	**Post-thymic (peripheral):**
Follicular lymphoma	Cutaneous T cell lymphoma
Small cleaved	Mycosis fungoides
Mixed	Sézary syndrome
Large cell[a]	Lennert's lymphoma
Mantle cell lymphoma	(lymphoepithelioid)
Nodular	Angioimmunoblastic
Diffuse	lymphadenopathy-like
Monocytoid B cell lymphoma	(AILD-like) lymphoma
MALT-oma[b]	Angiocentric immunoprolifera-
Intermediate–high-grade:	tive disorders
Diffuse large cell lymphoma[c]	Lethal midline granuloma
Small non-cleaved	Lymphomatoid
Burkitt	granulomatosis
Non-Burkitt	Ki-1 anaplastic large cell
	lymphoma
	Adult T cell lymphoma-leukemia
	Peripheral T cell lymphoma (not
	otherwise specified)

[a] May be classified as intermediate-high grade.
[b] Mucosa-associated lymphoid tissue
[c] Includes immunoblastic and diffuse mixed types of NHL.

hematogenous and noncontiguous spread, in sharp contrast to the distribution in HD. Extra-axial nodes, including epitrochlear and mesenteric nodes, are often involved, again in contradistinction to HD (see Table 21-1). Intermediate and high-grade NHLs often present in extranodal sites including Waldeyer's ring, the GI tract, skin, bone, and CNS.

C. B cell NHL: Low-grade

1. **Small lymphocytic lymphoma** is the tissue or nodal counterpart of chronic lymphocytic leukemia (CLL) and classically presents with diffuse lymphadenopathy and marrow involvement.

2. **Plasmacytoid lymphocytic lymphomas** include Waldenström's macroglobulinemia and other B cell lymphomas that may manifest monoclonal serum protein spikes. In **Waldenström's macroglobulinemia** the clinical picture may be dominated by the hyperviscosity syndrome caused by the IgM protein that forms asymmetric pentamers. The syndrome includes fatigue, confusion, tinnitus, and bleeding, which may be relieved by plasmapheresis. Bone marrow and lymph nodes are commonly affected. The cellular composition of plasmacytoid lymphocytic lymphoma is made up of lymphocytes, plasma cells, and hybridized forms with features of both.

3. **Follicular lymphoma.** The follicular lymphomas include the follicular small cleaved, mixed, and large cell types. Follicular small cleaved and mixed lymphomas are generally considered to be low-grade NHL, whereas the rarer follicular large cell type is considered to be intermediate grade by some authorities. Larger transformed cells constitute 25 to 50 percent of the cellular composition in mixed lymphomas, whereas follicular small cleaved lymphomas are composed of predominantly small cells.

    a. The follicular lymphomas tend to present as nodal disease. About 85 percent of cases are stage III–IV at presentation with frequent bone marrow involvement (>50% of cases). The liver, spleen, and mesenteric nodes are often involved.

   b. Follicular lymphomas often progress slowly and may not require immediate therapy. Temporary spontaneous regressions are observed in up to 30 percent of cases. Follicular lymphomas are highly responsive to therapy, but the impact of treatment on survival is modest and few patients are cured. Average survival varies between 6 and 10 years.

   c. Cytologic transformation to intermediate/high-grade NHL may occur at any point in the disease. A similar transformation may take place in some of the other forms of low-grade NHL.

4. Mantle cell lymphomas are presumably derived from cells surrounding the follicle of the germinal center and appear slightly irregular or cleaved. The nodal architecture may appear pseudofollicular or nodular because the normal germinal centers are compressed by the expanded neoplastic mantle cells.

   a. Other terms for mantle cell lymphoma include diffuse intermediate differentiated lymphocytic lymphoma, mantle zone lymphoma, and centrocytic lymphoma (Kiel classification). Many of these lesions were classified as diffuse small cleaved lymphomas in the Working Formulation.

   b. The **clinical presentation** of mantle cell lymphoma resembles follicular lymphoma though survival appears briefer. GI involvement (lymphomatous polyposis) may be seen throughout the GI tract. In some series, cases with a "nodular" pattern appear to survive longer than cases with a "diffuse" architecture.

5. Monocytoid B cell lymphomas have only been recently recognized, and the full spectrum of the disease awaits further description. The cells are predominantly small to medium size lymphocytes with irregular nuclei and abundant, clear cytoplasm (superficially resembling hairy cells). These lymphomas are believed to be derived from parafollicular or marginal zone cells that surround the mantle zone. Monocytoid B cell lymphomas and mucosa-associated lymphoid tissue (MALT)-omas (see **6**) may derive from a similar cell of origin.

6. MALT-omas (Mucosa-associated Lymphoid Tissue) are a group of extranodal lymphomas that frequently present as localized tumors in the stomach, lung, breast, thyroid, and other extranodal sites. In some cases, a preexisting organ-associated autoimmune disease is noted (e.g., Sjögren's syndrome or Hashimoto's thyroiditis). Many of these were designated as "pseudolymphomas" in the past. The natural history includes prolonged survival without widespread dissemination and suggests a role for RT or surgery in management.

D. B cell lymphomas: Intermediate/high-grade

1. Diffuse large cell, mixed and immunoblastic lymphomas of B cell origin can be considered together as aggressive lymphomas. Approximately 30 percent of cases originate in extranodal sites, particularly the GI tract and Waldeyer's ring, but also in sinuses, bone, CNS, and other sites. In contrast to most low-grade NHLs, localized presentations (stage I–II) are common and bone marrow involvement is less frequent (<25% of cases). Localized presentations (stage I–II) may be curable in up to 80 percent of cases, whereas disseminated disease (stage III–IV) is curable 30 to 40 percent of the time.

   a. AIDS-related NHLs are almost universally intermediate-high grade B cell lymphomas (see Chap. 37, sec. II). The majority of patients present with extranodal disease, often including the GI tract, bone, jaw, and CNS (as parenchymal disease), but almost any organ can be involved. Dissemination to bone marrow and meninges is characteristic.

   b. Organ transplant lymphomas are similar to the AIDS-related lymphoma. These lymphomas are associated with profound (iatrogenic) immunosuppression, and, like AIDS lymphomas, share similar histology, potential EBV pathogenesis, and a proclivity for primary parenchymal brain involvement. Reduction in immunosuppression may lead to regression of lymphoma in some patients.

2. **Small non-cleaved lymphomas** are rapidly proliferating lesions with an extremely high mitotic rate and doubling times as brief as 24 hours. Many lymphomas associated with AIDS or organ transplants are this type.

   a. The Burkitt variant has a distinctive natural history and behavior and is divided into African (endemic) and sporadic types. In the Burkitt lymphomas the cells are of nearly equal size and contain prominent small nucleoli and cytoplasmic lipid vacuoles. The non-Burkitt type is characterized by a less homogeneous cellular size and composition.

   b. The treatment strategy for Burkitt's lymphoma has become quite specialized. Clinicians disagree whether to treat the non-Burkitt type as Burkitt's lymphoma or in accordance with the general recommendations for intermediate/high-grade NHL.

E. **T cell NHLs** comprise approximately 20 percent of NHLs in Western societies. They have been poorly characterized in the Working Formulation and are made up of a number of clinical-pathologic entities. They are divided into prethymic and postthymic or peripheral T cell lymphomas.

   1. **Prethymic T cell lymphomas** are commonly called **lymphoblastic lymphoma,** are closely related to T-ALL, and are tumors of immature T cells that occur predominantly in adolescent and young male adults.

      a. The nuclei are often "convoluted" in appearance and the mitotic rate is very high. The cells have characteristic terminal deoxynucleotidyl transferase (TdT) activity. TdT positivity is generally restricted to lymphoblastic lymphoma, ALL (pre-B, T, null subtypes), and the lymphoid blast crisis of CML; it is not seen in other NHLs.

      b. Patients usually present with anterior mediastinal masses and often manifest pleural effusion, pericardial effusion, or superior vena cava syndrome. Bone marrow and peripheral blood involvement are frequent and the syndrome then merges with T-ALL. Meningeal involvement is anticipated unless CNS prophylaxis is employed. Therapy that is similar to that used for ALL may cure 40 percent of cases of lymphoblastic lymphoma.

   2. **Peripheral or post-thymic T cell lymphomas (PTCL)** refer to all NHLs of T cell origin except lymphoblastic lymphoma. The spectrum includes low-grade disorders such as the cutaneous T cell lymphomas and a variety of specialized clinical-pathologic syndromes. With the exception of the cutaneous T cell lymphomas, PTCLs tend to exhibit a high degree of clinical aggressiveness even if the morphology suggests a low-grade behavior. Although the higher grade PTCLs have not been directly compared with intermediate/high-grade B cell NHLs, it appears that they have a poorer prognosis, particularly with stage IV disease.

      a. The **pathologic manifestations** of PTCL often include primary infiltration of T lymph node regions (paracortical) and increased atypical epithelioid venules. The pleomorphic tumor cells often exhibit clear cytoplasm and occasionally resemble Reed-Sternberg cells. The tumors frequently contain an admixture of interdigitating cells, epithelioid cells, eosinophils, and plasma cells. Many peripheral T cell lymphomas would be placed in the "diffuse mixed" category in the Working Formulation.

      b. **Clinical aspects.** PTCL often develop in middle aged to elderly patients who present with constitutional symptoms (B symptoms). Most patients have nodal-based stage III–IV disease with frequent hepatosplenomegaly. Pulmonary and skin involvement are not uncommon. In some cases, eosinophilia and polyclonal hypergammaglobulinemia are observed.

   3. **Specific clinical-pathologic syndromes** of probable peripheral T cell origin include:

a. **Cutaneous T cell lymphomas (CTCLs).** Mycosis fungoides and the Sézary syndrome will be described separately (see sec. **VI.A**).

b. **Lennert's lymphoma** (or **lymphoepithelioid lymphoma**) refers to an uncommon subtype of lymphoma that was originally considered a variant of HD but more recently shown to be a T cell NHL. In this disorder small lymphocytes with an irregular "corkscrew" nucleus are associated with a marked infiltration by reactive epithelioid cells (activated histiocytes). The reactive cells are probably stimulated by lymphokines elaborated by the neoplastic T cells. Patients are often symptomatic (B symptoms) and manifest diffuse disease with splenic involvement. Prognosis is poor.

c. **Angioimmunoblastic lymphadenopathy-like lymphoma** (AILD-like lymphoma). Immunoblastic lymphadenopathy and angioimmunoblastic lymphadenopathy with dysproteinemia (AILD) were originally described as abnormal immune reactions clinically characterized by fever, skin rash, autoimmune hemolytic anemia, polyclonal hypergammaglobulinemia, and generalized lymphadenopathy. Pathology revealed diffuse effacement of lymph node architecture, involvement by immunoblasts and plasma cells, and often an abnormal vascular network. Some of these patients went on to develop clearcut, high-grade NHL. Immunohistochemistry and gene rearrangement studies have indicated that many such patients have underlying T cell lymphomas from the onset.

d. **Angiocentric immunoproliferative disorders** include the former **lethal midline granuloma** (malignant midline reticulosis) and **lymphomatoid granulomatosis.** The neoplastic cells in these disorders involve vessels and lead to an angiodestructive necrotizing process. Lethal midline granuloma involves the palate and sinuses, whereas lymphomatoid granulomatosis affects the lung, skin, and nervous system. Crossover syndromes have been described.

e. **Ki-I anaplastic large cell lymphoma** is a recently recognized lymphoma, usually of T cell origin. Occasional cases appear to be of B or undefined lineage. The large anaplastic cells mark positively for Ki-1 (CD30), an antigen initially described in HD but later found to be present in some neoplastic cells in a variety of aggressive NHL. Ki-1 appears to be a marker of lymphoid activation.

   (1) **Pathologically** the cases are frequently confused with epithelial tumors (carcinomas) or melanoma. The confusion is sometimes compounded by positive staining for epithelial membrane antigen and by a sinusoidal distribution (characteristic of carcinomas or melanomas).

   (2) **Clinically** patients may be children or adults. In some cases involvement is limited to skin and spontaneous regressions are noted. More advanced presentations may respond a bit better to standard chemotherapy than other PTCL.

f. **Adult T cell lymphoma-leukemia (ATLL)** was initially described in southwestern Japan, but has been subsequently seen throughout the world, including the United States. The disease is apparently caused by the HTLV-I virus. Antibodies to HTLV-I are found in more than 10 percent of clinically unaffected residents of endemic areas in Japan. ATLL is characterized by cutaneous involvement, lymphadenopathy, organomegaly, a leukemic blood picture, hypercalcemia with osteolytic bone lesions, and CNS involvement. The cells frequently show a remarkable "knobby" configuration. Immunologically, the cells are of T helper phenotype (T_4) but behave in vitro as suppressor cells. The response to treatment has been poor; death usually occurs within 8 to 10 months. A prodromal less aggressive phase of HTLV-I infection is also recognized.

F. Immunologic abnormalities

1. Hypogammaglobulinemia is typically seen in small lymphocytic lymphoma but may develop in other lymphomas, particularly following treatment.
2. Paraprotein spikes, often IgM, are seen particularly in plasmacytoid lymphocytic lymphomas but are also noted in other B cell malignancies.
3. Warm or cold antibody immune hemolytic anemias may be seen particularly in the small lymphocytic type.
4. Additional autoimmune phenomena, such as circulating anticoagulants (e.g., acquired von Willebrand's disease) may occur, especially in the small lymphocytic lymphomas.
5. Polyclonal hypergammaglobulinemia is commonly observed in patients with AIDS or in PTCL.
6. Defects in T cell function are prominent in ATLL and in other lymphomas following treatment.

G. Pathogenesis

1. **Monoclonal antibodies** can identify epitopes on lymphoid cells characteristic of developmental stages of B cell and T cell ontogeny. The antibodies are utilized with flow cytometry in cell suspensions and with **indirect immunoperoxidase labeling** in frozen sections. Some of the most useful antibodies are shown in Appendix C2, and leukocyte differentiation antigens are presented in Appendix C4. **Monoclonality** of B cell lymphomas is usually established by showing marked dominance of a single light chain (kappa or lambda) or heavy chain type.
2. **Gene rearrangements.** B and T cells must rearrange DNA to assemble antigen specific receptors. Each clone rearranges its genes in a unique way that can be differentiated from the germ line pattern by Southern blot techniques. Identification of gene rearrangements for immunoglobulin and T cell receptor loci can establish cellular lineage, monoclonality, and sometimes stage of differentiation for lymphoid neoplasms. The technique is sensitive enough to detect less than 5 percent involvement of a tissue by lymphoma-leukemia. The application of the polymerase chain reaction methodology may enable detection of one clonal cell in one million utilizing amplification of breakpoint regions by specific primers.
3. **Specific chromosomal translocations** (Table 21-6) have been associated with histologically distinct lymphoma types. The genetic material found at or near the breakpoint of each translocated chromosome is frequently highly informative and provides clues regarding pathogenesis. For example, in Burkitt's lymphoma, the transforming c-*MYC* cellular oncogene found on chromosome 8 is involved in a translocation within or adjacent to the heavy chain gene on chromosome 14 or to one of the light chain genes (kappa on chromosome 2 or lambda on chromosome 22).

   In the follicular lymphomas the translocation also involves the heavy chain gene on chromosome 14, which is this time juxtaposed with the so-called *BCL*-2 gene on chromosome 18. The *BCL*-2 gene appears to be significantly involved in the abrogation of **apoptosis** (programmed cell death). Thus, the activation of the *BCL*-2 gene by translocation in follicular lymphomas may result in the excessive longevity or accumulation of lymphoma cells, implying a defect in cell death rather than a pure problem of proliferation in that disease. In mantle cell lymphoma, the heavy chain gene on chromosome 14 and the *BCL*-1 gene on chromosome 11 are brought into proximity. The *BCL*-1 gene appears to encode a protein (cyclin-1) which is involved in the cell cycle.
4. **Production of lymphokines** by tumor cells may be related to the symptoms or manifestations of specific lymphomas. For example, production of IL-4 by T cells in Lennert's lymphoma may explain the exuberant proliferation of histiocytes in that disease, whereas in AILD-lymphomas, IL-6 production may result in plasmacytosis and hypergammaglobulinemia.

Table 21-6. Chromosomal translocations and immunophenotypic markers in lymphoma*

Lymphoma type	Translocation	Genes at breakpoint	Immunophenotype
B cell lymphoma			
Small lymphocytic	t(14;19)(q32;q13)	heavy chain; BCL-3	CD5(+), CD10(−), SIg+ (weak)
Plasmacytoid	t(9;14)(p13;q32)	heavy chain; —	CD5(−), CD10(−), CIg+
Mantle cell	t(11;14)(q13;32)	BCL-1; heavy chain	CD5(+), CD10(−), SIg+
Follicular	t(14;18)(q32;q21)	heavy chain; BCL-2	CD5(−), CD10(+), SIg+
Small noncleaved (including Burkitt's)	t(8;14)(q24;q32)	MYC; heavy chain	CD5(−), CD10(+), SIg+
	t(2;8)(p12;q24)	kappa; MYC	
	t(8;22)(q24;q11)	MYC; lambda	
Large cell	t(3;14)(q27;q32)	BCL-6	SIg+
	t(3;22)(q27;q11)		
	t(2;3)(p12;q27)		
T cell lymphoma			
Lymphoblastic	Variable involvement of T cell receptor genes	—	TdT(+)
Ki-1 anaplastic	t(2;5)(p23;q35)	—	CD30(+) or Ki-1 (+)

Key: CD5 = Leu-1 or T-101; CD10 = common acute lymphocytic leukemia antigen (CALLA); SIg = surface immunoglobulin; CIg = cytoplasmic immunoglobulin; TdT = terminal deoxynucleotidyl transferase.
*See Appendix C4 for leukocyte differentiation antigens and Appendix C3 for glossary of cytogenetic nomenclature.

5. The **pattern of surface antigens** (Table 21-6) found on lymphoma cells when flow cytometry is used may help identify or corroborate certain lymphoma types. For example, the CD5 antigen, a pan T cell antigen expressed by a small minority of B lymphocytes, is found on the neoplastic cells of patients with small cell lymphocytic lymphoma and mantle cell lymphoma but is absent from the cells of follicular lymphomas and monocytoid B cell lymphoma.

III. Staging system and prognostic factors

A. **The Ann Arbor system** is utilized for both HD and NHL, but histopathologic subtype is the prime determinant of survival in NHL.

B. **Survival** (see Figure 21-2 and Table 21-4)
   1. **Low-grade lymphomas** are rarely curable and appear to cause a steady percentage of deaths annually. It is possible that the rare, early stages of low-grade NHL (stage I or II) may be curable in some cases, but even this is uncertain. Survival averages between 6 and 10 years for follicular lymphomas but is less than 5 years in mantle cell lymphomas.
   2. **Intermediate–high-grade lymphoma** survival curves generally display two components: a rapid fall off in the first one to two years followed by an eventual plateau representing a presumptively cured population. Eighty to 90 percent of patients with stage I and early stage II and 30 to 40 percent with stage III/IV intermediate–high-grade lymphomas may be curable.

C. **Prognostic factors.** Extent of disease at presentation and survivals are shown in Table 21-4.
   1. **Low-grade lymphomas**
      a. **Sensitivity to therapy** is a prognostic sign in that the attainment of CR or an excellent PR identifies patients who are likely to do well.
      b. **Early stage.** Stage I/II cases constitute less than 15 percent of all patients with low-grade lymphoma. In a small series from Stanford, 80 percent of stage I/II patients under age 40 treated by RT were disease-free 10 years after diagnosis.
      c. **Follicular mixed (small cleaved and large cell) lymphomas.** Although these lymphomas are probably rarely curable, extremely long-term remissions have been reported by some institutions utilizing both Adriamycin and non-Adriamycin–based regimens. Other authorities believe that there is little difference, if any, in responsiveness to treatment or duration of remission between follicular small cleaved and mixed NHL.
   2. **Intermediate–high-grade lymphoma.** Stage I or II presentations comprising 30 to 40 percent of these lymphomas are highly curable (approximately 80%), although tumor bulk (>10 cm in largest diameter) adversely affects outcome. A recently published report by the International Non-Hodgkin's Lymphoma Prognostic Factors Project has identified a predictive model for outcome that has established five independently important prognostic factors. The five-year survival was 73 percent for patients manifesting none or one of the adverse risk factors and 26 percent for patients with four or five risk factors. These important risk factors are:
      a. age (>60 years adverse)
      b. stage I–II versus III–IV (III–IV adverse)
      c. number of extranodal sites (>1 adverse)
      d. performance status (low status adverse)
      e. serum LDH (elevated level adverse)
   3. **Newer biologic prognostic factors** under scrutiny include growth fraction (Ki-67 antigen expression), B versus T phenotype (T generally worse), Ia antigen expression, and drug-resistance phenotype (multiple drug resistance expression).

IV. Staging

A. **Clinical evaluation.** See *Evaluation of Suspected Lymphoma,* sec. I. Symptoms and signs, II. Differential diagnosis, III. Biopsy procedures, and IV. Clinical evaluation.

B. Initial staging evaluation

1. The staging evaluation as outlined in *Hodgkin's Disease*, sec. **III.A,** is generally applicable in NHL, but patients undergo two adequate bone marrow aspirations and biopsies.

2. Flow cytometry on the peripheral blood and bone marrow in low-grade lymphomas may define a clonal excess and suggest hematogenous involvement, even when circulating lymphoma cells are not seen.

3. Diagnostic spinal tap is indicated in lymphoblastic lymphoma, lymphomas occurring in AIDS, Burkitt's lymphoma, and probably in intermediate–high-grade lymphomas with marrow, sinus, or testicular involvement.

4. The LAG is usually not required. LAG is used in NHL when the discovery of retroperitoneal lymphadenopathy will change the treatment plan or when the CT scan is equivocal and there is no other disease to follow.

5. Upper GI and small bowel series should be performed in patients with GI symptoms and signs or involvement of mesenteric nodes or Waldeyer's ring because of the high association of these findings with GI involvement. Endoscopic evaluation is performed as indicated.

6. Staging laparotomy is rarely indicated in NHL.

C. Restaging evaluation
is performed to verify CR, particularly with potentially curable histologies. All abnormal studies are repeated including biopsies of accessible previously involved sites. Patients with intermediate–high-grade lymphomas and residual masses on CT scans or x-rays should be followed extremely closely with repeat studies; stable residual masses usually do not contain lymphoma.

V. Management

A. Surgery is limited to

1. **Biopsy** for diagnosis. Staging laparotomy is rarely conducted.
2. **Splenectomy** for very large spleens and significant hypersplenism.
3. **Resection of stomach or bowel** may be indicated in primary GI lymphoma (see sec. **VI.C**).

B. Therapy for indolent lymphomas

1. **True stage I/II disease** (15% cases): RT (3500–4000 cGy) may be administered to all known sites of disease (including draining lymph nodes in E presentation). Large RT fields do not increase cure rate and may decrease tolerance to chemotherapy later. Limited abdominal presentations of NHL may require whole abdominal radiation because of frequent involvement of mesenteric nodes or bowel.

2. **Stage III ("limited").** Although Stanford University has quoted long-term disease-free survival with total lymphoid radiation for highly selected stage III presentations (e.g., no bulky disease, asymptomatic, fewer than five involved sites), this approach is not generally accepted for most patients.

3. **Stage III/IV**

   a. **No treatment.** The majority of patients with advanced indolent disease may be observed with no therapy and without adverse influence on survival. Therapy is instituted in the presence of any systemic symptoms, rapid nodal growth, or imminent complications of the disease such as obstructive phenomena or effusions. The median times to "requiring therapy" vary from 16 months for the follicular, mixed group, to 48 months for the follicular, small-cleaved group, and to 72 months for the small lymphocytic group. Spontaneous remissions may occur during the period of no therapy.

   b. **Single agent therapy** with chlorambucil or cytoxan gives good responses that may develop slowly in indolent NHL. Chlorambucil, 4 to 6 mg/m^2 is given daily with careful monitoring of the CBC. Cytoxan has the disadvantages of alopecia and hemorrhagic cystitis. Recent data suggest that the purine analogs, fludarabine and 2-chlorodeoxyadenosine (2-CdA), may exhibit activity rivaling the alkylating agents, but relatively few previously untreated patients have been reported. Up to 40 to 50 percent of patients with previously treated low-grade lymphomas respond to these purine analogs.

c. **Combination chemotherapy.** Multiple agent therapy may be utilized if a rapid response is required. Chlorambucil or cyclophosphamide and corticosteroids in pulse doses, CVP (cyclophosphamide, vincristine, and prednisone), C-MOPP (cyclophosphamide, vincristine, prednisone, procarbazine) and CHOP (cyclophosphamide, Adriamycin, vincristine, and prednisone) are commonly used regimens (see Appendix A2 for dosages). Single agent or combination chemotherapy produces CR or excellent PR in 60 to 80 percent of patients. Adriamycin-containing regimens have no clear advantages and are often reserved for later stages of the disease. Treatment is generally continued until a maximum response is achieved. Maintenance therapy does not appear to prolong survival, may compromise further treatment, and is potentially leukemogenic.

d. **α-IFN** has demonstrable activity in the follicular lymphomas. No clear-cut dose schedule is superior, and doses as low as two to three million units three times weekly may produce responses in up to 40 to 60 percent of patients. The place of α-IFN in the routine management of follicular lymphoma is not clear. It may be used in patients who no longer respond to conventional chemotherapy. Recently it has been utilized in several randomized studies as either part of induction or maintenance therapy for previously untreated patients. To date, results of some of these series suggest a potentiation of response rates and a prolongation of remission duration, but the effect of α-IFN on survival is not known.

e. **RT.** Palliative RT is used for sites of bulky disease and to relieve obstruction or pain. RT alone may be used when the majority of disease sites do not require treatment but one or two areas are troublesome. However, multiple courses of RT exhaust the marrow and are discouraged since chemotherapy is an effective alternative.

f. **Histologic conversion.** Indolent lymphomas that transform to an aggressive cell type usually have a poor prognosis. Limited, relatively asymptomatic presentations, however, may respond very well to treatment used for intermediate-high grade NHL. The CNS is frequently involved (particularly the meninges) in transformed NHL and is rarely affected in the low-grade NHL. Many consultants advise high-dose chemotherapy and stem cell support for cases of transformed low-grade NHL. This treatment policy has met with variable success but should probably be considered in chemosensitive cases, especially with widespread symptomatic transformation.

4. **Experimental therapies**
   a. **Monoclonal antibodies** of several types have been recently employed in the treatment of low-grade (and some higher grade) NHL.
      (1) **Anti-idiotype antibodies** generated against the patient's own lymphoma idiotype have been difficult to prepare but are associated with occasional durable responses. **Shared idiotypes** (a panel of idiotypes that recognize up to 30% of low-grade B cell NHLs) have been under study to circumvent the difficulties in preparing custom idiotypes for each patient. **Idiotype vaccines** have been used in a limited fashion to produce a polyclonal antibody response against the idiotype, thereby circumventing the problems with somatic mutations observed in the idiotypes of low-grade NHL.
      (2) **Monoclonal antibodies to common lymphoma antigens** are also under study (see Chap. 4, sec. **VIII.B.5**). Targets include B cell antigens (e.g., anti-CD19, anti-CD20, etc.), HLA-Dr (Lym-1), and a site common to many lymphocytes and monocytes (CAMPATH-1H). High-doses of radiolabeled antibody (such as ^{131}I-labeled anti-CD20) have been very promising in studies at the University of Washington. Plant toxins (ricin) coupled to monoclonal antibodies ("immunotoxins") are under study at the Dana Farber Cancer Center. Monoclonal antibodies may eventually be useful not only for therapy but also for purging marrow or peripheral stem cells of contaminating tumor cells.

    b. Intensive multiagent chemotherapy regimens coupled with RT are being compared to a "watch and wait" policy in a randomized trial at the National Institutes of Health. The Southwest Oncology Group is also investigating aggressive treatment and examining α-IFN as a maintenance agent. The major question in such trials is the potential for long-term disease-free survival or cure.

    c. Bone marrow or peripheral stem cell support following high-dose chemoradiotherapy is undergoing extensive study in a number of institutions as a potential curative regimen for relapsed or newly diagnosed low-grade NHL. Some centers are purging marrow with monoclonal antibodies. Perhaps the most interesting data have been generated in the follicular lymphomas by the Dana Farber Cancer Center. Researchers have observed a striking correlation between disease-free survival and the ability to purge marrow of cells expressing the t(14;18) rearrangement (utilizing the sensitive polymerase chain reaction technique). At present, however, no convincing data support high-dose therapy in the routine management of low-grade NHL.

C. Therapy for intermediate–high-grade NHL excluding lymphoblastic lymphoma, AIDS-associated lymphoma, ATLL, and Burkitt's lymphoma, which are discussed in sections **D, E, F,** and **VI.D,** respectively.

  1. Localized presentations. Nonbulky (<10 cm) stages IA and IIA cases, including extranodal ("E") presentations, can be successfully managed by three cycles of an Adriamycin-containing regimen (CHOP) **followed by** involved field RT (equivalent to 3000 cGy in 10 fractions). Virtually all patients achieve CR and the actuarial relapse-free survival exceeds 80 percent. Other approaches include full course aggressive chemotherapy with or without subsequent RT and RT alone in carefully selected stage I cases (staging may include laparotomy). RT alone is not appropriate for stage II.

  2. Stage I-II (bulky) to IV disease. Despite claims to the contrary, there is currently no proof that any of the newer more complex and more toxic regimens is superior to CHOP (Table 21-7). The results of the recently published Intergroup Trial comparing CHOP with three of the purportedly more effective newer combinations showed CHOP to be equally active and less toxic. One can expect long-term disease control ("cure") in roughly 30 to 40 percent of patients with advanced stage intermediate–high-grade NHL treated with CHOP and similar programs. The claims for improved outcome reported in single-institution trials using other regimens are likely the result of incomplete follow-up and selection bias based on prognostic factors (see sec. **III.C.2**).

    a. Complete restaging to assess completeness of response is **mandatory.** Restaging is usually done after three to four cycles of CHOP and again after six cycles. Patients are generally given at least two additional cycles of therapy after attainment of CR (usually a total of eight cycles).

    b. CNS prophylaxis utilizing intrathecal chemotherapy, sometimes complemented by cranial irradiation, appears to be indicated in situations associated with a high risk of meningeal relapse. This strategy is particularly advised in cases of involvement of the paranasal sinuses and in the small noncleaved lymphomas (especially the Burkitt's type). Other indications may include primary testicular lymphoma, transformed lymphomas, and intermediate–high-grade lymphomas involving the bone marrow, although the latter indication is more controversial.

    c. Maintenance therapy is not advised because it has not been shown to enhance survival.

  3. Relapsed intermediate–high-grade lymphomas

    a. Salvage chemotherapy regimens (see Table 21-7) often employ high-dose cytosine arabinoside, corticosteroids, and cisplatin with or without etoposide (e.g., DHAP, ESHAP). Other combinations include ifosfamide, mitoxantrone, and etoposide (e.g., MINE). These programs generally produce significant but short-lasting remissions in 30 to 50 percent of patients. A small proportion of patients, probably under 10 percent, have prolonged responses.

    b. High-dose chemotherapy/RT with autologous bone marrow or stem cell support (see *Hodgkin's Disease*, sec. **V.D.3**). A similar strategy to that employed in HD has been adopted for intermediate–high-grade NHL following relapse from standard CHOP-like chemotherapy. A conditioning regimen based on high-dose chemotherapy, sometimes combined with total body irradiation, is used, followed by reinfusion of cryopreserved marrow or peripheral blood progenitor cells (stem cells) mobilized by growth factors and sometimes chemotherapy. The results of this strategy are best in chemosensitive recurrences, in which approximately 40 percent of patients may derive long-term, disease-free survival. The results are far less optimistic in patients who are chemoresistant or in patients who have never achieved remission. The relative merits of salvage chemotherapy are being compared with autologous BMT in an international, cooperative, randomized trial.

    c. Allogeneic BMT differs from autologous transplantation in that a potential graft versus lymphoma immune reaction may complement the effects of the conditioning regimen. The degree to which this effect exists in lymphoma is subject to debate. Allogeneic transplantation may be most reasonable in young patients with a suitable match who do not fall into the favorable categories for benefit from autologous transplantation.

  4. Experimental therapies. The purine analogs and interferon have limited value in intermediate–high-grade NHL. Monoclonal antibody approaches similar to those employed in low-grade NHL are under investigation. Other programs attempt to reverse multiple drug resistance as mediated by the *MDR*1 gene (using agents such as the calcium channel blockers, quinine, and cyclosporine) or intensify the dose of chemotherapeutic agents (using growth factors with repeated infusions of autologous, mobilized stem cells).

D. Therapy for lymphoblastic lymphoma is patterned after therapy for the closely related acute lymphocytic leukemia. Overall results of therapy indicate a 40 percent long-term, disease-free survival with the best prognosis seen in patients who have minimal or no marrow involvement, no CNS involvement, and normal serum LDH levels. Patients with poor prognostic presentations of lymphoblastic lymphoma are being considered for early autologous or allogeneic transplantation or more intensive primary chemotherapy programs. Stanford University reported a 94 percent freedom from relapse at five years for patients without the above adverse prognostic factors with a regimen that involves one month of induction therapy, one month of CNS prophylaxis, three months of consolidation, and finally seven months of maintenance therapy as follows:

Cyclophosphamide, 400 mg/m^2 PO for 3 days on weeks, 1, 4, 9, 12, 15, and 18
Adriamycin, 50 mg/m^2 IV on weeks 1, 4, 9, 12, 15, and 18
Vincristine, 2 mg IV on weeks 1, 2, 3, 4, 5, 6, 9, 12, 15, and 18
Prednisone, 40 mg/m^2 daily for 6 weeks (tapered off); then for 5 days on weeks 9, 12, 15, and 18
L-Asparaginase, 6000 units/m^2 IM (maximum 10,000 units) for 5 doses at the beginning of CNS prophylaxis
CNS prophylaxis consists of whole brain RT (2400 cGy in 12 fractions) and intrathecal methotrexate (12 mg for each of 6 doses) given between weeks 4 and 9
Maintenance therapy consists of methotrexate (30 mg/m^2 PO weekly) and 6-mercaptopurine (75 mg/m^2 PO daily) on weeks 23 to 52.

E. Therapy for AIDS-associated lymphoma. See Chap. 37, sec. **II**.
F. Therapy for ATLL is quite ineffective. Recently a combination of zidovudine (AZT) and α-IFN has been stated to show promise. Occasional patients may benefit briefly from combination chemotherapy programs utilized in intermediate–high-grade NHL or from 2-deoxycoformycin, a purine analog.
G. Therapy of peripheral T cell lymphomas has generally followed the treatment

Table 21-7. Combination chemotherapy regimens for intermediate-high grade non-Hodgkin's lymphomas (excludes lymphoblastic and Burkitt's lymphomas)

Regimen (cycle frequency)	Route	Dose	Days given
		INITIAL THERAPY	
CHOP (q21d)			
Cyclophosphamide	IV	750 mg/m^2	1
Adriamycin (hydroxy-daunorubicin)	IV	50 mg/m^2	1
Oncovin (vincristine)	IV	1.4 mg/m^2 (maximum 2.0 mg)	1
Prednisone	PO	100 mg (total)	1–5
M-BACOD (q21d)			
Methotrexate	IV	3000 mg/m^2	14
Leucovorin	IV/PO	10 mg/m^2 q6h × 12 doses*	
Bleomycin	IV	4 mg/m^2	1
Adriamycin	IV	45 mg/m^2	1
Cyclophosphamide	IV	600 mg/m^2	1
Oncovin (vincristine)	IV	1.0 mg/m^2	1
Dexamethasone	PO	6 mg/m^2	1–5
m-BACOD (q21d)			
Same as M-BACOD except:			
Methotrexate	IV	200 mg/m^2	8 and 15
Leucovorin	PO	10 mg/m^2 q6h × 8 doses*	
ProMACE/cytaBOM (q21d)			
Prednisone	PO	60 mg/m^2	1–14
Methotrexate	IV	120 mg/m^2	8
Leucovorin	IV	25 mg/m^2 q6h × 4 doses*	
Adriamycin	IV	25 mg/m^2	1
Cyclophosphamide	IV	650 mg/m^2	1
Etoposide (VP-16)	IV	120 mg/m^2	1
Cytosine arabinoside	IV	300 mg/m^2	8
Bleomycin	IV	5 mg/m^2	8
Oncovin (vincristine)	IV	1.4 mg/m^2	8
MACOP-B (for 12 wk total)			
Methotrexate	IV	400 mg/m^2	wk 2, 6, 10
Leukovorin	PO	15 mg (total) q6h × 6 doses	
Adriamycin	IV	50 mg/m^2	wk 1, 3, 5, 7, 9, 11
Cyclophosphamide	IV	350 mg/m^2	wk 1, 3, 5, 7, 9, 11
Oncovin (vincristine)	IV	1.4 mg/m^2 (maximum 2.0 mg)	wk 2, 4, 6, 8, 10, 12
Prednisone	PO	75 mg (total dose)	12 wk (taper over last 14 days)
Bleomycin	IV	10 mg/m^2	wk 4, 8, 12
(Cotrimoxazole DS ketoco-	PO	bid	12 wk
nazole 200)	PO	200 mg/day	12 wk
		SALVAGE THERAPY	
DHAP (q21–28d)			
Dexamethasone	IV	40 mg (total)	1–4
High-dose cytosine arabinoside	IV	2.0 gm/m^2 over 2 hr following cisplatin and 12 hr later (2 doses)	2
Cisplatin	IV	100 mg/m^2 as a 24-hr infusion	1

Table 21-7 (continued)

Regimen (cycle frequency)	Route	Dose	Days given
ESHAP (q21–28d)			
Etoposide	IV	60 mg/m²	1–4
Solumedrol (methyl-prednisone)	IV	500 mg (total)	1–4
High-dose cytosine arabinoside	IV	2.0 gm/m² over 2 hr following cisplatin (once)	5
Cisplatin	IV	25 mg/m²/day by 24 hr infusion (100 mg/m² total)	1–4
MINE (q21d)			
MESNA	IV	1.33 gm/m² mixed with ifosfamide over 1 hr and 500 mg PO 4 hr later	1–3
Ifosfamide	IV	1.33 gm/m² over 1 hr	1–3
Novantrone (mitoxantrone)	IV	8 mg/m²	1
Etoposide	IV	65 mg/m² over 1 hr	1–3

*Begin 24 hr after methotrexate.

for the more common B cell disorders. This approach may not be applicable in all cases but useful data based on multi-institutional, randomized trials are lacking. In selected cases specific management approaches may pertain.

1. **AILD-like lymphomas** have been managed with generally poor results by conventional chemotherapy or corticosteroids, although occasional long-term responses or spontaneous regressions have occurred. More recently, responses to α-IFN, cyclosporine, or high-dose chemotherapy with stem cell support have been described in small series or case reports.

2. **Angiocentric immunoproliferative disorders** with localized involvement of the palate and sinuses (lethal midline granuloma) may benefit from RT alone. Responses to cyclophosphamide and corticosteroids have been reported in lymphomatoid granulomatosis. Both syndromes may evolve into high-grade T cell lymphomas, however, and then require increasingly aggressive management.

VI. **Specialized lymphoma syndromes**

A. **CTCLs** encompass mycosis fungoides (MF) and Sézary syndrome (SS). Both are malignant cutaneous lymphoproliferative disorders of helper T cells (CD_4).

1. **Dermatologic presentation** is localized plaques evolving into tumor nodules in MF and diffuse exfoliative erythroderma associated with abnormal circulating cells in SS.

2. **Histopathology** shows atypical T cells with irregular cerebriform nuclei (MF cells) infiltrating the epidermis and a zone beneath it, forming characteristic Pautrier's microabscesses. Enlarged lymph nodes may not always show overt lymphomatous infiltration, but techniques such as T cell receptor gene arrangement may reveal early involvement.

3. **Natural history.** A long history of undiagnosed skin disease often precedes the specific diagnosis.

   a. **Cutaneous stages of MF**

   (1) Premycotic stage: nonspecific eczematoid or erythematous lesions may last many years.

   (2) Plaque stage.

   (3) Tumor stage.

    b. Lymph node involvement occurs with increasing skin involvement. Histologically confirmed lymph node involvement indicates a poor prognosis.

    c. Visceral involvement. Almost any organ can be involved late in the disease, particularly the liver, spleen, lung, and GI tract, but the marrow is relatively spared. A peculiar epitheliotropic pattern of dissemination may be observed.

4. Staging system. A variety have been proposed including a TNM system. One example is

Stage I
    Stage IA: Limited plaques without adenopathy.
    Stage IB: Generalized plaques without adenopathy.
Stage II
    Stage IIA: Limited or generalized plaques with adenopathy (but without histologic involvement of nodes).
    Stage IIB: Cutaneous tumors with or without adenopathy (but without histologic involvement of nodes).
    Stage III: Generalized erythroderma with or without adenopathy but without histologic involvement of lymph nodes or viscera.
    Stage IV: Histologic involvement of lymph nodes or viscera at any cutaneous stage.

5. Prognosis. The overall median survival is eight to nine years from time of diagnosis. Survival time is two to four years from onset of tumor stage or lymph node involvement and less than 18 months from visceral involvement.

6. Treatment for skin involvement

    a. Topical chemotherapy with nitrogen mustard is useful in the plaque stage. Cutaneous allergic reactions may develop.

    b. Electron beam RT is technically demanding and relatively unavailable, but has produced durable remissions particularly in early stages of disease.

    c. Psoralen with ultraviolet light (PUVA) repeated three times a week is effective for the plaque phase. Long-term benefits and side effects are poorly defined.

    d. Cis-retinoic acid has activity particularly in the plaque stage.

7. Systemic chemotherapy and investigational approaches

    a. Systemic therapy is recommended only for patients with extracutaneous disease. A variety of single agents (e.g., Adriamycin, cyclophosphamide, methotrexate, bleomycin, steroids) and combinations have provided temporary responses. Combinations produced more CR than single agents.

    b. The **purine analogues** 2-deoxycoformycin (Penostatin), 2-chlorodeoxyadenosine (2-CdA), and fludarabine have all shown activity; 2-deoxycoformycin and 2-CdA are perhaps more active than fludarabine.

    c. α-IFN has a response rate of 45 percent in CTCL.

    d. Antibody therapy. Transient responses to monoclonal T cell antibodies have been observed in CTCL, and radiolabeled monoclonal antibodies have demonstrated activity.

B. Primary CNS lymphoma is essentially always of high histologic grade (large cell, immunoblastic) and of B cell origin. Lesions are primarily parenchymal and involve deep periventricular structures. Multiple lesions occur in 20 to 40 percent of cases. The leptomeninges are involved in 30 percent of cases at diagnosis and in most cases at autopsy.

    1. Etiology and epidemiology

        a. Primary CNS lymphoma accounts for about 1 percent of brain tumors and 1 percent of extranodal lymphomas. The disease is associated with advanced age (>60 years), AIDS, drug-induced immunosuppression (e.g., for transplantation), and congenital immunodeficiency syndromes.

b. Primary CNS lymphoma accounts for roughly 50 percent of all lymphomas seen in transplant patients and occurs at a somewhat lesser frequency in AIDS.

c. Relationship to EBV infection is suggested by discovery of the EBV genome in some cases of CNS lymphomas arising in transplant and AIDS patients.

d. In AIDS cases primary CNS lymphoma appears in a setting of severe CD4 depression, with counts frequently less than $50/mm^3$.

2. Clinical presentations include headache, personality changes, and hemiparesis. Symptoms of meningeal infiltration or spinal cord compression are less common. Associated systemic lymphoma is rare. Ocular lymphoma (uveitis) may precede or follow the diagnosis of CNS lymphoma.

3. Evaluation. The diagnosis usually can be made with stereotactic biopsy and without formal surgical exploration.

a. CT scan. Deep periventricular lesion(s) often involve the corpus callosum, basal ganglia, or thalamus and often appear hyperdense prior to contrast dye. Contrast often produces generalized intense enhancement, unlike the picture of gliomas and metastases. In the AIDS patient, the precontrast scan may be hypodense.

b. MRI scan may reveal additional lesions not seen by CT scan.

c. Lumbar puncture (LP). Nonspecific elevation of CSF protein is common. Abnormal cells may be found in 25 to 35 percent of cases undergoing LP at diagnosis. Identification of malignant cells may be enhanced by immunofluorescent techniques with monoclonal antibodies.

d. Ophthalmologic examination, including slit-lamp examination.

e. HIV antibody.

f. Enumeration of the helper-suppressor cell ratio.

g. Abdominal CT scan, chest x-ray.

h. Bone marrow biopsy.

4. Therapy

a. Corticosteroids. Primary CNS lymphomas are extremely sensitive. Lesions may disappear on steroids alone and preclude histologic diagnosis after steroids are given.

b. Cranial RT. Doses of 4000 to 5000 cGy appear necessary with 1000 to 1500 cGy focal boost to the tumor bed.

c. Chemotherapy given before RT and using agents such as high-dose methotrexate with leucovorin rescue, high-dose cytosine arabinoside or intrathecal therapy is being investigated because of the penetration of those agents into the CNS and the poor prognosis observed with RT alone. Although survival advantages have been claimed in small institutional trials, formal proof of the superiority of this approach requires randomized study or at least multi-institutional confirmation.

5. Clinical course. Initial response is generally followed by relapse in the CNS, meninges, or intraocular contents. Systemic relapse is uncommon. Survival is usually less than two years, although longer survivals are occasionally observed. Primary CNS lymphoma complicating AIDS is associated with a median survival of less than three months.

C. Primary gastrointestinal lymphoma (PGL) is the most common form of solitary extranodal disease and may occur in the stomach and small and large bowel.

1. Associated diseases. The incidence of PGL is increased in patients with ulcerative colitis, regional enteritis, or celiac disease. Alpha heavy-chain disease is present in some patients with the Mediterranean type of PGL.

2. Histopathology is intermediate-high grade in the majority of patients with PGL in Western countries. Low-grade NHLs, including follicular lymphoma, usually involving small bowel, are also observed in the GI tract. Two less common low-grade NHL, MALT-omas and mantle cell lymphoma, are associated with gastric and bowel involvement (multiple lymphomatoid polyposis), respectively.

3. **Symptoms and physical findings.** Anorexia, nausea, vomiting, weight loss, GI bleeding, or abdominal pain is present in the majority of patients. An abdominal mass may be present, but peripheral lymphadenopathy is not common.

4. **Complications.** Obstruction may complicate the course of PGL. Perforation or hemorrhage may either be a presenting sign or more often, a complication of treatment for PGL. Therapy can cause perforation by the lysis of lymphomatosis involvement of the full thickness of the wall of the organ involved.

5. **Diagnosis.** Barium contrast radiographs usually show large mucosal folds, ulceration, masses, luminal narrowing, or annular strictures. Gastric lymphomas may be indistinguishable from peptic ulcer by both radiologic and endoscopic criteria. Undifferentiated carcinoma of the GI tract may be confused with intermediate- and high-grade lymphoma even after expert histologic evaluation; immunohistochemical verification of diagnosis is often necessary.

6. **Management of PGL**
   a. **Surgical management.** Laparotomy may be needed to establish diagnosis or treat complications. Many authorities advise resection of primary gastric lymphomas in the absence of widespread dissemination. This strategy has been justified in order to avoid treatment-related perforation but may not be necessary, because those patients developing perforation may be managed surgically as necessary. On the other hand, readily resectable lesions of the small or large bowel should be considered for surgical removal in view of the greater risks associated with spillage of their bacterial-laden intraluminal contents. If a total gastrectomy is required for gastric lymphoma, postsurgical morbidity may be excessive, and medical management is advised.
   b. **Medical management** should be based on histologic subtype and extent of disease. Intermediate–high-grade lesions are treated primarily with combination chemotherapy. Limited non-bulky stage IE–IIE presentations involving the stomach may be treated with shorter courses of chemotherapy followed by involved field radiation. Although we recommend a full course of chemotheapy. This approach is less applicable in the intestinal presentations because of anatomic considerations requiring large radiation ports. The localized low-grade MALT-omas in the stomach may be managed by involved field radiation. Recent reports suggest an association between *Helicobacter pylori* and gastric MALT-oma with possible response of the lymphoma to antibiotic therapy.

D. **Burkitt's lymphoma** (BL) is a specific subtype of the small noncleaved cell high-grade NHL. The cells in BL are very uniform with round-oval nuclei, two to five prominent nucleoli, and cytoplasm rich in RNA. The cells are of B lineage, expressing monoclonal IgM surface immunoglobulin. A consistent series of cytogenetic translocations (see sec. **II.C.3**) and explosive growth characterizes BL.

1. **Epidemiology and etiology**
   a. BL is endemic in certain regions of equatorial Africa and other tropical locations. A sporadic form of BL occurs in the United States and throughout the world. The disease occurs predominantly in childhood but can be seen in young adults, particularly in the sporadic form.
   b. **EBV** has been found in the genome of endemic BL but rarely in the sporadic form. Very high EBV antibody titers are seen in the endemic form.

2. Clinical features

	Endemic (Africa)	Sporadic
Association with EBV	Yes	Rarely
Chromosomal translocation	t(8;14) very common	t(8;14) very common
Involvement	Jaw, orbit	Abdomen, GI tract, marrow
Therapy	50% prolonged survival with cyclophosphamide	Requires multiple agents
Relapse	Survival possible	Poor prognosis

   a. Jaw and orbital involvement is typical in Africa, but abdominal (ileocecal) disease dominates in sporadic cases.
   b. Lymph node involvement is seen rarely in Africa but not infrequently in sporadic cases.
3. **Staging system.** A variety of systems have been proposed. The NCI system is shown.

Stage	Disease distribution
A	Single solitary extra-abdominal site.
B	Multiple extra-abdominal sites.
C	Intra-abdominal tumor.
D	Intra-abdominal plus one or more extra-abdominal sites.
AR	Intra-abdominal: more than 90% of tumor resected.

4. **Prognosis.** Prior to effective treatment only 30 percent of sporadic cases survived. Using combination chemotherapy and CNS prophylaxis, the survival rate is at least 60 percent. Patients with limited (A, B, AR) disease have an excellent prognosis with 90 percent survival. Bone marrow and CNS involvement carry a poor prognosis. Adult cases of BL, particularly those with advanced stage, do more poorly than childhood cases.
5. **Treatment**
   a. Cyclophosphamide therapy alone has been curative for many localized presentations in Africa.
   b. Multiagent, aggressive regimens are necessary for the sporadic form. One such program combines cyclophosphamide, Oncovin, methotrexate, and prednisone (COMP) with CNS prophylaxis. Limited RT to sites of bulky disease is sometimes used as adjunctive therapy but may be unnecessary.
   c. Because of the extremely rapid growth rate, massive acute destruction of tumor with initial chemotherapy usually results in **tumor lysis syndrome** (see Chap. 27, sec. **XIII**).
E. **Malignant histiocytosis** remains an extremely confusing category. True "histiocytic" lymphomas are extremely rare and make up less than 1 percent of NHLs. A syndrome of presumably benign proliferation by activated histiocytes is associated with fever, pancytopenia, jaundice, hyperlipemia, coagulopathy, and varying degrees of hepatosplenomegaly and lymphadenopathy. It is characterized pathologically by **hemophagocytosis** by histiocytes found in the sinuses of nodes and diffusely throughout the lymphoreticular system. Initially believed to be a histiocytic malignancy **(histiocytic medullary reticulosis),** many similar cases have been associated with viral and opportunistic infections **(viral-associated hemophagocytic syndrome or VAHS)** and with T cell malignancies (including T-ALL and T cell lymphomas). A familial hemophagocytic syndrome is also well described.
   Clinically, these cases manifest an often fulminant course and therapeutic strategy is unclear. The familial forms have been managed successfully in some cases by allogeneic BMT. Occasional responses to combination chemotherapy programs used in intermediate/high grade NHL have been noted. Etoposide

(VP-16) may have a particular role in management. However, an underlying concern regarding pathogenesis (infectious versus neoplastic) confuses the treatment approach.

F. Systemic Castleman's disease. Initially Castleman's disease referred to localized giant lymph node hyperplasia usually involving the mediastinum or abdomen. Recently a disorder exhibiting the histopathologic features of the plasma cell type of Castleman's disease but with a **generalized** presentation has been described.

  1. Clinical features
    a. Fever, malaise, and weakness
    b. Lymphadenopathy, usually generalized
    c. Organomegaly
    d. Edema, anasarca, and effusions
    e. Pulmonary and CNS involvement
    f. Anemia, thrombocytopenia, polyclonal hypergammaglobulinemia, and elevated erythrocyte sedimentation rate

  2. Histopathology shows preservation of lymph node architecture, but with prominent germinal centers, either hyperplastic or hyalinized, and diffuse marked plasma cell infiltration.

  3. Clinical course is either persistent or episodic with remissions and exacerbations. Lymphoma or Kaposi's sarcoma occasionally develops. The median survival is 30 months.

  4. Treatment. Responses to corticosteroids and antitumor agents used in NHL have met with occasional response. More recently, IL-6 has been implicated in the pathogenesis of this disorder with a reported clinical response to treatment with an anti-IL-6 antibody.

Selected Reading

Hodgkin's Disease

Bonnadonna, G., et al. Alternating non-cross resistant combination chemotherapy or MOPP in Stage IV Hodgkin's disease. A report of 8 year results. *Ann. Intern. Med.* 104:739, 1986.

Canellos, G. P., et al. Chemotherapy of advanced Hodgkin's disease with MOPP, ABVD or MOPP alternating with ABVD. *N. Engl. J. Med.* 327:1478, 1992.

Longo, D. L., et al. Twenty years of MOPP therapy for Hodgkin's disease. *J. Clin. Oncol.* 4:1295, 1986.

Reece, D. E., et al. Intensive therapy with cyclophosphamide, carmustine, etoposide ± cisplatin and autologous bone marrow transplantation for Hodgkin's disease in first relapse after combination chemotherapy. *Blood* 83:1193, 1994.

Urba, W. J., et al. Hodgkin's disease. *N. Engl. J. Med.* 326:678, 1992.

Non-Hodgkin's Lymphoma

Connors, J. M., et al. Brief chemotherapy and involved field radiation therapy for limited stage histologically aggressive lymphoma. *Ann. Intern. Med.* 107:25, 1987.

Fisher, R. I., et al. Comparison of a standard regimen (CHOP) with three intensive chemotherapy regimens for advanced non-Hodgkin's lymphoma. *N. Engl. J. Med.* 328:1002, 1993.

Gribben, J. G., et al. Immunologic purging of marrow assessed by PCR before autologous bone marrow transplantation for B-cell lymphoma. *N. Engl. J. Med.* 325:1525, 1991.

Jaffe, E. S., et al. Histopathologic subtypes of indolent lymphomas: caricatures of the mature B-cell system. *Semin. Oncol.* 20 (Suppl 5):3, 1993.

National Cancer Institute sponsored study of classifications of non-Hodgkin's lymphomas. Summary and description of a Working Formulation for clinical usage. *Cancer* 49:2112, 1982.

A predictive model for aggressive non-Hodgkin's lymphoma. *N. Engl. J. Med.* 329: 987, 1993.

Press, O. W., et al. Radiolabeled-antibody therapy of B-cell lymphoma wtih autologous bone marrow support. *N. Engl. J. Med.* 329:1219, 1992.

Phillip, T., et al. High-dose therapy and autologous bone marrow transplantation after failure of conventional chemotherapy in adults with intermediate-grade or high-grade non-Hodgkin's lymphoma. *N. Engl. J. Med.* 316:1493, 1987.

Rosenberg, S. A. Karnofsky Memorial Lecture. The low-grade non-Hodgkin's lymphomas. Challenges and opportunities. *J. Clin. Oncol.* 3:299, 1985.

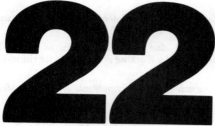

Plasma Cell Disorders

James R. Berenson and
Dennis A. Casciato

Immunoglobulins are produced by B lymphoctyes and plasma cells. A clone of cells producing immunoglobulins may proliferate to sufficient mass that a monoclonal protein (M protein) is detectable as a peak or "spike" on serum protein electrophoresis. Clonal growth may be progressive or stable for many years. Properties of normal serum immunoglobulins are shown in Table 22-1.

I. Epidemiology and etiology

A. Classification of diseases associated with monoclonal paraproteinemia

1. **Plasma cell neoplasms**
   a. Plasma cell myeloma (PCM)
   b. Waldenström's macroglobulinemia (WM)
   c. Heavy chain disease
   d. Amyloidosis
   e. Papular mucinosis

2. **Other neoplastic diseases**
   a. B lymphocyte neoplasms (malignant lymphoma, chronic lymphocytic leukemia)
   b. Neoplasms of cell types not known to synthesize immunoglobulins (solid tumors, monocytic leukemia)

3. **Non-neoplastic disorders**
   a. Monoclonal gammopathy of undetermined significance (MGUS)
   b. Autoimmune diseases (e.g., systemic lupus erythematosus)
   c. Hepatobiliary disease
   d. Chronic inflammatory diseases
   e. Immunodeficiency syndromes
   f. Miscellaneous diseases (e.g., Gaucher's disease)
   g. Pseudoparaproteinemia

B. Incidence. MGUS, PCM, and WM are the most common disorders associated with M proteins. The average age at the time of diagnosis is 60 years, and the incidence increases with age.

1. **MGUS** (formerly *benign monoclonal gammopathy*). The approximate incidence of MGUS is 0.2 percent for patients 25 to 49 years old, 2 percent for those 50 to 79 years old, and 10 percent for those 80 to 90 years old.

2. **PCM** develops in three persons per 100,000 population. Sixty percent of patients are men. More than 98 percent of patients are over 40 years old. PCM is the most common lymphohematopoietic malignancy in African Americans.

3. **WM** has an incidence which is approximately 5–10 percent of that of PCM. Two-thirds of cases occur in men.

4. **Lymphomas.** Excluding MGUS, PCM, and WM, approximately 50 percent of patients with monoclonal gammopathies have lymphocytic lymphoma or chronic lymphocytic leukemia. The paraprotein is nearly always either IgM or IgG, and patients are usually asymptomatic from the paraprotein. Patients with other types of lymphoma or Hodgkin's disease do not have an increased incidence of monoclonal proteins.

Table 22-1. Normal human serum immunoglobulins

Property	IgG*	IgA	IgM	IgD	IgE
Heavy chain class	γ	α	μ	δ	ε
Light chain type	κ or λ	κ or λ	κ or λ	κ or λ	κ or λ
Molecular weight	150,000	160,000	900,000	180,000	190,000
Proportion of total serum immunoglobulins	75%	15%	10%	0.2%	0.005%
Normal serum concentration (range)	1200 mg/dl (800–1500)	200 mg/dl (50–400)	100 mg/dl (40–180)	2 mg/dl	0.05 mg/dl
Proportion of immunoglobulin distributed intravascularly	52%	55%	75%	75%	40%
Serum half-life	20 days	6 days	5 days	3 days	3 days
Half-life decreases as serum concentration increases	Yes	No	No	No	No

*IgG comprises four subclasses. Approximately 70 percent of IgG is IgG₁, 17 percent IgG₂, 8 percent IgG₃, and 5 percent IgG₄. The data shown apply to all subtypes except IgG₃. IgG₃ differs from the other subclasses in that 65 percent is distributed intravascularly, its serum half-life is seven days and is not affected by high serum concentrations, it most avidly binds complement (other subclasses do so weakly, if at all), and it is most likely to produce hyperviscosity.

Note: Data are approximate. Normal ranges vary considerably among laboratories.

C. Etiology. No specific etiologic agent for the plasma cell dyscrasias has been found. Predisposing factors in humans appear to be

1. **Radiation exposure,** which slightly increases the risk of PCM.

2. **Chronic antigen stimulation.** Many M proteins have been shown to be antibodies directed against specific antigens such as bacterial and viral antigens, red cell antigens, lipoproteins, rheumatoid factors, neural antigens, and coagulation factors. Chronic antigenic stimulation (e.g., chronic osteomyelitis or cholecystitis) may predispose to the development of PCM or MGUS.

3. **Environmental exposure.** Exposure to benzene in the workplace and use of hair dye associated with an increased incidence of PCM.

D. Genetics

1. **PCM.** Multiple, complex karyotypic changes are observed in the malignant plasma cells of most patients.

   a. The most consistent changes are translocations involving either chromosome 14 at the site of the Ig heavy chain locus, chromosome 11 at the site of proto-oncogenes *BCL*-1 and Cyclin D, or chromosome 8 at the site of the c-*MYC* proto-oncogene.

   b. Mutations of *ras* genes occur in approximately 20 percent of myelomas and are associated with a poor prognosis. Similarly, mutations of p53 are found in 15 to 20 percent of cases and are associated with more advanced and clinically aggressive disease.

   c. Rearrangements of proto-oncogenes that are commonly rearranged in other B cell malignancies (c-*MYC*, *BCL*-1, and *BCL*-2) have been rarely found in myeloma.

2. **WM.** Complex karyotypes are also commonly observed in WM. Occasional patients have translocations involving the Ig heavy chain locus on chromosome 14 and either c-*MYC* on chromosome 8 or *BCL*-2 on chromosome 18.

II. Pathology and natural history

A. Bone marrow pathology is usually distinctive in PCM and WM. Plasma cells that constitute more than 20 percent of the nucleated marrow cells (*excluding erythroblasts*) are characteristic but not diagnostic of PCM.

1. **MGUS.** Normal plasma cells rarely exceed 10 percent of bone marrow cells.

2. **PCM.** Plasma cells usually constitute 20 to 95 percent of the marrow cells, have abundant basophilic cytoplasm, and eccentric nuclei with paranuclear clear zones. Immaturity of the plasma cells is evident with the presence of prominent nucleoli ("myeloma cells"). Bone marrow biopsy showing monotonous infiltration with plasma cells is the only diagnostic criterion for PCM accepted by many authorities. The presence of large, homogeneous infiltrates or nodules of plasma cells is highly suggestive of PCM. However, early in its course, marrow involvement is patchy and normal marrow particles may be obtained.

3. **WM** may closely resemble chronic lymphocytic leukemia. Bone marrow in WM contains 10 to 90 percent plasmacytoid lymphocytes or small mature lymphocytes; mast cells are often prominent.

4. **Reactive plasmacytosis.** Peripheral blood plasmacytosis occurs in many viral illnesses, serum sickness, and plasma cell leukemia (which is very rare). Bone marrow plasmacytosis, when not caused by myeloma, is characterized by a diffuse distribution (not infiltrative), and alignment of mature plasma cells along blood vessels or near marrow reticulum cells. Reactive bone marrow plasmacytosis is commonly seen in the following disorders:

   a. Viral infections

   b. Serum sickness

   c. Collagen vascular disease

   d. Granulomatous disease

   e. Liver cirrhosis

   f. Neoplastic disease

    g. Marrow hypoplasia

    h. A variety of other disorders

B. Natural history of MGUS. MGUS by definition is asymptomatic and diagnosed by exclusion. The only finding is monoclonal paraproteinemia. Transition of MGUS to a malignant disorder (usually PCM) occurs in about 20 percent of patients over 8 to 10 years. **Peripheral neuropathy** is not uncommon and has been observed in patients with a monoclonal immunoglobulin directed against a myelin-associated protein (see sec. **VII.B**).

C. Natural history of WM. The natural history of WM resembles lymphocytic lymphoma much more than PCM. Indeed, separating WM from MGUS, chronic lymphocytic leukemia, or lymphocytic lymphoma with IgM spikes may be more arbitrary than real. WM originates from clones of lymphocytes or plasma cells that synthesize μ chains. Lymphadenopathy, splenomegaly, and hyperviscosity are hallmarks of WM; skeletal lesions and impaired renal function are unusual. Concomitant macroglobulinemia and osteolytic lesions usually signify malignant lymphoma or solid tumor rather than primary WM. Glomerular lesions are frequent in WM, but renal failure is uncommon. Low levels of light chains in the urine occur in about 25 percent of patients.

D. Natural history of PCM. Three to 20 years of clonal growth may pass before PCM becomes clinically evident. The disease may be localized (7% of cases), indolent (3%), or disseminated and progressive (90%). Manifestations of disease progression arise from bone marrow and skeletal involvement, plasma protein abnormalities, and the development of renal disease.

    1. Plasmacytomas (plasma cell tumors) may develop anywhere in the skeleton or, rarely, in extraskeletal sites, such as the nasopharynx or paranasal sinuses. Localized plasmacytomas produce a monoclonal spike in the serum or urine protein electrophoresis in only 50 percent of cases. The median survival is more than 8 years. Most plasmacytomas that appear to be solitary become generalized in approximately three years, particularly those involving the skeleton. Extraskeletal plasmacytomas have a better prognosis than those of skeletal origin and less frequently progress to multiple myeloma.

    2. Hematopoiesis is often impaired. At the time of diagnosis, 60 percent of patients have anemia; 15 percent, leukopenia; and 15 percent, thrombocytopenia. Nucleated red cells and immature granulocytes may be present in the peripheral blood (leukoerythroblastic reaction).

    3. Skeletal disease that produces pain develops in about 70 percent of patients.

        a. Bone lesions. Multiple osteolytic lesions are present in about 70 percent of patients, single osteolytic lesions or diffuse osteoporosis in 15 percent, and normal skeletal x-ray films in 15 percent. Lesions are most commonly seen in the skull, vertebrae, ribs, pelvis, and proximal long bones. Osteoclast-activating factor (OAF) produced by neoplastic plasma cells probably accounts for the osteolytic lesions and demineralization. Interestingly, OAF's activity is largely mediated by tumor necrosis factor, IL-1, and IL-6. Osteoblastic lesions occur in less than 2 percent of patients, often in association with neuropathy; because of their rarity, the diagnosis of PCM should be doubted in the presence of osteoblastic lesions.

        b. Hypercalcemia develops in approximately one-third of patients because of the increased resorption of bone salts from areas of osteolysis. The incidence of hypercalcemia is increased in patients with renal dysfunction. Painful fractures often lead to bed rest and immobilization, producing a vicious cycle of worsening hypercalcemia, deteriorating renal function, nausea and vomiting, and dehydration. Serum alkaline phosphatase levels are usually normal but may be increased slightly with recalcification of fractures.

    4. Protein abnormalities

a. **Frequency.** The incidences of monoclonal immunoglobulins in PCM and compared to MGUS are

Paraprotein	PCM	MGUS
IgG	52%	65%
IgA	22%	25%
IgM	Very rare	10%
Light chains only	25%	Nil
Nonsecretory	<1%	—

b. **Increased excretion of κ or λ** light chains in the urine depends on the rate of unbalanced synthesis of excess light chains, plasma volume, degradation rate, renal catabolism, and urine volume. Monoclonal light chains in the urine are present in two-thirds of all patients with PCM and present without an M protein in the serum in 25 percent.

c. **Normal immunoglobulins** are usually decreased in the serum of patients with PCM and are occasionally decreased in patients with MGUS. The mechanism of inhibition of their synthesis is unknown. This suppression is responsible for the increased susceptibility to infections with encapsulated bacteria (*Haemophilus influenzae, Streptococcus pneumoniae,* and *Neisseria meningitidis*). However, sepsis caused by gram-negative bacteria is more frequent overall in PCM and is often a lethal complication late in the course of disease.

d. **Other plasma alterations** (see sec. **VII.A**). Hyperviscosity is unusual in PCM (<5% of patients).

5. **Renal dysfunction,** both acute and chronic, occurs at diagnosis in 15 to 20 percent of cases and develops during their course in about 50 percent of patients with PCM. Patients with light chain myeloma commonly present with renal failure. The most important causes of renal dysfunction in PCM are the following:

a. **Myeloma kidney** is generally attributed to the deposition of κ and λ chains in the distal and collecting tubules, which is where the light chains are catabolized. The tubules dilate, apparently obstructed by casts surrounded by multinucleated giant cells, and undergo cellular atrophy. Glomerular basement membrane disease also occurs in most patients with myeloma kidney. In most instances, proteinuria contains monoclonal light chains only. These abnormalities occur slightly more commonly in PCM producing λ chains.

PCM is the most common cause of the **adult Fanconi's syndrome** (aminoaciduria, glycosuria, phosphaturia, and electrolyte loss in the urine). Fanconi's syndrome may precede the recognition of PCM by many years.

b. **Amyloidosis** is common in PCM; it affects the glomeruli and results in nonselective proteinuria.

c. **Inconstant findings** that may aggravate renal function include pyelonephritis, metabolic abnormalities (hypercalcemia, nephrocalcinosis, and hyperuricemia), glomerulosclerosis, and focal myeloma cell infiltration. Renal tubular acidosis occasionally occurs. Nephrotic syndrome is rare in PCM unless amyloidosis supervenes.

d. **Intravenous contrast dye studies** should be done with caution since patients with PCM are more susceptible to renal dysfunction after such studies, particularly if they are dehydrated.

6. **Neurologic dysfunction** often develops in PCM and is the result of several pathogenetic mechanisms.

a. **CNS.** Spinal cord and nerve root compression develops in approximately 15 percent of patients and is usually caused by epidural plasmacytoma. Amyloidosis is a rare cause of epidural masses. Collapse of vertebral bodies may also cause spinal cord compression but, more likely, produces radicular symptoms secondary to nerve root compression. Cranial nerve palsies may develop from tumor occlusion of calvarial foramina. Intracerebral and meningeal plasmacytomas are rare.

   b. Peripheral neuropathy. The carpal tunnel syndrome, which is usually the result of amyloid infiltration of the flexor retinaculum of the wrist (causing entrapment of the median nerve), is a common peripheral neuropathy in PCM. Infiltration of nerve fibers and vaso nervorum with amyloid may also produce peripheral neuropathy. Additionally, peripheral neuropathy may be associated with monoclonal immunoglobulins to myelin-associated glycoproteins (see sec. **VII.B**). Rarely, patients with PCM and osteosclerotic lesions develop a characteristic peripheral neuropathy.

   c. Neurologic paraneoplastic syndromes (see Chap. 32, sec. **V**).

III. Diagnosis

   A. Symptoms. Fatigue, weakness, and weight loss are common in both PCM and WM. Skeletal pain occurs in 70 percent of patients with PCM at the time of diagnosis but is very rare in patients with WM.

   1. Symptoms of hypercalcemia (see Chap. 27, sec. **I**) are present in about 30 percent of patients with PCM at the time of diagnosis and develop in another 30 percent later in the course of the disease.

   2. Hyperviscosity syndrome symptoms (bleeding, neurologic dysfunction, visual disturbances, or congestive heart failure) are present in about 50 percent of patients with WM and in less than 5 percent of patients with PCM (see sec. **VII.A.1**).

   3. Cold sensitivity may occur in patients with cryoglobulins, especially in WM (see sec. **VII.A.2**).

   B. Physical findings

   1. Hepatosplenomegaly is present in 40 percent of patients with WM at the time of diagnosis and is very rare in PCM.

   2. Lymphadenopathy occurs in 30 percent of patients with WM but is rare in patients with PCM except late in the disease.

   3. Bone tenderness in patients with PCM often signifies recent fracture or subperiosteal infiltration with malignant cells.

   4. Neurologic abnormalities are frequent in PCM (see sec. **II.D.6**); neurologic abnormalities in WM are caused by hyperviscosity (see sec. **VII.A.1**) or demyelination (see sec. **VII.B**).

   5. Purpura signifies thrombocytopenia in PCM and hyperviscosity syndrome in WM.

   C. Laboratory studies. The following studies should be obtained in the investigation of patients with suspected plasma cell neoplasms:

   1. CBC. Anemia is variable in MGUS and WM and present in 60 percent of patients with PCM. Neutropenia or thrombocytopenia are absent in MGUS and present in 15 percent of patients with PCM and 5 percent of patients with WM.

   2. Biopsy. Bone marrow, solitary osteolytic lesion, masses, skin nodules, or enlarged lymph nodes. Bone marrow findings are discussed in sec. **II.A.**

   3. Serum biochemistry. BUN, creatinine, electrolytes, calcium, uric acid, total protein, and alkaline phosphatase.

   4. Serum proteins. Protein electrophoresis (PEP), immunoelectrophoresis (IEP), and quantitative immunoglobulins (QIG).

   5. Serum β-2 microglobulin (β2m) and C-reactive protein (CRP) may be useful prognostic indicators.

   6. urine. 24-hour excretion of protein and PEP and IEP of a concentrated specimen (urine dip sticks are usually not sensitive enough to detect light chains, and Bence-Jones protein assays are unreliable.)

   7. Skeleton studies

   a. Complete skeletal x-ray survey, including skull and long bones.

   b. MRI of spinal cord if there is a paraspinal mass or signs of cord or nerve root compression.

   c. Bone scans are of limited usefulness in PCM since most lesions are osteolytic, and bone scans require perilesional osteoblastic activity to be positive. Positive bone scans in PCM usually indicate regions of fracture or arthritis, except in the rare event of osteoblastic myeloma.

   d. Bone densitometry studies may be useful in following patients with PCM.

  8. Special studies. Serum viscosity, cryoglobulins, and rectal biopsy or analysis of joint effusions for amyloid are obtained when indicated.

D. Protein studies. Some serum immunoglobulin properties that have clinical relevance are listed in Table 22-1. Kinetic studies of protein synthesis in animals and humans show tumor burden to be closely correlated with the quantity of paraprotein in the blood (approximately 1 gm/dl of paraprotein corresponds to 100 gm of tumor and 1×10^{11} plasma cells).

  1. Protein electrophoresis is extremely valuable for recognizing cases of monoclonal gammopathies and for following quantitative changes in spikes. However, PEP is only a presumptive screening test; IEP must be done to establish the diagnosis of monoclonal gammopathy. Examples of serum and urine PEP patterns are shown in Figure 22-1.

    a. M protein spikes are usually located in the γ or γ-β region. Monoclonal peaks in the α or α-β region are usually not caused by paraproteins but by reactant proteins (see sec. **VII.C**).

    b. IgG spikes are usually tall, narrow, and located in the γ region. **IgA spikes** are usually broader as the molecule tends to form polymers of different sizes; they are located in the β region. **IgM spikes** are usually located near the point of origin. **IgD spikes** usually cause only slight deflections in the pattern because the protein is present in a relatively small concentration.

    c. Light chains are not ordinarily found in the serum since light chains are rapidly catabolized by the kidney or excreted in the urine. Light chain spikes may be found in the serum of patients with renal insufficiency or in instances in which polymerization of light chains has occurred. The normal ratio of κ to λ chains in humans is 2:1. This normal ratio is usually maintained when excretion of light chains is due to renal disease but is significantly altered when the excretion is due to malignant gammopathies. Urinary excretion of monoclonal light chains is found in 50 to 60 percent of patients with PCM, 10 to 20 percent of patients with WM, and rarely in MGUS.

  2. IEP determines the exact heavy chain class (γ, α, μ, δ, ε) and light chain type (κ, λ) of the M protein and distinguishes polyclonal and monoclonal increases in gammaglobulins. IEP is more sensitive than PEP for low concentration (e.g., IgD) or heterogeneous globulin mixtures.

  3. QIG estimations are excellent for measuring normal or decreased immunoglobulin levels and are useful for distinguishing MGUS from PCM, but are unreliable if levels are markedly increased or if protein aggregation has occurred.

  4. Serum viscosity. The rate of descent of serum at 37°C through a calibrated capillary tube is compared with that of distilled water. Plasma is not used because elevated levels of fibrinogen can markedly affect the results. Normal values for serum viscosity ratios range from 1.4 to 1.9. Symptoms usually do not develop unless the serum viscosity exceeds 4.

E. Differentiation of plasma cell dyscrasias. In the absence of biopsy proof of malignant disease, differentiating MGUS from early malignant disease may be impossible at the initial examination. To establish the diagnosis, serial evaluations of the patient and paraprotein level must be done for several months or years. Table 22-2 indicates the important data that need repeated observation. These data predict benign or malignant monoclonal gammopathy but none is diagnostic by itself; patients with MGUS may slowly progress to PCM. The most important findings that suggest malignant disease are significant (more than 25%) and sustained increase in the serum paraprotein or urinary light chain concentration.

  1. IgM monoclonal gammopathies may be benign or due to WM, lymphopro-

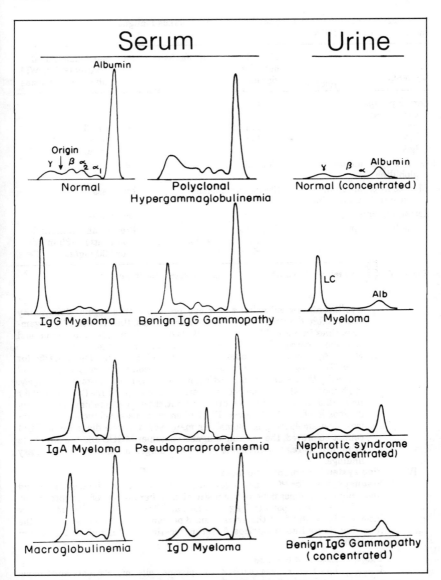

Fig. 22-1. Electrophoresis patterns (*Alb* = albumin). **Serum.** Normal: The point of application of serum is indicated. Benign IgG gammopathy: Normal levels of albumin and gamma globulins plus a peak in the γ region. Pseudoparaproteinemia: Small peaks in β or α regions (see sec. **VII.C**). Polyclonal hypergammaglobulinemia: Occurs in many conditions. **Urine.** Myeloma: Typical homogeneous peak of light chains (LC) in γ region. Nephrotic syndrome: Panproteinuria. Benign IgG gammopathy: Normal pattern in urine.

Table 22-2. Protein variables for predicting benign versus malignant monoclonal gammopathy

Variable	Monoclonal gammopathy of undetermined significance (MGUS)	Malignant monoclonal gammopathy (PCM, WM, B lymphocyte neoplasms)
Serum paraprotein concentration		
IgG	<2.0 gm/dl	>2.0 gm/dl
IgM	<2.0 gm/dl	>2.0 gm/dl
IgA	<1.0 gm/dl	>1.0 gm/dl
Other serum immunoglobulins	Normal or decreased	Decreased
Change in paraprotein concentration over time	Stable or transient	Increases
Serum albumin	Normal	Decreased
Urine light chains	Absent or normal κ/λ ratio and less than 300 mg/day	Present and abnormal κ/λ ratio (>30 mg/dl or 300 mg/day)

Key: PCM = plasma cell myeloma; WM = Waldenström's macroglobulinemia.

tive disorder or epithelial tumor can present with a serum abnormality years before the neoplasm becomes evident. Thus, the division of IgM gammopathies into MGUS, primary or Waldenström's macroglobulinemia, and secondary macroglobulinemia is at times arbitrary (see sec. II.C).

2. **IgG, IgA, and IgD monoclonal gammopathies: diagnostic criteria for PCM.** To establish the diagnosis of PCM, invasion or destruction of normal tissues by the uncontrolled growth of plasma cells must be proved by biopsy. High concentrations of monoclonal serum immunoglobulins (>3.5 gm/dl for IgG, >2.0 mg/dl for IgA) or urinary light chains (>1 gm/day) are nearly diagnostic of PCM. However, PCM often remains subclinical or indolent (so-called smoldering myeloma) for many years. If the diagnosis of PCM cannot be proved, the working diagnosis becomes MGUS and the patient is examined at regular intervals to detect changes in clinical or laboratory findings.

IV. **Staging system and prognostic factors**

A. **Staging system for PCM.** Distinguishing patients with low, intermediate, and high volumes of tumor mass before institution of therapy is useful for prognosis: 1×10^{12} cells correspond to 1 kg of tumor, and 3 to 5×10^{12} cells are usually incompatible with life in the average-sized patient. Some centers subdivide the following stages into **substages** A (serum creatinine <2 mg/dl) and B (serum creatinine ≥2 mg/dl).

Stage	Extent of disease
I	Low tumor mass (<0.6 × 10^{12} plasma cells/m²). Patients must have *all* of the following: 　Hemoglobin >10 gm/dl 　Serum calcium: normal or ≤12 mg/dl 　Low M-component production rates with 　　IgG value <5 gm/dl 　　IgA value <3 gm/dl 　　UPEP M-component light chain <4 gm/24 hr 　Skeletal x-ray: normal or with a solitary plasmacytoma
II	Intermediate tumor mass (0.6–1.2 × 10^{12} plasma cells/m²). Patients who qualify for neither stage I nor III

III   High tumor mass ($>1.2 \times 10^{12}$ plasma cells/m^2). Patients having *any one* of the following:
   Hemoglobin <8.5 gm/dl
   Serum calcium >12 mg/dl
   High M-component production rates
      IgG >7 gm/dl
      IgA >5 gm/dl
      UPEP M-component light chain >12 gm/24 hr
   Extensive lytic bone lesions

B. Prognostic factors
   1. MGUS. If a patient with the presumptive diagnosis of MGUS remains stable for two years, the chance for malignant disease is about 20 percent.
   2. WM. Median survival is about three to four years for patients who are unresponsive to treatment and about five to seven years for responsive patients. However, survival of 10 to 20 years is not rare. The development of complications, such as hyperviscosity, hemorrhage, or infection, contributes to death. Age more than 60 years, male gender, and hemoglobin less than 10 gm/dl are associated with shortened survival.
   3. PCM. The overall median survival rate of patients with PCM is two to three years. The prognosis in PCM is affected by tumor mass, response to therapy, renal function, and M protein type.
      a. Tumor mass. Patients with a low tumor mass have a median survival of 3.5 to 10.0 years. Patients with a high tumor mass can expect a median survival of 0.5 to 3.0 years.
      b. Response to therapy. Patients with a high tumor mass who have a reduction of the serum peak by more than 75 percent of the original value have a median survival of three years or more, while patients who have less than a 50 percent reduction in the peak have a median survival of less than one year. Paradoxically, patients who respond too rapidly to therapy with melphalan and prednisone (more than 50% reduction in less than 3 months) have a poor prognosis.
      c. Renal function previously was thought to be a very important prognostic factor. Increasing degrees of azotemia were associated with progressively shorter life expectancies. Recent advances in plasmapheresis, dialysis, and supportive care make this a less important prognostic factor.
      d. Immunoglobulin class. Patients with IgD myeloma or λ light chain myeloma have the worst prognosis (median survival is less than one year). Patients with IgG myeloma of κ light chain myeloma have the best prognosis (median survival is 2 to 3 years).
      e. (β-2m) is the light chain moiety of classical HLA antigens and is found on the surface membranes of most nucleolated cells. Patients with PCM and higher initial values of β-2m appear to have a worse prognosis. Despite the high correlation of β-2m levels with renal function, β-2m has emerged as an important independent prognostic factor. Elevated β-2m levels are also found in patients with acute or chronic myelocytic leukemia, lymphoproliferative disorders, myeloproliferative disorders, myelodysplastic syndromes, benign or malignant liver diseases, and autoimmune diseases.
      f. Labeling index (LI). The LI is indicative of the percentage of cells undergoing mitosis. A high LI (>3%) is associated with a poor prognosis in PCM.
      g. Other markers. Elevated IL-6 levels may possibly portend a poor prognosis. CRP levels appear to reflect IL-6 serum levels, but most patients with PCM do not have elevated CRP levels.
V. Prevention and early detection. The availability of PEP and of screening chemistry panels has probably resulted in earlier detection of monoclonal gammopathies. If IEP were used for screening populations, the incidence of MGUS might well double but survival would not be affected.
VI. Management

A. MGUS. Patients should have PEP studies every three months for the first year, every six months for the next two years, and then yearly thereafter. Patients with MGUS should not be treated with cytotoxic agents.

B. WM. The best management for WM has not been established. We recommend the following approach:

1. **Asymptomatic patients** without anemia, hyperviscosity, renal insufficiency, or neurologic abnormalities should be monitored for clinical status and PEP until disease progression is confirmed.

2. **Patients with symptoms of progressive disease** are treated with a single agent.
   a. Chlorambucil is used in moderate doses (6–8 mg/day for 1–3 months, followed by 2–4 mg/day for maintenance). The majority of patients improve with treatment.
   b. Patients unresponsive to chlorambucil may respond to fludarabine. Patients with WM should be treated with only several courses of fludarabine because responses can persist many months after discontinuing the agent.

3. **Patients with hyperviscosity syndrome** (see sec. **VII.A**).

C. PCM. Maximizing ambulation, administration of chemotherapy and RT are the mainstays of treatment.

1. **Surgery** in PCM is restricted to orthopedic procedures (see Chap. 33, sec. I). Fractures of long bones usually require fixation with a medullary pin and postoperative irradiation. Sometimes impending fractures with large osteolytic lesions of the femoral head are internally fixed prophylactically. If the diagnosis of the underlying disease is in doubt, acute spinal cord compression or vertebral fracture may make laminectomy necessary.

2. **RT** is very useful for palliation of lesions that are localized or cause spinal cord or nerve root compression. Small subcutaneous tumors or small painful lesions in bone may be treated with only a single dose of 800 cGy. Large osteolytic lesions in long bones should be irradiated before a fracture occurs. Large lytic lesions or paraspinous masses rarely need more than 2000 cGy in five days.
   a. **Solitary plasmacytomas** in bone or pharynx mandate more aggressive treatment, which may be curative.
   b. **Back pain** is relieved by RT unless the pain is due to compression fracture. Since spinal cord compression is a common complication in PCM, the physician should not hesitate to order an MRI or myelogram on patients with PCM with new or changes in back pain. This should be treated emergently if it occurs (see Chap. 32, sec. **III**).

3. **Chemotherapy.** Several alkylating agents (melphalan, cyclophosphamide, nitrosoureas, and chlorambucil) are equally effective in producing responses in about 30 percent of patients. Refractoriness to one alkylating agent is often associated with responsiveness to another alkylating agent.
   a. **Regimens**
      (1) **M&P** (cycle frequency is 4–6 weeks)
          (a) Melphalan: 10 mg/m^2 PO on days 1 through 4
          (b) Prednisone: 60 mg/m^2 PO on days 1 through 4
      (2) **VAD** (cycle frequency is 4 weeks)
          (a) Vincristine: 0.4 mg/day for 4 days by continuous infusion through a central venous line
          (b) Adriamycin: 9 mg/m^2/day for 4 days by continuous infusion
          (c) Dexamethasone: 40 mg PO on days 1 to 4, 9 to 13, and 17 to 21
      (3) **M-2 protocol** (cycle frequency is 5–6 weeks)
          (a) Melphalan: 0.25 mg/kg PO on days 1 through 4
          (b) Prednisone: 1.0 mg/kg PO on days 1 through 7
          (c) Vincristine: 0.03 mg/kg IV on day 1
          (d) BCNU: 1.0 mg/kg IV on day 1
          (e) Cyclophosphamide: 10 mg/kg IV on day 1

(4) VBAP (cycle frequency is three weeks)
  (a) Vincristine: 1 mg IV on day 1
  (b) BCNU (carmustine): 30 mg/m^2 IV on day 1
  (c) Adriamycin: 30 mg/m^2 IV on day 1
  (d) Prednisone: 100 mg PO on days 1 through 4
(5) Dexamethasone alone, 40 mg PO daily for four days every other week.
(6) High-dose chemotherapy. Recent efforts to improve the long-term survival of patients with myeloma have involved the infusion of autologous peripheral blood stem cells or allogeneic bone marrow. Treatment regimens have generally contained either myeloablative doses of intravenous melphalan with or without total body irradiation (TBI) or high doses of cyclophosphamide with either oral busulfan or TBI. Although response rates and disease-free survival are better with these more intensive regimens than with conventional chemotherapy, results of long-term follow-up are unavailable. Randomized trials comparing patients who received transplants to patients treated with conventional therapy have been initiated to address the utility of transplantation in myeloma.
b. Responses. The addition of prednisone to an alkylating agent regimen (e.g., M&P) increases the response rate to 40 or 50 percent. Response rates to daily low-dose, single-agent therapy appear to be equivalent to pulse therapy given every four to six weeks. Responses to VAD occur more rapidly and are somewhat more frequent than to M&P. Steroids alone (dexamethasone) may produce response and survival rates nearly equivalent to those achieved with infusional VAD or M&P. Other combination chemotherapy regimens have not been proved to improve survival when compared with M&P.
c. Recommendations. In patients considered to be candidates for high-dose chemotherapy with hematopoietic support, initial therapy should begin with either infusional VAD or high-dose oral dexamethasone alone. This approach avoids the permanent stem cell cytotoxic effect of alkylator therapy.
  Otherwise, patients should begin with pulse M&P therapy, particularly those with low or intermediate tumor masses. If a rapid response is desired (e.g., patients with hypercalcemia, marrow failure or renal dysfunction), initial therapy with VAD may be preferable.
  In patients who either relapse shortly after discontinuation of M&P therapy or are refractory to M&P, high-dose dexamethasone or VAD may be tried. If the relapse occurs late, another course of M&P may be effective therapy. In patients who fail VAD, M&P may help. IFN alone has been shown to be effective in only a small percentage of relapsing patients, especially those with IgA paraproteins.
d. Duration of therapy and maintenance. Patients should be treated until a plateau phase (stabilization of paraprotein levels for several months) is achieved. Continuation of chemotherapy beyond plateau phase has not been demonstrated to prolong survival but does increase the risk of secondary malignancies, especially acute leukemia. Although remissions are sustained longer with the addition of IFN, a significant survival benefit for maintenance therapy with this cytokine after conventional therapy has not been demonstrated, except for possibly those patients treated with high-dose chemotherapy.
4. Supportive care is extremely important in PCM. Bed rest is often necessary because of the painful bony lesions or fractures. However, bed rest further promotes bone demineralization, which may lead to hypercalcemia.
  a. Pain relief may be achieved with focal radiotherapy. Analgesics should be prescribed in a regimen that gives the most consistent pain relief.
  b. Ambulation should be maximized as early as possible following the onset

of fractures or pain. Corsets and braces are often effective in relieving back pain by stabilizing the spine until RT or chemotherapy becomes effective.

c. Hydration. Patients must be repeatedly reminded to drink two to three liters of fluids daily to promote urinary excretion of light chains, calcium, and uric acid. This simple reminder has been shown to greatly improve survival in some studies.

d. Infections are the foremost cause of death in patients with PCM because such patients have greatly suppressed normal immunoglobulins. Infections must be investigated and treated urgently.

e. Bone remineralization. Fluoride and vitamin D are not effective in increasing bone remineralization in patients with PCM; fluoride treatment results only in increased bone density because of fluorosis. Biphosphonates (particularly pamidronate) and gallium nitrate are promising agents that are being investigated for their potential ability to reduce bone pain and skeletal complications.

f. Renal failure is best prevented by hydration and treatment of hyperuricemia and hypercalcemia. Plasmapheresis may be a useful adjunct. When renal failure becomes severe, some patients may be candidates for hemodialysis treatment, especially if they have a reasonable prognosis and have not failed initial therapy. Azotemia improves slowly in these patients.

VII. Special clinical problems
A. Plasma alterations in patients with M proteins

1. Hyperviscosity syndrome. The blood cells normally contribute more to the whole blood viscosity than do plasma proteins. The development of hyperviscosity with M proteins depends on their concentration and their ability to aggregate or polymerize. WM is typically associated with hyperviscosity. Symptoms usually do not occur unless the serum paraprotein concentration exceeds 3 to 4 gm/dl and the serum viscosity index exceeds 4.

a. Complications of hyperviscosity include the following:

(1) Bleeding diathesis is manifested by spontaneous bruising, purpura, retinal hemorrhages, epistaxis, or mucosal bleeding. The hemorrhagic diathesis is compounded by thrombocytopenia. Bleeding in the hyperviscosity syndrome appears to be a result of:

(a) Interference with coagulation, especially the third stage of coagulation (polymerization of fibrin monomer), resulting in prolongation of clotting times

(b) Impaired platelet function resulting in abnormalities of bleeding times, clot retraction, and other platelet functions

(2) Retinopathy is manifested by venous dilatation and segmentation ("link-sausage" appearance), retinal hemorrhages, and papilledema.

(3) Neurologic symptoms develop in about 25 percent of patients and include malaise, focal neurologic defects, stroke, and coma.

(4) Hypervolemia develops with an increase of M protein concentration, resulting in distention of peripheral blood vessels and increased vascular resistance. Plasma volume expansion may actually lessen the viscosity but may also precipitate congestive heart failure (which occurs in about 10 percent of patients who have hyperviscosity).

b. Management. Hyperviscosity syndrome is treated by reducing the quantity of paraprotein in the serum. Reduction of paraprotein concentrations with cytotoxic agent therapy takes several weeks or months. Symptomatic patients should be treated with plasmapheresis, four to six units daily, until the viscosity index is less than 3. Patients with hyperviscosity caused by monoclonal IgM usually respond to plasmapheresis more rapidly than those with IgG or IgA gammopathies because IgM has a predominantly intravascular distribution (see Table 22-1). Additionally, there is an exponential relationship between serum viscosity and IgM level so that, for example, a 20 percent decrease in IgM concentration results in a 100 percent decrease in serum viscosity. Improvement should be monitored by noting changes in clinical findings, coagulation tests, and serum viscosity determinations.

2. **Cold sensitivity** may afflict patients with M proteins (especially IgM) that have physicochemical properties that permit cold precipitation. The cryoglobulins in plasma cell dyscrasias and lymphoproliferative disorders are monoclonal. The cryoglobulins in other disorders (such as collagen vascular diseases and viral infections) are circulating soluble immune complexes (IgM-IgG, IgA-IgG, IgG-IgG). Manifestations include cold urticaria, Raynaud's phenomenon, and vascular purpura in the absence of severe thrombocytopenia.

3. **Cold agglutinins** are IgMs with a specificity for specific red cell antigens (usually Ia) at temperatures less than 37°C. These proteins may be responsible for a mild extravascular complement-dependent hemolysis and acrocyanosis but not for other symptoms of cold sensitivity unless cryoglobulins are also present.

4. **Pseudohyponatremia** may be observed with high levels of M proteins (plasma water is displaced by the paraprotein).

5. **Anion gaps,** noted with measurement of serum electrolytes (serum concentration of [sodium−chloride−bicarbonate]), may be decreased in patients with cationic monoclonal proteins. The normal anion gap is about 12 mEq/L; in patients with monoclonal gammopathies of benign or malignant origin, the gap may be 8 mEq/L or less. The decreased gap is produced by the increase of chloride and bicarbonate anions.

B. **Peripheral neuropathy** occurs especially in patients with IgM monoclonal gammopathies. Approximately 5 percent of patients with a sensorimotor neuropathy have an associated monoclonal gammopathy. Nearly 10 percent of patients with WM and or with MGUS and an IgM paraprotein develop a demyelinating peripheral neuropathy. Sural nerve biopsies demonstrate monoclonal IgM deposition on the outer myelin sheath. The antibody can be shown to react with myelin-associated glycoprotein (MAG) in half of cases. These patients usually have a mostly sensory or ataxic polyneuropathy, whereas patients with non-MAG reactive antibodies usually have both a sensory and motor component to their neuropathy. Treatment with plasmapheresis may be effective in some cases. Other forms of treatment have included high doses of glucocorticosteroids or intravenous gammaglobulin.

C. **Pseudoparaproteinemia.** The PEP can detect serum proteins when the concentration exceeds 200 mg/dl. In certain situations, a nonimmunoglobulin homogeneous protein concentration may exceed 300 mg/dl and appear as a spike on PEP. The location of these spikes usually are in the α and β regions, but may be in the β-γ region. The differential diagnosis is clarified by review of the clinical picture, the location of the PEP spike, and IEP. Conditions that may produce pseudoparaproteinemia include

1. Hyperalpha$_1$-globulinemia (acute-phase reactant in many inflammatory and neoplastic diseases)
2. Hyperalpha$_2$-globulinemia (nephrotic syndrome or hemolysis)
3. Hemoglobin-haptoglobin complexes (intravascular hemolysis)
4. Hyperlipidemia
5. Hypertransferrinemia (iron deficiency)
6. Bacterial products
7. Desiccated serum
8. Fibrinogen (if plasma is measured)

D. **Pseudomyeloma.** Several malignancies, including lymphoma and cancer of the breast, bowel, or biliary tract, may be associated with the production of a monoclonal paraprotein. These same malignancies may produce lytic lesions in the skeleton and induce marrow plasmacytosis. Pseudomyeloma must be distinguished from true myeloma.

E. **Therapy-linked acute leukemia** is discussed in Chap. 34, *Cytopenia,* sec. **I.D.**

F. **Heavy chain diseases** (HCDs) are rare plasma cell–lymphocytic neoplasms characterized by secretion of abnormal heavy chains (γ, α, or μ) without light chains (κ, λ). α-HCD is the most common and μ-HCD chain disease is the rarest. The heavy chains may also be excreted in the urine and detected by UPEP. Normal immunoglobulin levels are usually suppressed. Diagnosis of these disorders necessitates detailed immunochemical investigation. IEP is the critical test; it should demonstrate reaction of antisera with the appropriate heavy chain but not with light chains.

   1. **α-HCD** nearly always involves only the α_1 subtype of heavy chain. α-HCD was discussed in reference to GI lymphomas in Chap. 21, *Non-Hodgkin's Lymphoma*, **VI.C.**

   2. **γ-HCD** usually affects elderly patients. Generalized lymphadenopathy, hepatosplenomegaly, involvement of Waldeyer's ring, fever, pancytopenia, and eosinophilia are common features of the disease. The illness initially resembles granulomatous disease or Hodgkin's disease. Biopsies of lymph nodes and bone marrow are rarely diagnostic. The disease has a variable course, from a few months to several years. A satisfactory treatment plan has not been established.

   3. **μ-HCD** nearly always occurs in patients with chronic lymphocytic leukemia, and the two disorders are treated in the same manner. However, in μ-HCD lymphadenopathy is infrequent and, in contrast with other HCDs, large amounts of κ light chains are excreted in the urine. The rare disease may be suspected when a patient with chronic lymphocytic leukemia has unusual vacuolated plasma cells (characteristic of μ-HCD) in the bone marrow.

G. Amyloidosis may be primary (with or without associated plasma cell or lymphoid neoplasms), secondary to a variety of chronic inflammatory diseases or hereditary disorders (familial Mediterranean fever), or associated with the aging process. The disease is characterized by organ deposition of fibrillar substances of many different types. The fibrils are mostly or exclusively composed of immunoglobulin light chains (especially the λ type) in amyloidosis associated with primary amyloidosis and myeloma, but the fibrils are composed of substances other than light chains in secondary amyloidosis.

   1. **Organ distribution of amyloid.** The various forms of amyloidosis overlap considerably. **Secondary amyloidosis** affects the kidneys, spleen, liver, or adrenal glands, and rarely involves the heart, GI tract, or musculoskeletal system. **Primary amyloidosis** and **amyloidosis associated with PCM** mostly affect the heart, GI tract, skeletal muscle, ligaments (carpal tunnel syndrome), and periarticular and synovial tissue (articular manifestations), as well as the tongue (macroglossia) and skin. Skin involvement most commonly is located in the periorbital and skin fold regions and is manifested by spontaneous purpura and ecchymoses, which may be aggravated by coagulation factor X deficiency, which occasionally accompanies amyloidosis; postproctoscopic eyelid ecchymoses are characteristic. Involvement of the respiratory tract, endocrine glands, and peripheral and autonomic nervous systems also occurs.

   2. **Diagnosis**

      a. **Biopsy** of an involved organ (especially the carpal ligament, sural nerve, rectum, or gingivae) must be performed to establish the diagnosis of amyloidosis; liver or renal biopsy may result in hemorrhage. Amyloid deposits have a homogeneous eosinophilic appearance on light microscopy. Confirmation is made by the demonstration of specific birefringence by polarized microscopy of specimens stained with Congo red.

      b. **Monoclonal light chains** in the urine are found in both the primary type and amyloidosis associated with PCM. Many patients with primary amyloidosis are found to have developed plasma cell disease if they survive long enough.

   3. **Treatment** of amyloidosis is unsatisfactory. Even if the underlying disease is treated, regression of amyloid deposits is usually slow and insignificant.

H. Papular mucinosis (lichen myxedematosus) is a dermatologic condition characterized by cutaneous papules and plaques that result from the deposition of a mucinous material. The disease is often preceded by chronic pyoderma. It demonstrates a monoclonal paraprotein, usually IgG-λ, with a characteristic mobility (slower than any other gamma globulin component) and a strong affinity for normal dermis. Other manifestations of PCM (plasmacytosis, osteolysis, and excretion of light chains) are rare. Treatment with melphalan is often beneficial.

Selected Reading

Alexanian, R., and Dimopoulos, M. The treatment of multiple myeloma. *N. Engl. J. Med.* 330:484, 1994.

Barlogie, B., Alexanian, R., and Jagannath, S. Plasma cell dyscrasias. *J.A.M.A.* 268:2946, 1992.

Case, D. C., et al. Combination chemotherapy for multiple myeloma with the M2 protocol. *Oncology* 42:137, 1985.

Dimopoulos, M. A., and Alexanian, R. Waldenström's macroglobulinemia. *Blood* 83:1452, 1994.

Duggan, D. A., and Schattner, A. Unusual manifestations of monoclonal gammopathies. *Am. J. Med.* 81:864, 1986.

Kyle, R. A. "Benign" monoclonal gammopathy—after 20 to 35 years of follow-up. *Mayo Clin. Proc.* 68:26, 1993.

Reidel, D. A., and Pottern, L. A. The epidemiology of multiple myeloma. *Hematol. Oncol. Clin. North Am.* 6:225, 1992.

van Dobbenburgh, O. A., et al. Serum beta-2-microglobulin: a real improvement in the management of multiple myeloma? *Brit. J. Haematol.* 61:611, 1985.

23

Chronic Leukemias

Kenneth A. Foon and
Dennis A. Casciato

Chronic Lymphocytic Leukemia

I. Epidemiology and etiology

A. Incidence. Chronic lymphocytic leukemia (CLL) is the most common type of leukemia in Western countries, accounting for one-third of cases. The disease is rare in Asians; 90 percent of patients are more than 50 years old. Men are affected more than women by a ratio of 2:1.

B. Etiology

1. **Genetic factors.** Familial clusters of CLL have been described. The incidence in relatives of patients with leukemia is two- to threefold greater than the general population. The great majority of cases are sporadic.

2. **Immunologic factors.** Inherited and acquired immunodeficiency syndromes are often associated with CLL and other lymphoproliferative neoplasms. These observations suggest that defective immunosurveillance may result in proliferation of malignant cell clones and increased susceptibility to potential leukemogens, such as viruses.

3. **Chromosomes, oncogenes, and viruses.** A variety of chromosome abnormalities have been described in patients with CLL. The most common abnormalities include trisomy 12 and 13q⁻ with deletions involving the retinoblastoma gene. Rearrangements of three oncogenes are rarely associated with CLL. The t(11;14) translocation with rearrangement of the *BCL*-1 oncogene is more common in mantle cell lymphomas. The t(14;18) translocation with rearrangement of the *BCL*-2 oncogene is associated with 90 percent of follicular lymphomas and rarely with CLL, although overexpression of *BCL*-2 is common in CLL. The t(14;19) translocation with rearrangement of the *BCL*-3 oncogene appears unique to CLL but is very rare.

4. **Radiation.** Populations exposed to radiation do not have an increased incidence of CLL.

II. Pathology and natural history

A. Pathology. CLL is a clonal disease of immunologically incompetent, long-lived lymphocytes. All cases involve CD5-B lymphocytes. CD5-B lymphocytes represent approximately 10 percent of normal B lymphocytes and appear to play a major role in autoimmunity.

B. Natural history

1. **Immunologic abnormalities in CLL**

   a. Advanced disease is associated with hypogammaglobulinemia and decreased humoral responses to antigens.

   b. A variety of in vitro lymphocyte function tests are abnormal, including mitogenic response to plant lectins, spontaneous cytotoxicity, and antibody-dependent cytotoxicity. Many studies have suggested decreased T-helper functions, and patients generally show an inversion of the normal T-helper cell to T-suppressor cell ratios.

   c. The leukemia cells have low levels of surface immunoglobulin and absence of immunoglobulin capping. Most cells display a single heavy chain class, typically μ; some cells display both μ and δ; less commonly γ, α, or no heavy chain determinant is found. The leukemia cells display either κ or λ light chains, but never both.

  d. Surface membrane antigens include the B cell antigens CD19, CD20, and CD23 (see Appendix C4, Leukocyte Differentiation Antigens). The CD11c and CD25 antigens are found on the cells in half of cases. The putative T cell antigen, CD5, is always present in B cell CLL.

  e. Monoclonal paraproteins are not routinely identified; however, when one uses more sensitive techniques, it appears that most patients with CLL secrete small amounts of paraproteins (usually IgM). These paraproteins rarely produce symptoms of hyperviscosity.

  f. Coombs'-positive warm antibody hemolytic anemia occurs in about 10 percent of patients and immune thrombocytopenia in about 5 percent. Immune neutropenia and pure red cell aplasia are rare.

  g. Compared with the general population, the incidence of skin carcinoma is increased eightfold and visceral cancers twofold in patients with CLL.

2. Clinical course. The natural history of CLL is highly variable. Survival is closely correlated with the stage of disease at the time of diagnosis. Since most patients are elderly, more than 30 percent will die of diseases unrelated to leukemia.

  a. Manifestations. In 25 percent of patients, CLL is first recognized at routine physical examination or by a routine CBC. Clinical manifestations develop as the leukemic cells accumulate in the lymph nodes, spleen, liver, and bone marrow.

  (1) Osteolytic lesions and isolated mediastinal involvement are unusual and suggest a diagnosis other than CLL.

  (2) Pulmonary leukemic infiltrates and pleural effusions are very common late in the course of disease.

  (3) Renal involvement is common in CLL, but functional impairment is unusual in the absence of obstructive uropathy, pyelonephritis, or hyperuricemia secondary to tumor lysis from therapy.

  (4) Skin involvement is rare.

  (5) Transformation into a diffuse histiocytic lymphoma (Richter's syndrome) or "prolymphocytoid" leukemia occurs in less than 10 percent of patients.

  b. Progressive disease is accompanied by deterioration of both humoral and cell-mediated immunity.

  (1) Herpes zoster is the cause of 10 percent of infections in CLL patients.

  (2) Bacterial pathogens associated with hypogammaglobulinemia include *Streptococcus pneumoniae, Staphylococcus aureus,* and *Haemophilus influenzae.*

  (3) *Pneumocystis carinii* may be the causative infectious agent in patients with pulmonary infiltrates.

  (4) As the disease progresses, patients develop progressive pancytopenia, persistent fevers, and inanition. During the latter stages of disease, cytotoxic chemotherapy is generally ineffective and dosages are restricted because of pancytopenia. Death is usually caused by infection, bleeding, or other complications of the disease.

III. Diagnosis

A. Symptoms and signs. Patients with CLL that was discovered by chance are usually asymptomatic. Chronic fatigue and reduced exercise tolerance are the first symptoms to develop. Advanced and progressive disease are manifested by severe fatigue out of proportion to the degree of the patient's anemia, fever, bruising, and weight loss.

Lymphadenopathy, splenomegaly, and hepatomegaly should be carefully assessed. Edema or thrombophlebitis may result from obstruction of lymphatic or venous channels by enlarged lymph nodes.

B. Laboratory studies

1. Hemogram

a. **Erythrocytes.** Anemia may be caused by lymphocyte infiltration of the bone marrow, hypersplenism, autoimmune hemolysis, as well as other causes. Red cells are usually normocytic and normochromic in the absence of prominent hemolysis.

b. **Lymphocytes.** The absolute lymphocyte count typically ranges from 10,000 to 200,000/μL, but may exceed 500,000/μL. Lymphocytes are usually mature-appearing with scanty cytoplasm and clumped nuclear chromatin. When blood smears are made, the cells are easily ruptured, producing typical "basket" or "smudge" cells.

c. **Granulocytes.** Absolute granulocyte counts are normal or increased until late in the disease.

d. **Platelets.** Thrombocytopenia may be produced by bone marrow infiltration, hypersplenism, or immune thrombocytopenia.

2. Other useful studies that should be obtained in patients with CLL are

a. Renal and liver function tests

b. Coombs' (antiglobulin) tests

c. Serum protein electrophoresis

d. Chest x-ray film

e. CT scans can be used to evaluate retroperitoneal, abdominal and pelvic lymph nodes.

3. Bone marrow examination is usually not necessary to establish the diagnosis in patients with persistent lymphocytosis. The bone marrow of all patients with CLL contains at least 30 percent lymphocytes. The pattern of bone marrow infiltration is an important prognostic factor. Patients with nodular or interstitial patterns of bone marrow involvement have longer survivals than patients with diffuse ("packed") involvement. The indications for bone marrow aspiration and biopsy are

a. Borderline cases of lymphocytosis when the diagnosis is in doubt

b. Thrombocytopenia, to distinguish immune thrombocytopenia from severe bone marrow infiltration

c. Coombs'-negative, unexplained anemia

4. Unhelpful studies in most cases of CLL include:

a. **Lymph node biopsy** in patients with CLL shows malignant lymphoma of the small lymphocytic type. A lymph node biopsy is not indicated in CLL unless the cause of the lymph node involvement is in doubt, particularly when Richter's transformation is suspected.

b. **Liver-spleen scans** are not accurate in assessing the size of these organs in patients with CLL. Physical examination is generally more accurate.

c. **Lymphangiography** is an invasive test and unnecessary in the staging or diagnosis of CLL.

C. Establishing the diagnosis of CLL. The NCI Working Group for CLL has established a minimum requirement for the diagnosis of CLL in *borderline cases.* Diagnostic criteria include:

1. Lymphocytosis (>5,000/μL) sustained for at least four weeks

2. Mature lymphocytes with no more than 55 percent atypical or immature lymphoid cells

3. More than 30 percent lymphocytes in the bone marrow (see III.B.3)

4. Cells with kappa or lambda light chain clonal excess, low-density cell surface immunoglobulin, and CD5 antigen.

D. Differential diagnosis

1. Benign causes of lymphocytosis in adults

a. Viral infections, especially hepatitis, cytomegalovirus, and EBV. Lymphadenopathy and hepatosplenomegaly are absent or mild in elderly patients with infectious mononucleosis. The presence of fever, LFTs compatible with hepatitis, and positive EBV serologies should distinguish mononucleosis from CLL.

b. Brucellosis, typhoid fever, paratyphoid, and chronic infections.

        c. Autoimmune diseases, drug and allergic reactions.

        d. Thyrotoxicosis and adrenal insufficiency.

        e. Postsplenectomy.

    2. Hairy cell leukemia must be differentiated from CLL because management of the two disorders is quite different. Diagnosis depends on recognizing the pathognomonic hairy cells.

    3. Cutaneous T cell lymphomas are suspected if skin involvement is extensive. Differentiation from CLL is made by identifying the convoluted nuclei and helper T-cells (with immunohistochemistry) that are characteristic of this disease.

    4. Leukemic phase of NHL is usually distinguished from CLL morphologically and immunologically. NHL cells are often cleaved, whereas CLL cells are never cleaved. In addition, NHL cells demonstrate intense surface immunoglobulins without the CD5 antigen, and the opposite is generally true for CLL cells.

    5. Prolymphocytic leukemia has large lymphocytes with prominent nucleoli. Lymphadenopathy is minimal, splenomegaly is massive (see sec. **VI.B**).

IV. Staging system and prognostic factors. Routine CBCs may detect asymptomatic cases of CLL, but this has no bearing on the overall survival of these patients. Early, aggressive, effective treatment of complicating infections in CLL probably has improved survival more than cytotoxic agents. Clinical staging is helpful for determining prognosis and deciding when to initiate treatment. Anemia and thrombocytopenia adversely affect prognosis when they are due to leukemic infiltration ("packing") of the bone marrow but not when due to autoimmune destruction of red cells or platelets. The pattern of bone marrow infiltration also appears to affect prognosis (see sec. **III.B.3**). The **Modified Rai classification** of CLL (see sec. **III.C.** for differences with the NCI Working Group criteria) is

Stage	Extent of disease	Risk	Median survival (years)
0	Lymphocytosis of bone marrow ($\geq$40% lymphocytes) and blood (>15,000/μL)	Low	10
I	Stage 0 plus lymphadenopathy	Intermediate	7
II	Stage 0 or I plus splenomegaly and/or hepatomegaly	Intermediate	7
III	Stage 0, I, or II plus anemia (hemoglobin <11.0/gm/dl)	High	2
IV	Stage 0, I, or II plus thrombocytopenia (platelets <100,000/μL)	High	2

V. Management

    A. Indications for treatment. CLL is usually indolent. Treatment of asymptomatic patients with stable disease is not warranted. The blood lymphocyte count does not indicate the need to start therapy and generally is not useful to monitor therapy. The indications for instituting therapy in CLL are

        1. Persistent or progressive systemic symptoms (fever, sweats, weight loss)

        2. Lymphadenopathy that causes mechanical obstruction or bothersome cosmetic deformities

        3. Progressive enlargement of the spleen

        4. Stage III or IV ("high risk") disease that results from the replacement of bone marrow with lymphocytes

        5. Immune hemolysis or immune thrombocytopenia

    B. Chemotherapy. Alkylating agents (especially cyclophosphamide and chlorambucil) represent the standard first-line treatment of CLL. Nucleosides as first-line therapy are currently being studied. Most patients respond to therapy, including at least one half of the patients with high-risk disease. Favorable response to therapy is manifested by decreased lymphadenopathy and hepatosplenomegaly and by improvement of the hematologic parameters. It is not clear that therapy leads to prolonged survival.

1. **Guidelines**
   a. **The initiation of therapy** with alkylating agents should be timed according to the clinically assessed pace of disease. Complete remission is not a necessary goal. Treatment is discontinued when the inciting problem has been controlled (after a few weeks to several months).
   b. **Pulse therapy** appears to be less toxic and at least as effective as continuous therapy.
   c. **Immune hemolysis or thrombocytopenia** should be treated with prednisone alone, 60 mg PO daily, which is then tapered following achievement of control of blood cell counts.
   d. **Resistant disease** should be treated with nucleosides. Third-line therapy includes combination chemotherapy regimens such as CVP or CHOP (see Appendix A2).

2. **Drug dosages**
   a. **Alkylating agents**
      (1) **Chlorambucil,** 0.1 to 0.2 mg/kg PO daily for three to six weeks as tolerated; the dose is usually tapered to 2 mg daily until the desired effect is achieved. Alternatively, 15 to 30 mg/m^2 PO may be given for one day (or divided over four days) every 14 to 21 days; the dose is adjusted to tolerance.
      (2) **Cyclophosphamide,** 2 to 4 mg/kg PO daily for 10 days; the dose is then adjusted downward for continued therapy until the desired effect is achieved.
   b. **Nucleosides**
      (1) **Fludarabine,** 25 to 30 mg/m^2 IV daily for five consecutive days every four weeks.
      (2) **Cladribine** (2-chlorodeoxyadenosine, 2-CdA), either 0.10 mg/kg daily by continuous IV infusion for seven days every four weeks, or 0.14 mg/kg daily IV over two hours for five consecutive days every four weeks.

C. **RT.** Local irradiation is recommended only for reduction of lymph node masses that threaten vital organ function and that respond poorly to chemotherapy. Splenic irradiation may result in improvement of disease elsewhere and may temporarily improve signs of hypersplenism; however, the clinical usefulness of splenic irradiation has not been established. TBI has been used in all phases of CLL but remains investigational and potentially dangerous.

D. **Surgery.** Splenectomy is indicated in CLL patients who have immune hemolytic anemia or thrombocytopenia that either fails to respond to corticosteroid therapy or must be treated with corticosteroids chronically. Splenectomy also may be helpful in patients with problematic hypersplenism.

VI. **Special clinical problems in CLL**

A. **Richter's syndrome.** Approximately 5 percent of patients with CLL develop a diffuse large cell lymphoma with rapid clinical deterioration, and death within 1 to 6 months. The clinical features include fever, weight loss, increasing localized or generalized lymphadenopathy, lymphocytopenia (as well as other cytopenias), and dysglobulinemia. Combination chemotherapy with CHOP is usually tried but is rarely effective.

B. **Prolymphocytic leukemia** is a rare variant of CLL. The main clinical features are massive splenomegaly without substantial lymph node enlargement. Leukocytosis usually exceeds 100,000/μL and is characterized by large lymphoid cells with single prominent nucleoli. Tissue sections show almost no mitotic figures despite the immature appearance of the leukemic cells. Splenectomy and standard chemotherapeutic regimens used to treat CLL do not appear to be effective. Fludarabine or cladribine used as single agents or combination therapy with CHOP may be useful.

Eighty percent of cases involve B cells that have different surface markers than typical CLL (the B cells of prolymphocytic leukemia show intense surface immunoglobulin, the CD19 and CD20 B cell antigens, but typically not the CD5 antigen). Twenty percent of cases are T cell, usually with the helper phenotype (CD3 and CD4 positive). Cytogenetic studies usually show an abnormal translocation in the B cell variety t(11;14) with rearrangement of the *BCL*-1 oncogene and an inversion of chromosome 14 in the T cell variety.

A small percent of CLL patients develop a "prolymphocytoid" transformation where more than 30 percent of the peripheral blood cells are prolymphocytic. This differs from de novo prolymphocytic leukemia in that the cells maintain the immune features of CLL and the clinical course resembles typical CLL.

Hairy Cell Leukemia

I. **Epidemiology and etiology**
Hairy cell leukemia (HCL) (leukemic reticuloendotheliosis, lymphoid myelofibrosis) acounts for about 2 percent of all leukemias. Men outnumber women 5:1. The median age of patients is 55 years; patients less than 30 years of age are unusual. The etiology is unknown.

II. **Pathology and natural history**
   A. **Pathology.** The pathognomonic hairy cell can be identified in the peripheral blood, bone marrow, liver, and spleen of affected patients. The hairy cells are B lymphocytes in virtually every case (rare T cell variants have been reported).
   B. **Natural history.** The natural history is extremely variable, ranging from a relatively fulminant course, to a waxing and waning course of exacerbations and spontaneous improvements, and to prolonged survival measured in decades. The vast majority of patients are able to function normally throughout most of their illness. Patients with HCL usually present with an insidious development of nonspecific symptoms, splenomegaly, and pancytopenia. Progression of disease is manifested by bleeding because of thrombocytopenia, anemia requiring transfusions, and recurrent infections. Death is caused by severe infection in more than half the cases and (uncommonly) by hemorrhage.

III. **Diagnosis**
   A. **Symptoms and signs.** Weakness and fatigue are the presenting complaints in about 40 percent of the cases. A bleeding diathesis, recent infection, or abdominal discomfort is present in approximately 20 percent of patients.

   Splenomegaly occurs in 95 percent of patients and is severe in the majority. Hepatomegaly is seen in about 40 percent of patients and is usually mild. Peripheral lymphadenopathy is rarely present in patients with HCL. However, CT scans of the abdomen may reveal retroperitoneal lymphadenopathy.
   B. **Preliminary laboratory studies**
      1. **CBC.** Anemia and thrombocytopenia occur in 85 percent of patients. Approximately 60 percent of patients have leukopenia with granulocytopenia; 20 percent have increased hairy cells with a leukocytosis in the peripheral blood, usually associated with an absolute granulocytopenia.
      2. **Blood chemistries.** Only 10 to 20 percent of patients have abnormal liver or renal function tests. Polyclonal hyperglobulinemia or decreased normal immunoglobulin concentrations occurs in 20 percent of patients.
   C. **Special diagnostic studies.** The diagnosis of HCL is made by identifying the pathognomonic mononuclear cells in the peripheral blood or bone marrow. The cells have irregular and serrated borders with characteristic slender hairlike cytoplasmic projections and round, eccentric nuclei with spongy chromatin. The cytoplasm is sky blue without granules.
      1. **Phase contrast microscopy** with supravital staining of fresh preparations is extremely valuable for demonstrating the cellular characteristics because the cytoplasm of hairy cells is often poorly preserved in films mixed with Wright's stain.
      2. **Tartrate-resistant acid phosphatase** (TRAP). HCL cells have a strong acid phosphatase activity, which is resistant to inhibition by 0.05 molar tartaric acid (due to the presence of isoenzyme 5 of acid phosphatase); the acid phos-

phatase in leukocytes from most patients with lymphomas and CLL is sensitive to tartrate. A strongly positive TRAP study is present in the majority of patients with HCL but is not required for the diagnosis and can be detected in patients with other lymphoid malignancies.

3. **Bone marrow aspiration** frequently is unsuccessful ("dry tap"). Marrow biopsy shows a characteristic loose and spongy arrangement of cells, even with extensive infiltration with hairy cells. Fibrosis of the marrow with reticulin fibers is also characteristic in areas of HCL infiltration and accounts for the high frequency of dry taps.

4. **Splenic morphology.** The spleen is the most densely infiltrated organ in HCL. The red pulp of the spleen may contain a unique vascular lesion: pseudosinuses lined by hairy cells.

D. **Differential diagnosis.** It is important to distinguish HCL from other diseases because management is substantially different. HCL is most often confused with CLL, malignant lymphoma, histiocytic medullary reticulosis, myelofibrosis, or monocytic leukemia. Differentiation is made by identifying the pathognomonic cell, TRAP test, and pathologic findings of the bone marrow biopsy.

IV. **Staging system and prognostic factors.** The natural median survival for HCL appears to be 5 to 10 years, but this has been dramatically altered by current therapies.

V. **Management**

A. **The decision to treat.** Many patients tend to have a very indolent course and have an excellent survival without therapy. Therapy may be deferred for asymptomatic patients until at least one of the following problems develop:

1. Anemia (hemoglobin < 10 gm/dl)
2. Granulocytopenia (< 1000/μL)
3. Severe thrombocytopenia (< 100,000/μL)

B. **Splenectomy** has achieved at least a partial response in 75 percent of patients and historically had been the standard therapy for HCL.

C. **Cladribine (2-CdA)** is now the treatment of choice for HCL. The drug is given by continuous IV infusion *once only* at a dose of 0.1 mg/kg/day for seven days. More than 95 percent of patients respond to treatment, and 80 percent are complete responders. Few patients have relapsed thus far, but the median follow-up time is less than five years. Toxicity has been limited to transient fevers that are usually associated with neutropenia.

D. **α-IFN** is a highly effective agent in reversing the pancytopenia and splenomegaly in HCL. Dosages of IFN ranging from 2 to 4 million units daily or three times weekly for one year achieve responses in 90 percent of patients with HCL. Complete responses with disappearance of hairy cells from the bone marrow however, are unusual. Immune parameters, such as natural killer cells and cell surface markers, normalize in association with the reversal in the hematologic parameters.

E. **Pentostatin (2′-Deoxycoformicin)** is also highly effective in the therapy of HCL. Most patients not only have normalization of their CBC but also a complete response with disappearance of hairy cells from their bone marrow (rarely seen with α-IFN). Complications include skin rash and neurotoxicity. The dosage is 4 mg/m^2 IV every two weeks for three to six months.

Chronic Myelogenous Leukemia

I. **Epidemiology and etiology.** Chronic myelogenous leukemia (CML) is classified with the myeloproliferative disorders (see Chap. 24.) The rate of transformation to acute leukemia and the presence of chromosomal markers and neutrophil alkaline phosphatase (NAP) abnormalities, however, clearly distinguish CML from the myeloproliferative disorders.

A. Incidence. CML constitutes about 20 percent of adult leukemias in Western countries. Individuals in their fourth decade are most often affected, although children and older adults are also affected.

B. Etiology. The cause of CML is unknown. Radiation exposure is related to an increased incidence of CML but accounts for only a small portion of cases.

II. Pathology and natural history

A. The Philadelphia chromosome (Ph^1), designated t(9;22), arises from the translocation of the C-*ABL* gene from the long arm of chromosome 9 (band q34) to the long arm of chromosome 22 (band q11). The C-*ABL* gene is juxtaposed with the *BCR* gene on chromosome 22 in a head-to-tail fashion, forming a chimeric *BCR-ABL* gene that produces a chimeric protein of 210 kd (p210$^{BCR-ABL}$). The mutation is somatic and is found in erythroblasts, megakaryocytes, granulocytes, monocytes, and most lymphocytes, but not in nonhematopoietic cells. This universal finding in CML can be detected by the polymerase chain reaction if it cannot be found by cytogenetics.

1. Ph^1-negative CML differs from typical CML and may be a different disease for the following reasons:

a. The prognosis is poorer.

b. The patient is usually a young child or an elderly person.

c. The leukocyte and platelet counts are frequently lower.

d. NAP scores tend to be higher.

e. The bone marrow shows more immaturity in the myeloid series.

2. Ph^1 chromosome in acute leukemia. The Ph^1 chromosome can be found in de novo acute leukemia. Approximately 25 percent of adults with ALL and 2 percent of adults with AML present with the Ph^1 chromosome. These cases generally have an overall worse prognosis than similar cases that do not have a Ph^1 chromosome. Some of these cases represent CML that was never diagnosed in the chronic phase; effective treatment may reverse some cases to a chronic phase.

B. Clonality. Clonal studies using the isoenzyme of glucose 6-phosphate dehydrogenase (G-6-PD) in African-American women who are heterogeneous for this enzyme have demonstrated that CML is a clonal disease of an abnormal stem cell. Myeloid, erythroid, megakaryocytic, and most lymphoid cells are involved in the malignant clone.

C. Clinical course. The major clinical manifestations in CML relate to the unrestrained growth of granulocytes. Chronic, accelerated, and acute phases are recognized. Death is usually caused by hemorrhage or infection.

1. Chronic phase. The chronic phase, which usually lasts about three to four years, is manifested by mild systemic symptoms, hepatosplenomegaly, and leukocytosis. Granulocyte production proceeds at a more or less steady rate; a few patients exhibit spontaneous cyclic fluctuations in the granulocyte count. The clinical and laboratory abnormalities are readily controlled by chemotherapy, and most patients are able to lead normal lives.

2. Accelerated phase. Approximately 15 percent of patients enter an accelerated phase, which is resistant to therapy. Cytopenias, increasing splenomegaly, osseous and extraosseous collections of leukemic cells, fever, anorexia, and weight loss are common. Patients may die of any of a variety of problems.

3. Acute phase. Approximately 85 percent of patients develop acute leukemia ("blast crisis"), either abruptly or after three to six months of an accelerated phase. The risk of developing blast crisis is 25 percent in each year, whether it be the first year or the tenth year since the time of diagnosis. Blast crisis is recognized when 30 percent or more of the myeloid cells in the bone marrow or blood are myeloblasts or promyelocytes.

a. Cytogenetic changes, other than the Ph^1 abnormality, develop in more than 75 percent of patients, often several months before clinical evidence of acute transformation.

b. Approximately 30 percent of cases of acute leukemic transformation occur as ALL. The **blasts** morphologically, immunologically, and enzymatically (terminal deoxynucleotidyl transferase [TdT] activity) are characteristic of lymphoid cells.

   c. The **clinical course** following acute transformation is virtually identical to that of de novo acute leukemia, except that the blast crisis phase of CML is usually refractory to treatment.

III. Diagnosis. The diagnosis of CML is usually made easily on the basis of a constellation of findings. No single test is pathognomonic of CML.

  A. Symptoms and signs

    1. Chronic phase

      a. Approximately 20 percent of patients are asymptomatic; disease is discovered by the incidental finding of leukocytosis.

      b. Fatigue, malaise, anorexia, or weight loss occur in about 80 percent of patients. Fever, sweats, and other manifestations of hypermetabolism are common and roughly proportional to the degree of anemia and organomegaly.

      c. Bone pain and sternal or other bony tenderness, from expanding leukemic mass in the marrow, is present in 80 percent of patients.

      d. Abdominal fullness or easy satiety usually reflect splenomegaly. Splenomegaly, which may be massive, is present in 95 percent of cases, and hepatomegaly in 50 percent.

      e. Unusual hemorrhagic or thrombotic episodes reflect abnormalities in platelet number and function. Easy bruisability and purpura are the most frequent manifestations.

    2. Acute phase

      a. Fever, which occasionally is high and spiking

      b. Rapid weight loss

      c. Recurrence of bone pain or tenderness after successful treatment

      d. Splenic pain because of a rapidly enlarging spleen or splenic infarcts

      e. Signs of infection or bleeding

      f. Lymphadenopathy

      g. Cutaneous infiltrations

      h. Meningeal leukemia

  B. Laboratory studies

    1. Erythrocytes. A mild to moderate normocytic, normochromic anemia is usually present. Erythrocytosis may occasionally occur. Often a few nucleated RBCs are seen on the peripheral blood smear. As myeloid overgrowth progresses, erythrocytes show considerable variation in size and shape.

    2. Leukocytes. The granulocyte count exceeds 30,000/µL and usually ranges from 100,000 to 300,000/µL at the time of diagnosis. The blood smear is dramatic and represents a shift of the cells out of the overcrowded marrow; it is often described as peripheral blood that looks like bone marrow. The granulocytes are normal in appearance and functional. The most mature neutrophil elements are present in greatest number, and the less mature in decreasing frequency. Myeloblasts and promyelocytes constitute less than 10 percent of the leukocytes. In contrast to acute leukemia, discontinuity of maturation in the granulocyte series is absent. Eosinophil and basophil counts are often elevated.

    3. Platelets. About 50 percent of patients have thrombocytosis, which may exceed 1,000,000/µL at presentation. Thrombocytopenia is unusual early in the disease. Platelet aggregation and other platelet function tests are commonly abnormal, especially with markedly elevated counts.

    4. Uric acid. Hyperuricemia and hyperuricosuria is the rule, both with and without treatment.

    5. Bone marrow. The marrow is markedly hypercellular as a result of massive granulocytic hyperplasia; consequently, the myeloid-erythroid ratio is markedly increased. Megakaryocyte numbers are occasionally increased. Fibrosis is present in variable amounts but is rarely profound. Maturation of the granulocytes is normal. Gaucherlike cells are seen in some patients because of the prominent phagocytic activity of marrow macrophages.

6. **Ph¹ chromosome** analysis should be performed at the time of bone marrow examination. However, if cells capable of division (myelocytes and less mature forms) are present in the circulation in sufficient numbers, chromosome analysis may be performed on peripheral blood samples.

7. **BCR-ABL rearrangement** can be detected by widely available sensitive techniques, such as Southern blotting or polymerase chain reaction.

8. **NAP activity** in circulating granulocytes is substantially decreased or absent. Five fresh blood smears are submitted for special staining. The intensity of staining of the neutrophils is graded on a scale of 0 to $4+$, and 100 neutrophils are scored and counted (normal range is 40 to 100). The NAP score in cases of CML usually is 0 to 10. The NAP score may occasionally be low in myelodysplastic syndromes (see Chap. 25, sec. I.C) and is usually elevated in myeloproliferative disorders.

9. **Helpful studies in special circumstances**
   a. **Serum vitamin B$_{12}$ concentrations and B$_{12}$ binding capacity** are markedly elevated because of increased levels of transcobalamin I, which is synthesized by granulocytes.
   b. **Chromosome analysis** by sensitive banding techniques may demonstrate a second Ph¹ chromosome, an extra chromosome number 8, or other changes in 75 percent of patients in an imminently acute phase.

C. **Differential diagnosis** mainly involves distinguishing CML from myeloproliferative disorders and leukemoid reactions (see Table 24-1 and Chap. 34, *Increased Blood Cell Counts,* sec. II.C).

IV. Staging system and prognostic factors

A. **Staging system.** No staging system is available for CML. Some research centers have adopted a staging system based on chromosomal analysis only.

B. **Unfavorable signs.** Patients with CML usually pursue a normal life-style during the chronic phase. Virtually anything that changes the stable pattern may signal transformation into the accelerated or acute phase. Changes that may herald blastic transformation include:

1. Signs or symptoms of the acute phase (see sec. III.A.2)
2. Anemia, thrombocytopenia, granulocytopenia, progressive basophilia, or more rapidly increasing leukocytosis in a patient whose disease was previously under control
3. Rising NAP score in the face of poor disease control
4. Myelofibrosis with nucleated red cells in the peripheral blood
5. Lytic bone lesions
6. Chromosome abnormalities other than a single Ph¹ chromosome (usually multiple Ph¹ chromosomes or aneuploidy)

C. **Survival.** The median survival for Ph¹-positive CML ranges from 30 to 45 months; survival for five or more years occurs in 20 percent of patients, and survival exceeding 10 years does occur. The median survival for Ph¹-negative CML is only 9 to 15 months. Survival after the development of blast crisis is usually two to four months.

V. Management

A. **Chemotherapy** has not been proved to increase survival in CML but does significantly improve the quality of life. The bone marrow remains hypercellular and the chromosome abnormality persists or only transiently disappears despite other evidence of improvement with therapy. Thus, the term *complete remission* is usually inappropriate for CML. The goal of therapy is to relieve symptoms and to control disease. All signs, symptoms, physical findings, and laboratory abnormalities usually parallel the leukocyte count; management of the patient as a whole is accomplished by managing the WBC.

1. **Chronic phase**
   a. **Choice of drugs.** Hydroxyurea, busulfan and α-IFN are the most effective and most widely used agents. Hydroxyurea has the advantage of a

more rapid onset of action, shorter period of activity, and fewer side effects than busulfan. α-IFN may control the chronic phase and may also have the advantages of inducing a Ph^1-negative status in a minority of patients and of possibly prolonging survival.

   b. Initiating treatment. Treatment is usually initiated when the WBC exceeds 50,000/μL and is discontinued when the WBC reaches 20,000/μL (the WBC will continue to fall after busulfan therapy ends but will rise again shortly after stopping hydroxyurea therapy). Estimating the WBC doubling time is often useful in planning patients' return visits, ordering blood counts, and predicting when therapy must be reinstituted.

   c. Starting daily doses are 4 to 8 mg PO for busulfan, and 2 to 4 g PO for hydroxyurea. As the patient demonstrates response to treatment, doses are decreased to 2 to 4 mg for busulfan, and to 1 to 2 g for hydroxyurea. α-IFN is typically initiated at 3 to 5 million units SQ daily; the dose may have to be adjusted downward because of toxicity or WBC counts.

   d. Indicators of response. Within a few weeks, in the vast majority of patients in the chronic phase of CML, a response to treatment is demonstrated by disappearance of symptoms, improving anemia, control of granulocytosis and thrombocytosis, reduction in spleen size, increase in the NAP score, and decreasing vitamin B$_{12}$ values.

   e. Allopurinol, 300 mg/day orally, is given to all patients continuously and should be instituted before chemotherapy is started.

   2. Accelerated phase. Once the accelerated phase has developed, the cytotoxic drug should be stopped. Other agents may be tried but without much hope of success. Patients usually require blood component therapy and other supportive measures. Extramedullary sites of symptomatic disease may be controlled with RT.

   3. Acute phase. Management of the myeloblastic acute phase of CML is virtually the same as for de novo adult acute leukemia. However, chances of durable complete remission are dim for all treatment regimens. Complete remissions are achieved in about 50 percent of patients with lymphoblastic transformation using vincristine (2 mg/week IV) and prednisone (daily, high-dose); The remissions rarely exceed 6 months, however, and eventually all patients relapse.

B. Leukapheresis rapidly decreases the granulocyte count for short periods of time but is time-consuming and expensive. This procedure is useful in
   1. Patients with priapism
   2. Patients with CNS or pulmonary symptoms from leukostasis
   3. Pregnant patients when cytotoxic agents are contraindicated

C. RT
   1. Splenic radiation may be transiently useful in patients with symptomatic splenomegaly.
   2. Radioactive phosphorus may be effective in CML but is rarely used.

D. Splenectomy during the chronic phase of CML may be beneficial for hypertension, but it neither delays the onset of blastic transformation nor prolongs survival. The complications (postoperative infections and thromboembolism) are formidable. Splenectomy during the accelerated phase is not indicated.

E. BMT is the treatment of choice and should be initiated as soon as possible for patients in the chronic phase who are less than 55 years old and have an HLA-identical allogeneic sibling donor. Disappearance of the Ph1 chromosome and long-term disease-free survival are reported in more than 50 percent of patients who are treated with BMT.

VI. Special clinical problems in CML

A. Leukostasis can result in profound CNS and pulmonary symptoms. While it is less common in the chronic phase, leukostasis is very common in the acute phase of CML and in de novo acute myelogenous leukemia when the WBC exceeds 100,000/μL. Leukapheresis and hydroxyurea should be implemented emergently.

B. False platelet counts. Patients with accelerated or acute phase CML usually develop severe, refractory thrombocytopenia. Platelet counts that incorrectly show improvement may be found in patients with marked leukocytosis and advancing disease. The false platelet count happens because the granulocytes become disrupted in the test tube and automatic platelet counting machines enumerate the larger leukocyte granules as platelets. The paradox is resolved by reviewing the peripheral blood smear and estimating platelet numbers.

C. Other false laboratory results. Pseudohyperkalemia, pseudohypoglycemia, and pseudohypoxemia are discussed in Chap. 24, sec. **VII.**

Chronic Myelomonocytic Leukemia

I. **Terminology.** Chronic myelomonocytic leukemia (CMML) has also been described as "smoldering leukemia." CMML is now classified with the myelodysplastic syndrome (see Chap. 25).

II. **Diagnosis**

   A. **Physical examination.** CMML most commonly affects the elderly. Splenomegaly is variably present and tends to increase as the disease progresses. Hepatomegaly is uncommon and lymphadenopathy is rare.

   B. **Blood studies.** Patients usually have unexplained monocytosis with granulocytosis or thrombocytopenia.

   1. **Erythrocytes.** Anemia is usually mild unless complicated by iron deficiency.

   2. **Platelets** are moderately decreased in the majority of patients, normal in 15 percent, and severely decreased in 15 percent.

   3. **Leukocytes.** Leukocytosis in the range of 11,000 to 50,000/μL (because of increased numbers of both granulocytes and monocytes) is present in the vast majority of patients; leukopenia occasionally occurs. The morphology of leukocytes is characteristically indeterminate and abnormal. Nucleolated cells in the peripheral blood are uncommon.

   4. **Serum lysozyme** levels are usually elevated.

   5. **NAP** values are variable but rarely as low as those in CML.

   C. **Bone marrow** aspirates in CMML are very hypercellular. Granulocytic hyperplasia with increased numbers of promyelocytes and myeloblasts (5 to 30% of nucleated cells) is prominent. The myeloid series in the marrow often has monocytoid features, but pure monocytosis is unusual. Features of myelodysplasia are also seen. In cytogenetic studies, the Ph^1 chromosome is absent but other noncharacteristic abnormalities are common.

III. **Clinical course.** Distinguishing CMML from acute myelomonocytic leukemia is essential. Patients with CMML often have an insidious onset and an indolent course. The majority live two years or longer, and about 30 percent survive more than five years. Eventually, the majority of patients die of acute monoblastic or myeloblastic leukemia.

IV. **Management.** Early treatment for CMML does not forestall the development of acute leukemia. Treatment is often not necessary at all. Tissue infiltration and marrow proliferation may be controlled with etoposide, beginning with a dose of 100 mg PO daily and then tapering to 50 mg every two or three days. Hydroxyurea, 6-thioguanine, and low-dose cytarabine may also be useful. Intensive therapy is best avoided until and unless acute leukemia becomes overt.

Hypereosinophilic Syndrome

Hypereosinophilic syndrome (HES) is a group of disorders marked by the sustained overproduction of eosinophils and a distinct predilection to damage multiple organs, including the heart.

I. Epidemiology and etiology

A. Epidemiology. More than 90 percent of patients with HES are men, usually between the ages of 20 and 50 years. Both pediatric and elderly patients have also been described.

B. Etiology. The etiology of HES is unknown. GM-CSF, IL-5, and IL-7 may be involved in the dysregulated overproduction of eosinophils. Furthermore, despite the major propensity of thrombosis development, no consistent systemic alterations in coagulation or fibrinolysis have been found.

II. Pathology and natural history.

Most authorities recognize HES to be part of a spectrum of disease characterized by blood and bone marrow eosinophilia, *tissue infiltration* by relatively mature eosinophils, and multisystem organ dysfunction. Debility is usually related to involvement of the blood, bone marrow, heart, lungs, and brain.

A. Hematopoietic system involvement

1. Leukocytes. All patients with HES have eosinophilic leukocytosis from the outset. The WBC count usually ranges from 10,000 to 35,000/μL with 30 to more than 70 percent being eosinophils. The eosinophils are usually mature but often contain decreased numbers of granules that are small in size or cytoplasmic vacuoles. Immature eosinophils are seen occasionally. Neutrophilia is frequently also present. Mild basophilia and blasts are observed in some patients.

    a. Neutrophil alkaline phosphatase values are usually normal but may be increased or decreased.

    b. Serum vitamin B_{12} levels are commonly elevated.

2. Erythrocytes. Half of the patients have a persistent normocytic, normochromic anemia, but teardrop and nucleated red cells can be found in peripheral blood smears.

3. Platelets are usually normal, but they may be decreased in about 30 percent of patients or increased in 15 percent.

4. Bone marrow cytology shows myeloid hyperplasia and 25 to 75 percent of these cells are eosinophils, which are shifted to the left in maturation. Increased numbers of myeloblasts are absent.

5. Chromosome analysis has demonstrated aneuploidy in a minority of mitoses in about 25 percent of cases; the Ph^1 chromosome is found occasionally.

B. Cardiac involvement

occurs in 55 to 75 percent of cases. Cardiac damage emanates from the presence of increased numbers of eosinophils (seen on endomyocardial biopsy) and other poorly defined factors in eosinophil physiology; this damage occurs identically whether the eosinophilia is caused by HES or many other etiologies.

1. Three stages of cardiac involvement in HES

    a. Acute, necrotic stage. Myocardial necrosis is of short duration (about 1.5 months). Echocardiography and angiography are normal, and diagnosis is made by endomyocardial biopsy.

    b. Thrombotic stage. Thrombosis in the ventricles or atria develops after a mean duration of eosinophilia of 10 months.

    c. Fibrotic stage. Mitral or tricuspid valvular regurgitation and restrictive cardiomyopathy due to endomyocardial fibrosis develop after a mean duration of eosinophilia of 24 months.

2. Clinical findings. Patients with HES usually present in the thrombotic or fibrotic stages with chest pain, mitral regurgitation, and congestive heart failure from restrictive cardiomyopathy. Frequently, echocardiograms are abnormal and show an increased left ventricular mass or thickening of the left ventricular free wall or interventricular septum.

C. Neurologic involvement

occurs in about 40 to 70 percent of cases with undefined etiology; biopsy and autopsy findings are inconsistent. The three clinical manifestations are

1. Cerebral thromboemboli originating in the heart or in local arterioles.

2. A distinct encephalopathy with behavioral changes, confusion, ataxia, memory loss, and upper motor neuron signs. Impaired cognitive abilities may persist for months. Seizures, dementia, and organic psychoses occur less frequently.

3. **Peripheral neuropathies** account for half of the neurologic abnormalities associated with HES and manifest as symmetric or asymmetric sensory polyneuropathies.

D. **Cutaneous involvement.** Skin rashes develop in more than 50 percent of cases. Three types of manifestations occur.

1. **Angioedematous and urticarial lesions.** Affected patients are likely to have a benign course without cardiac or neurologic complications. These cases usually respond to prednisone or require no treatment.

2. **Erythematous, pruritic papules and nodules** show a mixed cellular infiltrate in the skin and perivascular tissue devoid of vasculitis on biopsy. These tend to respond to PUVA, dapsone, or sodium chromoglycate.

3. **Mucocutaneous manifestations** may occur anywhere with incapacitating mucosal ulcers; these respond poorly to treatment.

E. **Lung involvement** occurs in about 40 to 50 percent of cases. The chest x-ray is usually clear despite a chronic nonproductive cough. Bronchial asthma is a rare occurrence in HES. Diffuse or focal infiltrations develop in 15 to 25 percent of patients with no predilection for the lung periphery. Pulmonary function test abnormalities are rare in the absence of congestive heart failure or pulmonary emboli arising from the right ventricle.

F. **Involvement of other organs**

1. **Splenomegaly,** which develops in 40 percent of cases, is caused by eosinophilic infiltrates.

2. **Ocular manifestations,** usually visual blurring, are caused by microemboli or local thrombosis.

3. **Rheumatologic manifestations** include arthralgias, effusions, and cold-induced Raynaud's phenomenon with digital ischemia or necrosis.

4. **Gastroenterologic manifestations.** Eosinophilic gastritis, enterocolitis, or colitis may occur. Chronic active hepatitis and the Budd-Chiari syndrome have also been observed in HES.

5. **Renal manifestations.** Pyuria or microscopic hematuria are apparent in about 25 percent of cases. Azotemia is a late event that is usually associated with congestive heart failure.

III. Diagnosis

A. **Diagnostic criteria for HES**

1. Persistently increased absolute eosinophil count greater than 1500/μL (the upper limit of normal is 600/μL) for longer than six months.

2. Absence of parasites, allergies, or other causes of eosinophilia.

3. Evidence of organ system involvement.

B. **Helpful studies**

1. Complete history and physical examination, CBC, liver and renal function tests, and urinalysis.

2. IgE levels and serologic tests for collagen vascular disorders

3. Chest x-ray film

4. Electrocardiogram and echocardiogram

5. Bone marrow aspirate, biopsy, and chromosome analysis

6. Several stool samples for ova and parasites

7. Duodenal aspirates and blood serology to exclude *Strongyloides* infection

8. Cultures for fungi, mycobacteria, and bacteria to exclude infection

9. Biopsy of skin lesions

C. **Differential diagnosis.** The differential diagnosis of eosinophilia is discussed in Chap. 34. *Increased Blood Cell Counts,* sec. **IV.**

1. **Eosinophilic leukemia** can be distinguished with a marked increase in immature eosinophils in the blood or marrow, more than 10 percent blasts in the marrow, infiltration of tissues with immature eosinophils, pronounced anemia, severe thrombocytopenia, chromosomal abnormalities described in other acute nonlymphocytic leukemias, and a clinical course similar to other acute leukemias.

2. **Myeloproliferative disorders.** Patients with HES rarely have expansions of other cell lines besides eosinophils to the extent seen in MPD and do not develop severe myelofibrosis.

3. **Eosinophilic syndromes limited to specific organs** characteristically do not extend beyond their own target organ and hence lack the multiplicity of organ involvement often found in HES.

4. **Churg-Strauss syndrome** is the major vasculitis associated with eosinophilia. It is characterized by asthma, pulmonary infiltrates, eosinophilia, paranasal sinus abnormalities, neuropathy, and blood vessels showing extravascular eosinophils. Asthma is usually absent in HES and may be the only feature that distinguishes it from Churg-Strauss syndrome.

5. **Episodic angioedema with eosinophilia** is characterized by recurring episodes of angioedema, urticaria, fever, and marked eosinophilia. This syndrome is distinguished from HES by its periodicity and its lack of associated cardiac damage.

6. **Other cutaneous diseases associated with eosinophilia** can usually be distinguished by biopsy.

7. **Eosinophilia-myalgia syndrome** caused by ingestion of contaminated L-tryptophan should be excluded.

8. **Parasites.** Helminthic parasites, particularly strongyloidiasis, filarial infections, and enteric protozoans, particularly *Isospora belli* and *Dientamoeba fragilis,* should be carefully excluded.

IV. **Prognostic factors.** Prior to 1975, the median survival of patients with HES was only nine months; less than 15 percent of patients survived more than four years. Since then more than 75 percent of patients have survived five years, and 40 percent survive 10 and 15 years. These contradictions reflect improvements in cardiac diagnosis and therapy. The original terrible prognosis associated with HES is no longer warranted. If the sequelae of organ damage, especially to the heart, can be managed, the course of HES can be prolonged over decades.

A poor prognosis is indicated by refractory congestive heart failure, WBC count greater than $90,000/\mu L$, and the presence of blasts in the peripheral blood. Those who develop cardiac disease are more likely to be males who are positive for HLA-Bw44 and have splenomegaly, thrombocytopenia, elevated B_{12} levels, abnormal eosinophil morphology, and abnormal early myeloid precursors in their blood. Those HES patients free of cardiac disease tend to be females with angioedema, hypogammaglobulinemia, elevated serum levels of IgE, and circulating immune complexes. Extremely elevated IgE levels portend a good prognosis with a requirement for no treatment or with a good response to prednisone.

V. **Prevention and early detection.** Early recognition, management, and close follow-up of cardiac disease can significantly prolong longevity.

VI. **Management**

A. **Observation.** Treatment should be withheld until there is evidence of progressive organ system involvement and dysfunction.

B. **Corticosteroids** have been the most effective agents. A suggested regimen is prednisone, 60 mg daily for one month, then every other day for three months. More prolonged therapy may be necessary. Therapy is discontinued if organ dysfunction improves and if the eosinophil count is reduced to or near the normal range. A good response to corticosteroids is associated with a better prognosis.

C. **Cytotoxic agents.**

1. **Hydroxyurea** is used in patients with organ involvement and eosinophilia that do not respond to prednisone.

2. **Vincristine** is especially useful for acutely reducing eosinophil counts and may be useful for controlling HES and thrombocytopenia.

3. **Other cytotoxic agents.** Chlorambucil has been useful in HES. Cyclosporin and α-IFN are also effective occasionally. Toxic regimens should be avoided.

D. **Leukapheresis** is not helpful because eosinophil counts rebound to pretreatment levels within one day.

E. **Antithrombotic agents,** such as aspirin or warfarin, have been frequently used because of the occurrence of thromboembolic disease, but their role has not been established.

F. Cardiac surgery is indicated for severe mitral regurgitation (bioprosthetic valve placement) and less commonly for thrombectomy or endomyocardectomy.

Selected Reading

Chronic Lymphocytic Leukemia

Dighiero, G., et al. B-cell chronic lymphocytic leukemia: Present status and future directions. *Blood* 78:1901, 1991.

Foon, K. A., Rai, K. R., and Gale, R. P. Chronic lymphocytic leukemia: New insights into biology and therapy. *Ann. Intern. Med.* 113:525, 1990.

Foon, K. A., et al. Genetic relatedness of lymphoid malignancies: Transformation of chronic lymphocytic leukemia as a model. *Ann. Intern. Med.* 119:63, 1993.

Hairy Cell Leukemia

Kraut, E. H., Bouroncle, B. A., and Grever, M. R. Pentostatin in the treatment of advanced hairy cell leukemia. *J. Clin. Oncol.* 7:168, 1989.

Piro, L. D., and Saven, A. Treatment of hairy cell leukemia. *Blood* 79:1111, 1992.

Ratain, M. J., et al. Durability of responses to interferon alpha-2b in advanced hairy cell leukemia. *Blood* 69:872, 1987.

Chronic Myelogenous Leukemia

Clift, R. A., Applebaum, F. R., and Thomas, E. D. Treatment of chronic myelogenous leukemia by marrow transplantation. *Blood* 82:1954, 1993.

Hehlmann, R., et al. Randomized comparison of interferon-α with busulfan and hydroxyurea in chronic myelogenous leukemia. *Blood* 84:4064, 1994.

Rowley, J. D. The Philadelphia chromosome translocation. A paradigm for understanding leukemia. *Cancer* 65:2178, 1990.

Schofield, J. R., et al. Low doses of interferon-α are as effective as higher doses in inducing remissions and prolonging survival in chronic myeloid leukemia. *Ann. Int. Med.* 121:736, 1994.

Talpaz, M., et al. Interferon-alpha produces sustained cytogenetic responses in chronic myelogenous leukemia. Philadelphia chromosome-positive patients. *Ann. Intern. Med.* 114:532, 1991.

Hypereosinophilic Syndrome

Fauci, A. S., et al. The idiopathic hypereosinophilic syndrome: Clinical, pathophysiologic, and therapeutic considerations. *Ann. Intern. Med.* 97:78, 1982.

Weller, P. F., and Bubley, G. J. The idiopathic hypereosinophilic syndrome. *Blood* 83:2759, 1994.

Myeloproliferative Disorders

Dennis A. Casciato

Comparative Aspects

The myeloproliferative disorders (MPDs) include polycythemia vera (PV), myelofibrosis with myeloid metaplasia (MMM), and essential thrombocythemia (ET). All bone marrow cells proliferate en masse, producing a "panmyelosis." The individual diseases are distinguished by the predominant proliferation of one of the marrow cell lines. Table 24-1 compares important clinical and distinguishing features of MPD and chronic myelogenous leukemia (CML), which is discussed in Chapter 23.

I. **Epidemiology and etiology**
   A. **Incidence.** The MPDs are uncommon illnesses; their frequencies in the general population are uncertain. Both PV and ET each affect approximately one person per 100,000 population. The peak incidences are in patients 50 to 60 years of age, but the diseases also occur in children and the elderly. The MPDs affect men and women equally, except in young patients with ET, where females predominate.
   B. **Etiology.** Radiation exposure is associated with an increased incidence of MMM but accounts for only a very small percentage of cases. No other etiologic factors have been determined for MPDs. Familial factors may be involved in PV and MMM.

II. **Pathogenesis.** The MPDs usually have insidious onsets and manifestations evolve at varying rates.
   A. **Clonality of MPDs.** The MPDs arise from a single hematopoietic stem cell. Thus, they are clonal and hence, neoplastic. The description of clonality is based on studies of women with these MPDs who were also heterozygous for isotypes A and B of glucose-6-phosphate dehydrogenase. Chromosome analyses have established that a clonal cytogenetic abnormality is present in erythroblasts, neutrophils, basophils, macrophages, megakaryocytes, and subsets of B lymphocytes, but not in fibroblasts.
   B. **Fibrosis** of the marrow, which develops in all patients with MMM, in many patients with PV, and in some patients with ET, is not an intrinsic part of clonal expansion in the MPDs. Rather, the fibroblastic proliferation and enhanced collagen synthesis develops as a secondary reaction to the abnormal hematopoiesis. Marrow fibrosis is most closely related with increased numbers of dysplastic megakaryocytes. The pathogenetic roles of released growth factors are incompletely understood.

   All three types of collagen present in normal marrow are increased in MMM, but type III is increased preferentially. The fine reticulin fibers that are visible with silver stains are principally type III collagen and do not stain with trichrome dyes.
   C. **Hematopoiesis** in the MPDs is generally characterized by autonomous growth and hypersensitivity of progenitor cells to growth factors.
      1. **Erythropoiesis** in vitro in semisolid media normally requires exogenous erythropoietin (EPO). Blood or bone marrow from patients with PV forms erythroid colony-forming units (CFUs) without exogenous EPO. Serum EPO levels are low in PV and are elevated in most cases of secondary polycythe-

Table 24-1. Clinical features of the myeloproliferative disorders

Feature	Polycythemia vera	Myelofibrosis with myeloid metaplasia	Essential thrombocythemia	Chronic myelogenous leukemia
Degree of Cellular Proliferation				
Erythrocytes	+ +	N or D	N	N
Megakaryocytes	+ → + + +	+ + → + + + +	+ + + +	+ → + + +
Granulocytes	+ → + + +	D → + + +	N → + +	+ + + +
Fibroblasts, fibrosis	+	+ + → + + +	N	N → +
Extramedullary hematopoiesis	Late stages	+ + → + + +	A → +	N → +
Giant platelets in peripheral blood	+	+ + +	+	+ + +
Proportion of Patients with				
Splenomegaly	75%	95%	30%	95%
Hepatomegaly	40%	75%	<15%	50%
Special Assays				
NAP score	N or I	N, I, or D	N or I	D or A
B_{12} and B_{12} binding capacity	I	I	N	2–4 times normal
Philadelphia chromosome	A	Rare	A	80%
Preeminent Clinical Features (Etiology)	Hyperviscosity (erythrocytosis)	Deformed RBC and splenomegaly (extramedullary hematopoiesis)	Recurrent hemorrhage and thrombosis (thrombocytosis)	Progressive granulocytosis and splenomegaly (leukemic infiltration)
Transition to Acute Leukemia	5–25%	5–10%	Very rare	80%

Key: + → + + + + = relative degrees of prominence; N = normal; D = decreased; I = increased; A = absent; NAP ≠ neutrophil alkaline phosphatase.

mia. In PV, erythropoiesis is either autonomous or excessively sensitive to extremely low levels of EPO. Increased erythroid burst-forming units are demonstrable in vitro for both ET and MMM as well.

2. **Granulocytopoiesis** is frequently increased in MPDs to varying degrees and is manifested by myeloid hyperplasia in the marrow and neutrophilia.

3. **Megakaryocyte** CFUs in ET are not only increased in number but also are able to grow autonomously without added growth factor.

4. **Extramedullary hematopoiesis** is consistently present in the liver and spleen in patients with MMM and contributes to organ enlargement. This *does not* result in quantitatively significant hematopoiesis outside of the marrow. The splenomegaly in patients with PV does not represent extramedullary hematopoiesis except in late stages of the disease.

D. **Interconversions** of the MPDs are probably uncommon. The only consistent transformation is the conversion of PV into MMM (5 percent of cases).

E. **Complications**

1. **Hemorrhagic phenomena** are common in PV, ET, and late MMM, and infrequent in early MMM. Easy bruisability and purpura are the usual manifestations. GI hemorrhage can be catastrophic, but the incidence of peptic ulcer disease has not proved to be increased in any of the MPDs.

2. **Thrombotic phenomena,** both venous and arterial, are common in uncontrolled PV and ET and are frequently the cause of death.

3. **Erythromelalgia,** the most characteristic vaso-occlusive manifestation in MPDs, is caused by the toxic effects of platelet arachidonic acid on arterioles. Localized painful erythema and warmth occurs in the distal portions of the extremities and may progress to cyanosis or necrosis of toes or fingers. Erythromelalgia is relieved by lowering the platelet count or using NSAIDs, particularly aspirin or indomethacin.

4. **Metabolic problems.** Fever, heat tolerance, and weight loss ensue when the disease becomes rapidly progressive. Hyperuricemia and hyperuricosuria are present in nearly all patients with active MPD. Treatment with allopurinol can prevent gouty arthritis, uric acid nephropathy, and nephrolithiasis, but its necessity is unproven and controversial. Pruritus is a frequent problem, particularly in PV.

5. **AML.** The chance that an MPD will convert to leukemia is almost nonexistent in ET, 0 to 15 percent in MMM (depending on the reported series), 5 to 25 percent in PV (depending on the form of treatment) and 20 percent of patients who convert from PV to MMM.

F. **The Polycythemia Vera Study Group** was founded in 1967 to study the natural history of MPDs and the effects of therapies on them. Over 1000 patients have been entered into protocols. Diagnostic criteria and therapeutic recommendations by the PV Study Group have been incorporated into this chapter.

III. **Diagnosis**

A. **Laboratory studies**

1. **Hemogram** results are discussed under each specific entity.

2. **Neutrophil alkaline phosphatase (NAP)** scores are normal or increased in MPDs and decreased in CML.

3. **Platelet function.** *Neither the severity of thrombocytosis nor the results of platelet function tests correlate with thrombotic or hemorrhagic events in the MPDs.* Platelet dysfunction is common in all MPDs and is manifested by lack of aggregation in response to epinephrine and in abnormal surface membrane properties. Template bleeding times are usually normal in PV and ET and prolonged only in CML and late MMM.

4. **Vitamin B_{12}.** Transcobalamins I and III are synthesized by granulocytes. The total body granulocyte mass, when increased, is reflected by increased serum levels of vitamin B_{12} and unsaturated B_{12}-binding capacity (UBBC). These levels are usually elevated in patients with MPD and CML and normal in other causes of erythrocytosis or granulocytosis. Transcobalamin I is increased in CML, and transcobalamin III is increased in PV.

5. **Bone marrow** examinations demonstrate hypercellularity. Megakaryocytes are greatly increased in ET and MMM at all stages of disease and to a lesser degree in PV. Bone marrow findings, however, are diagnostic of a specific disorder only in MMM. Reticulin is increased in all MPDs, but collagen fibrosis occurs only in MMM and in PV that has converted to MMM.

6. **Cytogenetics.** Many types of nonrandom structural and numeric chromosomal abnormalities are common in PV and MMM at any stage of disease, particularly in patients treated with myelosuppressive therapy. These abnormalities, however, are not useful in prognosis except possibly in post-polycythemic myelofibrosis in which karyotypic evolution may indicate transformation to acute leukemia.

7. **False laboratory results**
   a. **Pseudocoagulopathy.** Prolonged clotting times in patients with marked erythrocytosis are usually the result of excessive amounts of anticoagulant relative to the small plasma volume in the test tube. Accurate determinations can be made if the volume of anticoagulant is adjusted for the hematocrit.
   b. **Pseudohyperkalemia.** Marked thrombocytosis may result in elevated serum potassium concentrations because platelets release potassium during the clotting reaction. The true level is determined by reviewing the ECG for evidence of hyperkalemia and by measuring the potassium concentration in plasma rather than serum.
   c. **Pseudo-hyperacid-phosphatemia.** Platelets are rich in acid phosphatase. Marked thrombocytosis may result in spurious elevations of enzyme levels measured in serum and plasma.
   d. **Pseudohypoglycemia.** Leukocytes metabolize glucose from serum in test tubes. Dramatically low blood glucose concentrations may result from marked granulocytosis. More accurate glucose levels can be measured if the clot with entrapped leukocytes is removed immediately.
   e. **Pseudohypoxemia.** Oxidative respiration is used by monocytes and immature leukocytes to a greater extent than by mature leukocytes and platelets and is not used by mature erythrocytes. Falsely low oxygen tensions may be seen in patients with severe thrombocytosis or granulocytosis because of oxygen consumption within the test tubes. The presence of hypoxemia may be clarified if specimens are collected in test tubes containing fluoride and are immediately placed in ice.

B. **Differential diagnosis**
   1. **Elevated blood counts** (see Chap. 34, *Increased Blood Cell Counts,* sections I to V for discussion of polycythemia, neutrophilia, eosinophilia, basophilia, and thrombocytosis).
   2. **Marrow fibrosis** (see Chap. 34, *Cytopenia,* sec. I.B).
   3. **Differentiation of the MPDs** necessitates attention to the characteristics listed in Table 24-1 and the diagnostic criteria for each disorder discussed in this chapter. Long-term observation often clarifies the diagnosis. Patients must have iron and folate deficiencies corrected before the specific disorder can be accurately diagnosed.
   4. **MPD, undifferentiated type** is the best designation for patients who have leukoerythroblastic blood smears, normal red cell mass, and a hypercellular marrow that shows only mild fibrosis. The diagnosis of MPD is made by exclusion.

IV. **Staging system and prognosis.** No staging system exists for the MPDs. Prognosis depends on the pace of disease, the ability of treatment to control manifestations, and the development of complications. With modern therapy, survival for patients with PV and ET appears to be the same as for age-matched controls. Survival for patients with MMM, on the other hand, is clearly decreased.

Polycythemia Vera

See *Comparative Aspects* at the beginning of this chapter for epidemiology, etiology, pathogenesis, comparative laboratory results, false laboratory results, and differential diagnosis of the MPDs.

I. **Diagnosis.** The erythroid series is the predominant proliferating cell line in the panmyelosis of polycythemia vera (PV, polycythemia rubra vera).

   A. **Diagnostic criteria for PV** (according to the PV Study Group). The diagnosis of PV is made if all three variables from category A are present; or, in the absence of splenomegaly, if the remaining two variables of category A plus any two of category B are present.

      1. **Category A**

         a. **Increased red cell mass** measured with ^{51}Cr-labeled red cells: in males ≥ 36 ml/kg, in females ≥ 32 ml/kg (normal ranges should be established in each laboratory)

         b. **Normal arterial oxygen saturation** ≥ 92 percent

         c. **Splenomegaly**

      2. **Category B**

         a. **Thrombocytosis:** platelets $>400,000/\mu L$

         b. **Leukocytosis:** WBC $\geq 12,000/\mu L$ (in the absence of infection)

         c. **Elevated NAP** score >100 (in the absence of fever or infection)

         d. **Elevated vitamin B$_{12}$ or UBBC:** B$_{12}$ >900 pg/ml; UBBC >2200 pg/ml

   B. **Laboratory abnormalities**

      1. **Erythrocytes.** To establish the diagnosis of PV, an increased red cell mass must be demonstrated by using ^{51}Cr at some time during the course of disease unless the hematocrit is 60 percent or more. Erythrocytes are usually normocytic and normochromic unless iron deficiency is present. Poikilocytosis and anisocytosis reflect the transition into MMM late in the disease course. Some cases have increased amounts of fetal hemoglobin.

      2. **Granulocytes.** Granulocytosis in the range of 12,000 to 25,000/μL occurs in two-thirds of patients at presentation. Early forms may be present but are not prominent. Two-thirds of cases have basophilia.

      3. **Platelets.** Platelet counts usually are in the range of 450,000 to 800,000/μL occasionally with abnormal morphology.

      4. **NAP score** is increased (70% of patients) or normal.

      5. **Serum B$_{12}$ and UBBC.** The serum B$_{12}$ concentration is increased in 35 percent of patients. The UBBC is increased in 75 percent and is mostly transcobalamin III.

      6. **Bone marrow examinations** are not diagnostic of PV. Bone marrow findings show panhyperplasia with mildly increased numbers of megakaryocytes. Reticulin is increased in 10 to 20 percent of patients (100 percent in the "burned out" phase). Iron stores are decreased or absent in the vast majority of untreated patients.

      7. **Immunologic abnormalities** occur in one-third of PV patients.

   C. **Differential diagnosis** includes the other MPDs (particularly for patients with PV who are anemic secondary to blood loss) and relative and secondary erythrocytoses (see Chapter 34, *Increased Blood Cell Counts*, sec. I.). Although not necessary for the vast majority of cases, bone marrow biopsy, measurement of the serum EPO level, or assessment of CFU in semisolid media may be helpful in difficult cases.

II. **Clinical course.** The survival of patients with PV may be identical to that of a matched otherwise healthy population with modern therapy. Previously the mortality rate was 1.5 to 2 times the control population.

   A. **Predominant signs and symptoms** early in the disease are secondary to increased red cell mass that results in plethora and hyperviscosity. Modest splenomegaly is present in 75 percent of cases and hepatomegaly in 40 percent. Splenomegaly is caused by an increased splenic red cell pool and not by extramedullary hematopoiesis, which is absent early in the disease. Pruritus develops in 15 to 50 percent of cases, urticaria in 10 percent, and gout in 5 to 10 percent.

1. **Hyperviscosity** results in decreased blood flow and, consequently, in tissue hypoxia. Manifestations include headache, dizziness, vertigo, tinnitus, visual disturbances, stroke, angina pectoris, claudication, and myocardial infarction.

2. **Hemorrhagic manifestations** (10–20% of patients) include epistaxis, ecchymosis, and GI bleeding. Minor mucosal bleeding is most common. Acquired abnormalities of von Willebrand's factor and coagulation factors V and XII frequently occur in PV.

3. **Thrombotic manifestations** in patients treated with phlebotomy alone develop in 15 percent of patients during the first 2 years and in 33 percent during the first 7 years after diagnosis.

   a. **Types of events.** Both arterial and venous thrombosis occur in PV. Approximately two-thirds of thrombotic events are life-threatening and are associated with a 25 percent mortality rate. Half of these events are cerebrovascular accidents and half comprise myocardial infarction, pulmonary infarction, and axillary, hepatic, or mesenteric vein thrombosis. The remaining one-third of events are uncomplicated deep vein or other thromboses. PV accounts for half of the cases of hepatic, portal, splenic, or mesenteric vein thrombosis that occur.

   b. **Thrombosis-related risk factors** in PV include advanced age, history of prior thrombosis, treatment with phlebotomy alone, and the rate of phlebotomy, and *not the platelet count or platelet function tests*.

B. **Phases of disease**

   1. **Erythrocytic phase.** The phase of persistent erythrocytosis that necessitates regular phlebotomies lasts from 5 to 25 years. The manifestations of erythrocytosis and severity of complications depend on comorbid conditions.

   2. **"Burned-out" phase.** Eventually the patient enters a "spent" or "burned-out" phase; the need for phlebotomies is greatly reduced or the patient enters a long period of apparent "remission." Anemia eventually supervenes, but thrombocytosis and leukocytosis usually persist. The spleen increases in size, but little marrow fibrosis is present.

   3. **Myelofibrotic phase.** Myelofibrosis develops in 10 percent of patients and increases over the course of PV. When cytopenias and progressive splenomegaly develop, the clinical manifestations and course become similar to that of myelofibrosis with myeloid metaplasia.

   4. **Terminal phase.** In 35 to 50 percent of patients with PV, death results from thrombotic or hemorrhagic complications. Death is attributed to myelofibrosis in less than 15 percent of cases. The risk of acute leukemia is greatly increased when patients are treated with radioactive phosphorus or alkylating agents compared with treatment by phlebotomy alone.

C. **Pregnancy and PV.** Pregnant patients with PV have an increased incidence of premature births, fetal wastage, preeclampsia, and postpartum hemorrhage. Pregnancy does not affect the course of PV.

III. **Management**

A. **Principles of treatment**

   1. Reduction of blood volume and control of erythropoiesis with phlebotomy

   2. Avoidance of elective surgery

   3. Avoidance of overtreatment

   4. Avoidance of myelosuppressive agents in patients less than 50 years old, if possible

   5. Control of panmyelosis with hydroxyurea in patients less than 70 years old who have one of the following characteristics:

      a. A history of a prior thrombotic event, a high risk for thrombotic complications, or a very high requirement for phlebotomy (more frequently than every two months)

   b. Problematic splenomegaly
   c. Uncontrolled systemic symptoms (e.g., intractable pruritus, bone tenderness, weight loss) or poor venous access
   6. Control of panmyelosis with myelosuppressive drugs or radioactive phosphorus in patients more than 70 years old

B. Medical management
   1. Phlebotomy alone may be adequate for many years. The hematocrit is maintained between 42 and 47 percent.
      a. Initially, 500 ml of blood may be removed every other day (only 250 ml of blood should be removed in patients with serious vascular disease).
      b. Approximately 200 mg of iron is removed with each 500 ml of blood (the normal total body iron content is about 5 gm). Iron deficiency is a goal of chronic phlebotomy treatment. Symptomatic iron deficiency (glossitis, cheilosis, dysphagia, asthenia, pruritus) resolves rapidly with iron administration.
   2. Hydroxyurea, 15–30 mg/kg daily PO, is a noncarcinogenic myelosuppressive agent that has been shown to control the panmyelosis in 85 percent of patients within 12 weeks and to reduce the incidence of thrombotic events by 50 percent in patients with PV. This drug has not yet been shown to be leukemogenic or carcinogenic. The drug must be given continuously and patient compliance must be excellent. Occasional side effects of hydroxyurea include fever, rash, stomatitis, gastric discomfort, and possible renal dysfunction.
   3. Radioactive phosphorus (^{32}P), 2 to 5 mCi, controls panmyelosis in 80 percent of patients within two months and may be effective for two years or longer. Doses may be repeated every 12 weeks if necessary. Serious cytopenias are rare. Treatment with ^{32}P reduces the incidence of thrombotic complications, but also increases the incidences of acute leukemia (fivefold) lymphomas, and cancers of the skin and GI tract.
   4. Alkylating agents (chlorambucil, busulfan, and melphalan) successfully control panmyelosis within two to four months and reduce the incidence of thrombosis, but unacceptably increase the incidence of acute leukemia (13-fold) and other malignancies. These drugs are not recommended for the management of PV.
   5. α-IFN. 3 to 5 million units SQ three to five times weekly, can control both the red cell mass and platelet production. α-IFN, however, is costly and associated with problematic side effects.
   6. Anagrelide, an inhibitor of platelet function that does not suppress erythrocyte or granulocyte production, has successfully lowered platelet counts in MPD patients with problematic thrombocytosis when other available agents have failed. The dosage is 0.5 to 1.0 mg q.i.d. PO. The main side effects of anagralide are neurologic, GI, and cardiac.
   7. Antiplatelet drugs. Aspirin (900 mg/day) and dipyridamole (Persantine) (225 mg/day) used together do not prevent thrombotic complications in PV, occasionally result in serious hemorrhage, and are not recommended.
   8. Supportive care
      a. Hyperuricemia, if associated with complications, is treated with allopurinol (100 to 600 mg/day PO). Other measures are discussed in Chap. 27, sec. **IX.**
      b. Burned-out PV is managed as for MMM.
      c. Erythromelalgia is treated with cyclo-oxygenase inhibitors (aspirin, indomethacin) and cytotoxic drugs to reduce the platelet count.
      d. Platelet transfusions are given for important hemorrhage, even if the platelet count is normal or elevated, because platelet function abnormalities may be present and are not predictable by laboratory tests.
      e. Anticoagulation with heparin and then warfarin is used for acute thrombotic complications.
      f. Pruritus is multifactorial and often resistant to therapy.

(1) Histamine blockers, such as cyproheptadine (4 mg PO t.i.d.) or cimetidine (300 mg PO t.i.d.) should be tried initially.
(2) Combined histamine and serotonin blockage can be tried by using doxepin or trifluoroperazine and cyproheptadine.
(3) Low-dose ferrous sulfate supplementation to treat pruritus that may be caused by iron deficiency should be considered. In these cases, the hematocrit must be closely monitored for the expected increase in requirement for phlebotomy.
(4) Cholestyramine is helpful in some cases.
(5) Psoralens with ultraviolet A light (PUVA) are occasionally helpful.
(6) If the above measures fail, myelosuppressive agents may be necessary.

C. Surgery

1. **Elective surgery** should be avoided whenever possible in patients with PV. More than 75 percent of patients with uncontrolled PV who undergo surgery develop hemorrhagic or thrombotic complications, and approximately one-third of patients die as a result. The longer the disease is controlled, the fewer the complications. The following is recommended:

   a. **Phlebotomy.** The hematocrit should be reduced to 45 percent. If there is evidence of clinically significant arterial disease, reducing the hematocrit to 35 to 40 percent appears to be justified. The blood obtained by phlebotomy may be saved for autologous transfusion.

   b. **Prevention of perioperative thromboembolism**
      (1) **Mechanical devices** to speed blood flow through the calf (elastic stockings or pulsating boots) should be used.
      (2) **Low-dose heparin.** 5000 units SQ q8-12h, can be given, if there are no contraindications, until the patient returns to normal activity.

2. **Emergency surgery.** Aggressive phlebotomy with reinfusion of the patient's plasma or colloid may be lifesaving.

3. **Splenectomy** is extremely hazardous in all phases of PV and should be restricted to highly selected patients.

Essential Thrombocythemia

See *Comparative Aspects* at the beginning of this chapter for epidemiology, etiology, pathogenesis, comparative laboratory results, false laboratory results, and differential diagnosis of the MPDs.

I. **Diagnosis.** The megakaryocyte is the predominant proliferating cell line in the panmyelosis of ET (essential, hemorrhagic, idiopathic, or primary thrombocythemia or thrombocytosis). Distinguishing PV from ET may be difficult in the early stages of disease.

A. **Diagnostic criteria for PT** (according to the PV Study Group) are
   1. **Platelet counts** greater than 1,000,000/μL (some authorities accept 600,000/μL)
      a. No prior splenectomy
      b. Thrombocytosis is not secondary to other causes
   2. **Bone marrow** examination shows hypercellularity, markedly increased numbers of megakaryocytes, and clumps of platelets.
      a. Hemosiderin is present. If hemosiderin is absent or if there is a history of recent GI bleeding, thrombocytosis persists after replacement therapy with ferrous sulfate.
      b. Absence of tumor infiltration.

B. **Laboratory abnormalities**
   1. **Erythrocytes.** Hypochromic, microcytic anemia is present in more than 60 percent of patients. Other abnormalities of red cell shape and size are mild. Howell-Jolly bodies are found in 20 percent of patients and indicate splenic atrophy from repeated infarctions.

2. **Granulocytosis** is present in half of the cases, usually in the range of 15,000 to 30,000/μL. Myelocytes and earlier forms are rare and basophilia is mild.

3. **Platelet counts** always exceed 600,000/μL and are often present as clumps or megakaryocytic fragments. Counts may reach 15,000,000/μL.

4. **NAP scores** are nearly always normal. Elevated scores probably indicate that the patient will eventually manifest polycythemia vera. Low values are seen occasionally.

5. **Serum B$_{12}$ and UBBC** levels are usually normal.

6. **Bone marrow** examinations show markedly increased numbers of large megakaryocytes and often only massive clumps of platelets. Granulocytic hyperplasia is present, and fibrosis is usually absent.

C. **Differential diagnosis** of ET includes reactive thrombocytosis, the other MPDs, CML, and myelodysplastic syndromes. Myelodysplastic syndromes with thrombocytosis usually manifest more severe anemia, macrocytosis, ringed sideroblasts, or the 5q- chromosomal abnormality. Reactive thrombocytosis is discussed in Chapter 34, *Increased Blood Cell Counts*, sec. **III.**

II. Clinical course

A. **Predominant signs and symptoms.** Two-thirds of patients are asymptomatic when ET is discovered. The spleen may be enlarged (one-third of cases) or atrophic. Hepatomegaly is absent. Extramedullary hematopoiesis is not a major feature of ET; surgically removed spleens usually demonstrate only chronic passive congestion. Pruritus develops in 10 to 15 percent of patients.

B. **Thrombotic, embolic or hemorrhagic episodes** of varying severities are the most common spontaneous manifestations of ET. In spite of extensive study, it is not known why some patients bleed. Neither platelet counts nor platelet function tests correlate with clinical events. Cardiovascular risk factors, particularly smoking, appear to increase the risk of thrombosis.

1. **Thrombotic episodes** are most frequently venous, and the splenic vein or the extremities are particularly affected. Arterial thromboses most frequently result in distal ischemia or infarction or symptoms relative to occlusion of small and medium-sized vessels. CNS manifestations include recurrent or transient headaches, confusion, visual disturbances, hemiparesis, or seizures.

2. **Hemorrhage** most frequently occurs in the mucous membranes or skin. Life-threatening hemorrhage rarely occurs except after trauma or surgery.

C. **Survival** appears to be the same as matched otherwise healthy controls. The median survival exceeds 10 years, and the five-year survival rate is greater than 80 percent. Transformation of ET into acute leukemia is very rare if leukemogenic agents are avoided.

III. Management. The mainstays of treatment for ET are myelosuppression and avoidance of splenectomy. Asymptomatic young patients can do well without sequelae for many years and probably should be observed without initiating treatment. Severe thrombocythemia should always be treated in older patients, even in the absence of symptoms. All patients with ET and hemorrhagic or vaso-occlusive disease should be treated promptly to lower the platelet count.

A. **Medical management**

1. **Radioactive phosphorus** is probably the simplest form of therapy to administer, the most rapidly acting agent, and is associated with the longest duration of effect (see *Polycythemia Vera*, **III.B.3**).

2. **Cytotoxic agents** effectively reduce platelet counts; maintenance therapy is necessary in most cases. A recommended regimen is hydroxyurea given at a dose of 15 to 30 mg/kg/day until thrombocytosis is controlled (usually within 2–6 weeks). Melphalan, busulfan, chlorambucil, or thiotepa can also be used.

3. **Plateletpheresis** is indicated for emergency treatment of life-threatening complications of severe thrombocytosis and is nearly always associated with improvement in hemorrhagic and thrombotic symptoms.

4. **Antiplatelet drugs** are clearly indicated for patients with symptoms of digital or CNS ischemia; use in other situations is controversial. Aspirin alone,

0.3 to 1.8 gm/day, is effective, but may increase the risk of bleeding. Dipyridamole, 100 mg PO t.i.d. or q.i.d., has not been proved to be superior to aspirin when used alone or in combination with aspirin.

5. **Anagrelide and IFNs** may be useful in controlling thrombocytosis when other measures fail (see *Polycythemia Vera, sec. III.B.5* and **6**).

6. Treatment of pruritus and erythromelalgia are discussed above (see *Polycythemia Vera, sec. III.B.8*).

B. **Splenectomy** greatly aggravates thrombocytosis, often leads to death, and is absolutely contraindicated in patients with ET.

Myelofibrosis with Myeloid Metaplasia

See *Comparative Aspects* at the beginning of this chapter for epidemiology, etiology, pathogenesis, comparative laboratory results, false laboratory results, and differential diagnosis of the MPDs.

I. **Diagnosis.** Megakaryocytes and fibroblasts are the predominant proliferating cell lines in the panmyelosis of myeloid metaplasia (MMM, agnogenic myeloid metaplasia, osteosclerosis, myelosclerosis).

A. **Diagnostic criteria for** MMM (according to the PV Study Group) consists of
   1. Splenomegaly
   2. Leukoerythroblastic blood smear (nucleated red cells and granulocytosis) with prominent anisocytosis and poikilocytosis
   3. Normal red cell mass
   4. Bone marrow examination that demonstrates fibrosis involving more than one-third of the cross-sectional area and the fibrosis is not secondary to some identifiable cause (see Chap. 34, *Cytopenia, sec. I.B*).
   5. Absence of Ph^1 chromosome

B. **Diagnostic criteria for osteosclerosis** consist of sclerotic lesions demonstrated on roentgenograms of the pelvis, spine, and long bones plus the criteria for diagnosis of MMM. X-ray film evidence of patchy osteosclerosis occurs in 50 percent of patients with MMM and may resemble metastases from carcinoma.

C. **Laboratory abnormalities**
   1. **Erythrocytes.** At presentation, anemia is moderate in two-thirds of patients. Macrocytosis reflects the presence of folic acid deficiency. Dacrocytes (teardrop cells), ovalocytes, pronounced anisocytosis, polychromasia, and nucleated red blood cells make up the characteristic and nearly pathognomonic blood picture of patients with MMM. The anemia is usually due to ineffective erythropoiesis but may be caused by acquired versions of autoimmune hemolysis, hemoglobin H disease, or a paroxysmal nocturnal hemoglobinuria-like syndrome.
   2. **Granulocytes** usually range from 10,000 to 30,000/μL. Blasts and promyelocytes constitute less than 10 percent of the granulocytes. Granulocytopenia occurs in 15 percent of patients. Basophils are only slightly increased.
   3. **Platelet count** is increased in one-third, normal in one-third, and decreased in one-third of patients with MMM, depending on the stage of disease. Platelets usually have abnormal morphology.
   4. **NAP score** is normal or increased but may be decreased late in the course.
   5. **Serum B_{12} and UBBC** are slightly increased in many patients but not to the degree observed in patients with PV or chronic myelogenous leukemia.
   6. **Bone marrow** examination shows decreased fat content, granulocytic hyperplasia, and markedly increased numbers of dysplastic megakaryocytes. Fibrosis is patchy and variable in distribution. The extent or progression of fibrosis is *not correlated* with the duration of disease, splenic size, or degree of splenic myeloid metaplasia. Marrow sinusoids are characteristically distended and contain clumps of hematopoietic cells intravascularly. Reticulin is always increased and is striking in 50 percent of patients.

7. **Immunologic abnormalities,** such as monoclonal antibodies (10%), positive direct Coombs' tests (20%), polyclonal hyperglobulinemia, rheumatoid factor, antinuclear antibodies, antiphospholipid antibodies, or circulating immune complexes are found in more than 50 percent of patients with MMM.
   D. **Differential diagnosis** of MMM includes the other MPDs, CML, hairy cell leukemia, metastatic carcinoma associated with marrow fibrosis (desmoplastic reaction), and disseminated mycobacterial infection. A long list of other disorders associated with secondary myelofibrosis include collagen vascular diseases and are discussed in Chapter 33, *Cytopenias,* **I.B.**

II. **Clinical course**
   A. **Predominant signs and symptoms** relate to the severity of anemia and splenomegaly. Virtually all patients have splenomegaly, which may be massive in one-third of cases, and three-quarters of patients have enlarged livers. One-quarter are asymptomatic at the time of diagnosis. Progressive disease is commonly manifested by fever, weight loss, and debilitating bone pain from periostitis.
   B. **Chronic myelofibrosis.** The clinical course of MMM is extremely variable. Some patients are asymptomatic for long periods without treatment. Hemorrhagic manifestations rarely develop until late in the disease.

   Poor prognostic indicators are fever, ecchymosis, worsening anemia, or thrombocytopenia; splenic size and bone marrow findings do not affect prognosis. The median survival is three years when the hemoglobin is less than 10 gm/dl or granulocytosis is present (particularly if immature cells account for more than 10% of these cells). The median survival rate is seven years without those findings. Death is due to infection, hemorrhage, postsplenectomy mortality, or transformation to acute leukemia. The transition rate of MMM into acute leukemia ranges from less than 5 to 10 percent.
   C. **Associated syndromes**
      1. **"Acute myelofibrosis"** is now recognized to be acute megakaryocytic leukemia (type M7).
      2. **Portal hypertension and varices** in MMM are caused by massive increases in splenoportal blood flow and decreased hepatic vascular compliance. The decreased compliance is due to extramedullary hematopoiesis and its secondary collagen deposition.
      3. **Extramedullary hematopoietic tumors** can develop in any organ and are most problematic in the epidural space. Foci of these tumors on serosal surfaces can result in massive effusions containing immature hematopoietic cells.
      4. **Neutrophilic dermatoses,** which are skin lesions with intense polymorphonuclear neutrophil infiltration, can be a presenting or complicating feature of MMM. The resultant raised tender plaques can progress to bullae or pyroderma gangrenosum.

III. **Management.** Therapy for MMM has not been shown to significantly improve survival. Treatment is therefore postponed until patients develop problems.
   A. **Medical management**
      1. **Transfusions** of packed red cells are given often enough to maintain tissue oxygenation above levels that produce symptoms.
      2. **Androgens,** such as danazol (200 mg PO q6–8h), may improve the anemia in many patients (see Chap. 4, sec. **VII.C**). Several months of treatment are necessary before improvement is evident.
      3. **Chemotherapy** with low doses of busulfan, hydroxyurea, or 6-thioguanine has been used in patients with very high leukocyte and platelet counts, symptomatic splenomegaly, or symptoms of hypermetabolism (fever, sweats, or weight loss). The response to treatment is unpredictable. Cytotoxic agents must be used cautiously because these patients have marginal hematopoietic reserves.
      4. **α- and γ-IFN** may prove to be useful in MMM.
      5. **Glucocorticoids** sometimes ameliorate systemic symptoms and are useful for immunologic complications.

6. **Radioactive phosphorus** has an uncertain role in the management of MMM.
7. **Folic acid,** 1 mg/day PO, is usually prescribed for all patients, particularly for those with weight loss or marked splenomegaly.
8. **BMT** should be considered for patients who are less than 40 years old and who have a histocompatible sibling.

B. **Splenectomy,** when decided upon cautiously in a timely fashion, is beneficial in nearly all patients who have painful splenomegaly and in about 40 percent of patients who have serious cytopenias. The expected survival after successful splenectomy is two years. The mortality rate is less than 10 percent if the procedure is performed by experienced surgeons; postoperative morbidity exceeds 30 percent. Progressive hepatomegaly develops in less than 15 percent of patients after splenectomy. The indications for splenectomy in medically suitable patients with MMM are

1. Persistent discomfort because of a grossly enlarged or infarcted spleen
2. Refractory hemolytic anemia as manifested by severe anemia that must be treated with increasingly frequent transfusions
3. Refractory, serious thrombocytopenia in the absence of evidence of disseminated intravascular coagulation
4. Portal hypertension associated with bleeding varices. Based on circulatory dynamic studies performed at the time of surgery, the following procedures should be performed:
   a. Splenectomy alone for portal hypertension secondary to markedly increased blood flow from the liver to the spleen
   b. Splenorenal shunt for portal hypertension secondary to intrahepatic block of blood flow

C. **RT**
1. Small doses (15–650 cGy per course) or RT to the spleen can relieve pain and early satiety secondary to massive splenomegaly in MMM when splenectomy is contraindicated. Blood counts must be monitored very carefully during splenic RT, because severe cytopenias may develop rapidly.
2. Focal areas of periostitis, extramedullary fibrohematopoietic tumors, and ascites secondary to myeloid metaplasia of the peritoneum may also be palliated by RT.

Selected Reading

Polycythemia Vera

Berk, P. D., et al. Therapeutic recommendations in polycythemia vera based on Polycythemia Vera Study Group protocols. *Semin. Hematol.* 23:132, 1986.

Dai, C. H., et al. Polycythemia vera. II. Hypersensitivity of bone marrow erythroid, granulocyte-macrophage, and megakaryocyte progenitor cells to interleukin-3 and granulocyte-macrophage colony stimulating factors. *Blood* 80:891, 1992.

Kaplan, M. E., et al. Long-term management of polycythemia vera with hydroxyurea: a progress report. *Semin. Hematol.* 23:167, 1986.

Silver, R.T . A new treatment for polycythemia vera: recombinant interferon alpha. *Blood* 76:664, 1990.

Essential Thrombocythemia

Anagrelide Study Group. Anagrelide, a therapy for thrombocythemic states: Experience in 577 patients. *Am. J. Med.* 92:69, 1992.

Colombi, M., et al. Thrombotic and hemorrhagic complications in essential thrombocythemia. A retrospective study of 103 patients. *Cancer* 67:2926, 1991.

McIntyre, K. J., Hoagland, H. C., and Silverstein, M. N. Essential thrombocythemia in young adults. *Mayo Clin. Proc.* 66:149, 1991.

Wadenvik, H., et al. The effect of α-interferon on bone marrow megakaryocytes and platelet production rate in essential thrombocythemia. *Blood* 77:2103, 1991.

Watson, K. V., and Key, N. Vascular complications of essential thrombocythemia: a link to cardiovascular risk factors. *Br. J. Haematol.* 83:198, 1993.

Myelofibrosis with Myeloid Metaplasia

Rozman, C., et al. Life expectancy of patients with chronic nonleukemic myeloproliferative disorders. *Cancer* 67:2658, 1991.

Weinstein, I. M. Idiopathic myelofibrosis: historical review, diagnosis and management. *Blood Rev.* 5:98, 1991.

Wolf, B. C., and Neiman, R. S. Myelofibrosis with myeloid metaplasia: pathophysiologic implications of the correlation between bone marrow changes and progression of splenomegaly. *Blood* 65:803, 1985.

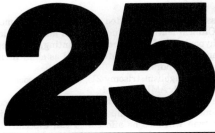

Acute Leukemia

Kenneth A. Foon and
Dennis A. Casciato

I. Epidemiology and etiology
  A. Incidence. Acute leukemia afflicts three to four per 100,000 population annually (11,000 new cases per year) in the United States. Children account for 25 percent of cases. Acute leukemia is the most common malignant disease of childhood (see Chap. 18, *Incidence, Leukemia, and Lymphoma*, sec. II).
  1. **Cell type.** Eighty percent of cases of acute lymphoblastic leukemia (ALL) occur in children, and 90 percent of cases of acute myelogenous leukemia (AML) occur in adults.
  2. **Age.** The peak incidence of ALL occurs at three to four years of age; the incidence steadily decreases after nine years of age and is rare after 40 years of age. The incidence of AML gradually increases with age; the median age of patients is 60 years.
  3. **Sex.** Acute leukemia shows a male predilection only in the very young and the elderly.
  B. Etiology
  1. **Radiation** is the leukemogenic factor in human beings that has been best documented. Increased incidences of leukemia proportional to the cumulative radiation dose have been demonstrated in populations exposed to atomic bombs, in patients irradiated for ankylosing spondylitis, and in radiologists (prior to current protective precautions). Doses of less than 100 cGy are not associated with the development of leukemia. The types of leukemia induced by radiation are ALL, AML, and chronic myelogenous leukemia (CML), but not chronic lymphocytic leukemia.
  2. **Viruses** have not been associated with acute leukemia in humans.
  3. **Chemicals.** The ability of chemicals to produce acute leukemia and pancytopenia is likely related to their ability to mutate or ablate the bone marrow stem cells.
     a. Benzene and toluene are well-documented causes of acute leukemia. Acute leukemia develops one to five years after exposure and is often preceded by bone marrow hypoplasia and pancytopenia.
     b. Drugs. Drug-induced acute leukemia is usually preceded by myelodysplasia. Alkylating agents given for prolonged periods are associated with a markedly increased risk of AML (see Chap. 34, *Cytopenia*, sec. I.D). Other drugs that have been implicated include arsenicals, phenylbutazone, and chloramphenicol.
  4. **Heredity**
     a. Hereditary syndromes that are associated with chromosomal abnormalities and very high risks for acute leukemia include
        (1) **Bloom's syndrome,** which is a recessively transmitted disease occurring predominantly in persons of Jewish ancestry. Chromosome breaks are readily found in cytogenetic studies. The syndrome is characterized by short and thin stature, delicate features, telangiectatic lesions over the malar eminences of the face, photosensitivity, and a variety of other cutaneous abnormalities (acanthosis nigricans, hypertrichosis, ichthyosis, and café-au-lait spots). AML is the type of leukemia that develops in these patients.
        (2) **Fanconi's congenital pancytopenia** (Fanconi's aplasia), which is an

autosomal recessive disease associated with multiple chromosomal abnormalities. Clinical features include skeletal abnormalities (absence of radii, hypoplasia of the thumbs), squinting, microcephaly, small stature, and hypogonadism. AML, as well as skin carcinoma, often complicates this syndrome.

(3) **Down's syndrome** (mongolism, trisomy 21), which is associated with an increased risk of both AML and ALL.

b. **Siblings** of patients with acute leukemia have a fivefold increased risk. If one member of a monozygotic twinship develops acute leukemia, the risk that the other twin will also be affected is 1:4, especially if the patient is less than eight years old and it is within one year of the first diagnosis of leukemia.

5. **Hematologic diseases.** CML transforms into acute leukemia ("blast crisis") in over 80 percent of cases. Patients with myelodysplastic syndromes (see sec. I.C), clearly have an increased likelihood of developing acute leukemia. The incidence of acute leukemia in myeloproliferative disorders, myeloma, and certain solid tumors is increased by the use of chemotherapy.

C. **Idiopathic myelodysplastic syndromes** ("preleukemia," "refractory anemias"). Patients who have idiopathic myelodysplastic syndromes (MDSs) have a high risk of developing AML. Theoretically, defects in stem cells account for ineffective hematopoiesis and for the wide variety of abnormalities. The diagnosis of a primary MDS may be made only in the absence of conditions that produce *secondary myelodysplasia,* namely, radiation exposure and cytotoxic agent therapy. Folic acid and vitamin B_{12} deficiencies produce a reversible myelodysplastic picture.

1. **Clinical features.** MDSs usually affect patients more than 50 years old, particularly men. Symptoms are absent or nonspecific and usually reflect the degree of anemia. Physical examination is usually normal. Various cytopenias, usually including anemia, may persist for months to years. The bone marrow is *always abnormal.*

2. **Dyspoiesis** is manifested by cytopenias in the presence of a normocellular or hypercellular bone marrow. Components and features of dyspoiesis, which occur in various combinations for each syndrome, are as follows:

a. **Dyserythropoiesis**

(1) **Peripheral blood.** Anemia and reticulocytopenia from ineffective erythropoiesis; anisocytosis, poikilocytosis, basophilic stippling; macrocytosis (when megaloblastoid maturation is present); dimorphic (normocytic, normochromic, and microcytic, hypochromic) red cell populations (when ringed sideroblasts are present)

(2) **Bone marrow.** Erythroid hyperplasia or hypoplasia; ringed sideroblasts; megaloblastoid maturation (multinuclearity, nuclear fragments, or cytoplasmic abnormalities)

(3) **Other assays.** Positive Ham test (paroxysmal nocturnal hemoglobinuria-like defect) and increased fetal hemoglobin levels may be detected

b. **Dysgranulocytopoiesis**

(1) **Peripheral blood.** Neutropenia; decreased or abnormal neutrophil granules; neutrophil nuclear changes with hyposegmentation (pseudo-Pelger-Huët anomaly), hypersegmentation, or bizarre shapes

(2) **Bone marrow.** Granulocytic hyperplasia; abnormal or decreased granules in neutrophil precursors; increased numbers of blast cells

(3) **Other assays.** Decreased NAP score; if monocytosis is present, increased serum lysozyme levels; decreased myeloperoxidase activity

c. **Dysmegakaryocytopoiesis**

(1) **Peripheral blood.** Thrombocytopenia; large platelets with abnormal and decreased granularity

(2) **Bone marrow.** Reduced numbers of megakaryocytes; micromega-

Table 25-1. Distinguishing features of the idiopathic myelodysplastic syndromes

Abnormality	RA	RA-S	RAEB	RAEB-T	CMML
DYSERYTHROPOIESIS	+	+ +	+	+	+
Ringed sideroblasts	–	+ +	+	+	+
DYSMEGAKARYOCYTOPOIESIS	–	–	+ +	+ +	+ +
DYSGRANULOCYTOPOIESIS	–	–	+ +	+ +	+ +
Auer rods	– –	– –	– –	+	– –
Proportion of blasts in bone marrow*	<5%	<5%	5–20%	20–30%	5–20%

Key: + = may be present; + + = prominent; – = usually absent; – – = always absent. RA = refractory anemia and/or cytopenia; RA-S = refractory anemia with ringed sideroblasts; RAEB = refractory anemia with excess blasts; RAEB-T = RAEB in transformation; CMML = chronic myelomonocytic leukemia.
*The diagnosis of AML is established with more than 30 percent blasts in the bone marrow.

karyocytes; megakaryocytes with large, single nuclei or multiple, small nuclei

    (3) Other assays. Abnormal platelet function tests

  3. Classification of the MDSs into one of five groups (on the basis of the French-American-British Cooperative Group Criteria) is accomplished by assessing the spectrum of hematologic abnormalities. Distinguishing features are shown in Table 25-1. In general, the risk of transformation to AML is proportional to the number of cell lines affected by cytopenia, the percentage of blasts in the marrow, and the complexity of chromosomal abnormalities.

    a. Refractory anemia (RA) applies to patients who do not fit precisely into any of the groups below. They present with anemia, neutropenia, or thrombocytopenia and a normocellular or hypercellular bone marrow. Dyserythropoiesis is present but ringed sideroblasts are either absent or less than 15 percent of nucleated cells in the marrow. The incidence of infection and hemorrhage depends on the severity of neutropenia and thrombocytopenia. The incidence of AML is not defined.

    b. Refractory anemia with ringed sideroblasts (RA-S) differs from **RA** by having more ringed sideroblasts (more than 15% of all nucleated cells in the bone marrow). Neutropenia and thrombocytopenia are uncommon. Less than 10 percent of cases develop AML.

    c. Refractory anemia with excess blasts (RAEB) shows conspicuous abnormalities in all three cell lines and cytopenias in at least two cell lines. Blast cells are increased in the marrow. AML develops in about 30 percent of cases. Some patients die from bone marrow failure caused by ineffective myelopoiesis, or from unrelated causes since this disorder affects the elderly.

    d. RAEB in transformation (RAEB-T) includes cases, often with a brief period of symptoms, which cannot clearly be classified as RAEB or AML. Auer rods or increased numbers of blasts are seen. Nearly all cases develop into AML.

    e. Chronic myelomonocytic leukemia (CMML) must have at least 1,000/μL total monocytes by definition. CMML is often accompanied by increased numbers of qualitatively abnormal granulocytes and a hypercellular bone marrow with similar morphology to RAEB, but with less than 3 percent blasts (this disease is discussed in Chap. 23, *Chronic Myelomonocytic Leukemia*).

  4. Cytogenetic abnormalities are nonrandom and occur in 40 to 60 percent of patients. Most combinations include whole or partial losses of chromosomes 5, 7, or 20 (5q–, –7, 20q–) or gains of chromosomes 1 or 8 (+1,

+8). The unbalanced translocation between chromosomes 1 and 7 [t(1; 7) (p11;p11)] results in trisomy for the long arm of chromosome 1 and monosomy for the long arm of chromosome 7 and may be causally related to therapy-related MDS. *RAS* oncogene activation occurs early in the pathogenesis of MDS in about 15 percent of patients. The development of cytogenetic abnormalities in patients with MDS and previously normal karyotypes portends rapid transformation to AML.

5. **The 5q− syndrome** is a unique MDS that is characterized by macrocytosis, hypolobulated micromegakaryocytic hyperplasia, and a clonal interstitial deletion of the long arm of chromosome 5 (5q−). The platelet counts are normal or increased, and granulocytopenia is rare. Patients have a median age of 68 years, and females predominate by a ratio of 2:1. Survival tends to be better than for other MDS types because of the lower occurrence of hemorrhage and infection, but 15 percent develop AML.

6. **Management.** MDSs must be managed conservatively unless and until acute leukemia supervenes. AML should become evident in a relatively short time, whereas the MDSs remain stable for months or years with only supportive treatment.

   a. Supportive care includes packed red cell transfusion as necessary, platelets for thrombocytopenic bleeding, and broad-spectrum antibiotics for neutropenic fever.

   b. Iron chelation therapy should be considered for patients who require red cell transfusions frequently and whose MDS has an indolent course.

   c. Androgens, pyridoxine, folate, and derivatives of vitamins A and D have been effective very rarely and have not improved survival. G-CSF and GM-CSF may increase neutrophils but have the theoretical disadvantage of stimulating growth of AML cells.

   d. BMT should be considered in patients less than 45 years of age who have an HLA-compatible sibling (less than 10% of MDS patients).

   e. Cytotoxic agents are usually not recommended in these patients. Some patients have benefited temporarily from "low-dose cytarabine" therapy (3–20 mg/m^2/day for 14–21 days).

II. Pathology and natural history

A. **Classification.** The French-American-British Cooperative Group classification of acute leukemia is summarized in Table 25-2.

   1. **Auer rods** are abnormal condensations of cytoplasmic granules. Their presence in the immature cells distinguishes AML from ALL; their absence is not diagnostically helpful.

   2. **Cytochemistry.** Identifying the type of early cell may be difficult but is facilitated by readily available histochemical techniques and measurement of serum lysozyme concentration (Table 25-3).

   3. **Quantitative bone marrow differential** based on a 500-cell count differentiates M1, M2, M4, M5, and M6 subtypes of AML (Table 25-4).

   4. **Immunologic markers** distinguish subsets of ALL with similar morphologies (usually L1 or L1/L2) and usually distinguish ALL and AML. These markers are summarized in Table 25-5). Anti-platelet antibodies (e.g., to CD41 or CD42a) are useful in differentiating megakargoblastic (M7) leukemia.

B. **Pathology.** Bone marrow examination in acute leukemia shows hypercellularity with a monotonous infiltration of immature cells. Normal marrow elements are markedly decreased. Erythroblast maturation is commonly megaloblastoid in all types of AML, especially subtypes M6.

C. **Natural history.** Leukemic cells generally replicate more slowly than their normal counterparts. Hematopoiesis is abnormal even before the proportion of blast cells in the marrow is conspicuously increased. Immature and malfunctioning leukocyte progenitors progressively replace the normal bone marrow and infiltrate other tissues. Unless complete remission following therapy lasts four or more years, relapse is inevitable. Relapse is associated with progressively poorer response to therapy and progressively shorter duration of remission. Unsuccess-

Table 25-2. Classification of acute leukemias

Subtype	Morphology	Incidence in adults (%)	Characteristics of immature cells						
			Cell size	Cytoplasm-nucleus ratio	Nucleoli	Cytoplasmic granules	Auer rods	Comments	
M1[a]	Myeloblastic leukemia without maturation	20	Small to large	About equal	Distinct	Scarce	Occasional	Easily confused with M7 or L2 without special studies	
M2	Myeloblastic leukemia with maturation	30	Large	About equal	Distinct	Present	Occasional	Predominant cells are blasts and early promyelocytes	
M3	Hypergranular promyelocytic leukemia	10	Large	Increased	Distinct	Large, abundant, and atypical	Common	Associated with a high incidence of disseminated intravascular coagulation	
M4	Myelomonocytic leukemia[b]	30	Large with monocytoid features	Increased	Distinct	Present	Occasional	Requires assessment of both peripheral blood and bone marrow	
M5	Monocytic leukemia; poorly (M5a) or well (M5b) differentiated	10	Large; monocyte lineage	About equal	Large	Present	Rare	Confirmation of diagnosis is necessary using fluoride-inhibited esterase reactions (see Table 24-3)	
M6	Erythroleukemia (usually progresses to M1, M2, or M4)	<5						Florid megaloblastoid erythroid hyperplasia, and bizarre multinucleated erythroblasts	
M7	Megakaryoblastic leukemia	<5	Small to large	Heterogeneous	Distinct	Scarce	Absent	Platelet peroxidase reaction by electron microscopy or monoclonal antibodies against platelet glycoproteins confirms diagnosis; marrow fibrosis is prominent	
L1	Lymphocytic leukemia, childhood form	20	Small	Scant	Indistinct	Absent	Absent	Homogeneous cell population	
L2	Lymphocytic leukemia, adult form	80	Intermediate to large	Heterogeneous	Distinct	Absent	Absent	Heterogeneous cell population	
L3	Burkitt-type cell leukemia	Rare						See Chapter 21, *Burkitt's Lymphoma*	

[a]MO represents myeloblastic leukemia without cytologic maturation. These cells have myeloid antigens (CD13 and CD33) and are myeloperoxidase-negative.
[b]A subtype of M4 is characterized by bone marrows that contain abnormal eosinophils (M4$_{EO}$). These eosinophils have large basophilic granules, single-lobed nuclei, or a positive reaction to PAS and chloracetate esterase (normal eosinophils stain negatively).

Table 25-3. Cytologic reactions in acute leukemia[a]

Reaction	Degree of reaction		
	Absent or weak	Moderate	Strong
Nonspecific esterase[b]	M0, M1, L	M2, M3	M4, M5
Nonspecific esterase with fluoride inhibitor[b]	M0, M1, M5, L	M2, M3, M4	—
Peroxidase or Sudan black	M0, M5, M7, L	M1, M4	M2, M3
Lysozyme (muramidase)[c]	M0, M1, M2, M3, L	M4	M5
PAS	M0, M1, M2, M3, L	M4, M5, L	L

[a]M0 through M7 types of myelogenous leukemia are described in Table 24-2. M6 is excluded. The three types of lymphocytic leukemia (L) are not distinguished by these studies.

[b]Sodium fluoride is a potent inhibitor of the predominant esterase in precursors of monocytes but not in precursors of granulocytes or lymphocytes; it is most useful to identify type M5 leukemias.

[c]Increased lysozyme levels are measured in the serum and characterize mixed (M4) or pure (M5) monocytic leukemias.

Table 25-4. Quantitative bone marrow differential counts in AML[a]

Subtype	Blasts		Nonerythroid cells		Erythroblasts (ANC)
	ANC	NEC	Granulocytes[b] (NEC)	Monocytes (NEC)	
M1		>90%	<10%	<10%	
M2	>30%	30–89%	>10%	<20%	<50%
M4[c]	>30%	>30%	>20%	>20%[c]	<50%
M5		>80%[d]	<20%	>80%[d]	
M6	< or >30%	>30%	Variable	Variable	>50%

Key: ANC = all nucleated cells; NEC = nonerythroid cells.
[a]M3 and M7 subtypes are classified by other criteria.
[b]Promyelocytes, myelocytes, metamyelocytes, and neutrophils.
[c]Also requires absolute monocyte count in peripheral blood greater than 5000/μl and/or lysozyme concentration greater than 3 times normal in serum or urine.
[d]Monoblasts in M5a; predominantly promonocytes and monocytes in M5b.

ful therapy is usually followed by death within two months. Death in acute leukemia is usually due to either infection or hemorrhage.

III. Diagnosis
A. Symptoms
1. **Nonspecific** fatigue and weakness are the most common symptoms. Bruising, fever, and weight loss are also frequent.
2. **CNS** involvement may be manifested by headaches, nausea, vomiting, blurred vision, or cranial nerve dysfunction.
3. **Bone pain** is more common in ALL than in AML.
4. **Abdominal fullness** usually reflects hepatosplenomegaly, which is more common in ALL.

Table 25-5. Immunologic cell surface markers in acute leukemias*

| Markers | Acute lymphoblastic leukemia | | Acute myeloblastic leukemia |
	Non-T cell	T cell	
Ia (HLA-DR)	100%	10%	90%
CD19	90%	0%	<5%
CD20	70%	0%	<5%
CD10	70%	10%	0%
Cytoplasmic μ	10%	0%	0%
Surface membrane Ig	<5%	0%	0%
LCD7	0%	100%	<5%
LCD3	0%	75%	0%
CD13	<5%	<5%	80%
CD33	<5%	<5%	80%

*The percentage of patients with leukemic cells that are positive for the respective markers are indicated. See Appendix C4. Leukocyte Differentiation Antigens.

   5. **Oliguria** may result from dehydration, uric acid nephropathy, or disseminated intravascular coagulation (DIC).
   6. **Obstipation** may signify disorders of calcium or magnesium metabolism.
B. **Physical findings**
   1. **Pallor, petechiae, and purpura** are the most frequent findings in acute leukemia.
   2. **Sternal tenderness** to palpation, **lymphadenopathy,** and **hepatosplenomegaly** are much more common in ALL than in AML.
   3. **Meningismus** may indicate CNS involvement. CNS leukemia is most common in ALL, less common in M4 (particularly with abnormal bone marrow eosinophils) and M5 AML, and rare in the other subtypes of AML.
   4. **Leukemic infiltrates in the optic fundus** appear as Roth-like spots with flame hemorrhages.
   5. **Gingival enlargement** is seen in ALL and M5 AML. Extranodal masses, especially involving the skin, orbits, breasts, or testes, are also most likely to occur in monocytic leukemias and ALL.
   6. **Other organs.** At the time of diagnosis, the kidneys are clinically involved in about 25 percent of cases, the lung, joints, or GI tract in 5 percent of cases, and the heart in 2 percent of cases. At postmortem examination virtually all organs are infiltrated with leukemic cells.
   7. **Bleeding** out of proportion to the degree of thrombocytopenia suggests the presence of DIC, especially in type M3 acute leukemia.
   8. Signs of **infection** should be carefully sought.
C. **Laboratory studies.** The diagnosis of acute leukemia is established by bone marrow examination. Borderline cases are observed and the diagnosis of acute leukemia deferred until progressive bone marrow infiltration and clinical deterioration are demonstrated.
   1. **Bone marrow** findings are discussed in sections **II.A** and **II.B.** Blasts must account for more than 30 percent of the nucleated cells to establish the diagnosis. Cytochemistries should be performed in all cases of acute leukemia. Immunologic cell surface markers should be evaluated in all cases suspected of being ALL.
   2. **Cytogenetic abnormalities** associated with the various subtypes of AML are as follows:
      a. M2—t(8;21)

     b. M3—t(15;17)

     c. M4 with eosinophilia—del(16)(q22) or inv(16)(p13q22)

     d. M5—11q⁻

3. Hemogram

  a. Erythrocytes. Ninety percent of patients have a normocytic, normochromatic anemia, which is usually severe. Reticulocytes are nearly always decreased. Macrocytosis usually reflects megaloblastoid maturation. Nucleated red blood cells are often observed in the peripheral blood.

  b. Leukocytes. The WBC is elevated in 60 percent of cases, normal in 15 percent, and decreased in 25 percent. Circulating blasts are demonstrable in virtually every case of acute leukemia. Blasts account for most of the circulating cells in patients with elevated WBCs.

  c. Platelet counts are decreased in 90 percent of cases and are less than 50,000/μL in about 50 percent.

4. Biochemical tests that should be obtained include

  a. Serum uric acid, calcium, phosphorus, and magnesium levels

  b. Serum renal and liver function tests

  c. Serum lysozyme concentration with M4 and M5 types of AML

  d. Coagulation tests for DIC (see Chap. 34, *Coagulopathy,* sec. II).

5. Radiologic studies that should be obtained include

  a. Chest x-ray film to look for leukemic or infectious infiltrates

  b. Bone x-ray study of painful or tender areas to look for periosteal elevation or bony destruction

6. CSF examination should be performed in patients with meningismus or CNS abnormalities. The fluid should be cultured routinely for acid-fast bacilli, fungi, and bacteria. Meningeal involvement with leukemia is associated with decreased sugar and increased protein concentrations, pleocytosis, and leukemic cells found by cytologic examination. Cytarabine (100 mg) or methotrexate (10 mg/m²) should be injected into the CSF at the completion of the exam because of the possibility of leukemic contamination from blood.

7. Surveillance bacterial cultures of the nose, pharynx, axillae, and perianal regions identify organisms that may have colonized the patient. These cultures, however, are not commonly helpful in predicting etiologic organisms for serious infection.

IV. Staging system and prognostic factors. A staging system for acute leukemia does not exist. Complete remission (CR) is the paramount prognostic factor in all forms of acute leukemia. A CR is defined as

A bone marrow containing less than 5 percent blasts

Normalization of erythrocyte, granulocyte, and platelet counts

Resolution of organomegaly

Return to normal performance status

A. Adverse prognostic factors in AML

  1. Secondary AML (following cytotoxic drugs, benzene, or radiation)

  2. AML following a prolonged MDS

  3. Age more than 60 years

  4. Presence of the Philadelphia chromosome, t(9;22)

B. Adverse prognostic factors in ALL

  1. Age less than three years or more than seven years (prognosis is poorer in older children and poorest in adults)

  2. Male sex

  3. WBC count greater than 20,000/μL in children, or 30,000/μL in adults

  4. Morphologic types L2 and L3

  5. True B cell L3 ALL (surface Ig positive) has the worst prognosis. T cell and CD10-negative B cell ALL have a less favorable pronosis than CD10-positive B cell ALL.

  6. The presence of any of the following:

    a. Hepatosplenomegaly, lymphadenopathy, or mediastinal mass

    b. CNS leukemia

c. Ph^1 chromosome (10% of children and 30% of adults with ALL)

C. Survival rates

1. **AML.** The median survival is 12 to 24 months for patients who achieve CR; the median duration of first remission is 10 to 12 months. About 15 to 25 percent of patients who achieve CR (5 to 15% of all patients) survive five or more years and many of these patients may be cured. Most relapses occur within three years.

2. **ALL**
   a. **Adolescents and adults** have a median first CR duration of about 12 to 18 months and a median survival of about 18 to 24 months.
   b. **High-risk children** (those with adverse prognostic factors) have remission duration and survival similar to that of adults.
   c. **Low-risk children** (age two to nine years, WBC less than 20,000/µL, common cell subtype, and without other adverse prognostic factors). Less than one-third of cases relapse if properly treated. Relapse or death is unusual in these patients after four years of continuous CR. More than 50 percent of cases have a five-year disease-free survival. Approximately 50 to 60 percent are cured of their disease.

V. Management. All patients should be begun on treatment with *allopurinol,* 300 to 600 mg daily, 12 to 48 hours before starting antileukemic therapy.

A. Treatment of AML

1. **Remission induction.** Intensive chemotherapy nearly always to the point of severe bone marrow aplasia (which generally occurs about 12 days after treatment is begun) is necessary to achieve CR in patients with AML. A typical regimen is

   > Cytarabine, 100 mg/m^2 by *continuous IV infusion* for seven days, *and*
   > Idarubicin, 12 mg/m^2 IV push on either days 1, 2, and 3, *or* days 5, 6 and 7 (daunorubin at a dose of 45 to 60 mg/m^2 may be substituted for idarubicin)

   a. The **combination therapy is repeated** once or twice more if the blasts are not cleared from the blood and bone marrow and if the patient can tolerate such intensive treatment. A CR is achieved in 60 to 75 percent of patients with good medical support, usually about one month after initiating treatment.
   b. **Toxicity of induction therapy**
      (1) Severe marrow depression with life-threatening pancytopenia
      (2) Nausea, vomiting, severe stomatitis
      (3) ECG changes, arrhythmias, congestive heart failure
      (4) Self-limited alopecia; tissue necrosis if the anthracycline is infiltrated outside the vein
   c. **Promyelocytic (M3) leukemia**
      (1) **All-*trans* retinoic acid** (45 mg/m^2/day PO divided into two doses for up to two months) induces a nonmyelosuppressive remission in virtually all cases of type M3 AML. To sustain a remission, however, some form of intensive chemotherapy is required after remission is induced.
      (2) **Coagulopathy** occurs in more than 90 percent of patients with subtype M3 AML, and it results in severe hemorrhagic manifestations in excess of that expected for the degree of thrombocytopenia. Laboratory abnormalities include not only features associated with DIC (decreased fibrinogen and increased fibrin/fibrinogen degradation products) but also evidence of increased fibrinolysis (acquired deficiency of the fibrinolysis inhibitor, α_2-antitrypsin).

      Patients should be monitored closely for the development of DIC (see Chap. 34, *Coagulopathy,* sec. II), and treated either prophylactically or at the first sign of DIC. Continuous infusion of heparin has been the mainstay of treatment (10,000 to 30,000 units/day). Transfusions with platelets, cryoprecipitate, or fresh-frozen plasma are usually also indicated. Heparin may be discontinued after induction therapy is completed provided there is no evidence of DIC. An alternative to heparin therapy is the use of antifibrinolytic agents such as tranexamic acid. When the coagulopathy is successfully managed, affected patients have the same or better CR rate as patients with other types of AML and may even have a more lasting remission.

   d. Elderly patients. The treatment of patients 65 years of age or older is controversial. Some authorities argue that intensive chemotherapy should be used because the rate of CR is the same as for younger patients. Other experts disagree. An antecedent MDS is often seen in elderly patients, who cannot tolerate the toxic effects of intensive induction therapy as well as younger patients; the death rate due to hematotoxicity in these patients is approximately 30 percent with intensive regimens.

   Less intensive treatment using attenuated dosages of drugs, oral agents (hydroxyurea or etoposide) or "low-dose cytarabine" (see sec. **I.C.6.e**) have been shown to be associated with less myelosuppression, fewer early deaths, and longer quality (outpatient) survival than standard intensive induction therapy. The use of supportive care alone is a reasonable option for many elderly patients with AML, particularly for patients who are not in good general medical condition. Two useful less intensive regimens for elderly patients who are in good general medical condition are:

   (1) Cytarabine, 100 mg/m^2 q12h for five days given by continuous IV infusion; and idarubicin, 12 mg/m^2 IV for one dose only.

   (2) Cytarabine, 100 mg/m^2 IV push or SQ b.i.d. for five days; and mitoxantrone, 10 mg/m^2 IV for one dose only.

2. Postremission therapy. After CR is achieved, the most important goal is to prevent recurrence. Leukemic cells that are not clinically apparent remain. Therapy to eradicate residual leukemia is required or recurrence is inevitable.

   a. Postremission chemotherapy. Relatively high doses of drugs are given shortly after the patient has achieved CR, has regained normal hematologic function, and has clinically completely recovered. High dose cytarabine alone is commonly used; doses range from 1.5 to 3.0 g/m^2 IV every 12 hours for seven days for two or three courses to 3.0 g/^{2} IV every 12 hours on Monday, Wednesday, and Friday only for each of four courses. Other regimens that are used include cytarabine with other drugs (such as idarubicin or mitoxantrone), or combinations of noncross-resistant agents (such as high-dose etoposide and cyclophosphamide).

   b. Autologous BMT with intensive chemotherapy and RT followed by infusion of bone marrow that is either untreated or "purged" with drugs or antibodies may be used rather than chemotherapy alone.

   c. Allogeneic BMT is considered when an HLA-identical sibling donor can be identified in a patient less than 50 years of age. Results are best in teenagers and young adults.

3. Controversial therapies

   a. Maintenance therapy. Low-dose prolonged maintenance therapy has not been shown to prolong survival.

   b. CNS prophylaxis with cranial irradiation and intrathecal chemotherapy may be effective in preventing meningeal leukemia but has not prolonged the length of remission as nearly all of these patients will relapse in the bone marrow. CNS relapse is most common in the M4 and M5 subtypes. CNS therapy *is indicated* when AML cells are detected in the CSF.

   c. Cycling AML cells with G-CSF or GM-CSF prior to cytarabine to make then more susceptible is under investigation.

B. Treatment of ALL
  1. Remission induction
    a. Children. Vincristine (V) and prednisone (P) are effective for producing CR in less than 50 percent of cases when used alone but in 85 to 90 percent of cases when used together. The addition of L-**asparaginase** produces CR in more than 90 percent of children with ALL. Most children achieve CR within four weeks of therapy; if CR is not achieved within six weeks, there is no value in continuing the drugs. Children often achieve CR without prolonged myelosuppression. Those who experience the least morbidity and achieve CR most often have the longest remissions.
      (1) Low-risk patients are treated with V + P for four to six weeks:

      Vincristine, 1.5 mg/m^2 (maximum 2 mg) IVP weekly, and
      Prednisone, 40 mg/m^2 PO daily

      (2) Intermediate-risk patients are treated with V + P and L-asparaginase, 6000 units/m^2 (maximum 10,000 units) IV or IM three times weekly for a total of 9 doses.
      (3) High-risk patients are treated with V + P and daunorubicin, 30 mg/m^2 IV weekly for a total of four to six doses.
    b. Adults. The combination of V and P result in CR in 45 percent of adults with ALL. The addition of an anthracycline with or without L-asparaginase increases the CR rate to 70 to 80 percent. Complex multiagent protocols may be more effective.
    c. Toxicity of induction therapy
      (1) V + P
        (a) Intestinal colic and constipation (bulk laxatives should be used prophylactically).
        (b) Peripheral neuropathy (usually reversible).
        (c) Hematosuppression and alopecia are uncommon.
      (2) V + P and an anthracycline. Same as (1) along with nausea, vomiting, stomatitis, alopecia, hematosuppression, and cardiac toxicity
      (3) V + P and L-asparaginase. Same as (1) with the addition of coagulation defects, allergic reactions, and encephalopathy
  2. Consolidation treatment with intermittent pulses of V + P, with or without other drugs, has not been shown to improve remission duration or survival in ALL.
  3. CNS prophylaxis prevents early CNS relapse and is mandatory in children with ALL after CR is induced. The CNS is the initial site of relapse in more than 50 percent of patients unless prophylaxis is given. However, this treatment has not been shown to improve remission duration or survival in adolescents or adults.
    a. Regimens. The form of CS prophylaxis is controversial. Many authorities recommend intrathecal methotrexate (6–12 mg/m^2 up to a maximum of 15 mg/dose of preservative-free methotrexate, twice weekly for 5–8 doses) combined with craniospinal irradiation (about 2400 cGy in 12 fractions over 2.5 weeks) for patients more than one year old. Intrathecal methotrexate alone is recommended by some authorities for patients at low risk for relapse (age two to nine years, WBC less than 10,000/μL, and CD10-positivity).
    b. Toxicity of CNS prophylaxis
      (1) Transient, but sometimes fatal, **encephalopathy** develops in up to 67 percent of patients for four to eight weeks after completion of cranial irradiation, especially if methotrexate is given in the maintenance program. Symptoms of encephalopathy include somnolence, headache, vomiting, and low-grade fever. Spinal fluid examination shows pleocytosis with neutrophils and mononuclear cells. The differential diagnosis includes CNS infection, cerebrovascular acci-

dents, and leukemic meningitis, which should be distinguishable by CT scans and by spinal fluid culture and cytology.
- **(2)** Self-limited **alopecia** after cranial irradiation.
- **(3)** **Headache** after intrathecal drug administration.
- **(4)** Chemical **arachnoiditis** with meningismus and back pain on account of epidural extravasation of methotrexate.
- **(5)** **Leukoencephalopathy** may develop in patients given large doses of IV methotrexate after brain irradiation.
- **(6)** **Neuropsychologic effects** of treatment are common, especially in children less than six years of age. Memory and mathematical and motor skills may be impaired. CNS prophylaxis and the drugs that have activity in the CNS (methotrexate, prednisone, vincristine, and L-asparaginase) are thought to cause these problems. However, the disease itself may contribute: ALL disrupts the patient's family, social, and school life, and alters attitudes of others toward the patient.
- **4. Maintenance therapy** for two to three years is *mandatory* in childhood ALL.
    - **a. Effective drugs.** Methotrexate (20 mg/m^2 PO weekly) and mercaptopurine (50 mg/m^2 PO daily) are the cornerstones of maintenance therapy in ALL. The addition of other drugs has not improved remission duration or survival. It is important that the drugs be given in dosages sufficient to produce hematosuppression; otherwise the risk of relapse is substantially increased.
    - **b. Toxicity of maintenance therapy.** Late side effects of maintenance therapy in patients cured of ALL are not established. All of the following side effects resolve after therapy is stopped.
        - **(1)** **Therapy is interrupted** if any of the following occur:
            - **(a)** Significant hematosuppression (which is dose-limiting but is a necessary goal)
            - **(b)** Abnormal LFTs
            - **(c)** Stomatitis, diarrhea
            - **(d)** Renal tubular necrosis because of methotrexate (renal function is closely monitored)
        - **(2)** **Immunosuppression** (increased susceptibility to infection, particularly varicella and *Pneumocystis carinii*)
        - **(3)** **Growth inhibition**
        - **(4)** **Skin disorders**
        - **(5)** **Osteoporosis** with long-term methotrexate treatment
- **C. Treatment of meningeal leukemia**
    - **1. Manifestations.** Meningeal leukemia is manifested by a variety of neurologic signs (see also Chap. 32, sec. II) and by blast cells that are identified by cytologic evaluation of the cerebrospinal fluid.
    - **2. Treatment.** Optimal treatment has not been determined. Most patients are given cranial or craniospinal irradiation over a three-week period plus intrathecal chemotherapy. Intrathecal therapy alone may be insufficient.
        - **a. Drugs.** Preservative-free methotrexate (6–12 mg/m^2, maximum of 15 mg) or cytarabine (50–100 mg) is used for intrathecal therapy. Toxic effects of methotrexate may be prevented by giving citrovorum factor (leucovorin, 1 mg per each mg methotrexate) IM, 24 hours after intrathecal administration.
        - **b. Diluent.** Artificial spinal fluid (Elliott's B solution) is available at some institutions to dilute the cytotoxic agents.
        - **c. Technique.** Intrathecal chemotherapy is given isovolumetrically by serial withdrawal and injection of spinal fluid with a syringe containing the chemotherapeutic agent; the drug is thereby given gradually. The drugs may be administered by lumbar puncture, by cisternal puncture, or through an inserted intraventricular reservoir.
        - **d. Duration.** Intrathecal chemotherapy is given at three- to seven-day intervals until abnormal cells and excess protein are cleared from the

spinal fluid. Therapy is often continued at one- to two-month intervals for a period thereafter.

D. Treatment of relapses

1. **AML.** Relapses in AML are typically systemic (i.e., in the marrow and elsewhere). Some cases are heralded by extramedullary relapse (e.g., chloromas in skin or lymph nodes) but are followed by systemic relapse. Up to 50 percent of patients achieve a second CR using either the same drugs as were used to induce first remission or investigational drugs. Investigational drugs (see **F.4**) are often prescribed because the second remission is so short, usually less than six months, and is so difficult to achieve with agents that are available commercially.

2. **ALL** may relapse systemically or in sanctuary sites (testicle or CNS).

   a. **Extramedullary relapse.** Without CNS prophylaxis, relapse in just the CNS is common. Relapse in only the testis occurs, but is unusual. Patients who have solitary extramedullary relapse and an absolutely normal bone marrow may be treated with local therapy alone (i.e., CNS irradiation plus intrathecal chemotherapy for CNS relapse or radiation to the testicle for testicular relapse).

   b **Systemic relapse.** In 50 percent of cases, systemic relapse may be successfully treated with the agents used to induce the original remission.

   c. **Subsequent remissions.** Each subsequent remission becomes progressively shorter and drugs available for maintenance therapy are progressively limited. Patients who relapse after cessation of maintenance therapy have a better prognosis than those who relapse during continuous therapy.

E. When to stop maintenance therapy

1. **Children.** Prolonged chemotherapy is of greatest consequence in children because adverse, very late, side effects may develop. Most children in remission are treated for 30 to 36 months; 20 percent of children taken off treatment relapse, most within the first year. Elective testicular biopsy of boys prior to stopping maintenance therapy has been shown to be of no clinical value.

2. **Adults.** The vast majority of adults with ALL or AML relapse despite maintenance therapy. There are very little data to support the use of maintenance therapy for AML. Currently, we recommend maintenance therapy for three years in adults with ALL based on the experience with children.

F. Investigational therapies, which have not been proved to improve CR duration or survival (not recommended except in research protocols), include

1. **Intensification therapy,** which uses high doses of new drugs that the patient has not previously received. "Early" intensification is given within a few months of achieving CR. "Late" intensification is given to patients who have been in continuous CR for one or more years.

2. **Immunotherapy,** which has most often been studied in patients who achieve CR. It theoretically preferentially kills leukemic cells and spares normal cells. Immune stimulation has been attempted with agents such as BCG, *Corynebacterium parvum,* levamisole, or specific leukemic cells. The overwhelming data suggest that these forms of immunotherapy do not benefit patients with AML or ALL. IL-2 stimulates killer cells and is currently under investigation.

3. **BMT.** Results of allogeneic BMT are disappointing for patients with resistant acute leukemia but are most promising in patients undergoing BMT during CR (during the first CR for patients with AML and adults with ALL and during the second or subsequent CR for children with ALL). The major limitations of BMT are

   a. Only about 25 percent of patients have *compatible donors.*

   b. The best survivals are in patients *less than 22 years of age;* the vast majority of patients with AML are older.

   c. The *complications* of BMT in surviving patients remain substantial.

   d. The results of investigations of BMT are still *preliminary.*

   4. Cytotoxic drugs that show promise in the treatment of resistant acute leukemia include 5-azacytidine, podophyllin derivatives, AMSA, high-dose cytarabine, and mitoxanthrone.
G. **Supportive care**
   1. **Indwelling silastic right atrial catheters** are used during the induction phase to facilitate the administration of IV therapies and the sampling of blood for laboratory tests (see Chap. 5, sec. **XI**).
   2. **Blood component therapy**
      a. **Packed red cell transfusions** are used to treat symptomatic anemia and active hemorrhage (see Chap. 34, *Cytopenia,* sec. **VI**).
      b. **Platelet transfusions** are clearly indicated for patients with thrombocytopenia of any severity when there is active hemorrhage. If the patient is not actively bleeding but petechiae are present, then platelet transfusions should be given with platelet counts of 20,000/μL or less. Without petechiae or bleeding, platelets are transfused "prophylactically" when counts are 50,000/μL or less.
      c. **Granulocyte transfusions** are not recommended. The chance of survival depends on recovery of the patient's own granulocytes.
      d. **G-CSF or GM-CSF** is not routinely used to accelerate granulocyte recovery because of the possibility of stimulating the AML clone. This complication rarely occurs in practice.
   3. **Fever in patients with acute leukemia.** Early empiric treatment of fever with antibiotics in neutropenic patients with acute leukemia (see Chap. 35, sec. **I**).
   4. **Prophylaxis against infection** (see Chap. 35, sec. **I.E.3**).
   5. **Tumor lysis syndrome.** See Chap. 27, sec. **XIII**.
VI. **Special clinical problems**
A. **Leukostasis** is more common in AML than ALL and frequently occurs in patients with WBC greater than 100,000/μL. Sludging impairs circulation and results in organ dysfunction. The circulating blast count can be rapidly reduced with leukopheresis, thereby reducing the risks of leukostasis, DIC, and metabolic abnormalities associated with tumor lysis. Hydroxyurea (3 g daily) should be instituted with leukapheresis.
B. **Ocular and gingival involvement.** Blindness may be prevented by irradiating eyes involved with leukemic infiltrates. Gingival enlargements in patients with monocytic leukemia does not require special treatment because it should resolve with induction chemotherapy.
C. Patients exposed to **varicella zoster infections** should be given zoster immune globulin (see Chap. 35, sec. **IV.C**).
D. **Acute leukemia during pregnancy** (see Chap. 26.)

Selected Reading

Myelodysplastic Syndromes

Bennett, J. M., et al. Proposals for the classification of the myelodysplastic syndrome. *Br. J. Haematol.* 51:189, 1982.

Hirst, W. J. R., and Mufti, G. J. Management of myelodysplastic syndromes. *Br. J. Haematol.* 84:191, 1993.

Mathew, P., et al. The 5q- syndrome: A single institution study of 43 consecutive patients. *Blood* 81:1040, 1993.

Acute Myeloblastic Leukemia

Avvisati, G., Wouter Ten Cate, J., and Mandelli, F. Acute promyelocytic leukemia. *Br. J. Haematol.* 81:315, 1992.

Bennett, J. M., et al. Proposal revised criteria for the classification of acute myeloid leukemia. A report of the French-American-British Cooperative Group. *Ann. Intern. Med.* 103:626, 1985.

Berman, E., et al. Results of a randomized trial comparing idarubicin and cystosine arabinoside with daunorubicin and cytosine arabinoside in adult patients with newly diagnosed acute myelogenous leukemia. *Blood* 77:1666, 1991.

Johnson, P. R. E., and Liu Yin, J. A. Acute myeloid leukemia in the elderly: Biology and treatment. *Brit. J. Haematol.* 83:1, 1993.

Warrell, R. P., Jr., et al. Differentiation therapy of acute promyelocytic leukemia with tretinoin (all-trans retinoic acid). *N. Engl. J. Med.* 324:1385, 1991.

Wiernik, P. H. Diagnosis and treatment of acute nonlymphocytic leukemia. In Wiernik, P. H. ed. *Neoplastic Diseases of the Blood.* 2nd. ed. New York: Churchill Livingstone, 1991. Pp 285–302.

Wiernik, P. H., et al. Cytarabine plus idarubicin or daunorubicin as induction and consolidation therapy for previously untreated adult patient with acute myeloid leukemia. *Blood* 79:313, 1992.

Acute Lymphoblastic Leukemia

Champlin, R., and Gale, R. P. Acute lymphoblastic leukemia: Recent advances in biology and therapy. *Blood* 73:2051, 1989.

Foon, K. A., and Todd, R. F. Immunologic classification of leukemia and lymphoma. *Blood* 68:1, 1986.

Hoelzer, D. F. Diagnosis and treatment of adult acute lymphoblastic leukemia. In Wiernik, P. H. ed. *Neoplastic Diseases of the Blood.* 2nd. ed. New York: Churchill Livingstone, 1991. Pp 253–274.

Linker, C. A., et al. Treatment of adult acute lymphoblastic leukemia with intensive cyclical chemotherapy: A follow-up report. *Blood* 78:2814, 1991.

IV

Specific Complications of Cancer

26

Mimi Mott-Smith and
Lawrence Stolberg

I. Sexual function in patients with cancer

A. Background. The ability to enjoy intimate relationships and to express oneself as a sexual being is a prominent determinant of quality of life for many survivors of cancer. Pretreatment sexual function strongly influences post-treatment status. The desire phase of the sexual response cycle is highly sensitive to a variety of adverse conditions. Orgasmic response is much more resistant to damage than are desire and arousal. Factors affecting sexual function in cancer patients are:

1. **Depression,** which is the most common reason for loss of interest in sex.
2. **Guilt.** Some patients experience cancer as punishment for past behavior and resolve to give up sex and other pleasures in exchange for survival.
3. **Anxiety and fear.** Fears of contagiousness, pain, disability, death, or financial disaster may overwhelm the patient.
4. **Self-image changes.** Hair loss, loss of body parts or function, appliances, colostomy, or tracheostomy may result in loss of self-esteem or loss of one's sense of femininity or masculinity. Losses of earning power and roles in the family and community also threaten self-esteem.
5. **Personal philosophy and style of coping with disaster.** Responses vary from determination and positive attitude to resignation and despair.
6. **Concomitants of chronic disease.** Pain, other systemic symptoms, and side effects of drug and cancer therapy.

B. Sexual problems specific to women

1. **Germ cell depletion** is discussed in sec. III. Indirect indicators of menopause are amenorrhea, increased serum follicle-stimulating hormone (FSH) and luteinizing hormone (LH) levels, and symptoms of estrogen deficiency. Symptoms include hot flashes, loss of vaginal lubrication, atrophy of genital structures, and discomfort with intercourse.
2. **Tamoxifen therapy,** commonly used in women with breast cancer, may have a positive estrogenic effect on the vaginal mucosa or may contribute to vaginal atrophy and dyspareunia. Patients who are taking tamoxifen often experience hot flashes or vaginal discharge. Tamoxifen does appear to have a somewhat proestrogenic effect on serum lipids and bone density.
3. **Chemotherapy** may cause ovarian failure (see III.B). Emotional and physical changes also can adversely affect sexual function. The effect of chemotherapy on ovarian androgen output is unknown. Diminished androgen production affects libido.
4. **RT.** Effects of ionizing radiation on sexual function depend on age, field, and dose (see sec. III.B). RT for cervical cancer leads to vaginal fibrosis, dyspareunia, and ovarian failure. Symptoms may not become apparent until one year after treatment.
5. **Pelvic surgery**
   a. **Cervical conization** does not impair desire, arousal, or orgasm.
   b. **Radical hysterectomy** results in a shallower vagina. Women may need to experiment with different positions to experience comfortable penetration.
   c. **Radical cystectomy** leads to decreased vaginal lubrication and dyspareunia.

   d. Abdominal-perineal (A-P) resection commonly causes dyspareunia, but orgasmic function is preserved.
   e. Total pelvic exenteration with vaginal reconstruction results in loss of vaginal lubrication, loss of some erotic zones, dyspareunia, decreased intensity of orgasm, and the need to relearn how to achieve orgasm.
 6. Mastectomy. Women often feel less feminine and less physically attractive after mastectomy. Twenty-five percent experience significant anxiety or depression, and 33 percent are unable to enjoy or tolerate making love. About 30 percent of patients' partners reported decreased sexual activity after mastectomy and fears of causing pain during intercourse. Men's reactions to seeing their partner's incision and chest wall area appear to have prognostic value: if the reaction is primarily empathic rather than negative, the prognosis for good sexual adjustment appears favorable. Women treated with lumpectomy and breast irradiation have improved self-image compared with mastectomy. Women who undergo breast reconstruction have a better body image than those who do not.
C. Sexual problems specific to men. Men treated for testicular cancer, prostate cancer, and Hodgkin's disease are particularly at risk for sexual dysfunction (see **II.A**). Twenty percent of surviving testicular cancer patients have reported that they have been sexually inactive; many have reported decreased sense of pleasure with orgasm, anxiety, and marital unhappiness.
 1. Germ cell depletion. Clinical indicators of germ cell depletion include decreased testicular size, severe oligospermia or azoospermia, infertility with elevated serum LH and FSH levels, and decreased testosterone level.
 2. Impotence. The reported incidence of impotence in the general population is approximately 10 percent: 8 percent at age 50, 20 percent at age 60, and 80 percent at 80. The incidence of impotence in men treated for cancer is increased, particularly for men with tumors involving the pelvis and genital tract. Often, men emotionally relate impotence to a loss of masculinity with attendant fear, anxiety, depression, and feelings of diminished self-worth.
   Temporary or permanent erectile impotence is the most common symptom of sexual dysfunction in men with cancer. Recovery of erectile function is more likely in men less than 60 years of age and may take months to years. Preexisting conditions such as diabetes, cardiovascular disease, and antihypertensive medication exacerbate the risk of erectile dysfunction. Ejaculatory dysfunction occurs less frequently and may be due to retrograde ejaculation or dry orgasm. The presence of nocturnal tumescence is helpful in differentiating nonorganic from organic causes of impotence.
 3. Systemic therapy. Fatigue, nausea, alopecia, anxiety, and other general effects of chemotherapy interact to diminish libido during treatment.
   a. Chemotherapy is thought to suppress Leydig cell function resulting in decreased serum testosterone, increased serum LH levels, and resultant loss of desire and erectile function. Chemotherapeutic agents associated with neuropathy (e.g., vinca alkaloids) can cause dry orgasm with preservation of pleasurable sensation. The effect of chemotherapy on spermatogenesis is discussed in sec. **II.D.**
   b. Hormonal therapy for prostate cancer can impair all phases of the sexual response cycle. Gonadotropin-releasing hormone agonists (leuprolide acetate, flutamide, DES) all reduce serum testosterone to prepubertal levels, and lead to loss of libido, difficulty with arousal, and diminished intensity of orgasm. Hot flashes may occur. In addition, DES and flutamide can cause gynecomastia.
 4. RT
   a. Prostate cancer. RT can result in loss of erectile function in 20 to 80 percent of patients treated for prostate cancer. Younger men with intact sexual function prior to RT are most likely to regain adequate erectile function. Semen volume is also reduced with RT, leading to little or no ejaculatory fluid.
   b. Testicular cancer. Patients who receive radiation to the pelvis and ret-

roperitoneum have an increased incidence of erectile dysfunction. The effects of RT on sperm count is discussed in sec. **II.C.**

   c. Testicular shielding should be used if the distance between the testes and the radiation field boundary is less than 30 cm. Radiation dose to the testes is reduced to less than 10 percent of the total dose if this method is used.

5. Surgery. After the recovery period from pelvic surgery itself, the desire phase generally remains intact. Orgasmic function may be normal or reduced.

   a. Radical prostatectomy causes impotence or impaired erection in the vast majority of patients, although partial recovery of erectile function is possible. Parasympathetic stimulation causes tumescence; sympathetic stimulation causes detumescence. One or both of these autonomic bundles are at risk during radical prostatectomy.

   b. Nerve sparing techniques during radical prostatectomy allow a greater percentage of men to recover erectile function (reportedly up to 85%). However, closer analysis has disclosed that many men do not have erections firm enough for vaginal penetration.

   c. Radical cystectomy results in erectile dysfunction and dry orgasm. With nerve-sparing procedures up to 67 percent may recover erectile function.

   d. A-P resection leads to problems with erection (55%) and dry orgasm due to nerve damage.

   e. Total pelvic exenteration results in permanent impotence and dry orgasm.

   f. Retroperitoneal lymph node dissection (RPLND) leads to retrograde ejaculation. With *modified* RPLND in clinical stage I nonseminomatous germ cell tumor patients, ejaculatory function can be preserved in approximately 90 percent of cases.

D. Guidelines for treatment of sexual problems

1. Initial history should include information about the patient's sexual function prior to diagnosis. Patients at particular risk of dysfunction include couples in relationships characterized by conflict and poor emotional adjustment, younger individuals, those who want more children, and those with a history of rape or incest.

2. Brief counseling can alleviate most problems. Physicians should include the sex partner in discussions and recognize and deal with feelings and fears. In addition, clinicians should specifically tell patients that it is all right to resume sexual activity and that cancer is not contagious.

3. Refer for expert assistance if needed: occasionally, patients need the services of a sex therapist, marital counseling, or referral to a urologist. An invaluable resource is the pamphlet *Sexuality and Cancer* (separate pamphlets for women and men) available from the ACS.

4. Control pain and treat depression.

5. For men with erectile dysfunction

   a. Intracavernous injections of papaverine and phentolamine, or prostaglandin E (fibrosis may result from long term use).

   b. Vacuum erection device or penile prosthesis.

6. For men with testicular cancer

   a. Depotesterone, 200 to 300 mg IM every three weeks for hypotestosteronism (check serum testosterone levels).

   b. Imipramine, 25 to 50 mg daily PO, may induce antegrade ejaculation in those who have undergone RPLND.

7. For women with dyspareunia and vaginal fibrosis

   a. Vaginal dilators of graduated sizes can help women learn to relax voluntary muscles progressively until penetration can be achieved without pain.

   b. Water-based lubricants and vaginal moisturizers can be used.

8. **For women with dyspareunia and vaginal dryness,** administer estrogen replacement therapy or creams.
9. **For women with breast cancer**
   a. The dictum that estrogen replacement therapy is contraindicated is being seriously challenged. A decision for such replacement therapy must be individualized.
   b. Early discussion of the option of breast reconstruction may alleviate feelings of loss and poor self-image. A prosthesis should be fitted as soon as feasible for a normal silhouette in clothing. The "Reach to Recovery" program of the ACS exposes the patient to women with breast cancer who have made successful adjustments.

II. Reproductive function in men with cancer
A. Pretreatment hypogonadism in cancer patients
1. **Testicular cancer.** More than 80 percent of men with disseminated germ cell tumors are oligospermic or azoospermic prior to therapy, probably due to effects of the disease itself and abnormalities of the malignancy-prone testis.
2. **Hodgkin's disease.** More than 50 percent of men with Hodgkin's disease have low sperm counts and poor motility before treatment.
3. **Metastatic cancer** of any type may be associated with low levels of testosterone in up to two-thirds of male patients. Malnutrition is believed to play a significant role.

B. Effects of RT in men.
The testes are exquisitely sensitive to radiation (see sec. I.C.4). Doses as low as 15 cGy result in transient suppression of spermatogenesis. The duration of azoospermia is proportional to the magnitude of the RT dose. At 200–300 cGy, recovery takes three years, and at 400–600 cGy, azoospermia can persist for five years. A dose of 600 cGy or more results in permanent sterility.

C. Effects of chemotherapy in men.
Spermatogenesis is highly susceptible to toxic effects of certain chemotherapeutic agents.
1. **Alkylating agents** cause germ cell depletion in a dose-related fashion. Drugs reported to be definitely associated with azoospermia include chlorambucil (possibly reversible if total dose is <400 mg), cyclophosphamide (possibly reversible if total dose is <6 to 10 gm), nitrogen mustard, busulfan, procarbazine, and nitrosoureas.
2. **Other drugs** probably associated with germ cell depletion include doxorubicin, vinblastine, cytosine arabinoside, and cisplatin. Effects of methotrexate, 5-fluorouracil, 6-mercaptopurine, vincristine, and bleomycin are either unknown or unlikely to cause damage.
3. **Combination regimens.** MOPP therapy for Hodgkin's disease leads to testicular atrophy in 80 percent of patients. ABVD is an alternative to MOPP with a reported 35 percent occurrence of azoospermia during therapy but eventual return of spermatogenesis in nearly 100 percent of cases (NOVP shows similar results). Approximately 50 percent of patients treated with cisplatin, vinblastine, and bleomycin for nonseminomatous testicular cancer regain spermatogenesis within two to three years.

D. Measures to protect reproductive function in men
1. **Sperm banking** can be offered to men who are likely to suffer prolonged or permanent sterility. Unfortunately, 50 to 80 percent of patients with Hodgkin's disease or testicular cancer have low sperm counts (<20 million/ml) with poor motility (<50%) before treatment. Candidates for sperm banking should have adequate numbers of normal, motile sperm. Collection of two or three ejaculates over several hours may be required to achieve these criteria. Even several specimens, however, may be inadequate because of poor postthaw quality of the sperm.
2. **Artificial insemination** may be tried in women whose partner's posttreatment sperm quality is good despite low sperm count.
3. **In vitro fertilization (IVF)** techniques in men with very low sperm counts

can result in successful creation of an embryo with relatively few sperm. In addition, IVF can be carried out prior to cancer therapy with cryopreservation of embryos.

4. Nerve-sparing procedures for prostatectomy, modified RPLND to reduce retrograde ejaculation, and testicular shielding for RT are discussed in sec. I.C.4. and I.C.5.

III. Reproductive function in women with cancer

A. Effects of RT in women. The effects of radiation on fertility are strongly influenced by age as well as by RT field and total dose. Cessation of menses for variable periods of time occurs at doses above 150 cGy. A dose of 500 to 600 cGy to the ovaries usually results in permanent ovarian failure. After total nodal irradiation 70 percent of women under 20 years of age resume normal menses, whereas 80 percent of women over 30 do not.

Oophoropexy, or sequestering the ovaries surgically in midline behind the uterus, reduces the risk of infertility in 50 percent of women undergoing inverted-Y field irradiation. Sparing one ovary in women under 40 years of age prevents premature menopause.

B. Effects of chemotherapy in women. The likelihood of permanent ovarian failure after chemotherapy increases with age. Menses rarely return after age 35 to 40 years.

1. **Alkylating agents.** Cyclophosphamide, nitrogen mustard, alkeran, busulfan, and procarbazine are clearly associated with ovarian failure.

2. **Other drugs.** Methotrexate, 5-fluorouracil, and 6-mercaptopurine are unlikely to cause ovarian dysfunction. Agents with unknown effects on the ovary include: doxorubicin, bleomycin, vinca alkaloids, cisplatin, nitrosoureas, cytosine arabinoside.

3. **Combination regimens.** MOPP leads to ovarian dysfunction in 40 to 50 percent of women treated for Hodgkin's disease. Nearly all patients under 25 years of age experience a return of normal menses. ABVD is associated with a much lower incidence of infertility than MOPP.

IV. Pregnancy and cancer

A. Background

1. **Epidemiology.** Cervical cancer is the most common malignancy complicating pregnancy, occurring in 1 in 1000 pregnancies, followed by breast cancer (1/3000), melanoma and ovarian cancer (1/10,000), and colon cancer, leukemia, and lymphoma (1/50,000–100,000).

2. **Natural history.** The incidence of malignancy is not increased in pregnancy. Pregnancy neither alters the biologic behavior or prognosis of cancer nor reactivates cancer in remission. Metastasis to the placenta or fetus is very rare.

3. **Teratogenesis.** The definition of teratogenesis has been broadened to encompass not merely morphologic abnormalities readily apparent at birth, but also other types of malformation, growth retardation, fetal death, and developmental disability. The incidence of major malformations apparent at birth in the general population is about 3 to 4 percent. Damage from chemotherapeutic agents in the first trimester is more likely to cause morphologic abnormalities and spontaneous abortion. Exposure during the second and third trimesters is more likely to cause intrauterine growth retardation, microcephaly, and developmental delay with attendant risks of mental retardation and learning problems.

B. Diagnostic studies during pregnancy

1. **Biopsies** under local anesthesia carry essentially no risk to the fetus. Biopsy procedures using general anesthesia present minimal risk to the fetus.

2. **Studies to avoid:** Radionuclide scans, contrast studies of the GI and urinary tracts, abdominal and chest CT scans, pelvic and lumbosacral spine films, and full lymphangiograms. In general, studies should only be done if results would have a significant impact on treatment decisions.

3. **Mammograms** lack sensitivity in pregnancy due to breast engorgement and

histologic changes. Up to 50 percent of pregnant women with a breast mass have a negative mammogram.

4. **Chest x-rays** can be done safely with proper abdominal shielding. The dose of ionizing radiation to the fetus is approximately 0.008 cGy.

5. **Bone scans** are relatively contraindicated in pregnancy. The fetus receives a dose of approximately 0.1 cGy. Due to low yield, bone scans are not justified in asymptomatic stage I and II breast cancer patients and can be deferred until postpartum.

6. **Sonography** does not involve ionizing radiation and is safe.

7. **Other permissible radiologic studies.** Brain CT scans and x-rays of the cervical spine or long bones are probably associated with radiation doses to the fetus of less than 0.5 cGy if the abdomen and uterus are properly shielded.

8. **MRI** has unknown effects on the fetus. Because of theoretical risks of increased temperature during organogenesis, MRI is not recommended during the first trimester and is used with caution in the second and third trimesters.

C. **Principles of cancer therapy during pregnancy**

1. Pregnancy prevention should be emphasized in all women of childbearing age with cancer and in the context of the patient's personal goals. All options, including pregnancy termination, should be discussed.

2. Accurate determination of gestational age should be made before commencing diagnostic studies or therapy.

3. When maternal cure is possible and delay would compromise this goal, institute therapy as soon as possible. If feasible, delay chemotherapy until the second or third trimester or after delivery.

4. Therapeutic abortion (TAB) may be performed up to the 24th week of gestation. TAB should be offered to the patient if her fetus has received a dose of ionizing radiation in excess of 10 cGy during the first trimester.

5. Breast-feeding is usually contraindicated, because chemotherapeutic agents are excreted into human milk and have caused neutropenia in infants.

D. **Surgery during pregnancy.** Surgical treatment is far less likely to adversely affect pregnancy than is chemotherapy or RT. General anesthesia is an uncommon cause of teratogenesis. The fetus is exquisitely sensitive to hypoxia: the anesthesiologist and surgeon must take special precautions to ensure adequate oxygenation.

E. **RT during pregnancy**

1. A dose of 10 cGy to the fetus during the first trimester carries a substantial risk of fetal damage. No increase in the incidence of spontaneous abortion, growth retardation, or congenital malformations has been noted when the dose of radiation is less than 5 cGy at any time during pregnancy.

2. Defects most commonly seen with radiation damage include microcephaly, growth retardation, and ocular abnormalities. Late effects of radiation in early pregnancy include an increased incidence of thyroid cancer and leukemia.

F. **Chemotherapy during pregnancy**

1. **Pharmacokinetics.** Absorption, distribution, and metabolism of chemotherapeutic agents are undoubtedly altered by the multiplicity of physiologic changes accompanying pregnancy. Because the effects of pregnancy on pharmacokinetics are unknown, standard drug dosages are used. It can be assumed that most antineoplastic drugs cross the placenta.

2. **First trimester exposure.** When folic acid antagonists and concomitant radiation therapy are excluded, single agents lead to congenital defects in 6 percent of infants exposed in the first trimester.

   a. **Antimetabolites.** Folic acid antagonists are the agents most frequently associated with teratogenesis and should not be used in the first trimester. Aminopterin and methotrexate are abortifacient and teratogenic. The aminopterin syndrome consists of facial anomalies, bone and limb deformities, and variable intellectual impairment. Although other anti-metabolites, including cytarabine and 5-fluorouracil, have been associated with fetal malformation, 6-mercaptopurine has not.

b. Alkylating agents are less frequently associated with fetal malformation than antimetabolites. A 14 percent overall occurrence rate has been reported in one series; cyclophosphamide was associated with congenital defects in three of seven exposed infants.

c. Vinca alkaloids. Vinblastine resulted in malformation in one in 14 exposed infants. No data are available for vincristine.

d. Others. Procarbazine is associated with fetal malformation. DES has been linked to clear cell vaginal cancer in offspring.

e. Combination chemotherapy regimens are associated with a 25 percent rate of fetal malformation. MOPP was linked to congenital defects in four of seven exposed infants.

3. Second and third trimester exposure. Forty percent of fetuses exposed to a variety of antineoplastic agents in the second and third trimesters have exhibited low birth weight, with its attendant risk for developmental delay. Other potential adverse effects include prematurity, spontaneous abortion, and major organ toxicity.

G. Recommendations concerning TAB

1. TAB not recommended

a. Treatment does not jeopardize the pregnancy (e.g., surgery for breast cancer).

b. Refractory malignancies for which treatment has no significant impact.

2. TAB considered, but not strongly recommended

a. Treatment may be delayed with reasonable safety until fetal maturity allows delivery.

b. Treatment may be delayed into the second or third trimester, when the fetus is relatively resistant to the effects of chemotherapy (e.g., acute leukemia) or RT.

3. TAB strongly recommended

a. Cancers in which curative therapy cannot be delayed or accomplished during pregnancy (e.g., most gynecologic malignancies).

b. Treatment that is likely to cause abortion or fetal malformation is required in the first trimester (e.g., MOPP, methotrexate).

V. Management of specific cancers and pregnancy

A. Cervical cancer

1. Screening. Papanicolaou's (Pap) smears should be done on all prenatal patients.

2. Evaluation of cervical dysplasia. Colposcopy can be done. Endocervical curettage biopsy is contraindicated. In the absence of invasive disease, there is no urgency to treat cervical dysplasia during pregnancy. Cervical conization should be avoided, but it may need to be done to rule out invasive disease. In pregnancy, conization is associated with cervical hemorrhage and a high incidence of incomplete resection.

3. Staging and treatment. The extent of invasive disease is often underestimated because of limitations on physical examination and diagnostic procedures. Treatment of invasive cervical cancer, using either surgery or radiation, is incompatible with fetal survival.

B. Breast cancer

1. Screening. A delay in diagnosis of five months or more has been observed in gravid patients with breast cancer, resulting in node-positive disease in 74 percent of patients as compared to 37 percent in nonpregnant patients. Physiologic changes in the breasts during pregnancy hamper adequate physical examination. Serial breast exams should be done throughout pregnancy, and masses should be investigated promptly. Clinicians have tended to observe breast masses two months longer in pregnant than in nonpregnant patients.

2. Diagnosis. Mammograms are not helpful during pregnancy. Fine-needle aspiration may be inaccurate, and excisional biopsy is the procedure of choice. Estrogen and progesterone receptor studies may be falsely negative or difficult to interpret.

3. **Treatment.** Modified radical mastectomy is the procedure of choice. Lumpectomy with radiation results in unacceptable radiation exposure to the fetus. Tamoxifen is contraindicated during gestation. Adjuvant chemotherapy should be delayed until at least the second or third trimester, or, if possible, until after delivery.

C. **Hodgkin's disease**
   1. Limit staging procedures that may expose the fetus to radiation. When lymphangiography would affect treatment, it may be performed after the first trimester; the important modification is that only one abdominal film is taken 24 hours after injection of dye (fetal dose is less than 1 cGy).
   2. If the disease is diagnosed during the first trimester, either perform a TAB and proceed as usual or delay chemotherapy or RT until later in the pregnancy.
   3. If the disease is diagnosed during the second or third trimester:
      a. Try to delay therapy until delivery if the mother's outcome will not be adversely affected.
      b. If therapy is necessary, proceed with proper counseling regarding possible growth and developmental abnormalities.
      c. Very limited field RT has been largely successful. Internal scatter from standard mantle field RT can result in fetal exposure of 50 to 250 cGy.

D. **Non-Hodgkin's lymphoma** is generally a more virulent disease and poses a greater risk to the mother and secondarily to the fetus than Hodgkin's disease. Therapeutic recommendations parallel Hodgkin's disease, except for the possibility of protracted delay of treatment with indolent lymphomas.

E. **Genetic counseling.** Retrospective studies and case reports of patients who were treated for malignancy in childhood or adolescence and bore children later show a 4 percent rate of major malformations in offspring. This rate is similar to the risk borne by the general population. The late effects of cancer treatment on infants exposed *in utero* are unknown. Female survivors of cancer who later became pregnant, particularly those who have had abdominal radiation, have an increased rate of preterm delivery and low-birth-weight infants.

Selected Reading

Costabile, R. A. The effects of cancer and cancer therapy on male reproductive function. *J. Urol.* 149:1327, 1993.

Gallenberg, M. M., and Loprinzi, C. L. Breast cancer and pregnancy. *Semin. Oncol.* 16:369, 1989.

Jacob, J. G., and Stringer, C. A. Diagnosis and management of cancer during pregnancy. *Semin. Perinatol.* 14:79, 1990.

Myers, S. E., and Schilsky, R. L. Prospects for fertility after cancer chemotherapy. *Semin. Oncol.* 19:597, 1992.

Nicholson, M. S., and Byrne, J. Fertility and pregnancy after treatment for cancer during childhood or adolescence. *Cancer* (supplement) 71:3392, 1993.

Schover, L. R. The impact of breast cancer on sexuality, body image, and intimate relationships. *CA* 41:112, 1991.

Walsh, P. C., and Schlegel, P. N. Radical pelvic surgery with preservation of sexual function. *Ann. Surg.* 208:391, 1988.

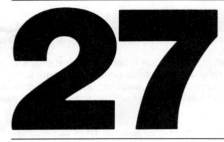

Metabolic Complications

Harold E. Carlson and
Dennis A. Casciato

I. Hypercalcemia

A. Mechanisms. Cancer is the most common cause of hypercalcemia in hospitalized patients. Hypercalcemia usually results from excessive bone resorption relative to bone formation.

1. **Bone metastases.** Most tumors capable of bone metastasis (see Chap. 33, sec. I) can also produce hypercalcemia. Some tumors, such as breast cancer (de novo or with "flare" following hormonal therapy), produce hypercalcemia only in the presence of bone involvement. Local production of various substances by tumor cells may stimulate osteoclastic bone resorption.

2. **Ectopic parathyroid hormone** (PTH) appears to be very rare.

3. **Humoral hypercalcemia of malignancy** is caused by production of a PTH-like substance called PTH-related peptide (PTH-RP) by a variety of carcinomas (squamous tumors of many organs, hypernephroma, parotid gland tumors). PTH-RP has bone-resorbing activity and interacts with the renal PTH receptor to stimulate renal calcium resorption. PTH-RP is not measured in serum PTH assays.

4. **Vitamin D metabolites** (e.g., 1,25-dihydroxyvitamin D) may be produced by some lymphomas; these metabolites promote intestinal calcium absorption.

5. **Prostaglandins and IL-1** produced by various tumors may occasionally cause hypercalcemia, perhaps by enhancing bone resorption.

6. **Tumors rarely or never associated with hypercalcemia** despite high frequencies of bone metastases
   a. Small cell lung cancer
   b. Prostate cancer
   c. Colorectal cancer

B. Diagnosis

1. **Symptoms of hypercalcemia** depend on both the serum level of ionized calcium and how fast the level rises. Rapidly rising serum calcium levels tend to produce obtundation and coma with only moderate elevated serum calcium levels (e.g., 13 mg/dl). Slowly rising serum calcium levels may produce only mild symptoms even with serum levels exceeding 15 mg/dl.

   a. **Early symptoms**
      (1) Polyuria, nocturia, polydipsia
      (2) Anorexia
      (3) Easy fatigability
      (4) Weakness

   b. **Late symptoms**
      (1) Apathy, irritability, depression, decreased ability to concentrate, mental obtundation, coma
      (2) Profound muscle weakness
      (3) Nausea, vomiting, vague abdominal pain, constipation, obstipation, increased gastric acid secretion, acute pancreatitis
      (4) Pruritus
      (5) Abnormalities of vision

2. **Differential diagnosis of hypercalcemia.** Idiopathic hypercalcemia is not a tenable diagnosis in adult patients. More and more often, benign causes of hyper-

calcemia are recognized to occur in patients with cancer. The possible etiologies of hypercalcemia include:

- **a.** Malignancy
  - **(1)** Metastases to bone
  - **(2)** Secretion of PTH-like or other humoral factors
  - **(3)** Production of vitamin D metabolites
- **b.** Primary hyperparathyroidism
- **c.** Thiazide diuretic therapy
- **d.** Vitamin D or vitamin A intoxication
- **e.** Milk-alkali syndrome
- **f.** Familial benign hypocalciuric hypercalcemia
- **g.** Others
  - **(1)** Immobilization of patients with accelerated bone turnover (e.g., Paget's disease or myeloma)
  - **(2)** Sarcoidosis, tuberculosis, and other granulomatous diseases
  - **(3)** Hyperthyroidism
  - **(4)** Lithium administration
  - **(5)** Adrenal insufficiency
  - **(6)** Diuretic phase of acute renal failure
  - **(7)** Severe liver disease
  - **(8)** Theophylline intoxication

3. Laboratory studies. All patients with cancer and polyuria, mental status changes, or GI symptoms should be evaluated for hypercalcemia.

- **a. Routine studies**
  - **(1) Serum calcium, phosphate, and albumin levels**
    - **(a)** Ionized calcium constitutes about 47 percent of the serum calcium and is in equilibrium with calcium bound to proteins, especially to albumin. Roughly 0.8 mg of calcium is bound by 1 gm of serum albumin. An alkaline pH (e.g., resulting from repeated vomiting because of hypercalcemia) tends to decrease the fraction of ionized calcium. When serum albumin is low, the measured serum calcium can be corrected (to a "normal" albumin concentration of 4.0 g/dl) using the following formula:

      Corrected serum calcium (mg/dl)
      = measured calcium + 0.8(4.0 − measured albumin)

    - **(b)** Long-standing hypercalcemia with hypophosphatemia suggests primary hyperparathyroidism.
  - **(2) Serum alkaline phosphatase.** Elevated levels may be due to either hyperparathyroidism or metastatic disease to the bone or liver. Normal levels are typical in cases of hypercalcemia produced by myeloma.
  - **(3) Serum electrolytes.** Serum chloride concentrations are frequently elevated in primary hyperparathyroidism. Renal tubular acidosis may complicate chronic hypercalcemia.
  - **(4) BUN and serum creatinine.** The direct effect of hypercalcemia on the kidneys can result in azotemia and defective renal tubular water conservation (i.e., symptoms of polyuria).
  - **(5) ECG.** Hypercalcemia results in relative shortening of the Q–T interval and prolongation of the P–R interval. The T wave widens at blood levels above 16 mg/dl, paradoxically lengthening the Q–T interval.
  - **(6) Roentgenograms** of the abdomen and bones
    - **(a) Nephrolithiasis** is rare in hypercalcemia caused by malignancy and suggests hyperparathyroidism.
    - **(b) Nephrocalcinosis** and other ectopic calcifications are common in long-standing hypercalcemia.
    - **(c) Subperiosteal reabsorption** is pathognomonic of hyperparathyroidism, but osteopenia is the most common radiologic finding.

      b. Further studies. Results from preliminary evaluation may indicate the need for measuring serum PTH levels, or performing other tests.

        (1) Evidence for concomitant primary hyperparathyroidism

          (a) Documented long history of hypercalcemia or renal stones

          (b) X-ray evidence of hyperparathyroid bone disease (subperiosteal reabsorption, osteitis fibrosa cystica, or salt-and-pepper skull)

          (c) Hyperchloremic acidosis, particularly with a serum chloride to phosphate ratio equal to or greater than 34

          (d) Elevated serum PTH level in the presence of hypercalcemia

        (2) Evidence for humoral hypercalcemia of malignancy

          (a) Low or low-normal serum PTH levels in the presence of hypercalcemia

          (b) Elevated level of PTH-RP

          (c) Metabolic alkalosis

          (d) Low serum level of 1,25-dihydroxyvitamin D

4. When should neck exploration be considered? Both primary hyperparathyroidism and humoral hypercalcemia of malignancy are characterized by hypercalcemia and, with many cancers, elevated urinary excretion of cAMP. Neck exploration is justified *if all of the following apply:*

    a. Clinical and laboratory findings (above) suggest hyperparathyroidism.

    b. The malignancy is under control and the patient's expected survival is reasonably long.

    c. The general condition of the patient makes the risk of surgery acceptable.

    d. The hypercalcemia is severe enough to warrant treatment. Mild hypercalcemia (e.g., ≤11.5 mg/dl) caused by primary hyperparathyroidism may remain stable and asymptomatic for many years and may never produce clinically significant complications during the patient's remaining life span.

C. Management

    1. Acute, symptomatic hypercalcemia should be treated as an emergency.

      a. Hydration and saline diuresis. Achieving and maintaining intravascular volume and hydration are the cornerstones of promoting calcium excretion. Normal saline containing KCl (10 mEq/l) is given IV at 2 to 3 l/day. Calciuresis may be enhanced by administering furosemide, 40 to 80 mg IV bid, after fluid and volume deficits have been corrected.

        (1) Fluid intake and output and body weight are carefully monitored. Patients are evaluated for evidence of congestive heart failure two or three times daily. Patients with a history of congestive heart failure or renal insufficiency should be monitored with central venous pressure measurements.

        (2) Blood levels of calcium, potassium, and magnesium are measured every 8 to 12 hours, and concentrations of cations in the IV solutions are adjusted.

        (3) Treatment is continued until the blood calcium concentration is below 12 mg/dl. CNS manifestations in elderly or comatose patients may not improve until normal blood calcium levels are maintained for several days.

        (4) More vigorous administration of fluids (e.g., 12–14 liters over 24 hr) and diuretics (e.g., every 1–2 hr) requires excellent cardiac and renal functions and necessitates close monitoring in an intensive care unit. Treatment at this intensity is rarely necessary for patients with malignancies.

      b. Diphosphonates are potent inhibitors of osteoclast activity and are effective in the treatment of hypercalcemia of malignancy. These drugs are relatively free of significant adverse effects. Pamidronate (Aredia) is the most effective of the available drugs; it is given as a single IV infusion of 60 to 90 mg in 1000 ml of normal saline over 24 hours.

Studies currently in progress suggest shorter infusions of the same doses may be equally safe and effective. Significant reductions in serum calcium occur in one to two days and generally persist for several weeks. About 20 percent of patients develop transient fever after receiving the drug.

Etidronate (Didronel), which is also available, is given IV in 500 ml of normal saline over three hours at a dose of 7.5 mg/kg daily for five days. Three liters of normal saline is also infused daily. Significant reduction of serum calcium levels are usually achieved by the third day of treatment. Oral maintenance therapy with etidronate is investigational, but a dose of 20 mg/kg/day or more may be helpful.

c. Gallium nitrate (Ganite), a potent inhibitor of bone resorption, is given IV in a dose of 200 mg/m^2 daily for five days. Serum calcium falls within a few days and remains normal for about one week. Renal function may worsen during gallium nitrate therapy, and the drug should not be given if the serum creatinine is over 2.5 mg/dl.

d. Mithramycin. Patients who have congestive heart failure, fluid overload, or unresponding calcium levels during saline diuresis can be treated with mithramycin. The drug inhibits bone resorption by reversibly poisoning osteoclasts. Mithramycin, 25 μg/kg, is given by rapid infusion into a well-established IV line; serum calcium levels are lowered in 24 to 48 hours. The dose may be repeated every three to four days. Hypocalcemia is averted by measuring blood calcium levels every day or two or when mental status changes or tetany develops. Other important toxicities of mithramycin are discussed in Chapter 4, sec. **IV.G.** The drug is contraindicated in the presence of severe thrombocytopenia or severe hepatocellular dysfunction. In patients with renal failure, mithramycin may be given in lower doses (10 μg/kg), but calcitonin is preferred.

e. Calcitonin is useful for rapid reduction of blood calcium levels. Calcitonin can be given when mithramycin or saline diuresis is contraindicated or ineffective (e.g., in severe thrombocytopenia, renal failure, congestive heart failure). The drug inhibits bone resorption and increases renal calcium clearance. Blood calcium levels are decreased within two to three hours of administration. The effect is transient, but may be prolonged to four or more days by concurrent administration of prednisone, 10 to 20 mg t.i.d. Allergy is the only important complication of therapy. Synthetic salmon calcitonin is given in a dose of 3 Medical Research Council (MRC) units/kg as a 24-hour infusion, or 100 to 400 units given SQ q8–12h.

f. Dialysis. Peritoneal and hemodialysis rapidly lower blood calcium levels but are rarely used.

g. Dangerous therapies that have little clinical usefulness and are not recommended
   (1) Intravenous phosphates (extraosseous calcification).
   (2) Intravenous sodium sulfate (hypernatremia, heart failure)
   (3) Calcium chelating agents (severe renal damage)

2. Chronic hypercalcemia. Ambulation is encouraged to minimize bone resorption that accompanies immobilization. Liberal fluid intake (two to three liters per day) is prescribed. Foods containing large amounts of calcium, such as milk products, are avoided. Thiazide diuretics aggravate hypercalcemia and should not be taken.

a. Glucocorticoids. Prednisone, 20 to 40 mg PO daily, or hydrocortisone, 100 to 150 mg IV every 12 hours, may be used for patients with tumors that are sensitive to glucocorticoids (e.g., lymphoma, multiple myeloma).

b. Phosphates given orally lower blood levels by binding calcium in the gut. Since this may compromise renal function, effects of therapy should be monitored. Diarrhea nearly always accompanies phosphate therapy and is treated with diphenoxylate (Lomotil), 2 to 5 mg PO, with each

dose of phosphate. Diarrhea may also be reduced by diluting the liquid or powder forms. The daily dose is 1.0 to 6.0 gm of phosphate. *One gram of inorganic phosphate* is supplied by the following preparations:
  (1) Fleet Phospho Soda, liquid, 6.7 ml
  (2) Neutra-Phos, four capsules or 1 teaspoon of powder (Neutra-Phos-K contains no sodium)
  (3) K-Phos Original Formula, six tablets (contains no sodium)

  c. **Prostaglandin inhibitors,** such as aspirin and indomethacin, produce variable and inconsistent lowering of calcium levels but may be tried in patients with refractory hypercalcemia.
  d. **Mithramycin,** 10 μg/kg IV every three to seven days, may be given until drug toxicity develops.

II. Hypocalcemia
A. Mechanisms
  1. **Paraneoplasia.** Hypocalcemia is an extremely rare paraneoplastic syndrome.
    a. **Rapid uptake of calcium.** Patients with bone metastases from prostate or breast cancer and who are treated with hormonal agents may develop hypocalcemia, supposedly because of rapid bone healing. Calcifying chondrosarcoma is a rare tumor, which has been associated with hypocalcemia.
    b. **Oncogenic osteomalacia** appears to be caused by tumor products that interfere with the production of 1,25-dihydroxycholecalciferol and promote phosphaturia. This entity has been associated with mesenchymal neoplasms and prostate cancer.
    c. **Calcitonin** production by medullary carcinoma of the thyroid rarely causes hypocalcemia.
  2. **Magnesium deficiency.** Magnesium is necessary for both the release of PTH and its peripheral action. Hypomagnesemia results in hypocalcemia that does not respond to calcium replacement therapy. Magnesium deficiency occurs in
    a. Patients who have prolonged nasogastric drainage
    b. Patients who receive parenteral hyperalimentation without magnesium replacement
    c. Cisplatin therapy
    d. Chronic diuretic therapy or diuresis due to glycosuria
    e. Chronic alcoholism (alcohol interferes with renal conservation of magnesium)
    f. Chronic diarrhea
  3. **Other causes of hypocalcemia**
    a. Therapy for hypercalcemia, especially if with mithramycin or IV phosphates
    b. Hypoalbuminemia
    c. Hyperphosphatemia (see sec. III)
    d. Pancreatitis
    e. Renal disease
    f. Hypoparathyroidism
    g. Pseudohypoparathyroidism
    h. Rickets and osteomalacia
    i. Sepsis
B. Diagnosis
  1. **Symptoms and signs** are aggravated by hyperventilation or other causes of alkalosis.
    a. Tetany is the most prominent symptom of hypocalcemia and is manifested by paresthesias (especially numbness and tingling of the face, hands, and feet), muscle cramps, laryngospasm, or seizures. Other problems include diarrhea, headache, lethargy, irritability, and loss of recent memory.

b. Dry skin, abnormal nails, cataracts, and papilledema may develop in long-standing cases.

c. **Chvostek's sign:** Twitching of muscles around the mouth, nose, or eyes after tapping the facial nerve.

d. **Trousseau's sign:** Spasm of the hand during three to four minutes of exercise while a blood pressure cuff on the arm is inflated midway between systolic and diastolic pressures.

2. **Routine laboratory studies.** Serum levels of calcium, phosphate, magnesium, electrolytes, urea nitrogen, creatinine, and albumin should be obtained. The ECG may show a prolonged Q–T interval; the ECG is monitored during therapy.

3. **Differential diagnosis of hypocalcemic therapy**

   a. Severe alkalosis resulting from prolonged nasogastriç suction, vomiting, or hyperventilation.

   b. Severe muscle cramps resulting from vincristine or procarbazine therapy

C. **Management**

1. **Severe hypocalcemia** (blood calcium 6 mg/dl or less) must be managed in an intensive care setting.

   a. **Calcium gluconate or calcium chloride.** 1 gm by rapid IV injection, is given every 15 to 20 minutes as long as tetany persists.

   b. **Magnesium sulfate,** 1 gm IV or IM q8–12h is also administered if the blood magnesium level is unknown or less than 1.5 mg/dl until the calcium or magnesium blood levels have normalized.

   c. **Hyperventilating** patients should breathe into a paper bag to decrease respiratory alkalosis.

   d. **Serum calcium levels** are obtained every one to two hours until the serum calcium level exceeds 7 mg/dl.

2. **Moderate hypocalcemia** (blood calcium between 7 and 8 mg/dl).

   a. **Calcium gluconate,** 2 gm IV in 500 ml of 5% dextrose in water, is given q8h. Blood levels should be measured twice daily until they exceed 8.5 mg/dl for 48 hours.

   b. **Hypomagnesemia** (less than 1.5 mg/dl) is treated with magnesium sulfate, 1 gm IM or IV once or twice daily, until the blood level is normal.

   c. **Patients recovering from hypercalcemia** who were treated with mithramycin are in jeopardy of recurrent life-threatening hypocalcemia for as long as four days after treatment is stopped.

   d. Patients with **oncogenic osteomalacia** can be treated with oral calcium lactate, 2 gm q.i.d. PO. Control of the underlying tumor resolves the problem.

   e. Patients with **postthyroidectomy hypoparathyroidism** are discussed in Chapter 15, sec. **III.F.1.**

III. **Hyperphosphatemia**

A. **Mechanisms.** Hyperphosphatemia (>4.5 mg/dl) is a rare complication of treatment of certain tumors, notably leukemia and lymphoma (especially Burkitt's lymphoma). Rapid tumor lysis releases large amounts of uric acid, potassium, and phosphate. Elevated blood phosphate levels may not be observed until two days after beginning tumor therapy; elevations may persist for four to five days and can exceed 20 mg/dl.

B. **Diagnosis.** The serum phosphate level itself does not cause symptoms. Renal damage or acute renal failure results from precipitation of calcium phosphate in the kidneys. Tetany may develop if ionized calcium concentration becomes inordinately reduced (e.g., with alkalosis from bicarbonate administration or vomiting).

1. **Laboratory studies.** Serum phosphate, calcium, and other electrolyte levels should be measured regularly in susceptible patients during the initial course of antitumor therapy.

    2. Differential diagnosis
        a. Hypoparathyroidism
        b. Renal failure
        c. Rapid tissue breakdown following muscle trauma or burn
        d. Tumor lysis syndrome (see sec. **XIII**)
        e. Large oral doses of phosphates
  C. Management. High phosphate levels must be lowered rapidly to avoid or re-verse renal damage. Serum chemistries are monitored every four to six hours. The following methods are used *simultaneously* until the phosphate concentra-tion reaches 5 mg/dl:
    1. An **intravenous infusion** of 20 percent dextrose containing 10 U/L regular insulin is administered at a rate of 50 to 100 ml/hr until the blood phosphate level falls below 7 mg/dl. The extracellular volume is expanded by infusing half-normal saline at 100 to 200 ml/hr. Potassium is added to the solution if the serum level is less than 4 mg/dl.
    2. An **aluminum hydroxide gel preparation** (e.g., Amphojel), 30 to 60 ml PO, q2–6h, is given to bind phosphate in the intestine.
    3. Oral fluids are given at a rate of two to four liters every 24 hours.
    4. Dialysis may be necessary for patients with renal failure.
IV. Hypophosphatemia
  A. Mechanism. Hypophosphatemia (<3.0 mg/dl) is occasionally associated with rapidly growing tumors (such as acute leukemia), presumably because tumor cells consume phosphate. Severe hypophosphatemia (<1.0 mg/dl) may result in rhabdomyolysis or hemolysis. Hypokalemia may be associated with hypophos-phatemia, the reasons for which are unclear. In patients with cancer, hypophos-phatemia more commonly accompanies marked nutritional deprivation or cachexia.
  B. Diagnosis
    1. Laboratory studies. Hypophosphatemia is usually recognized by routine serum electrolyte studies in patients with nutritional disturbances.
    2. Differential diagnosis of hypophosphatemia
        a. Renal phosphate wasting accompanies certain syndromes associated with malignancies, including myeloma (Fanconi's syndrome), multiple endocrine neoplasia (hyperparathyroidism), and oncogenic osteomalacia (hypocalcemia, see sec. **II**)
        b. Therapy with phosphate-binding antacid gels
        c. Starvation or malabsorption (decreased phosphate intake)
        d. Cachexia
        e. Alcoholism
        f. Nutritional recovery (e.g., during hyperalimentation) without adequate phosphate supplementation
        g. Massive, rapid tumor growth
        h. Alkalosis
        i. Diabetic ketoacidosis
  C. Management
    1. Patients with phosphate levels less than 1 mg/dl are given 30 to 40 mmol/l of neutral sodium phosphate or sodium potassium phosphate administered IV at a rate of 50 to 150 ml/hr. Doses and precautions are about the same as for IV potassium preparations.
    2. Patients with blood phosphorus levels of 1 to 2 mg/dl may be given oral inorganic phosphate supplements (see sec. **I.C.2.b.**). One bottle of Neutra-Phos (64 gm of phosphorus) is dissolved in four liters of water, and two to three oz of the solution are given q.i.d. PO.
    3. Patients with *simultaneous hypokalemia* are treated with 20 mEq of KCl in 10% solution t.i.d. or with potassium-containing phosphate preparations. Neutra-Phos-K and Phos-Tabs both contain 50 to 57 mEq of potassium per gram of phosphate.
V. Hypernatremia
  A. Mechanisms. Hypernatremia nearly always is due to a loss of water from the

body fluids. Any hypotonic fluid loss (e.g., sweating, hyperventilation, fever, vomiting, nasogastric suction) causes mild hypernatremia if not treated. *Extreme* elevations of plasma sodium concentrations (>160 mEq/L) are usually encountered in only three clinical situations:

1. **Decreased or absent fluid intake** is the most common cause of hypernatremia, especially in patients who have disabilities that impair normal fluid intake.

2. **Diabetes insipidus** (insufficient production of antidiuretic hormone [ADH]) is usually caused by head trauma (accidental or neurosurgical) or pituitary or hypothalamic neoplasms (primary or metastatic). Breast and lung cancer seems to have a special propensity for metastasizing to the hypothalamus. Although there are other rare causes of diabetes insipidus, nearly half of all cases are idiopathic. Diabetes insipidus is an exceptionally rare paraneoplastic syndrome. Nephrogenic diabetes insipidus occurs when the kidney is unable to respond to normal circulating levels of ADH.

3. **Osmotic diuresis,** and often osmotic diarrhea, is encountered in obtunded patients who receive a massive urea load from high-protein nasogastric tube feedings. Progressive dehydration develops and the osmotic diuresis produces an apparently normal urine output. Daily weighing and twice-weekly measuring of serum electrolytes and urea nitrogen are necessary to detect or prevent this problem.

B. **Diagnosis**

1. **Signs and symptoms.** Most patients with severe hypernatremia are already seriously ill. The specific contribution of hypertonicity is frequently difficult to distinguish from the underlying disease. Polyuria draws attention to the problem in most cases. However, if the solute intake is low, urine output may not exceed two to three liters per day.

2. **Laboratory studies.** To make a diagnosis of diabetes insipidus, a water deprivation test is performed. Baseline body weight, serum sodium concentration, serum osmolality, urine specific gravity, and urine osmolality are measured. Water intake is completely restricted; however, these patients should *never* be deprived of water without continuous observation. Beginning in the morning, urine volume and the baseline studies are determined hourly. The test must be *terminated* if the patient's weight decreases by more than 3 percent or serum osmolality exceeds 310 mOsm/kg. Pending results of direct measurement, the serum osmolality can be rapidly and accurately estimated from serum concentrations of sodium, urea nitrogen, and glucose by the following formula:

$$\text{Serum osmolality} = 2\,(\text{sodium}) + \frac{\text{BUN}}{2.8} + \frac{\text{glucose}}{18}$$

a. **Criteria for diagnosing diabetes insipidus**
   (1) Urine osmolality never exceeds 200 mOsm/kg unless there is severe dehydration.
   (2) The initial serum osmolality determination exceeds 280 mOsm/kg.
   (3) Serum osmolality rises above the initial determination.
   (4) The urine flow rate consistently exceeds one ml/min.

b. **Differentiating pituitary diabetes insipidus.** Significant diabetes insipidus is excluded if the urine osmolality is greater than 600 mOsm/kg after water deprivation in the absence of glycosuria or recently injected contrast media. Urine osmolality between 200 and 600 mOsm/kg suggests partial diabetes insipidus. It is necessary to distinguish pituitary (central) diabetes insipidus from nephrogenic diabetes insipidus. To do this, the kidney's response to ADH is assessed. Desmopressin, 0.5 μg, is given SQ at the conclusion of the water deprivation test, and hourly urine specimens are collected for an additional three hours. Urine osmolality exceeds 400 mOsm/kg in patients with ADH deficiency and 800 mOsm/kg in normal subjects; values are lower in patients with nephrogenic diabetes insipidus.

C. Management

1. **Severe hypernatremia** is life-threatening and must be carefully managed. Correcting the water deficit too rapidly precipitates fatal cerebral edema. Therapy should not lower the serum sodium level by more than two to four mEq/hr. Emergency therapy for patients in shock consists of plasma volume expansion with normal saline solution (200–250 ml boluses IV over 10 minutes until the systolic blood pressure exceeds 90 mmHg); volume expansion itself induces a saluresis and initiates reduction of the serum sodium level. When the patient is hemodynamically stable, 5% dextrose in water (5% D/W) is given according to the following formula:

$$\text{Total volume (liters of 5\% D/W/24 hours)} = \frac{\text{serum sodium concentration} - 140}{140}(0.6 \times \text{body weight in kg})$$

2. **Therapy for chronic ADH deficiency**

   a. **Chlorpropamide,** 250 to 500 mg PO each morning, appears to be effective only in patients with incomplete pituitary diabetes insipidus. The drug is not approved for this purpose by the FDA. Serious and prolonged hypoglycemia or hyponatremia may complicate therapy with chlorpropamide.

   b. **Desmopressin** (desamino-D-arginine vasopressin; DDAVP), 5 to 10 μg by nasal insufflation or 0.5 to 1.0 μg by SQ injection, produces 6 to 18 hr of antidiuresis. To avoid water intoxication, the next dose is not given until thirst and polyuria redevelop.

VI. Hyponatremia: syndrome of inappropriate antidiuretic hormone

A. Mechanisms

1. **ADH** is normally released from the posterior pituitary gland in response to increased osmolality or decreased volume of plasma. The release of ADH is normally inhibited by decreased plasma osmolality and increased plasma volume. The hormone acts by increasing water resorption from the renal collecting tubules.

2. **Syndrome of inappropriate ADH** (SIADH). Unregulated tumor production of ADH results in increased water retention by the kidney, increased total body water, and moderate expansion of plasma volume. Plasma hypotonicity fails to suppress the tumor source of ADH. Hyponatremia, plasma hypoosmolality, and inability to excrete maximally diluted urine are the consequences of SIADH.

3. **Associated tumors.** Ectopic production of ADH may occur with any malignancy but is most frequently associated with bronchogenic carcinoma, especially the small cell type, and mesothelioma.

   a. About one half of patients with small cell lung cancer are unable to excrete an exogenous free water load normally; however, only a small portion of these will develop severe hyponatremia (<120 mEq/l).

   b. Abnormalities of serum electrolytes, other than hyponatremia and (occasionally) hypouricemia, do not occur in SIADH. However, some tumors produce multiple ectopic hormones. Concomitant hypokalemia suggests a complicating ectopic ACTH syndrome. Concomitant hypercalcemia suggests the presence of a paraneoplastic disorder of calcium metabolism.

4. **CNS disease** (e.g., mass lesions, hemorrhage, infection) and pulmonary infection (e.g., pneumonia, tuberculosis, abscess) may result in excessive ADH release from the posterior pituitary.

5. **Drugs associated with hyponatremia**

   a. **Diuretics** commonly produce hyponatremia, particularly in patients with unrestricted fluid intake.

   b. **Vincristine** may produce SIADH and profound hyponatremia. Manifestations develop one to two weeks after treatment in about two weeks.

Table 27-1. Hyponatremia: Differential diagnosis and laboratory results

Condition	BUN	Osmolality S	Osmolality U	Urine Na concentration
SIADH	D,(N)	D	I	N,I
Edematous states	D,N,I	D	I	D
Myxedema	N	D	N,I	(D),N,I
Salt-wasting states				
Mineralocorticoid deficiency	I	D	I	I
Glucocorticoid deficiency	N	D	(N),I	N,I
Diuretics	N	D	I	(D),N,I
Chronic renal failure	I	D	D,N,I	D,N,I
GI loss with hypotonic replacement	N,I	D	D	D
Compulsive water drinking	N,D,	D	D	N
Hypothalamic osmoregulatory defect	N	D	N	D,N,I
Pseudohyponatremia				
Hyperglycemia	N,I	I	D,N,I	N
Mannitol	N,I	N	D,N	D,N
Marked hyperlipidemia or paraproteinemia	N	N	N	N

Key: BUN = blood urea nitrogen; S = serum; U = urine; SIADH = syndrome of inappropriate antidiuretic hormone; GI = gastrointestinal; D = decreased; N = normal; I = increased; ( ) = slight or occasional.

   c. **Cyclophosphamide,** when given IV, may produce SIADH. Mild hyponatremia develops 4 to 12 hours after a dose, persists for about 20 hours, and is usually asymptomatic.
   d. **Chlorpropamide** occasionally causes SIADH; other oral hypoglycemics rarely do so.
   e. **Carbamazepine** induces ADH secretion.
   f. **IV narcotics** have been associated with SIADH.
   g. **Psychotropic agents,** amitriptyline (Elavil) and thioridazine (Mellaril), have been rarely associated with SIADH.
B. **Diagnosis**
   1. **Symptoms and signs.** Lethargy, nausea, anorexia, and generalized weakness are common symptoms in patients with hyponatremia; however, the symptoms may be related more to comorbid conditions than to the serum sodium concentration. Confusion, convulsions, coma, and death may ensue if the hyponatremia is severe or rapid in onset.
   2. **Laboratory studies.** Laboratory results in conditions associated with hyponatremia are shown in Table 27-1. Measurements that should be obtained in patients with hyponatremia are as follows:
      a. **In all patients with hyponatremia**
         (1) Serum electrolytes, creatinine, urea nitrogen, calcium, phosphate, glucose, total protein, and triglycerides
         (2) Urine sodium
      b. **In patients with hyponatremia and without an elevated BUN**
         (1) Blood and urine osmolality.
         (2) Chest x-ray film to look for evidence of lung cancer.
         (3) Patients who meet the diagnostic criteria for SIADH but in whom there is no obvious cause should have a bone marrow biopsy performed to look for metastases from small cell lung cancer (some patients have normal chest x-ray films).
      c. **In patients with evidence of endocrine hypofunction**
         (1) Thyroid function tests

        (2) Adrenal function tests

        (3) Pituitary gland function tests as necessary

3. Diagnostic criteria for SIADH include *all* five of the following:

  a. Hyponatremia with a disproportionately low BUN (often <10 mg/dl)

  b. Absence of intravascular volume contraction

    (1) Volume contraction is a potent stimulus for ADH secretion and will override the suppressive effect of hypotonicity.

    (2) Persistent urinary excretion of sodium constitutes indirect evidence of volume expansion (urine sodium concentration >30 mEq/l; fractional excretion of sodium [FE_{Na}] >1).

  c. Absence of abnormal fluid retention, such as peripheral edema or ascites.

  d. Normal renal function

  e. Serum hypotonicity along with urine that is not maximally dilute. A normal adult should be able to dilute urine to an osmolality of 50 to 75 mOsm/kg in the presence of decreased plasma osmolality; higher values are presumptive evidence for ADH activity at the renal tubules. Urine must be less than maximally dilute, but need not be hypertonic relative to serum. Urine osmolality greater than 75 to 100 mOsm/kg (or urine specific gravity >1.003) with plasma osmolality less than 260 mOsm/kg is usually diagnostic of SIADH.

C. Management, Control of the responsible cancer usually corrects the problems associated with ectopic SIADH.

  1. Severe hyponatremia (serum sodium <110 mEq/L). Comatose or seizing patients with severe hyponatremia must receive aggressive management. Lowering the plasma volume is essential to promote proximal tubular reabsorption of sodium. Administering saline solutions without diuresis to patients with SIADH does not correct the problem; saline increases plasma volume and results in further loss of sodium in the urine.

    a. An IV infusion of 3% NaCl at a rate of one liter q6–8h is started.

    b. Furosemide (Lasix), 40 to 80 mg IV q6–8h, is administered simultaneously.

    c. The central venous pressure (CVP) is monitored every 15 to 30 minutes; serum sodium and potassium concentrations are obtained hourly. Give additional doses of furosemide, 20 to 40 mg IV, or decrease the saline infusion rate if the CVP exceeds 18 cm of water or if congestive heart failure becomes evident on physical examination.

    d. Furosemide and saline are discontinued when the serum sodium concentration exceeds 110 mEq/l. More rapid treatment increases the risk of cerebral herniation. The hyponatremia should then be further corrected more slowly as described in **C.2.**

    e. The development of mental status changes or seizures after partial correction of severe hyponatremia is prima facie evidence of cerebral herniation; dexamethasone, 10 to 20 mg IV, *and* mannitol, 50 gm IV, are given immediately.

  2. Moderately severe hyponatremia (serum sodium >110 mEq/L)

    a. Fluid restriction is of paramount importance in therapy of all patients with SIADH and should result in correction of hyponatremia within three to five days. Patients with serum sodium levels less than 125 mEq/l should be restricted to 500 to 700 ml/day. Patients with higher serum sodium levels can be restricted to 1000 ml/day.

    b. Demeclocycline (Declomycin), 150 to 300 mg PO q.i.d., induces renal resistance to ADH and facilitates free water excretion. The drug is useful in patients who cannot tolerate chronic fluid restriction or who have insufficient improvement of hyponatremia with fluid restriction. The only significant toxicity of the drug is azotemia, which may be a problem in patients who receive the higher doses or simultaneous nephrotoxic agents.

    c. Lithium salts are less reliable than demeclocycline.

VII. Hyperkalemia
A. Mechanisms
1. Hyperkalemia in patients with or without cancer usually develops as a consequence of renal failure.
2. Hyperkalemia may result from rapid tumor lysis following therapy, especially in Burkitt's lymphoma.
3. Adrenal metastases are common in patients with many types of cancer, but clinical adrenal insufficiency from metastases is unusual.
4. Pseudohyperkalemia occurs in patients with persistent thrombocytosis, especially in the myeloproliferative disorders (see Chap. 24, *Comparative Aspects,* sec. **III.A.7.b**).

B. Diagnosis
1. **Symptoms** mostly consist of weakness and other neuromuscular complaints.
2. **Laboratory studies**
   a. Serum potassium concentration.
   b. The severity of the ECG abnormalities corresponds to the severity of hyperkalemia; as hyperkalemia gets worse, the ECG shows increased T wave amplitude, decreased R wave amplitude and increased S wave depth, prolongation of P–R intervals and widening of the QRS complex, and then a "sine wave" pattern eventuating in asystole or ventricular tachyarrhythmias.
3. **Differential diagnosis**
   a. Renal insufficiency
   b. Excessive potassium intake, especially with renal insufficiency
   c. Potassium-sparing diuretics
   d. Adrenal insufficiency
   e. Acidosis
   f. Cell destruction (e.g., tumor lysis, rhabdomyolysis)
   g. Angiotensin-converting enzyme inhibitors

C. Management
1. Immediate lowering of the potassium is achieved by IV administration of 10 units of regular insulin plus 50 to 100 ml of 50% dextrose solution. If the patient is acidotic, 150 to 300 mEq (1–2 ampules) of sodium bicarbonate is given IV.
2. Removal of potassium from the body can be achieved with cation exchange resins like Kayexalate, 20 to 30 gm every six hours. Sorbitol, 20 ml of 70% solution PO t.i.d. or q.i.d., or 100 gm in a water retention enema, is given to expel the resin from the bowel.
3. Hemodialysis is necessary for management of chronic or refractory hyperkalemia.
4. Hyperkalemia due to adrenal insufficiency may be corrected with the synthetic mineralocorticoid, fludrocortisone, 0.05 to 0.20 mg daily.

VIII. Hypokalemia: ectopic secretion of ACTH
A. Mechanism.
A variety of tumors may ectopically synthesize ACTH and produce Cushing's syndrome. Biologically active ACTH is secreted in varying proportions with biologically inactive prohormone and pre-prohormone. All of these substances possess antigenic activity for ACTH. Thus assays based on ACTH antigenic activity do not prove the presence of Cushing's syndrome.
1. **Tumors commonly producing ectopic ACTH syndrome**
   a. Small cell lung cancer
   b. Malignant thymoma
   c. Pancreatic cancer, especially islet cell tumors
   d. Bronchial carcinoids
2. **Tumors uncommonly or rarely producing ectopic ACTH syndrome**
   a. Ovarian cancer
   b. Thyroid cancer
   c. Pheochromocytoma
   d. Prostate cancer

e. Renal cancer
f. Sarcomas
g. Hematologic malignancies

B. Diagnosis

1. **Symptoms and signs.** The most common malignant causes of ectopic ACTH syndrome are rapidly fatal. The typical features of adrenal or pituitary Cushing's syndrome are often absent. Presenting signs usually are cachexia, weakness, and hypertension. Slower-growing cancers and benign tumors give rise to the characteristic rounded facies, truncal obesity, purple striae in skin stretch areas, and overt diabetes mellitus.

2. **Laboratory studies**
   a. Cancer patients who complain of weakness should have serum electrolytes measured. Hypokalemia and metabolic alkalosis may be severe (serum potassium as low as 1.0 mEq/L, bicarbonate >30 mEq/L) in patients with ectopic ACTH syndrome.
   b. The diagnosis of ectopic ACTH syndrome may be quickly made by demonstrating the failure of dexamethasone to suppress ACTH levels (see Chap. 15, sec. **V.C.2**).

3. **Differential diagnosis**
   a. GI losses associated with alkalosis (vomiting, prolonged nasogastric suctioning, colonic neoplasms [villous adenoma], chronic laxative abuse)
   b. GI losses associated with acidosis (chronic diarrhea, ureterosigmoidostomy, Zollinger-Ellison syndrome)
   c. Potassium-wasting drugs (e.g., diuretics, cisplatin, corticosteroids)
   d. Hyperaldosteronism
   e. Hypercortisolism
   f. Licorice ingestion
   g. Renal tubular acidosis
   h. Hypercalcemia, hypomagnesemia
   i. Hypophosphatemia in anabolic states (e.g., rapid tumor growth)
   j. Respiratory therapy in patients with chronic carbon dioxide retention
   k. Correction of nutritional anemias

C. Management. Control of the underlying tumor is the most effective method. Hypokalemia per se is often very difficult to correct. Potassium replacement consists of PO or IV doses of 80 to 150 mEq/day. Severe symptoms may occasionally improve using adrenal suppressant medications, such as various combinations of mitotane, metyrapone, ketoconazole, and aminoglutethimide. The toxicity of these drugs may be worse than the symptoms from the underlying disease. Spironolactone, 100 to 400 mg daily, may be useful. Adrenalectomy is a consideration in the rare patient with a very indolent, unresectable tumor that causes the ACTH syndrome.

IX. Hyperuricemia

A. Mechanisms. Hyperuricemia and hyperuricosuria pose a major problem for patients with myeloproliferative disorders, lymphomas, myeloma, or leukemias, but usually not for patients with solid tumors.

1. **Hyperuricosuria.** Urinary uric acid excretion is increased in untreated patients who have myeloproliferative disorders, acute or chronic myelocytic leukemia, or acute lymphoblastic leukemia. Patients with lymphoma have normal or slightly increased uric acid excretion. During treatment with either cytotoxic agents or radiation, massive tumor lysis results in excess production of uric acid, especially in patients with lymphoma or leukemia.

2. **Uric acid nephropathy** results from the precipitation of uric acid crystals in the concentrated, acidic urine of the renal medulla, distal tubules, and collecting ducts. The resultant sludge leads to intrarenal obstructive nephropathy and distinct inflammatory interstitial changes. Hyperuricemic nephropathy comprises four types of renal disease.

   a. Acute hyperuricemic nephropathy is seen in patients treated for hematologic malignancies. It is characterized by acute renal failure with a rapidly rising serum creatinine. Blood uric acid levels more than 20 mg/dl are consistently associated with acute renal functional impairment or failure. Lower levels may acutely compromise renal function if the patient is dehydrated or acidotic.

   b. **Gouty nephropathy** is usually mild to moderate and is characterized by the deposition of uric acid crystals (tophi) in the medulla or pyramids and a surrounding giant cell reaction.

   c. **Uric acid nephrolithiasis** develops in gouty and nongouty subjects with or without hyperuricemia. Symptomatic uric acid calculi are usually manifested by renal colic. Acute or chronic renal failure may develop secondary to obstructive uropathy.

   d. **Interstitial nephritis** of hyperuricemia may lead to chronic renal failure after 20 to 30 years. This condition is almost always associated with hypertension and is questioned as an isolated cause of renal failure.

3. **Xanthine stones,** resulting from the inhibition of xanthine oxidase by allopurinol in the setting of purine hypermetabolism rarely complicates malignancies.

4. **Oxypurinol stones** have rarely developed after therapy with massive doses of allopurinol.

B. **Diagnosis** is established by measurement of serum and urine uric acid concentrations. The normal excretory rate for uric acid is 300 to 500 mg/day.

C. **Management**

1. **Prevention** is the cornerstone for management.

   a. **Vigorous hydration** is essential for increasing uric acid clearance and diluting the concentration of uric acid in the renal tubules. Urinary flow should be at least 100 ml/hr.

   b. **Alkalinization of the urine.** The urine pH should be maintained between 7.0 and 7.5 (by dipstick). Sodium bicarbonate is given (one to three tablets PO q4h) while the patient is awake. Acetazolamide (Diamox), 250 to 500 mg PO, is given at bedtime to maintain urine alkalinization. Other preparations that contain sodium or potassium citrate are also available.

   c. **Allopurinol** should be given continuously to patients with myeloproliferative disorders, and at least 12 hours before starting antitumor therapy to patients with the other hematologic malignancies. The usual dose is 300 to 600 mg PO daily; larger doses may be required. Allopurinol can be discontinued when remission is obtained.

2. **Renal failure** because of uric acid nephropathy

   a. **Ureteral lavage** through nephrostomies and **surgical removal** of stones may be necessary to relieve acute renal pelvis and ureteral obstructions.

   b. **Hemodialysis** should be used if the measures in **a** fail to improve renal function because uric acid nephropathy is usually a complication of effective antitumor therapy. Hemodialysis is superior to peritoneal dialysis for clearing uric acid.

X. **Hypouricemia**

A. **Mechanisms.** Hypouricemia is usually caused by defects in proximal renal tubular reabsorption of uric acid. Hypouricemia has also been reported to be associated with a variety of tumors, especially Hodgkin's disease and myeloma.

B. **Diagnosis**

1. **Symptoms.** Patients are asymptomatic.

2. **Laboratory studies.** Blood uric acid levels identify the abnormality.

3. **Differential diagnosis**

   a. Proximal renal tubular disease

      (1) Falconi's syndrome (myeloma is a common cause in adults)

      (2) Wilson's disease

      (3) Isolated defect in otherwise healthy individuals

   b. Uricosuric agents

      (1) Aspirin

           (2) X-ray contrast agents

           (3) Glyceryl guaiacolate

        c. Xanthine oxidase inhibitors (allopurinol)

        d. Hereditary xanthinuria

        e. Neoplastic diseases, especially Hodgkin's disease

        f. Liver disease

        g. SIADH

    C. Management. Treatment of hypouricemia is not necessary.

XI. Hyperglycemia

    A. Mechanisms

        1. Diabetic glucose tolerance curves with relative insulin deficiency are present in many patients with cancer. Paradoxical hypersecretion of growth hormone from the pituitary gland occurs in the majority of these patients. Nutritional replenishment seems to improve the abnormal glucose tolerance, hyperinsulinemia, and paradoxical growth hormone secretion.

        2. Hyperglycemia occurs in patients with glucagonoma, somatostinoma, pheochromocytoma, and hypercortisolism.

        3. Nonketotic hyperosmolar coma can be a complication of treatment with cyclophosphamide, vincristine, or prednisone in patients with even mild diabetes mellitus. Hyperosmolar coma also occurs as a result of hyperalimentation therapy.

    B. Diagnosis. Random or two-hour postprandial blood glucose determinations disclose the abnormality in most patients.

    C. Management

        1. Nutritional status should be improved in cancer patients with glucose intolerance, if feasible. Management of substantial hyperglycemia on account of tumor is effected by control of the neoplasm and by administration of insulin or oral hypoglycemics as needed.

        2. Hyperosmolar coma must be vigorously treated with fluid replacement of volume losses with IV saline until the blood pressure is stable. Insulin infusion (1 to 4 U/hr) usually controls the hyperglycemia.

XII. Hypoglycemia

    A. Mechanisms. Insulinlike substances may be produced by some tumors, especially large retroperitoneal sarcomas and (occasionally) other cancers. Hepatocellular carcinomas and extensive liver metastases from a variety of primary sites may deplete glycogen stores and impair gluconeogenesis. Insulinoma is discussed in Chap. 15, sec. **VI.C.**

        1. Etiologies of hypoglycemia

            a. Malignant tumors

                (1) Insulinoma

                (2) Large retroperitoneal tumor

                (3) Hepatocellular carcinoma

                (4) Extensive hepatic metastasis

            b. Drugs

                (1) Surreptitious or therapeutic insulin administration

                (2) Oral hypoglycemic agents

                (3) Alcohol

                (4) Salicylates

                (5) Jamaican vomiting sickness (akee fruit)

                (6) Quinine (in antimalarial doses)

            c. Metabolic disorders

                (1) Starvation

                (2) Chronic liver disease

                (3) Hypoadrenalism

                (4) Hypopituitarism

                (5) Myxedema

                (6) Glycogen storage diseases

                (7) Reactive hypoglycemias (e.g., prediabetes, postgastrectomy)

        2. Pseudohypoglycemia. False low glucose levels may occur in patients with marked granulocytosis, especially patients with myeloproliferative disorders, because of in vitro consumption of glucose.

B. Diagnosis

1. **Symptoms and signs.** Tumor-associated hypoglycemia produces mental status change, fatigue, convulsions, or coma. Some patients show features of fasting hypoglycemia, such as an altered morning personality that improves after breakfast. Tremors, sweating, tachycardia, and hunger pangs are suggestive of acute decrease in blood sugar level.

2. **Laboratory studies.** A blood glucose concentration less than 40 mg/dl establishes the presence of hypoglycemia. Further evaluation of fasting hypoglycemia is discussed in Chap. 15, sec. **VI.C.** Patients who surreptitiously abuse insulin should have C peptide and insulin serum levels measured. Absent C peptide with elevated insulin level suggests the diagnosis of exogenous insulin administration.

C. Management

1. **Intravenous glucose.** Any patient with suggestive signs, symptoms, or unexplained coma should have a blood sample drawn for glucose determination, followed immediately by rapid IV infusion of 50 ml of 50% dextrose solution. Serum glucose can remain low even while concentrated glucose solutions are being administered. All patients with glucose levels less than 40 mg/dl and symptomatic patients with glucose levels less than 60 mg/dl should be treated by continuous infusion of 20% glucose at 50 to 150 ml/hr; rates are adjusted to maintain glucose levels higher than 60 mg/dl. Blood glucose levels are measured every three to four hours until stabilization occurs.

2. **Glucagon,** 1 mg IM, also raises blood glucose by promoting glycogenolysis and gluconeogenesis.

3. **Octreotide,** a somatostatin analogue, can decrease insulin hypersecretion (see Chap. 15, sec. **VI.A.2.b**).

4. **Other measures.** If the blood glucose cannot be increased to safe levels with infusions, prednisone or diazoxide should be administered (see Chap. 15, sec. **VI.C.2.d**).

XIII. Tumor lysis syndrome

A. Mechanisms. Effective chemotherapy of several malignancies may result in the massive release into the blood of potassium, phosphate, uric acid, and other breakdown products of dying tumor cells. Hypocalcemia may occur with severe hyperphosphatemia. Tumor lysis syndrome develops within hours to a few days of treatment for the underlying neoplasm.

1. **Associated tumors** most commonly are acute leukemia, Burkitt's lymphoma, and occasionally other lymphoreticular malignancies. The syndrome rarely occurs following the treatment of solid tumors.

2. **Life-threatening complications** include renal failure from hyperuricemia and cardiac arrhythmias from hyperkalemia or hypocalcemia.

B. Diagnosis

1. **Physical examination.** Oliguria may call attention to the metabolic disorders. Tetany may be a presenting feature. Cardiac arrhythmias or cardiopulmonary arrest develop if the process is not controlled.

2. **Laboratory studies.** Patients treated for acute leukemia or Burkitt's lymphoma should have measurements of serum levels of potassium, calcium, phosphate, uric acid, and creatinine performed daily for one week and every few hours if the syndrome develops.

C. Management. Vigorous intravenous hydration with half-normal saline is initiated. Severe metabolic problems are treated as follows:

1. Hypocalcemia. See sec. **II.C.**

2. Hyperphosphatemia. See sec. **III.C.**

3. Hyperkalemia. See sec. **VII.C.**

4. Hyperuricemia. See sec. **IX.C.**

5. Hemodialysis may be necessary on an emergency basis for patients who do not respond to treatment or who develop renal insufficiency.

Selected Reading

Bajorunas, D. R. Clinical manifestations of cancer-related hypercalcemia. *Semin. Oncol.* 17:16, 1990.

Barton, J. C. Tumor lysis syndrome in nonhematopoietic neoplasms. *Cancer* 64:738, 1989.

Gucalp, R., et al. Comparative study of pamidronate disodium and etidronate disodium in the treatment of cancer-related hypercalcemia. *J. Clin. Oncol.* 10:134, 1992.

Orloff, J. J., and Stewart, A. F. Disorders of serum minerals caused by cancer. In F. L. Coe and M. J. Favus (eds.). Disorders of Bone and Mineral Metabolism. New York: Raven Press, 1992. Pp. 539–562.

Richardson, D. W., and Robinson, A. G. Desmopressin. *Ann. Intern. Med.* 103:228, 1985.

Ritch, P. S. Treatment of cancer-related hypercalcemia. *Semin. Oncol.* 17:26, 1990.

Silverman, P., and Distelhorst, C. W. Metabolic emergencies in clinical oncology. *Semin. Oncol.* 16:504, 1989.

Sterns, R. H. The treatment of hyponatremia: first, do no harm. *Am. J. Med.* 88:557, 1990.

Warrell, R. P., et al. A randomized double-blind study of gallium nitrate compared with etidronate for acute control of cancer-related hypercalcemia. *J. Clin. Oncol.* 9:1467, 1991.

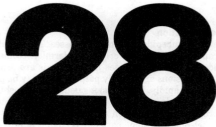

Cutaneous Complications

Richard F. Wagner, Jr., and
Barry B. Lowitz

I. Metastases to the skin

A. Incidence and pathology. Skin metastases occur in 25 percent of patients with breast carcinoma, in 7 percent of patients with lung cancer, 5 percent of patients with renal cancer, 3 percent of patients with colon cancer, and 1 to 2 percent of patients with other solid tumors. Tumor extension or metastasis to the skin also commonly occurs with oral cavity carcinoma or malignant melanoma. Iatrogenic metastases as a result of invasive procedures are exceedingly rare. T cell lymphoma characteristically involves the skin.

B. Natural history. Metastases to the skin may be delayed 10 to 15 years after the initial surgical treatment of primary melanoma, breast carcinoma, and renal cancer or may be the first indication of an internal malignancy. Draining fistulae may connect the skin to serosal surfaces; peritoneocutaneous fistulae may result in abdominal sepsis, and pleurocutaneous fistulae in atelectasis and empyema. Large, bulky, malodorous masses may form (see sec. II). Tumors developing near major vessels may result in vascular erosion and exsanguination.

  1. Distribution. Skin involvement most often occurs in a region near the primary tumor but may occur anywhere.

   a. Breast cancer that metastasizes to the skin typically involves the chest wall and scalp.

   b. Lung cancer. Cutaneous metastases most commonly appear on the chest wall or scalp. The small cell type of lung cancer tends to metastasize to the skin of the back. Lung cancer also has a rare but peculiar tendency to metastasize to the anal area, finger tips, or toes.

   c. GI tract cancers most commonly metastasize to the skin of the abdominal wall, often as closely grouped nodules around the umbilicus (see f). Anal cancer metastases to skin involve unusual sites, such as the scalp, eyelid, nose, or legs.

   d. Urinary tract cancers. Renal and bladder cancers most commonly metastasize to the skin of the lower abdominal wall, genitalia, or scalp, often in closely grouped clusters. Renal cancer may metastasize to unusual areas, such as the nose, eyelids, or finger tips. Prostate cancer may produce a zosterlike distribution of lesions over the flank because of lymphatic spread.

   e. Melanoma typically produces multiple skin metastases with some sparing only of anal areas. The face, scalp, torso, and proximal extremities may be diffusely involved with multiple nodular tumors. Placental and fetal metastases are known to occur.

   f. Umbilical metastases ("Sister Joseph's nodules") are nearly always adenocarcinomas. The primary site is most likely to be the GI tract, but it may be the ovary or endometrium. Umbilical masses must be considered malignant until proved otherwise.

  2. Prognosis. The prognosis of patients with skin metastases depends on the type of tumor and what other areas are involved. The average survival time from the recognition of skin metastases is three months and ranges from two months for lung cancer to 12 months for renal cancer.

C. Diagnosis
  1. History and physical examination
  a. Nodular lesions begin as subepidermal mobile masses. The nodules enlarge gradually or rapidly, invade the overlying epidermis, become fixed, and occasionally ulcerate. Nodular masses in the dermis are firm, rubbery, or stony-hard. The lesions are usually painless but may be painful and tender if they evolve rapidly. Early lesions usually are fleshtone to pink. Invasion of the overlying epidermis is associated with purplish discoloration and progressive induration that expands radially. Melanoma lesions may be jet-black. In some patients, ecchymoses or hair loss develops over subepidermal tumor masses.
  b. Diffuse lesions are most liable to develop in T cell lymphomas and are characterized as diffusely indurated and erythematous skin. Diffuse infiltration of subcutaneous tissues by solid tumors is frequently manifested by tender swellings without nodularity or discoloration.
  c. Inflammatory metastatic carcinoma (carcinoma erysipelatoides) is associated most frequently with breast cancer but also occurs with cancers of the lung, ovary, uterus, vulva, pancreas, stomach, rectum, and with melanoma.
  2. Biopsy. In patients with known solid malignancy, biopsy may be necessary to exclude treatable diseases with a similar morphology, such as opportunistic infection. If visceral malignancy was not known, cutaneous metastasis initiates further evaluation.
  a. Small nodules can be readily excised in toto.
  b. Diffuse skin masses can be evaluated by punch biopsy.
  c. Subcutaneous spreading solid tumors may be incised deeply without locating an identifiable mass; histologic examination demonstrates cancer in grossly normal tissue.
D. Management
  1. Tumors involving large areas of skin may be treated with cytotoxic or hormonal agents; the regimen is determined by the kind of primary tumor.
  2. Localized skin metastases are treated with RT, local excision, or cryotherapy.
  3. Intralesional thiotepa may be used *if only a few nodules exist* and other therapy is unavailable, contraindicated, or fails to cause tumor regression. Thiotepa is absorbed and should not be used if other myelosuppressive therapy is being administered. Injection of thiotepa is done as follows:
  a. Thiotepa, 30 mg (two vials), is dissolved in 5 to 10 ml of normal saline in a Luer-lok syringe equipped with a 21-gauge needle.
  b. The skin is anesthetized with a generous spray of ethylene chloride.
  c. The thiotepa is forcibly injected into the tumor nodule until it appears white and uniformly infiltrated. The injections may be repeated weekly if the CBC permits.
  d. Eventually the tumor becomes blackened and necrotic and sloughs. Healing with normal skin usually occurs after about six to eight weeks.
II. Paraneoplastic cutaneous diseases. The etiology of paraneoplastic cutaneous disease is unknown. Some syndromes may be mediated by immune mechanisms.
A. Bowen's disease is intraepithelial squamous carcinoma (in situ squamous cell carcinoma). The lesions typically appear as eczematous, scaly, red-brown plaques. Recent studies have questioned earlier work that linked Bowen's disease to internal malignancy.
  1. Associated tumors include cancer of the hypopharynx, larynx, lung, prostate, breast, ovary, esophagus, stomach, kidney, and bladder.
  2. Diagnosis. Biopsy of the scaling lesion must be done, and if it proves to be Bowen's disease arising on sun-protected skin, a search for a possible underlying malignancy should be considered.
  3. Therapy. Local therapy is the same as for other squamous skin cancers (Chap. 16, *Basal Cell and Squamous Cell Carcinoma*, sec. **V**).
B. Paget's disease presents as an erythematous patch on the breast areola, vulva,

or other skin area. Patients with unilateral nipple eczema are suspected of having Paget's disease if topical therapy fails to resolve the patch.

1. **Associated tumors**
   a. Mammary Paget's disease is almost invariably associated with an *underlying ductal cancer* of the breast.
   b. Extramammary Paget's disease is associated with *genital or visceral cancer* in about 50 percent of cases.
2. **Diagnosis**
   a. Bilateral nipple eczema is usually benign and should be treated with topical steroid creams and avoidance of possible allergens in clothing. If the rash persists, a biopsy is indicated. All patients with suspected Paget's disease should have a biopsy. If Paget's disease is proven, it is necessary to evaluate both breasts for underlying malignancy.
   b. Biopsy proof of extramammary Paget's disease mandates search for a primary tumor.
3. **Therapy.** Excision of extramammary Paget's disease is done whenever possible. Mammary Paget's disease with underlying cancer is managed the same way as is primary breast cancer.

C. **Acanthosis nigricans** is a black-to-brown warty eruption occurring in intertriginous areas (the axillae, groins, under the breast) as well as on the palms and soles. The lesions resemble dirty skin during the early phases.
   1. **Associated tumors.** Acanthosis nigricans resulting from a malignancy is associated with abdominal cancer in 80 percent of patients; primary gastric cancer constitutes 60 percent of these patients. Other tumors include cancers of the pancreas, liver, colon, ovary, lung, and breast. The dermatosis precedes evidence of the malignancy in 20 percent of cases. Malignant causes of acanthosis nigricans are associated with rapid progression of the skin lesions and an 80 percent mortality in the first year after diagnosis.
   2. **Benign causes of acanthosis nigricans**
      a. Acromegaly, gigantism
      b. Adrenal insufficiency
      c. Hyperthyroidism, hypothyroidism
      d. Lipodystrophy
      e. Diabetes mellitus
      f. Syndrome of hirsutism, obesity, amenorrhea, and acanthosis nigricans
      g. Inherited abnormality in humans (and Swedish dachshunds)
   3. **Diagnosis** is established by inspection of the lesions. Biopsy is not essential.
   4. **Therapy** must control the underlying tumor. The dermatosis may regress or temporarily disappear when the cancer is removed.

D. **Erythema gyratum repens** is a very rare condition manifested by undulating bands of urticarial eruptions over the entire body. Alternating bands of red and white streaks give the appearance of tiger stripes or knotty pine.
   1. **Associated tumors.** Erythema gyratum repens is nearly always associated with malignancy, usually rectal, esophageal, head and neck, lung, breast, or uterine cervical cancers.
   2. **Therapy** is directed at control of the underlying disease and treatment of pruritus.

E. **Dermatomyositis** (DMS) presents with symmetrical proximal muscle weakness and a violaceous rash that is most prominent in sun-exposed areas. In the beginning, periorbital changes develop, such as edema, erythema, and bluish red discoloration ("heliotrope ring"). Later, purplish plaquelike lesions appear over the knuckles (Gottron's papules), elbows, and other stretch areas of the skin. Some patients have muscle weakness without the skin rash (polymyositis) or the rash without myositis.
   1. **Associated tumors.** Approximately 25 percent of patients with DMS have, had, or will develop underlying cancer. Breast cancer is the tumor most commonly associated with DMS. Lymphoma, melanoma, and cancers of the nasopharynx, lung, stomach, bowel, urinary bladder, and ovary are also associated with DMS. The cancer is diagnosed before DMS occurs in one-

third of patients, concurrently in one-third, and months to years afterward in one-third.

2. **Diagnosis.** The characteristic skin rash or progressive proximal muscle weakness suggests the diagnosis of DMS. Diagnostic features of myositis include elevated serum creatine phosphokinase and aldolase, an inflammatory pathology on muscle biopsy, and myopathic features on EMG studies.

3. **Therapy.** The myopathy tends to be progressive unless the underlying tumor is controlled. Cyclophosphamide, 50 mg PO b.i.d., with prednisone, 40 mg/m^2 PO daily, may retard symptoms in some patients.

F. **Circinate erythemas.** Erythema figuratum perstans is a circular elevation of the skin that remains stable for weeks to months. Initially, erythema annulare centrifugum is a small erythematous area that slowly enlarges, leaving a central circle of normal-appearing skin. Lesions may be pruritic.

1. **Associated tumors** include lymphoma and, occasionally, visceral cancer. Circinate erythemas are associated less commonly with tumors than with nonmalignant diseases (especially collagen vascular syndromes, angiitides, and infections). Many cases are idiopathic.

2. **Diagnosis** is made by inspection.

3. **Therapy** is directed at control of the underlying illness.

G. **Hyperkeratosis,** particularly of the palms and soles, occurs as a result of tylosis palmaris et plantaris, chronic arsenic exposure, or as an idiopathic paraneoplastic syndrome.

1. **Associated tumors**

   a. Tylosis is a hereditary syndrome associated with esophageal cancer.

   b. Arsenical keratoses and idiopathic hyperkeratoses are associated with squamous skin cancer and a large variety of visceral tumors, including cancers of the lung, stomach, ovary, and genitourinary tract.

2. **Diagnosis.** Hyperkeratosis is usually obvious on inspection.

3. **Therapy.** Propylene glycol-salicylic acid (Keralyt gel) may help to remove excess skin.

H. **Acquired ichthyosis** is a condition of the skin appearing as fish-scale-like patches. Lesions appear over the body surface, particularly on the extremities; palms and soles are relatively spared.

1. **Associated tumors.** Hodgkin's disease is the malignancy most frequently associated with acquired ichthyosis. It also occurs with breast cancer, non-Hodgkin's lymphoma, and multiple myeloma.

2. **Diagnosis.** Ichthyosis in childhood is not rare. The onset of ichthyosis in a previously normal adult, however, suggests a possible underlying cancer. Acquired ichthyosis is not a specific sign for cancer because it may be seen in a variety of other conditions such as leprosy and sarcoidosis.

3. **Therapy.** Effective antitumor therapy often eliminates the ichthyosis. A urea cream is applied liberally to the affected areas and wiped off while showering. Patients are advised to keep their environment humidified and to use skin emollients.

I. **Pachydermoperiostosis** exhibits thickening of skin and creation of new skin folds (leonine facies). The scalp, forehead, lids, ears, and lips are the typical sites. The tongue, thenar and hypothenar eminences, elbows and knees may be enlarged. The fingers are clubbed.

1. **Associated tumors.** The familial form of pachydermoperiostosis is not usually associated with malignant tumors. The acquired variety occurs almost exclusively in patients with undifferentiated lung cancer. Clubbing and hypertrophic osteoarthropathy are also associated with a variety of nonmalignant disorders.

2. **Diagnosis** is made by inspection. Biopsy shows thickening of the horny layer and hypertrophy of the sweat and sebaceous glands.

3. **Therapy.** No specific management is available other than control of the underlying cancer.

J. **Vitiligo** is the hypopigmentation of skin due to the loss of melanocytes.

1. **Associated tumors.** Melanoma is most common; patients with metastatic

melanoma and vitiligo tend to survive longer than patients with metastatic melanoma without vitiligo.

2. **Diagnosis** is made by inspection. Vitiligo or a halo nevus may rarely be a sign of an occult melanoma.

3. **Therapy.** No specific therapy can be recommended except control of the malignancy. Vitadye lotion can be used to provide cosmetic camouflage.

K. **Sweet's syndrome** (acute febrile neutrophilic dermatosis) manifests as suddenly appearing, painful, erythematous plaques or nodules or both, typically on the upper extremities, head, and neck. Fever and elevated peripheral neutrophils are usually present.

1. **Associated tumors.** Acute myelogenous leukemia (most common malignant association); lymphoma, myelodysplastic syndromes, myeloproliferative disorders; genitourinary, breast, and GI cancers.

2. **Diagnosis.** Skin biopsy shows a neutrophilic dermatosis without vasculitis, often with karyorrhexis and endothelial swelling.

3. **Therapy.** Systemic corticosteroids dramatically resolve fever and skin lesions.

L. **Glucagonoma syndrome** (necrolytic migratory erythema) is caused by tumors of the pancreatic alpha cells. The skin disease, initially localized to the groin, waxes and wanes. Glucagonomas are discussed in Chap. 15, sec. **VI.D.**

M. **Miscellaneous skin diseases associated with visceral cancers**

1. **Alopecia mucinosa** may develop during the course of lymphoreticular neoplasms as a consequence of mucinous degeneration of collagen around hair follicles and sebaceous glands. The resultant alopecia is unrelated to therapy.

2. **Bazex's syndrome** (acrokeratosis paraneoplastica) is the psoriasiform changes of the face and extremities associated with malignancy of the upper respiratory or GI tracts.

3. **Erythema multiforme** is rarely associated with cancer and is usually caused by medications or infectious processes such as herpes simplex. The typical "bull's eye" lesions may appear anywhere, but they are most noticeable on the palms, extremities, and torso.

4. **Erythromelalgia** presents as painful, warm extremities that appear erythematous. Myeloproliferative diseases are the most common associated malignancies. Limb elevation and cooling provide relief.

5. **Florid cutaneous papillomatosis** is a very rare warty eruption of the extremities and trunk. All reported instances have been linked to internal malignancy, predominantly gastric adenocarcinoma.

6. **Gardner's syndrome** is familial intestinal polyposis with various anomalies and excessive numbers of cystic lesions, mostly on the face and extremities. Epidermal inclusion cysts are more common than sebaceous cysts (see Table 9-2.)

7. **Leser-Trélat sign** is defined by the sudden appearance and rapid increase in the number and size of seborrheic keratoses on previously normal skin. It is usually a rare manifestation of GI cancer.

8. **Malignant down** (acquired hypertrichosis lanuginosa). Extensive, sudden growth of lanugolike hair, at first over the face but later over the entire body, has been most frequently observed in association with cancer of the lung, colon, and rectum. Hair may grow to be 10 to 15 cm in two months.

9. **Multicentric histiocytosis** appears as cutaneous papules and nodules associated with arthritis. It is associated with a variety of solid and nonsolid tumors in 28 percent of presentations.

10. **Paraneoplastic pemphigus,** which is most commonly associated with lymphoid tumors, is a bullous disease that usually presents with painful oral erosions and flaccid cutaneous blisters. In contrast to other forms of pemphigus, IgG antibodies bind to columnar and transitional epithelia during indirect immunofluorescence. Other immunoprecipitants are also unique. The skin disease is usually resistant to treatment and fatal.

11. **Peutz-Jeghers syndrome** is familial intestinal polyposis and intestinal car-

cinoma associated with cutaneous manifestations. Within the first year of life, brown-to-black pigmented spots appear on the vermilion border of the lip, in the oral cavity, around the eyes, nose, and mouth, and on the fingers and toes. The spots usually disappear between puberty and 20 years of age (see Table 9-2.)

12. **Pityriasis rosea-like eruptions, erythroderma, and exfoliative dermatitis** may complicate a variety of tumors, mostly lymphoma. Prednisone, 40 mg/m^2 PO daily, usually controls life-threatening exfoliation until the underlying cause is managed. In erythroderma and exfoliative dermatitis, a skin biopsy should be considered to exclude cutaneous T cell lymphoma.

13. **Pityriasis rotunda** is a circular scaly patch appearing on the buttocks, trunk, and thighs. It is associated with hepatocellular carcinoma, gastric cancer, and other malignancies.

14. **Porphyria cutanea tarda** (PCT) is a blistering disease that appears in skin exposed to sunlight. Hepatocellular carcinoma and metastatic liver tumors are occasionally associated with paraneoplastic PCT.

15. **Pruritus.** Generalized pruritus is most frequently associated with Hodgkin's disease, lymphocytic leukemia, mycosis fungoides, and polycythemia rubra vera. Localized pruritus has been associated with brain tumors (nostrils) and squamous cell carcinoma (vulva).

16. **Pyoderma gangrenosum** appears as painful skin ulcers with a necrotic base and a purplish undetermined border. Of all malignant associations, it is most commonly found with acute myelogenous leukemia. It is also associated with myeloma, lymphoma, myeloproliferative diseases, and solid tumors.

17. **Scleroderma** is associated with diffuse bronchoalveolar carcinoma of the lung.

18. **Tripe palms** resembles bovine foregut and appears as thickened palmar skin with exaggerted dermatoglyphics. More than 90 percent of patients with tripe palms have associated malignancy, most frequently of the lung, stomach, and genitourinary tract.

19. **Urticaria pigmentosa** usually presents with reddish brown papules that produce urtication when rubbed (Darier's sign). This condition is due to increased mast cells in the skin. It is rarely associated with systemic mastocytosis and mast cell proliferation in the bone marrow and viscera.

20. **Vasculitis,** mainly leukocytoclastic angiitis or polyarteritis nodosa, is associated with hematologic malignancy.

III. **Adverse effects of radiation to the skin.** Modern equipment has greatly decreased both acute and late skin damage. The severity of skin changes is dependent on treatment site, dose, dose-rate, beam energy, beam quality, and beam direction. Beams passing through the skin tangentially or through skin folds result in focal areas of more severe reaction.

A. **Early side effects**

1. **Types of skin reactions**

   a. **Erythema** is a transient early response to RT.

   b. **Pigmentation** rarely is permanent and gradually disappears within three to four months.

   c. **Dry desquamation** (peeling) heals within two to four weeks after treatment.

   d. **Moist desquamation** (weeping) is often a desirable end point for treatment, particularly with primary skin tumors or dermal involvement by others tumors. Moist desquamation most commonly occurs around intertriginous areas and usually heals in four to eight weeks after treatment.

   e. **Skin necrosis.** Focal epidermal and dermal loss can result from moist desquamation or from chronic compromise of connective tissue or blood vessels.

2. **Management of skin reactions.** Severe erythema and moist desquamation are managed with cool water compresses for 10 minutes and are permitted

to air-dry. Dry desquamation is treated with unscented lubricating ointments.

3. Precautions to prevent skin damage

   a. Avoid local irritants, such as antiperspirants and lotions containing alcohol.

   b. Do not apply tape within the current radiation portal because the epidermis may be removed with the tape.

   c. Be sure that no physical irritants (such as straps, belts, or collars) are rubbing against the irradiated skin.

   d. Avoid direct sun on the treatment field, both during irradiation and even years afterward. Hats, protective clothing, and sunscreen lotions are advised.

   e. Skin lubricants and moisteners may offer long-term protection against fragility.

B. Late skin changes

   1. Mild late (benign) changes. Even minimal, transient RT-induced changes result in some late, often clinically inapparent, skin damage. Biologically and histologically, the skin never completely recovers. The skin may always show altered pigmentation, decreased natural oils, or woody subcutaneous fibrosis (less than 5% of patients).

   2. Severe late (benign) changes (marked atrophy, hyperkeratosis, fissures, telangiectasis, ulceration, and fragility) are rare with modern equipment and techniques. Atrophy is best treated by the avoidance of trauma and the use of ointments. Late irradiation skin ulcers may have to be treated by surgical excision and repair.

   3. Radiation-induced skin cancer is a problem that arose in the early years of RT development, especially among patients who were occupationally exposed or treated for benign skin conditions. The likelihood of a new skin cancer arising in an RT portal is greater than normal, but less than 0.1 percent of all skin cancer has occurred in these patients. Squamous cell carcinoma, basal cell carcinoma, and melanoma are all reported.

IV. Adverse cutaneous effects of chemotherapy

   A. Skin and nail changes associated with cytotoxic agents

      1. Acne. Actinomycin D, methotrexate (uncommon), steroids

      2. Bullous pemphigoid. Fluorouracil (rare)

      3. Dermatitis, nonspecific (uncommon). Methotrexate, mercaptopurine, thioguanine, fluorouracil, chlorambucil, nitrogen mustard, actinomycin D, mithramycin, mitomycin C; mitotane, hydroxyurea, procarbazine

      4. Erythroderma. Bleomycin

      5. Hyperpigmentation. Busulfan, fluorouracil, bleomycin ("flagellate"); rarely, Adriamycin, cyclophosphamide

      6. Local irritation following infiltration. Actinomycin D, Adriamycin, daunorubicin, mithramycin, mitomycin C, vinblastine, vincristine, nitrogen mustard, dacarbazine, carmustine

      7. Nails (dark bands or loss). Bleomycin, fluorouracil, busulfan; rarely, Adriamycin, cyclophosphamide

      8. Photosensitivity. Fluorouracil, methotrexate, vinblastine

      9. Pressure area vesiculation or ulceration. Fluorouracil, methotrexate

      10. Radiation recall (erythema or moist desquamation over a previous radiation port). Adriamycin, daunorubicin, bleomycin, actinomycin D, methotrexate, procarbazine

      11. Sclerodermoid changes. Bleomycin

      12. Telangiectasis. Topical nitrogen mustard, topical nitrosoureas, topical fluorouracil, L-asparaginase

      13. Urticaria, angioedema. Adriamycin, daunorubicin, L-asparaginase, chlorambucil, cyclophosphamide, nitrogen mustard, melphalan, methotrexate, procarbazine

   B. Extravasation of antitumor agents. Subcutaneous infiltration of vesicant cytotoxic agents (particularly anthracyclines, vinca alkaloids, and nitrogen mustard) usually causes immediate and intense pain. Edema and painful erythema develop within a few hours, and marked induration within a few days. Necrosis with ulceration usually develops within 1 to 4 weeks if it is to occur (approximately 25% of cases). Spontaneous healing of ulceration almost never occurs. The necrosis may involve periosteum, paratenon, and fascia. The prognosis is relatively unfavorable if extravasation on the dorsum of the hand or volar aspect of the wrist is not recognized early.

1. **Any questionable swelling or pain** around the IV site mandates that drug administration be immediately stopped.
2. **Acute treatment** for erythema, pain, or induration at injection site is as follows:
   a. **Infiltration of vinca alkaloids.** Apply hot packs and infiltrate the affected area with hyaluronidase.
   b. **Infiltration of other vesicant drugs.** Elevation of the extremity with intermittent ice packs for 48 hours may be sufficient, followed by physical therapy. Local injection of any medication has not been proved to be beneficial.
3. **Surgery.** If after 48 hours the condition worsens or the patient experiences increasing pain, the involved tissue should be excised and covered with a skin graft. Physical therapy is resumed in one week. Surgical repair of established ulceration is difficult. Amputation of the extremity is necessary in severe cases.

V. Other cutaneous complications
A. Skin pigmentation
1. **Gray discoloration** of the skin because melanosis may develop in patients with extensive malignant melanoma.
2. **Periorbital purplish discoloration** can develop in patients who have amyloid deposition in the eyelids from infiltration and purpura. The syndrome of postproctoscopic palpebral purpura is well described in these patients.
B. Skin infections may be caused by bacteria, fungi, or viruses in cancer patients. Nonspecific rashes may be the only cue for infection and thus a skin biopsy may be necessary.
C. Pruritus is discussed in Chap. 5, sec. VII.A.
D. Preventive skin care in the dying patient is discussed in Chap. 5, sec. VII.B.
E. Alopecia is discussed in Chap. 5, sec. VII.C.
F. Necrotic, malodorous tumor masses are discussed in Chap. 5, sec. VIII.
G. Cutaneous flushing is associated with carcinoid syndrome (see Chap. 15, sec. II) and mastocytosis.

Selected Reading

Allen, U., Smith, C. R., and Prober, C. G. The value of skin biopsies in febrile, neutropenic, immunocompromised children. *A.J.D.C.* 140:459, 1986.

Callen, J. P. Dermatomyositis and malignancy. *Clin. Dermatol.* 11:61, 1993.

Cohen, P. R., and Kurzrock R. Sweet's syndrome and cancer. *Clin. Dermatol.* 11:149, 1993.

Lee, M., and Wick, M. M. Bowen's disease. *Clin. Dermatol.* 11:43, 1993.

Wagner, R. F., Jr., and Nathanson, L. Paraneoplastic syndromes, tumor markers, and other unusual features of malignant melanoma. *J. Am. Acad. Dermatol.* 14:249, 1986.

Wolfson, J. S., Sober, A. J., and Rubin, R. H. Dermatologic manifestations of infections in immunocompromised patients. *Medicine* 64:115, 1985.

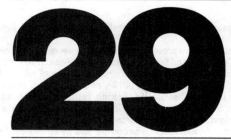

Thoracic Complications

Hassan J. Tabbarah and
Dennis A. Casciato

I. Superior vena cava (SVC) obstruction

A. Epidemiology and etiology

1. **Malignant etiologies**
   a. **Lung cancer** (most often the small cell type) accounts for 80 percent of cases of SVC obstruction. SVC syndrome develops in about 5 percent of patients with lung cancer.
   b. **Malignant lymphoma** accounts for 15 percent of cases of SVC obstruction. Nearly all cases have high-grade histology. Hodgkin's disease or low-grade nodular lymphomas rarely cause SVC obstruction.
   c. **Other etiologies.** Metastatic disease (most commonly the result of breast adenocarcinoma or testicular seminoma), sarcomas, and other malignancies account for the small remainder of cases.

2. **Benign etiologies** (rare)
   a. **Mediastinal fibrosis**
      (1) Idiopathic
      (2) Histoplasmosis (in endemic regions), actinomycosis
      (3) Tuberculosis and pyogenic infections
      (4) Associated with Riedel's thyroiditis, retroperitoneal fibrosis, sclerosing cholangitis, and Peyronie's disease
      (5) Following radiation therapy to the mediastinum
   b. **Thrombosis of vena cava**
      (1) Idiopathic
      (2) Behçet's syndrome
      (3) Polycythemia vera, paroxysmal nocturnal hemoglobinuria
      (4) Long-term central venous catheterization, transvenous pacemakers, balloon-tipped pulmonary artery catheters, peritoneal venous shunting
   c. **Benign mediastinal tumors**
      (1) Aneurysm of aorta or right subclavian artery
      (2) Dermoid tumors, teratomas, thymoma
      (3) Goiter, sarcoidosis

B. Pathogenesis

1. **Obstruction and thrombosis.** Tumors growing in the mediastinum compress the thin-walled vena cava, leading to its collapse. Venous thrombosis because of stasis or vascular tumor invasion appears often to be responsible for acute onset SVC syndrome.

2. **Collateral circulation.** Vena cava obstruction caused by malignancy usually progresses too rapidly to develop sufficient collateral circulation, which might alleviate the syndrome. If the obstruction occurs above the azygous vein, the obstructed SVC could then drain into the azygous system. The azygous vein, however, is frequently obstructed by malignancy below its origin.

3. **Incompetent internal jugular vein valves,** a rare occurrence, is a dire emergency that is manifested by filling of these veins. Patients who present with this finding die within hours or days of massive cerebral edema unless treatment is immediately instituted.

C. Diagnosis. The diagnosis is usually based on the clinical findings and the pres-

ence of a mediastinal mass. *SVC syndrome rarely has to be treated before a histologic diagnosis is made.*

1. **Symptoms** of SVC syndrome are present for less than two weeks prior to diagnosis in 20 percent of patients and for more than eight weeks in 20 percent.
   a. The most common presenting symptoms are shortness of breath (50% of patients), neck and facial swelling (40%), and swelling of trunk and upper extremities (40%). Sensations of choking, fullness in the head, and headache are also frequent complaints. Chest pain, cough, lacrimation, dysphagia, hallucinations, and convulsions are less frequent.
   b. SVC obstruction may occasionally be **accompanied by spinal cord compression,** usually involving the lower cervical and upper thoracic vertebrae. The SVC syndrome consistently precedes spinal cord compression in these cases. The coexistence of these two complications should be seriously suspected in patients with upper back pain.
2. **Physical findings.** The most common physical findings are thoracic vein distention (65%), neck vein distention and edema of face (55%), tachypnea (40%), plethora of the face and cyanosis (15%), edema of upper extremities (10%), and paralysis of vocal cords and Horner's syndrome (3%). Veins in the antecubital fossae are distended and do not collapse when elevated above the level of the heart. Retinal veins may be dilated on funduscopic examination. Dullness to percussion over the sternum may be present. Laryngeal stridor and coma are grave signs.
3. **X-ray films**
   a. **Chest x-ray** film demonstrates a mass in more than 90 percent of patients. The mass is located in the right superior mediastinum in 75 percent of cases and is combined with a pulmonary lesion or hilar adenopathy in 50 percent. Pleural effusions are present in 25 percent of cases, nearly always on the right side.
   b. **Lung CT scan** findings have little bearing on management decisions and thus generally are not recommended.
   c. **Superior venacavograms** demonstrate the exact site of the SVC obstruction but this information is rarely needed for RT port localization. It shows compression or thrombosis without clinical evidence of a mass in less than 10 percent of patients with SVC syndrome. Superior venacavography would be useful in patients suspected of having incompetence of the internal jugular valves.
   d. **Radionuclide scintigrams** have less predictive value than contrast radiography and are not recommended.
   e. **MRI scans** of the cervical and upper thoracic vertebrae should be planned in patients with SVC syndrome and back pain, particularly in the presence of Horner's syndrome or vertebral destruction on plain films.
4. **Histologic diagnosis** is important for identifying malignancies that must be treated with cytotoxic agents to improve survival (e.g., lymphoma, small cell lung cancer). Once RT is started, tissue diagnosis becomes exceptionally difficult, if not impossible; biopsies of masses within radiation portals usually demonstrate nondescript necrosis shortly after irradiation is begun. Histologic diagnosis should be sought in all cases of SVC syndrome; the procedure selected should be associated with the least possible morbidity. Invasive biopsy procedures can be performed safely if there is no tracheal obstruction.
   a. **Cytology** of sputum is positive in 67 percent of patients and of pleural effusion fluid in nearly all patients with SVC syndrome.
   b. **Bone marrow biospy** is helpful in patients suspected of having small cell lung cancer or lymphoma, especially in patients with cytopenia or leukoerythroblastic blood smear.
   c. **Bronchoscopy** and bronchial brushings are positive in 60 percent of patients. Bronchoscopy and bronchial biopsy are rarely associated with serious complications when performed by experienced endoscopists.

d. **Lymph node biopsy** of palpable nodes below the level of obstruction is desirable; biopsy of supraclavicular lymph nodes is associated with a substantial risk of bleeding. Biopsy of *palpable* scalene nodes in patients with SVC syndrome reveals tumor in 85 percent of cases; biopsy of non-palpable, scalene nodes reveals tumors in only 30–40% of cases.

e. **Minithoracotomy** nearly always results in a definitive histologic diagnosis. Bleeding points are usually visualized and can be controlled. Limited anterior thoracotomy should be considered in patients with early SVC syndrome and without productive cough, diagnostic bone marrow evaluation, pleural effusion, or palpable lymphadenopathy.

f. **Mediastinoscopy** with biopsy is not recommended and may be contraindicated because of the high incidence of severe hemorrhage, neck edema, and failure of wound healing. When mediastinoscopy is performed on a highly selected group of patients, positive results are obtained in 80 percent of cases.

D. **Management.** There is little clinical or experimental evidence that unrelieved SVC syndrome is life-threatening. Emergency treatment is indicated only in the presence of cerebral dysfunction, decreased cardiac output, or upper airway obstruction.

1. **Supportive therapy.** Airway obstruction should be corrected and hypoxia treated by oxygen administration. Corticosteroids reduce brain edema and improve the obstruction by decreasing the inflammatory reaction associated with the tumor and early RT. Diuretics may be helpful.

2. **RT.** The total dose of RT varies between 3000 to 5000 cGy, depending on the general condition of the patient, severity of the symptoms, anatomic site, and histologic type of underlying malignant tumor. Symptoms may resolve dramatically even without establishment of patency of the SVC.

   a. **Response.** Improvement is evident within three to seven days for most patients. Complete response is observed in about 75 percent with lymphoma, and in 25 percent with lung cancer. Virtually all patients with lymphoma have at least a partial response, whereas about 15 percent of patients with lung cancer experience no real benefit from treatment.

   b. **Median survival** is about 10 months for small cell lung cancer, and 3 to 5 months for other types of lung cancer.

   c. **Local relapse** and recurrent SVC syndrome occur in 20 percent of patients with small cell lung cancer, and 10 percent of those with other types of lung cancer. SVC obstruction rarely recurs after RT for lymphoma.

3. **Chemotherapy** is indicated in patients with malignant lymphoma or with small cell lung cancer. Chemotherapy is invariably used in combination with RT in these conditions.

4. **Anticoagulants** and antifibrinolytic agents rarely result in disappearance of caval thrombosis.

5. **Surgical decompression** of acute SVC obstruction and incompetence of jugulosubclavian valves consists of reconstructing or bypassing the SVC using a spiral saphenous vein graft or left saphenoaxillary vein bypass, which can be done under local anesthesia.

6. **Management of SVC obstruction refractory to RT and chemotherapy** is fruitless; only symptomatic care is indicated. Dehydration techniques (such as vigorous administration of diuretics plus fluid restriction) and surgical bypass grafts add to the misery of patients without providing palliation.

II. **Pulmonary metastases**

A. **Epidemiology and etiology**

1. **Incidence.** The lungs are the most frequent site of distant metastases for nearly all malignant tumors except those arising in the gastrointestinal tract (see Table 1-2).

2. **Dissemination.** Malignant melanoma, bone and soft tissue sarcomas, trophoblastic tumors, and renal cell, colonic, and thyroid carcinomas tend to spread to vascular routes and usually produce discrete metastatic lung nod-

ules. Malignant tumors of the breast, pancreas, stomach, and liver may spread directly through lymphatic channels, involve mediastinal lymph nodes, and produce diffuse interstitial or lymphangitic infiltration, focal or segmental atelectasis, and pleural metastasis or effusion. Germ cell tumors and sarcomas may also involve the mediastinum.

   3. Metastatic sites
   a. **Endobronchial metastasis** is not uncommon in Hodgkin's disease, hypernephroma, and breast adenocarcinoma.
   b. **Solitary pulmonary metastasis** is relatively uncommon but can occur in patients with carcinoma of the breast, uterus, testis, kidney, or urinary bladder, or with malignant melanoma.
   c. **Isolated pulmonary metastasis.** Osteogenic sarcoma, soft tissue sarcoma, and testicular carcinoma are the tumors that are most likely to have lung metastases without involvement of other organs. Renal and uterine carcinomas may also produce isolated lung metastases. Colonic adenocarcinoma and malignant melanoma rarely have pulmonary metastases without other organ involvement as well.

B. Natural history and prognostic factors
   1. Nodular lung metastases have a highly variable course ranging from slow-growing cystic adenoid carcinoma to rapidly growing teratocarcinoma and osteogenic sarcoma.
   a. **Symptoms.** The majority of patients with solitary or multiple pulmonary metastases are asymptomatic; the presence of symptoms portends a poor prognosis.
   b. **Histology.** Well-differentiated tumors have a better prognosis than undifferentiated tumors. Melanoma has a worse prognosis than breast, colonic, or renal cell carcinoma.
   c. **Hilar lymphadenopathy** worsens the prognosis.
   d. **Tumor doubling time (TDT)** is calculated by plotting tumor volumes against time on semilogarithmic graph paper. Doubling times vary greatly among different patients with the same type of primary tumor; for example, the TDT in breast carcinoma varies from 11 to 800 days. All metastases in a patient do not grow at the same rate. Pulmonary metastases with a TDT of less than 40 days are associated with a distinctly poorer prognosis than those with a TDT of more than 60 days.
   e. **Disease-free interval (DFI)** is the time that elapses from resection of the primary tumor to detection of metastases. DFI would seem to be directly proportional to the TDT, but this is not invariably true; a tumor with a long DFI may have a short TDT. Patients with long DFIs have a better prognosis than patients with short DFIs.
   f. **Multiple metastases.** Multiple or bilateral pulmonary nodules usually, but not invariably, have a worse prognosis than single or unilateral metastases.
   g. **Amenability to chemotherapy.** Responsive tumors (e.g., trophoblastic and testicular tumors) obviously have a better prognosis.
   2. Lymphangitic pulmonary metastases are rapidly lethal. Median survival is less than two to three months for patients without effective treatment.
   3. Central pulmonary metastases. Malignant tumors that invade hilar or mediastinal structures may result in SVC obstruction, major airways obstruction, postobstructive pneumonia, and invasion of the pericardium, myocardium, or esophagus. Consequently, this type of pulmonary metastases is associated with a poorer prognosis than nodular metastases.

C. Differential diagnosis of solitary pulmonary nodules in patients with resected *extrapulmonary* malignant tumor can follow a statistical probability. Table 29-1 depicts the probability that a *solitary* pulmonary nodule is metastatic compared to the likelihood that it is a new primary lung cancer in patients with known malignant disease.

D. Diagnosis
   1. Symptoms and signs. Most patients with solitary pulmonary metastasis

Table 29-1. Solitary pulmonary nodule in patients with known malignant disease

	Most likely diagnosis of nodule	
Type of primary tumor	New primary lung cancer	Metastatic disease
By histologic type		
Squamous cell carcinoma	X	
Lymphoma	X	
Adenocarcinoma	50%	50%
Sarcoma		X
Melanoma		X
By primary site		
Head and neck	X	
Stomach	X	
Colon	15–50%	50%
Kidney, testicle	15–50%	50%
Urinary bladder, prostate	X	
Uterine cervix	X	
Breast	0–70%	30–100%

Key: X = most probable diagnosis.
Data summarizes the results reported in several series. Reports on solitary nodules in patients with breast cancer are conflicting.

are asymptomatic. Patients with multiple pulmonary metastases, central, hilar, or mediastinal metastatic involvement, or lymphangitic metastasis are more often asymptomatic with cough, chest pain, hemoptysis, or progressive dyspnea. Physical examination may be absolutely negative.

2. **X-ray studies.** No current imaging modality can distinguish a benign tumor from a malignant tumor or a primary tumor from a metastasis. Plain films do not detect lesions less than 1 cm in diameter. CT scans can detect nodules as small as 0.5 mm in diameter, however. About 50 percent of patients with lymphangitic lung metastases have normal chest x-ray films; the remainder of patients have interstitial changes that are indistinguishable from radiation fibrosis, chemotherapy-induced lung disease, or a variety of infectious processes.

3. **Sputum cytologies** are positive in only 5 to 20 percent of patients with nodular metastases.

4. **Pulmonary function studies.** *Lymphangitic* pulmonary metastases characteristically produce a restrictive defect with hypocapnia but without hypoxemia. Restrictive lung disease can be confirmed by finding impaired diffusing capacity for carbon monoxide DL_{co} and low residual and total lung volumes.

5. **Bronchoscopy.** Bronchoscopy with biopsy or brushings of the lesion identified on chest film may be necessary to establish the diagnosis in patients with a history of malignancy (especially with tumors that do not typically metastasize to the lung), pulmonary lesions appearing four to five years after the original tumor was resected, or lesions that are very likely a new primary lung carcinoma. Bronchoscopy is contraindicated in patients with bleeding tendency or in the presence of definitive evidence of carcinomatous recurrence at other organ sites.

E. **Management**
   1. **Nodular lung metastases**
      a. **Surgery.** Approximately 5 to 15 percent of patients with solid tumors

become candidates for resection of pulmonary metastases at some time during the course of their disease. The type of histology, number of lesions, and whether they are bilateral does not appear to contraindicate resection or adversely influence the survival if the selection criteria discussed here are adhered to. Bilateral pulmonary nodules can be resected in one operation using a median sternotomy. The five-year survival of patients who undergo successful resection is 30 percent. Resection (preferably wedge resection) is the recommended treatment of pulmonary metastases in patients who meet *all* of the following criteria:

(1) The patient's general medical condition and pulmonary function status are suitable for surgery.

(2) The primary tumor is under control (no evidence of local recurrence).

(3) Metastases are limited to the lung.

(4) Pulmonary metastases are encompassable and resectable.

(5) TDT is prolonged (more than 41–60 days).

(6) There is no other effective treatment.

   b. RT is useful for palliation of local complications of metastatic tumors, such as bronchial obstruction, vena cava obstruction, hemoptysis, or pain caused by tumor invasion of the chest wall.

   c. Chemotherapy or hormonal therapy has proved very useful in responsive tumors and is curative in trophoblastic and nonseminomatous testicular tumors.

  2. Lymphangitic lung metastases represent an emergent problem in diagnosis and management. Symptomatic relief of dyspnea can often be rapidly achieved with prednisone, 60 mg PO daily. Chemotherapy is effective in responsive tumors. Hormonal manipulation is usually ineffective or achieves a response too slowly to be helpful. Symptoms from refractory lymphangitic lung metastases may be palliated by low-dose lung irradiation.

  3. Terminal problems in patients with lung cancer such as hemoptysis and air hunger are discussed in Chap. 5, sec. **VI.C.**

III. Malignant pleural effusions

  A. Pathogenesis

    1. Etiology. Malignant tumors causing pleural effusions are as follows (in order of decreasing frequency): lung cancer (especially adenocarcinoma), breast carcinoma, ovarian carcinoma, gastric carcinoma, lymphoma, melanoma, and sarcoma.

    2. Types of malignant effusions. Pleural effusions are usually caused by direct involvement of the pleura by tumor ("peripheral") or by lymphatic or venous obstruction ("central"). Peripheral and central effusions may be combined. Central effusions, particularly those caused by lymphoma or nerve tissue tumors, may be chylous and have high triglyceride and low cholesterol concentrations. Atelectasis, pneumonia, and severe hypoalbuminemia that complicates malignancy may also cause pleural effusion.

  B. Natural history. Malignant pleural effusion is a sign of widespread metastases. The pleural space is progressively obliterated by fibrosis and serosal tumor. Patients with carcinomatous pleural effusions have a mean survival of 3 months from the time of diagnosis; 50 percent die by 1 month, 80 percent by 6 months, and 95 percent by 12 months.

  C. Differential diagnosis of pleural effusions is shown in Table 29-2. The differentiation of pleural fluid from pleural fibrosis or pulmonary consolidation may not be possible by physical examination or chest x-ray films. Aspiration of fluid may be difficult because of loculation. Ultrasonography is helpful for identifying and sampling small pockets of effusion.

    1. Symptoms and signs. Cough and dyspnea are the most common symptoms of pleural effusion. Dullness to percussion, decreased breath and voice sounds, decreased vocal fremitus and egophony are the classic physical findings. The trachea may be shifted to the side opposite the effusion. Skodaic resonance to percussion above a pleural effusion is due to air trapping above

Table 29-2. Pleural effusion characteristics

Etiology	Appearance	Cytology	Cell count*	Glucose ratio (effusion/serum)	LDH ratio (effusion/serum)	pH	Protein (gm/dl)	Specific gravity	Other
Cancer	Serosanguineous or bloody	Positive in 50%	Variable	0.5–.75	>0.6	< or >7.32	>3.0	>1.018	
Chylous effusion	Cloudy, yellow	Negative	Variable	>0.5	>0.6	>7.32	>3.0	>1.018	High triglycerides, low cholesterol
Postradiation effusion	Serosanguineous or serous	Dysplastic MC	Variable with atypical MC	>0.5	>0.6	>7.32	>3.0	>1.018	
Pulmonary infarction	Serosanguineous or bloody	Negative	RBC, some PMN	>0.5	>0.6	>7.32	>3.0	>1.018	
Heart failure	Serous	Negative	Few MC	>0.5	<0.6	>7.32	<2.5	<1.015	
Empyema	Purulent or cloudy	Negative	PMN	≤0.5	>0.6	<7.32	>3.0	>1.018	Cultures usually positive
Tuberculosis	Serofibrinous or cloudy-serous	Negative	>1000 mononuclear cells is suggestive	≤0.5	>0.6	>7.32	>3.0	>1.018	Cultures usually positive
Rheumatoid arthritis	Serous to cloudy	Negative	Variable	<0.5	>0.6	< or >7.32	>3.0	>1.018	

Key: LDH = lactic dehydrogenase; MC = mesothelial cells; RBC = erythrocytes; PMN = neutrophils.
*Eosinophilia is nonspecific in pleural effusions and can be associated with cancer, infection, trauma, pulmonary embolism, and even prior thoracentesis.

the compressed lung. Thickened pleura from fibrosis or neoplastic involvement also produce dullness and decreased vibration.

2. **Thoracentesis** should be performed in any patient with a suspected malignant, infectious, or empyematous pleural effusion. Pleural fluid should be assayed for LDH, protein, specific gravity, glucose, cell count, cytology, pH, and stained and cultured for bacteria (especially mycobacteria) and fungi. If the effusion appears chylous, triglyceride and fatty acid concentrations should be measured. Malignant effusions are usually exudative but may be transudative. Results of fluid examination frequently are nonspecific.

    a. **Discrimination.** Effusions are considered to be *exudates* rather than transudates if (1) *total protein* is greater than 3.0 gm/dl or the pleural-serum protein ratio is greater than 0.5, (2) LDH is greater than 225 IU or the pleural-serum LDH ratio is greater than 0.6, or (3) WBC is greater than 2500/μl (counts less than 2500/μl are not definitive).

    b. **Leukocyte counts** in malignant pleural fluid may be low or several thousand per cubic millimeter, and the predominant cells may be either polymorphonuclear leukocytes or lymphocytes.

    c. **CEA** levels greater than 12 ng/ml are probably pathognomonic of malignancy.

    d. **pH.** In patients with bronchopneumonia, a pH less than 7.2 at the initial thoracentesis may be predictive for the development of an empyema that has to be drained by tube. However, in patients with malignancy and collagen vascular disease, values less than 7.2 are not predictive.

3. **Pleural biopsy.** Pleural needle (Cope) biopsy is painful and should be done only if the diagnosis cannot be made by other means. Fiberoptic pleuroscopy may be very useful; the entire costal pleura and a good portion of the diaphragmatic and mediastinal pleura can be visualized, thus allowing direct biopsy of any pleural lesion.

D. **Management.** Respiratory insufficiency caused by malignant effusion may be relieved by removing 1000 ml of fluid by needle aspiration. The effusion should be later tapped dry if possible. In about 10 percent of patients, no recurrence of the effusion develops after a single evacuation. In the majority of cases, the effusion recurs, and more definitive methods of therapy are required.

1. **Chemotherapy.** Pleural effusion secondary to metastatic tumors that are sensitive to chemotherapy (lymphoma, breast or ovarian carcinoma) should be treated with appropriate combinations of agents. The results may be dramatic if the effusion presented early in the disease before resistance to the chemotherapeutic drugs developed. Pleural effusions that occur in the late or terminal stage are usually resistant to chemotherapy.

2. **RT.** Central pleural effusions are best treated with RT to the central or mediastinal regions.

3. **Pleurodesis** (visceroparietal pleural symphysis) is accomplished with tube thoracostomy.

    a. **Patient selection.** Pleurodesis should be performed in patients who meet the following conditions:

        (1) The malignant pleural effusion is "peripheral" and does not respond to appropriate chemotherapeutic combinations.

        (2) The pleural effusion recurs after repeated needle aspirations (2–3 times) or rapidly reaccumulates (within a few days).

        (3) The patient's symptoms (shortness of breath) are caused by the pleural effusion and not by lymphangitic or intrapulmonary metastasis (i.e., symptoms improve after aspiration of fluid).

        (4) The patient's life expectancy is estimated to be more than one month (pleurodesis should not be done in terminally ill patients).

        (5) The pleural effusion is peripheral and has positive cytology and no evidence of central mediastinal mass lesion.

    b. **Drainage procedure**

        (1) The chest tube is inserted in the most dependent location, preferably at the anterior axillary line. The pleural fluid is first allowed to drain

Table 29-3. Drugs used for pleural and pericardial instillation

Drug	Dosage
Bleomycin	1 unit/kg (40 units maximum in the elderly)
Cisplatin	100 mg/m^2 (pleural)
Cytarabine	1200 mg (pleural)
Doxorubicin	30 mg
Doxycycline	500 mg (may be repeated)
5-Fluorouracil	750–1000 mg
Thiotepa	30–45 mg
^{32}Phosphorus	5 mCi (pericardial)
Talc, dry powder or 50-ml suspensions	1–2 gm (pericardial) 2–6 gm (pleural)

through a water-seal gravity drainage system. Negative suction may be later applied to ensure completeness of drainage.

   (2) When less than 50 ml drains in 24 hours, a chest x-ray is obtained to assess the amount of residual fluid and the extent of reexpansion of the underlying lung.

   (3) The evacuation of pleural fluid may take one to three days. The expansion of the underlying lung is necessary to bring the visceral and parietal pleural surfaces in close proximity in preparation for symphysis. Injecting sclerosing agents without apposition of the pleural surfaces is ineffective and may result in loculation.

  c. Instilling sclerosing agents

   (1) The chest tube is first cross-clamped and is cleaned with antiseptic solution. Morphine is given to prevent pain.

   (2) The sclerosing agent in 30 ml of normal saline is injected into the chest tube, which is then flushed with 50 ml of saline. Changing the patient's position to distribute the agent throughout the pleural space is not necessary except with nitrogen mustard, which is rarely used.

   (3) The chest tube should remain clamped for six hours for all other drugs. The pleural fluid is then allowed to drain, preferably with negative suction, until less than 50 ml drains in 24 hours.

   (4) After a drug has been instilled, there may be a great deal of drainage because of pleural weeping from drug irritation. A nonfunctioning or blocked tube may produce complications (pain, atelectasis, and infection) and should be removed.

  d. Choice of sclerosing agents. Drugs and doses used for the treatment of malignant effusions are shown in Table 29-3. These agents are successful in 70 to 85 percent of cases.

   (1) Doxycycline is the preferred agent from the viewpoints of effectiveness, cost, and toxicity.

   (2) Antineoplastic agents act by causing both tumor lysis and irritation of the pleural surfaces. These drugs are well absorbed from the pleural cavity and cause systemic effects. Although bleomycin is frequently used, it is substantially more expensive and appears to be less effective than doxycycline.

   (3) Other agents

   (a) Radioactive isotopes (^{198}Au and ^{32}P) are not recommended for malignant pleural effusions because isolation and disposal of radioactive fluid pose problems.

(b) Talcum powder instillation may be the most effective method, especially if good insufflation (very impractical with a chest tube) over the entire pleural surfaces can be accomplished. Video-assisted thoracoscopy with talc poudrage provides excellent results in skilled hands, but has disadvantages such as the need for general anesthesia and the expense of thoracoscopy.

e. Complications of pleural sclerosis .

  (1) Pneumothorax. Suction may be applied to the chest bottles to reexpand the lung if the chest tube is not blocked. If the chest tube is obliterated (no fluid oscillation), insertion of a new chest tube is indicated.

  (2) Cough may result from reexpansion of an atelectatic lung after the compressing pleural fluid is removed. This symptom is self-limited and may be advantageous because it further clears atelectasis.

  (3) Chest pain may be secondary to the chest tube insertion or the instillation of drugs. Pain usually dissipates within five days.

  (4) Fever may be caused by atelectasis or pneumonitis or by the sclerosing agent.

  (5) Loculation of fluid may be caused by inadequate drainage or the instillation of sclerosing agents before the lung has completely reexpanded. Injection of radiopaque material (Hypaque) into the pleural space followed by upright and lateral decubitus chest films may confirm this problem. Trying to break the loculation by tube manipulation is not recommended.

  (6) Empyema and pleurocutaneous draining sinus may occur when tumor seeds the chest tube site. Empyema may be the result of either contamination or bronchopleural communication.

4. Pleurectomy is a hazardous, bloody, major operative procedure that is rarely indicated.

IV. Other pulmonary complications

A. Chemotherapy lung

1. Etiology

a. Associated drugs. Bleomycin, methotrexate, cytarabine, nitrosoureas, mitomycin C, and busulfan are well-documented causes of pulmonary toxicity (Table 29-4). The pathogenesis of these reactions is unknown.

b. Association with RT. Cytotoxic drugs and thoracic RT, administered concomitantly or sequentially, may produce pulmonary toxicity. The interaction of RT with bleomycin has been particularly well documented in patients with testicular carcinoma. Severe pulmonary irradiation reactions have been associated with concurrent Adriamycin therapy, prior busulfan therapy, and concurrent or prior actinomycin D therapy; Adriamycin and actinomycin D have not been associated with pulmonary disease in the absence of RT.

2. Differential diagnosis.
Chemotherapy lung has no characteristic radiographic pattern, may be associated with a normal chest x-ray film, and is usually diffuse. Hilar or mediastinal lymphadenopathy or a purely segmental or lobar pattern should make other diagnostic possibilities more likely. Establishing the diagnosis of drug pulmonary toxicity is often difficult because cancer patients may also have pulmonary abnormalities caused by

a. Chronic lung disease

b. Opportunistic pulmonary infection

c. Lymphangitic lung metastases

d. RT of the thorax

e. Pulmonary hemorrhage, collagen disease, vasculitis, or granulomatous angiitis

f. Pulmonary toxicity from oxygen therapy

g. Pulmonary toxicity from non-antineoplastic drugs (heparin, warfarin sodium, aspirin, phenylbutazone, chlorpropamide, hydrochlorothiazide,

Table 29-4. Chemotherapy lung

Drug[a]	Incidence	Dose-dependent	Onset after therapy	Reaction type[b]	Reversibility (Steroids[c])	Risk factors[d]
Bleomycin	1–10%	Yes	Immediate to-months	A, BO, F, H	Possible (0)	Age >70, RT, CT, O_2, Renal insufficiency
Busulfan	1–10%	Yes	At least 1 yr (usually 4 yr)	F	Occasional (+)	RT, CT
Carmustine (BCNU)	2–30%	Yes	2 mo to 17 yr	A, F	Rare (0)	Pre-existing lung disease, Younger age, RT, CT
Cytarabine	20%	Yes	2 to 21 days (usually <6 days)	E	— (?)	Total dose
Mitomycin C	3–10%	Possible	2 to 6 wk	A, F	50% recover partially (++)	RT, CT, FA, O_2
Methotrexate	Occasional	No	10 days to 5 yr	E, F, H, P	Common (++)	CT, FA, Steroid tapering, Previous adrenalectomy
Chlorambucil	Rare	Possible	6 to 9 mo	A, F	Occasional (+)	CT
Cyclophosphamide	Rare	Possible	3 wk to 3 yr	E, F, H	Common (++)	CT, RT (?)
Procarbazine	Rare	No	2 to 6 mo	H	Possible (0)	

[a]Cases of chemotherapy lung have also been rarely associated with azathioprine, lomustine (CCNU), melphalan, mercaptopurine, nitrogen mustard, teniposide (VM-26), vinblastine, vindesine, and zinostatin. This complication occurs more frequently when vinblastine or vindesine is given with mitomycin C.
[b]A = acute pneumonitis; B = bronchospasm; BO = bronchiolitis obliterans; E = pulmonary edema; F = pulmonary fibrosis; H = hypersensitivity pneumonitis; P = pleuritis.
[c]Corticosteroid therapy: 0 = no or questionable value; + = occasionally helpful; ++ = may be helpful.
[d]CT = combination chemotherapy regimens; RT = radiation therapy; FA = frequency of administration; O_2 = oxygen administration.

carbamazepine; the penicillins, sulfonamides, erythromycins, or tetracyclines; and contrast dyes, such as during lymphangiography)

h. Pulmonary toxicity from blood component therapy

i. Graft-versus-host disease

3. **Diagnosis.** Drug-induced pulmonary toxicity may be insidious or acute in onset, and it rarely develops after the drugs have been discontinued. Clinical features are similar regardless of the specific drug involved.

   a. Symptoms. Dry cough and dyspnea are prominent.

   b. Signs. Fever, tachypnea, and rales are common. Incomplete or asymmetric chest expansion (respiratory lag) may be an early finding. Skin eruptions are common with methotrexate pulmonary toxicity.

   c. WBC. Eosinophilia occurs if methotrexate or procarbazine is the cause.

   d. Chest x-ray films may be normal. The most typical abnormalities are bibasilar linear densities. Nodular, interstitial, alveolar, and mixed patterns also occur. Pleural effusions are distinctly uncommon.

   e. Pulmonary function tests usually show hypoxemia, a decreased DL_{co}, and a restrictive ventilatory defect (decreased vital and total lung capacities).

   f. Lung biopsy may be necessary. Histology reveals acute and organizing interstitial pneumonia with hyaline membranes, atypical epithelial desquamation, and nodular inflammation or fibrosis. Busulfan lung toxicity may result in atypical, malignant-appearing cells on sputum cytology.

4. **Management.** Prospective measurement of pulmonary function has not clearly decreased the incidence or severity of drug toxicity problems. The drugs should be discontinued in any patient who develops symptoms, signs, or abnormalities in pulmonary function tests or chest x-ray films that suggest drug toxicity. Pulmonary toxicity may progress even after the drug is stopped. Treatment is mostly for control of symptoms. Administration of glucocorticoids has not been shown to be beneficial except possibly for shortening the course of toxicity for some drugs.

B. Radiation pneumonitis

1. **Acute radiation pneumonitis.** An acute alveolar infiltrate can develop 3 to 10 weeks after the completion of RT. Withdrawal of corticosteroids while the lungs are being irradiated or soon thereafter may precipitate this process. Pneumonitis is more frequent the higher the radiation dose and the greater the portal size.

   a. Manifestations. The patient is usually asymptomatic although a dry cough, dyspnea, fever, and leukocytosis may be present. Symptoms usually subside within two weeks. On x-ray film the infiltrate is the shape of the RT portal, which is usually sharply outlined. Pneumonitis may progress to interstitial fibrosis.

   b. Management is symptomatic, particularly with nonsteroidal antiinflammatory agents. Prednisone, 20 mg t.i.d. PO, may be effective. Antibiotics are used for superimposed infections.

2. **Pulmonary interstitial fibrosis** may appear as early as four months after RT. Patients may develop restrictive lung disease, alveolar-capillary block, or cor pulmonale. Corticosteroids have an uncertain role in preventing progression of fibrosis.

C. Pulmonary tumor thrombotic microangiopathy with pulmonary hypertension is characterized by fibrocellular intimal proliferation of small pulmonary arteries and arterioles in patients with metastatic carcinoma, particularly adenocarcinoma. This condition develops when microscopic tumor cell embolism induces both local activation of coagulation and fibrocellular proliferation of intima, but does not occlude the affected vessels. The increased vascular resistance results in pulmonary hypertension. This complication should be considered in the differential diagnosis in patients with known carcinoma who develop acute or subacute cor pulmonale.

D. Pulmonary infections are discussed in Chapter 35, sec. **II.A.**

V. Pericardial and myocardial metastases

A. Epidemiology and etiology

1. Malignant pericardial effusion is usually a preterminal event. Approximately 10 to 15 percent of patients dying of carcinoma have metastases in the heart or pericardium at autopsy. The epicardium is involved in 75 percent of metastatic lesions, and pericardial effusions are associated with 35 percent of epicardial metastases.

2. Carcinomas of the lung and breast constitute about 75 percent of all cases of malignant pericardial effusion. Melanoma, leukemia, and lymphoma also commonly affect the heart. Pericardial effusion, which is usually insignificant, occurs in 20 percent of patients with non-Hodgkin's lymphoma at the time of presentation.

B. Natural history

1. Most myocardial and pericardial metastases are clinically silent; approximately two-thirds are not diagnosed antemortem. Prognosis appears to be related to tumor type.

2. Pericardial metastases produce symptoms by causing pericardial effusion with tamponade, constrictive pericarditis, or arrhythmias.

3. Myocardial metastases produce symptoms by causing conduction blocks and arrhythmias. Metastases infrequently cause myocardial rupture, valvular disease, or emboli to other organs.

C. Diagnosis of pericardial effusion. Clinical manifestations arise from decreased cardiac output and venous congestion.

1. **Symptoms.** Frequently, pericardial tamponade develops slowly, and symptoms resemble those of congestive heart failure.

2. **Signs of pericardial tamponade**
   a. Neck vein distention that increases on inspiration (Kussmaul's sign)
   b. A fall in systolic pressure of more than 10 mm Hg at the end of inspiration (pulsus paradoxus)
   c. Distant heart sounds
   d. Localized dullness and tubular breath sounds at the angle of the left scapula, caused by compression of the left lung (Ewart's sign)
   e. Pulmonary rales, hepatosplenomegaly, ascites

3. **Differential diagnosis.** The differential diagnosis of malignant pericardial effusion includes SVC syndrome, radiation pericarditis, and a variety of nonmalignant causes of pericarditis, including myocardial infarction, connective tissue disorders, acute and chronic infections, uremia, myxedema, trauma, and drugs (hydralazine, procainamide).

4. **Diagnostic studies**
   a. **Chest film** may show enlargement of the cardiac silhouette or a "water bottle" configuration.
   b. **ECG** abnormalities are generally not specific. Total electrical alternans involving both the P wave and QRS complex is almost pathognomonic of pericardial tamponade. Alternans of only the QRS complex is suggestive of but not specific for cardiac tamponade.
   c. **Echocardiography** is the most effective method of making the diagnosis. False-positive echocardiograms may be secondary to tumor infiltration or encasement of the heart rather than fluid accumulation.
   d. **Cardiac catheterization.** The diagnosis of pericardial fluid or thickening may be confirmed by cardiac catheterization or angiocardiography
   e. **Pericardiocentesis.** A small catheter should be introduced through the needle into the pericardial sac and attached to water-seal gravity drainage to prevent the recurrence of effusion until the final diagnosis is made and definitive therapy can be delivered.
   f. **Fluid analysis.** Malignant pericardial fluids are usually exudative and often hemorrhagic. Fluid analysis and interpretation are the same as

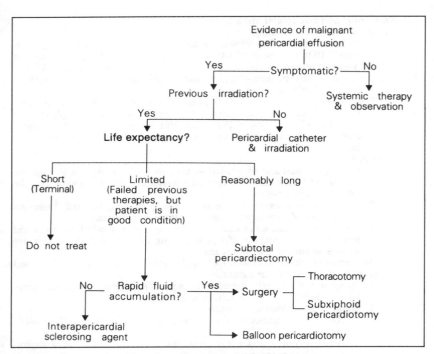

Fig. 29-1. Therapeutic options for malignant pericardial effusions.

for pleural effusions (see sec. **III.C.3**). Cytologic findings may be difficult to interpret in patients who have received RT. Negative cytologic results do not exclude the diagnosis of malignant effusion (e.g., cytologic findings are often negative in patients with lymphoma).

D. **Management.** Selection of therapeutic modalities for malignant pericardial effusions is diagrammed in Figure 29-1.

1. **RT.** The treatment of choice for malignant pericardial effusion appears to be RT. Overall response rates are reported to be 60 percent with a dose of 3500 cGy given in three to four weeks. Short- and long-term control of the effusion may result, but many radiotherapists are pessimistic.

2. **Pericardiocentesis and catheter drainage.** Conservative treatment of malignant pericardial effusion using pericardiocentesis or short-term catheter drainage as needed (with or without instillation of intrapericardial chemotherapeutic drugs) may be effective treatment for some patients. Serious complications of pericardial aspiration through a left parasternal or xiphosternal approach are rare, but they include laceration of the internal mammary vessels, lung, coronary vessels, right ventricle, liver, or stomach, and (very rarely) a dramatic shocklike reaction. Emergency subxiphoid pericardial decompression under local anesthesia, however, is reported to be associated with no operative mortality.

3. **Sclerosing agents.** Chemotherapeutic drugs or doxycycline may be instilled intrapericardially to include pericardial sclerosis and obliterate the pericardial space in patients with slowly recurrent effusions. The dose and method of administration of intrapericardial drugs are similar to those for malignant pleural effusion (see Table 29-3). Drug instillation should be performed with ECG monitoring and an IV line in place in case arrhythmia develops.

4. **Pericardiectomy.** The length of hospital stay for any surgical procedure represents a major portion of the life expectancy of these patients. Surgery should be reserved for patients with (1) rapidly accumulating pericardial effusions that cannot be controlled conservatively and (2) radiation-induced constrictive pericarditis.

   a. **Subtotal pericardiectomy** (resection of entire pericardium anterior to the phrenic nerves) is the surgical procedure of choice in patients whose expected survival is reasonably long. Subtotal pericardiectomy is superior to the pericardiopleural window, which usually seals off shortly after surgery.

   b. **Alternative interventions for pericardial tamponade**

      (1) **Percutaneous balloon pericardiotomy,** which recently proved successful in relieving the cardiac tamponade in more than 90 percent of cases.

      (2) **Subxiphoid pericardiotomy,** which is safe and effective.

      (3) **Laparoscopic** pericardial fenestration and pericardioperitoneostomy, which are effective and enable patients to be discharged within 24 hours.

5. **Myocardial metastases.** Patients with disseminated malignancy and new, unexplained cardiac arrhythmias that are refractory to treatment should be considered for cardiac irradiation, particularly if there is known mediastinal or pericardial involvement

VI. Other cardiac complications

A. **Nonbacterial thrombotic endocarditis** is most common in patients with mucinous adenocarcinoma of the lung, stomach, or ovary, but it can complicate any systemic cancer. Fibrin vegetations appear on heart valves that are otherwise normal. Heart murmurs and other stigmata of bacterial endocarditis usually are not present. Endocarditis is manifested by embolic peripheral or cerebral vascular occlusions that may become clinically apparent as acute peripheral arterial insufficiency, progressive encephalopathy, acute focal neurologic defects suggesting a stroke, or acute multifocal neurologic disease. Treatment with anticoagulants or antiplatelet drugs may be reasonable in some cases, but the results of such treatment are not encouraging.

B. **Bacterial endocarditis** is not more frequent in cancer patients than in the general population.

C. **Radiation pericarditis and pancarditis**

   1. **Acute pancarditis or pericarditis** is dependent on the volume of heart irradiated and the radiation dose. This complication develops in about 3 percent of patients who have received more than 4000 cGy to the internal mammary chain for breast carcinoma or to the mantle for Hodgkin's disease. Pancarditis or pericarditis can occur weeks, or even years, after treatment is completed.

      a. **Manifestations.** Symptoms and signs resemble acute or chronic pericarditis that have other etiologies: pleuritic chest pain, pericardial friction rub, ECG abnormalities, and enlargement of the cardiac silhouette on x-ray films. Most patients, however, are asymptomatic. Cytologic findings from irradiated mesothelium may suggest malignancy and obfuscate the cause of the effusion.

      b. **Management.** Treatment in the acute phase includes giving corticosteroids and antipyretics and doing pericardiocentesis. The disease is usually self-limiting, but may become chronic. In the chronic phase, a pericardial window for symptomatic effusions or pericardiectomy for constrictive pericarditis may become necessary.

   2. **Myocardiopathy** is a rare sequela of large doses of irradiation to the heart, particularly with concomitant or prior use of Adriamycin. Refractory heart failure may result.

D. **Anthracycline-induced cardiomyopathy.** A major dose-limiting toxicity of the anthracyclines (Adriamycin and daunorubicin) is cardiomyopathy. Proposed mechanisms of cardiac toxicity involve the generation of free radicals, which damages cell membranes through peroxidation of membrane lipids, the binding of drug to a variety of membrane sites (including cardiolipin and spectrim), which can cause alterations in membrane structure and ion transport, and the selective inhibition of cardiac muscle gene expression.

1. **Types of cardiac toxicity**
    a. **Acute myocardiopathy** is not related to total dose. Manifestations include
        (1) Arrhythmias, especially sinus tachycardia, which do not correlate with subsequent development of chronic cardiomyopathy.
        (2) Nonspecific ST-T wave changes.
        (3) Pericardial and pleural effusions (after 1–2 days).
        (4) Clinically inapparent decrease in left ventricular ejection fraction. Reversible congestive heart failure may develop after the first dose.
        (5) "Myocarditis-pericarditis syndome." Decreased myocardial function can be persistent in these patients.
        (6) Rarely, sudden death or myocardial infarction.
    b. **Chronic myocardiopathy** is related to the total dose and method of administration. The overall incidence of congestive heart failure related to Adriamycin use is about 1 to 2 percent. The incidence is less than 1 percent for total dose less than 500 mg/m^2, 10 percent for 500 to 600 mg/m^2, and 30 percent for more than 600 mg/m^2. The heart becomes dilated and may contain mural thrombi. Microscopy is nonspecific and reveals interstitial edema, cytoplasmic vacuolization, muscle fiber degeneration, and deformed mitochondria. Manifestations include:
        (1) Subclinical left ventricular dysfunction
        (2) Overt congestive heart failure, which usually develops within two months of the last dose but can occur six months to seven years later
2. **Evaluation of cardiac injury.** Symptoms, physical findings, and ECG abnormalities (reduction of QRS voltage by 30%) occur too late to be helpful. Abnormalities of systolic time intervals (determined by phonocardiograms) and abnormal ejection fractions (determined by echocardiograms) are associated with too many false-positive and false-negative results and occur too late to be helpful.
    a. **Endomyocardial biopsy** is the most specific method for determining anthracycline cardiotoxicity (short of waiting for overt heart failure). Semiquantitative scoring systems reveal a linear correlation of abnormalities with cumulative dose. This technique can be safely performed in an outpatient setting. However, only specially trained personnel can perform the biopsies and interpret the results.
    b. **Radionuclide angiography** with calculation of the ejection fraction (REF) is the only noninvasive method that has shown reasonable correlation with endomyocardial biopsy results.
3. **Prevention.** The development of cardiac toxicity is related to peak serum levels of Adriamycin. Weekly administration (20 mg/m^2) is associated with a lower incidence of cardiotoxicity when compared with monthly administration (60 mg/m^2). Continuous infusion over 24 to 96 hours through a central venous catheter also is less cardiotoxic than bolus administration; cumulative dosages much greater than 500 mg/m^2 have been administered by this technique without significant cardiac toxicity. Prophylaxis with cardiac glycosides, free-radical scavengers (tocopherol and acetylcysteine), histamine blockers, and catecholamine blockers is investigational.
4. **Recommendations**
    a. Recognize patients who are at high risk of developing cardiac toxicity; risk factors are the following:
        (1) Age greater than 70 years
        (2) Preexisting heart disease or hypertension
        (3) Prior chest or mediastinal RT (especially if more than 4000 cGy)
        (4) Concurrent treatment with cyclophosphamide or mitomycin C
    b. Limit the total cumulative dose of Adriamycin to 450 to 500 mg/m^2.

   c. Consider altering the schedule of administration (weekly or infusion).

   d. If one or more risk factors **(a)** are present, measure REF before starting treatment and after every 100 mg of Adriamycin. Discontinue the drug if the REF is less than 45 percent of predicted value or if REF decreases by 15 percent on subsequent measurements.

   e. If expertise in endomyocardial biopsy and interpretation are available, interpret abnormal REFs in the light of biopsy results.

   f. Discontinue the drug at the first sign of an unexplained tachycardia, cough, dyspnea, or S_3 gallop. Manifestations of congestive heart failure often do respond to therapy with cardiac glycosides and diuretics, but there are still a large number of patients with refractory symptoms.

E. Other chemotherapy-induced cardiotoxicity

   1. 5-Fluorouracil can cause cardiac ischemia with angina, hypotension, or congestive heart failure. The incidence of such toxicity is uncertain, but has been reported to occur in 2 to 8 percent of patients, particularly when the drug is given by continuous IV infusion in patients with a prior history of cardiac disease. These manifestations are reversible when the drug is stopped; patients respond well to conventional cardiac treatments.

   2. Cyclophosphamide, when given in very high doses (e.g., preparation for BMT), can cause hemorrhagic myocarditis.

   3. Taxol commonly results in asymptomatic bradycardia but can also occasionally cause conduction defects, cardiac ischemia, and ventricular tachycardia.

   4. α-IFN has been associated with reversible cardiac dysfunction.

Selected Reading

Campbell, P. T., et al. Subxiphoid pericardiotomy in the diagnosis and management of large pericardial effusions associated with malignancy. *Chest* 101:938, 1992.

Carlson, R. W. Reducing the cardiotoxicity of the anthracyclines. *Oncology* 6:95, 1992.

Comis, R. L. Detecting bleomycin toxicity: a continued conundrum. *J. Clin. Oncol.* 8:765, 1990.

Klatt, E. C., and Heitz, D. R. Cardiac metastases. *Cancer* 65:1456, 1990.

Krause, T. J., Margiotta, M. and Chandler, J. J. Pericardio-peritoneal window for malignant pericardial effusion. *Surg. Gynecol. Obstet.* 172:487, 1991.

Miles, D. W., and Knight, R. K. Diagnosis and management of malignant pleural effusion. *Cancer Treat. Rev.* 19:151, 1993.

Robbin, N. C., et al. The syndrome of 5-fluorouracil cardiotoxicity. *Cancer* 71:493, 1993.

Tabbarah, H. J., and Casciato, D. A. Is resection of pulmonary metastases really justified? In T. X. O'Connell (ed.), *Surgical Oncology: Controversies in Cancer Treatment.* Boston: G. K. Hall, 1981. Pp. 216–232.

Twohig, K. J., and Matthay, R. A. Pulmonary effects of cytotoxic agents other than bleomycin. *Clin. Chest Med.* 11:31, 1990.

Walker-Renard, P. B., et al. Chemical pleurodesis for malignant pleural effusions. *Ann. Intern. Med.* 120:56, 1994.

Ziskind, A. A., et al. Percutaneous balloon pericardiotomy for the treatment of cardiac tamponade and large pericardial effusions: description of technique and report of the first 50 cases. *J. Am. Coll. Cardiol.* 21:1, 1993.

30 Abdominal Complications

Hassan J. Tabbarah and
Barry B. Lowitz

I. GI bleeding

A. Etiology

1. **Benign causes.** GI bleeding in patients with active cancer is usually caused by erosive gastritis, peptic ulcer disease, esophageal or gastric varices or other benign diseases, and only 20 percent is caused by direct tumor bleeding. Hemorrhage is often related to the use of aspirin or glucocorticoids.

2. **Malignant causes.** Most primary GI cancers produce slow blood loss; massive hemorrhage is not common. Melanomas and leiomyosarcomas involving the GI tract, on the other hand, are likely to result in extensive hemorrhage. Blood or clots from ostomies or mucous fistulae usually signify recurrent cancer.

B. Management

1. **Benign conditions causing GI bleeding** in patients with advanced cancer should be managed the same as for patients without cancer with the following exceptions:

   a. Surgery should not be undertaken in patients who have a life expectancy of less than two months even if the bleeding is correctable.

   b. Nonsurgical therapy to control benign causes of bleeding is preferred for patients who have advanced cancer and a prognosis of more than two months even if surgery is usually indicated. However, surgery should generally be considered for large gastric peptic ulcers or recurrent peptic ulcer bleeding.

2. **Patients with persistent GI bleeding from unresectable tumors** are managed with RT. Resection of local tumor recurrences may be used if permitted by the patient's general condition.

II. Bowel obstruction

A. Etiology.
Bowel obstruction in patients with a history of cancer is due to the original tumor or its metastases in 70 percent of cases. Approximately 20 percent of patients have a benign cause of obstruction and 10 percent have a new, and often resectable, primary lesion. Bowel obstruction caused by malignancy occurs most often as a complication of ovarian carcinoma or GI tumors.

1. **Mechanisms** of bowel obstruction in malignancy

   a. External pressure on the intestine

   b. Obstructing masses in the bowel lumen

   c. Invasion of the intestine's neural plexus causing localized or diffuse ileus clinically indistinguishable from mechanical obstruction

   d. Intussusception with certain tumors, notably melanoma

   e. Pseudo-obstruction as a paraneoplastic syndrome (see sec. **VIII.B**).

2. **Differential diagnosis.** Diagnostic considerations in cancer patients include

   a. **Vinca alkaloid neurotoxicity** may produce constipation. Particularly in elderly patients, paralytic ileus or decreased bowel tone may lead to high fecal impaction with bowel obstruction. Impaction is better prevented than treated (see Chap. 5, sec. **IV.A**).

  b. Radiation injury of small bowel (see sec. **VI.C**) may be seen on small
  bowel x-ray films as mucosal effacement, ulcers, rigidity, narrowing,
  adhesions, bowel wall thickening, and bowel dilatation.
  c. Diverticulitis may produce tightly narrowed areas in the distal colon
  that are often radiologically indistinguishable from constricting carcinoma. In the absence of metastatic disease elsewhere, these lesions must
  be resected regardless of coexistent tumor.
  d. Other nonmalignant causes of ileus and obstruction include adhesions, hernia, inflammatory bowel disease, volvulus, spontaneous intussusception, acute pancreatitis, and bowel infarction.
B. Management of bowel obstruction caused by cancer
  1. Decompression. Patients with evidence of intestinal obstruction should
  have decompression by placement of a nasogastric tube and intermittent
  suction. The eventual outcome does not depend on whether a gastric or long
  (Miller-Abbot) tube is used.
  2. Operative intervention
    a. A history of cancer or even the presence of active tumor is not necessarily
    a contraindication to surgery. Approximately 75 percent of patients with
    a bowel obstruction resume normal bowel function that is maintained
    until death in 45 percent of patients. About 25 percent of these patients
    do not experience some improvement of symptoms with surgery. About
    30 percent of patients with a history of cancer are found to have a new
    disease or new primary cancer.
    b. Surgical intervention should be considered if the obstruction does not
    improve after four to five days of decompression and if the following
    conditions are met:
      (1) The patient's medical condition makes the operative risk low.
      (2) The patient does not have malignant ascites.
      (3) The patient's life expectancy is greater than two months if the bowel
      obstruction were relieved.
      (4) The patient underwent no more than one surgical intervention for
      obstruction during the previous year and was significantly palliated
      by that operation for more than four months.
      (5) The most recent operative intervention revealed no evidence of tu-
      mor in the abdomen and did not disclose multiple or widespread
      tumor sites causing obstruction.
    c. End-stage disease and poor performance status are obvious contraindica-
    tions to surgery.
  3. Other modalities of management
    a. Chemotherapy may be tried in patients with obstruction caused by car-
    cinomatosis. Specific regimens depend on the type of primary tumor.
    b. RT to relieve bowel obstruction may be beneficial in patients who have
    peritoneal carcinomatosis from ovarian carcinoma or extensive abdomi-
    nal lymphoma that is resistant to chemotherapy. Abdominal irradiation
    produces severe side effects and is not recommended for other types of
    malignant bowel obstruction.
    **c. Treatment of preterminal patients with refractory obstruction caused
    by cancer**
      (1) Nasogastric suction is used to alleviate abdominal pain. Intravenous
      fluids are given to maintain hydration.
      (2) In some situations, the abdominal pain is treated with appropriate
      analgesics, and the patient is allowed to eat whatever he or she
      wants and then vomits as necessary. The risk of intestinal rupture
      is not a consideration in terminal situations.
      (3) Parenteral hyperalimentation only prolongs misery in these patients
      and should not be given.
III. Metastases to the liver and biliary tract
  A. Incidence and pathology
    1. Liver. The liver is a common site of metastases (see Table 1-2). Liver metas-

tases account for over 50 percent of the deaths in certain malignancies, such as colorectal cancer.

   a. The relative risks of tumor metastasizing to the liver during the course of advanced disease are as follows:

   (1) Liver commonly involved: GI tract cancers (including carcinoids, pancreatic adenocarcinoma, and islet cell tumors), lung cancer (especially small cell), breast cancer, choriocarcinoma, melanoma, lymphomas, and leukemias

   (2) Liver occasionally involved: carcinoma of the distal esophagus, kidney, prostate, endometrium, adrenal gland, and thyroid; testicular cancers, thymoma; angiosarcoma

   (3) Liver rarely involved: carcinoma of the proximal esophagus, ovary, and skin; plasma cell myeloma; most sarcomas

   b. Types of metastases

   (1) Nodular metastases are the most common type and occur with all tumors capable of metastasizing to the liver, including lymphoma.

   (2) Diffuse metastases most frequently occur with lymphomas. Breast cancer, small cell lung cancer, poorly differentiated GI tumors, and, rarely, other types of tumors can also produce diffuse metastases.

   2. Extrahepatic biliary obstruction can occur from lymph node metastases in the porta hepatis, particularly from GI cancers and lung cancers (especially small cell type).

B. Natural history. The clinical course of liver metastases depends on the tumor's behavior and responsiveness to chemotherapy. In patients with solid tumors, death commonly occurs within six months with nodular metastases and more rapidly with diffuse metastases. A liver that appreciably increases in size in less than eight weeks is typical in small cell lung cancer and high-grade lymphoma; both of these tumors respond well to treatment. Rapid liver enlargement in patients with other tumor types is less common.

C. Diagnosis

   1. Symptoms and signs. Any combination of pain or discomfort in the right upper quadrant, weight loss, fatigue, anorexia, jaundice, or fever should raise the possibility of liver metastases, particularly in patients with a history of cancer. Symptoms are present in 65 percent of patients and hepatomegaly in 50 percent when liver metastases are discovered.

   2. Laboratory studies

   a. LFTs are obtained in all patients suspected of having liver metastases. An elevation of the alkaline phosphatase level out of proportion to that of the transaminases suggests either a mass lesion or biliary obstruction.

   b. Liver imaging is obtained in all patients with history, physical findings, or laboratory values suggestive of hepatic metastases. Hepatic CT scans or MRI are the most sensitive techniques. Ultrasonography and technetium 99 colloid liver scans have lower diagnostic accuracy. The evaluation of a single focal lesion in the liver is discussed in Chap. 9, *Liver Cancer.*

   3. Selective hepatic angiography is the most predictive diagnostic test to assess the presence, number, and distribution of hepatic metastases.

   4. Liver biopsy should be performed to confirm the presence and type of tumor in the following circumstances:

   a. There is *no primary history of cancer* and the liver is the only obvious site of disease.

   b. There has been *a long disease-free interval* (more than two years) since the removal of the primary tumor.

   c. The liver abnormality is *not typical* of the natural history of the primary cancer. Suggestive evidence for hepatic metastases in patients with primary tumor type that does not usually metastasize to the liver (see sec. **A.1.a.(3)**) indicates biopsy *if the results are likely to affect therapeutic decisions.*

  d. Contraindications for liver biopsy are
    (1) Coagulation protein or platelet abnormalities
    (2) Evidence of a vascular tumor (e.g., angiosarcoma) or vascular mal-
       formation (e.g., birth control pill–induced hemangiomas)
  5. Extrahepatic biliary obstruction. Patients with extrahepatic biliary ob-
    struction may have liver scans with no defects, or diffuse abnormalities, or
    vague focal defects. These patients must have special studies to exclude
    benign causes of obstruction, such as gallstones or bile duct strictures.
    a. CT scan or Disida scan of the liver is performed to look for parenchymal
       or porta hepatis masses and obstruction of the biliary tree.
    b. Percutaneous transhepatic cholangiogram or retrograde contrast
       study of the biliary tree is performed, depending on the availability of
       experienced radiologists and gastroenterologists.
    c. Laparotomy is indicated for both definitive diagnosis and treatment if
       the other studies suggest extrahepatic obstruction and if other sites of
       tumor are well controlled or not evident.
D. Management. *No treatment modality for hepatic metastases involving large cell
  carcinoma or adenocarcinoma has been clearly shown to improve survival in a
  significant percentage of patients.*
  1. Surgery
    a. Resection of hepatic metastases has been used in very few, highly
       selected patients. The surgical mortality from this procedure is 20 per-
       cent; very rarely, a patient will survive five years. Success is usually
       limited to patients with solitary metastases from low-grade, slow-
       growing tumors; the disease-free interval has typically been more than
       two years. However, patients with such indolent tumors may survive for
       several years with minimal or no treatment. Routinely exposing such
       patients to a 20 percent surgical mortality is questionable practice.
    b. Extrahepatic biliary tract obstruction may be decompressed surgically
       if pruritus is severe. Jaundice per se is generally not an indication for
       surgery unless the patient must have a laparotomy for diagnosis. Biliary
       cirrhosis occurs only after six to eight months of total obstruction, a
       period that exceeds the life expectancy of most patients with malignant
       obstructive jaundice.
       (1) Percutaneous drainage through internal or external catheter place-
          ment offers reasonable palliation. Drainage is achieved in 40 to 85
          percent of cases. This procedure has a 25 to 85 percent morbidity
          rate and a 2.5 to 30 percent mortality rate. The most frequent compli-
          cation is cholangitis, which seems to relate to multiple sites of ob-
          struction or inadequate drainage. Further intervention with tube
          manipulation, tube replacement, or surgery is required in 20 to 75
          percent of patients. The success rate for palliation is about 80 percent
          and similar to that achieved with **cholecystojejunostomy.**
       (2) Endoscopic placement of prostheses is another option that is suc-
          cessful in about 80 percent of patients. The difficulties of cholangitis
          from inadequate drainage result in a 15 percent mortality rate. Mor-
          bidity rates are similar to those associated with percutaneous proce-
          dures.
    c. Hepatic artery ligation or hepatic dearterialization alone or in combi-
       nation with perfusion produces no significant benefit.
  2. RT in low doses (less than 2400 cGy) is useful to palliate refractory pain from
    liver metastases. RT to portal masses may relieve biliary tract obstruction.
  3. Chemotherapy
    a. Oral and IV chemotherapy is useful for treating responsive tumors such
       as lymphomas, breast cancer, and small cell lung cancer. The primary
       tumor determines the selection of drugs. Prednisone, 60 mg PO daily,
       may be helpful to control pain from liver metastases that do not respond
       to chemotherapy.
    b. Direct perfusion of chemotherapy into the liver through hepatic artery

cannulation is used by some physicians to treat isolated liver metastases when no other organs are involved. The most extensively used drugs are fluorouracil, floxuridine, and Adriamycin. Compared with systemic chemotherapy (including continuous peripheral venous infusion), hepatic artery infusion is associated with more responses, less systemic drug toxicity, significantly greater development of extrahepatic metastases, and no difference in survival. Complications of hepatic artery infusion include hospitalization for catheter placement and perfusion (if a portable pump is not used), hemorrhage, thrombosis of the perfused vessels, embolization, catheter displacement or breakage, catheter sepsis, GI bleeding, chemical hepatitis, acalculous cholecystitis, and biliary sclerosis.

IV. Malignant ascites

A. Pathogenesis

1. **Peritoneal carcinomatosis** with malignant ascites is most often caused by colonic, gastric, biliary tract, pancreatic, and ovarian carcinomas. Breast cancer, lung cancer, and lymphomas less frequently produce massive peritoneal seeding. Mesothelioma is a rare cause.

2. **Hepatic venous obstruction** from hepatocellular carcinoma or extensive hepatic metastases from other tumors may result in ascites. Hyperviscosity states, particularly polycythemia vera, may result in the Budd-Chiari syndrome. Patients with hepatic venous obstruction have large, tender livers and rapidly evolving ascites.

3. **Chylous ascites** may result from obstruction or rupture of the major abdominal lymphatic passages. Over 80 percent of cases in adults are caused by abdominal neoplasms, usually lymphoma.

4. **Peritonitis** caused by *Streptococcus bovis* may be a presenting feature for right-sided colon carcinoma. Ascites from any cause may become infected.

B. Diagnosis

1. **Differential diagnosis of ascites.** Neoplastic diseases that cause ascites include liver metastases, peritoneal metastases, pseudomyxoma peritonei, and primary mesothelioma. The etiologies of ascites can be best classified by the "serum-ascites albumin gradient," which is the difference between serum and ascitic fluid albumin concentration. This gradient predicts the presence or absence of portal hypertension, and in parallel, the responsiveness to treatment with diuretics.

High albumin gradient (≥1.1 g/dl) (portal hypertension likely)	Low albumin gradient (<1.1 g/dl) (portal hypertension unlikely)
Massive hepatic metastases	Peritoneal carcinoma
Chronic liver disease	Peritoneal inflammation (fungal, tuberculous, vasculitic)
Hepatic vein obstruction (Budd-Chiari syndrome)	Oncotic (hypoalbuminemia): nephrotic syndrome, protein-losing enteropathy, chronic disease
Hepatic veno-occlusive disease	
Cardiac failure	Hollow organ leak: pancreatic, biliary, ureteric, chylous
Hemodialysis with fluid overload	
Myxedema (?)	Idiopathic

2. **Paracentesis** should be done in all patients with presumed malignant ascites to rule out complicating infections. Ascites from carcinomatosis is usually exudative and often bloody. Ascitic fluid should be studied for the following:

   a. **Culture** for bacteria (including acid-fast bacilli) and fungi.

   b. **Albumin** should be measured to calculate the gradient.

   c. **Exudates** are associated with **total protein** values more than 2.5 gm/dl, **WBC** more than 250/μL (lymphocytosis suggests tuberculous peritonitis), and **LDH** more than 50 percent of serum values.

   d. Values in ascitic fluid significantly greater than in serum of **amylase** or **triglyceride** indicate a pancreatic etiology or chylous content, respectively.

   e. Glucose level is often less than 60 mg/dl in carcinomatosis.

   f. Fibronectin levels greater than 75 μg/ml in the absence of infection or pancreatic disease or **CEA** levels greater than 12 ng/ml are nearly pathognomonic of malignancy.

   g. Cytology is positive in more than 50 percent of cases of peritoneal carcinomatosis.

C. Management of malignant ascites is principally directed toward palliation of symptoms rather than improving the patient's appearance. Furosamide and spironolactone may be helpful in ascites caused by hepatic metastases, but they are usually ineffective for ascites that is chylous or caused by peritoneal carcinomatosis. If paracentesis must be done more than once a month, more aggressive therapy is warranted.

   1. Drainage. A 14- to 16-gauge plastic catheter or a peritoneal dialysis catheter can be used; the latter is preferred for removing a large volume of fluid. A single suture should hold the catheter in place.

      a. Removal of large volumes of peritoneal fluid should not be done if a hepatic cause, such as cirrhosis or Budd-Chiari syndrome, is suspected.

      b. If cancer is suspected, as much fluid as possible should be removed; nonpalpable abdominal masses may later become evident. Removal of large volumes of ascites fluid that is a result of peritoneal carcinomatosis does not usually cause dangerous fluid shifts.

   2. Chemotherapy is the treatment of choice for responsive tumors.

   3. Intraperitoneal chemotherapy. Instillation of chemotherapy directly into the abdomen may control some malignant effusions. The abdomen is drained to be as dry as possible, preferably using a peritoneal dialysis catheter. The chosen drug is dissolved in 100 ml of normal saline, injected into the catheter and followed by another 100 ml of normal saline for flushing. The patient's position is shifted every few minutes for an hour to disperse the drug. If treatment is effective, the dose may be repeated at intervals. Fever or abdominal pain or tenderness may develop after the procedure, may persist for up to one week, and may require paracentesis to confirm that the peritonitis is sterile.

      a. Effective agents include bleomycin (15 units), 5-fluorouracil (1000 mg), thiotepa (45 mg), Adriamycin (30 mg), cisplatin, and α-IFN. Mitoxantrone (10 mg) palliates 60 percent of patients with gynecologic malignant ascites.

      b. Radioactive phosphorus may be tried, but leakage of the radioisotope through the needle tract is a major problem. Radioactive gold and vesicant drugs, such as nitrogen mustard, are extremely hazardous and can cause bowel necrosis, especially if the fluid is loculated.

   4. Peritoneovenous shunts (LeVeen and Denver) may be used to treat refractory cases if the patient has a life expectancy of greater than one month and does not have significant cardiac or renal disease, disseminated intravascular coagulation (DIC), liver metastases, or mesothelioma. The ascitic fluid should not be hemorrhagic, infected, or loculated, and should not contain large numbers of malignant cells. Complications of these shunts include DIC (virtually 100%), sepsis (20%), pulmonary edema (15%), pulmonary emboli (10%), upper GI bleeding, fever without sepsis, superior vena cava thrombosis, pneumonia, shunt displacement, seromas around the catheter (10%), and neoplastic seeding to the superior vena cava on adjacent subcutaneous tissues. Thrombocytopenia is caused by both DIC and hemodilution.

   5. Pseudomyxoma peritonei. Mucinous adenocarcinomas, "benign" mucin-producing tumors, and appendiceal mucoceles can produce abundant gelatinous material which is impossible to remove by paracentesis. Recurrent bowel obstruction and progressive ascites develop. Laparotomy with removal of as much of the jellylike substance as possible is indicated; 60 mg of thiotepa is instilled over as much of the serosal surface as possible. The procedure may be repeated if there is recurrence, depending on the changing anatomy and formation of adhesions.

V. Pancreatitis and metastases to the pancreas

A. **Etiology.** Pancreatitis rarely complicates primary or metastatic cancer of the pancreas. If abdominal carcinomatosis with secondary pancreatic involvement were excluded, metastases to the pancreas are rare. Small cell lung cancer metastasizes to the pancreas most commonly, but lymphoma and carcinomas of the breast, colon, and kidney do also.

B. **Diagnosis** of pancreatitis depends on signs and laboratory findings. CT scan of the abdomen is the best technique to demonstrate a mass in the pancreas. Differential diagnosis includes:

1. Pancreatitis associated with hypercalcemia
2. Drug-induced pancreatitis from
   a. Alcohol
   b. Glucocorticoids, indomethacin, salicylates
   c. L-Asparaginase, mercaptopurine, azathioprine
   d. Isoniazid, thiazides, oral contraceptives, certain antibiotics

C. **Management.** Pancreatitis complicating metastatic cancer should be treated with analgesics. IV fluids should be administered to replace losses.

VI. Adverse effects of radiation to the liver and alimentary canal

A. **Radiation hepatitis.** Clinical hepatitis is uncommon at doses of less than 2500 cGy to the liver. This dose is usually not exceeded except in the treatment of Wilms' tumor. Acute hepatitis from radiation can be mild to severe and may result in cirrhosis.

1. **Manifestations.** Signs and symptoms become evident two to six weeks after irradiation. Hepatomegaly and ascites develop. Enzyme abnormalities are indistinguishable from those in viral hepatitis. Decreased uptake of ^{99}Tc in the treatment portal is observed on liver scan. Liver biopsy demonstrates endophlebitis with thickening and obstruction of central veins and mild cellular necrosis or atrophy, findings similar to those found with veno-occlusive disease induced by chemotherapy.

2. **Management** is symptomatic. Corticosteroids may help.

B. **Radiation esophagitis**

1. **Acute esophagitis.** Transient esophageal dysphagia may occur toward the end of a course of RT to the mediastinum. Analgesics or viscous lidocaine solution might be helpful, but treatment is usually not required.

2. **Esophageal stricture** is a rare late complication that is more common when chemotherapy, particularly Adriamycin or methotrexate, is given concomitantly. Dilation is performed in symptomatic patients.

C. **Radiation enteritis**

1. **Acute radiation enteritis**
   a. **Manifestations** are usually related to the volume of the bowel irradiated and to the daily dose. Most injuries involve the terminal ileum.
      (1) Nausea, vomiting, and anorexia usually do not persist more than three days after RT is stopped.
      (2) Diarrhea is more severe in patients who have had laparotomies. Symptoms can occur after the second week of RT and disappear within two weeks after its completion.
   b. **Management**
      (1) **Antiemetics** are given regularly throughout the day for patients with persistent vomiting. If symptoms are severe, parenteral hyperalimentation and reduction of the daily dose of radiation may be necessary.
      (2) **Diarrhea** is managed by eliminating alcoholic beverages, roughage, and milk products from the diet. Paregoric (tincture of opium), cholestyramine, or diphenoxylate-atropine (Lomotil) may be useful.

2. **Chronic radiation enteritis.** Abdominal pain syndromes, malabsorption, bowel strictures, hemorrhage, perforations, and fistulae usually occur with

doses to the abdomen of more than 4500 cGy and are more frequent in the presence of postsurgical adhesions. Symptoms may develop months to many years after completion of therapy. Parenteral hyperalimentation may be necessary while the bowel abnormality is being corrected.

- **a. Abdominal pain syndromes** are treated with analgesics, bulk laxatives, and dietary modifications.
- **b. Perforations and fistulae** indicate a poorer prognosis than strictures and hemorrhage; malignancy recurs in 70 percent of these patients.
- **c. Bowel obstruction.** Tube decompression may lead to resolution. Laparotomy should be avoided if possible. If the obstruction progresses, intestinal bypass (10% mortality) rather than bowel resection should be performed in the absence of gangrenous bowel (75% mortality).
- **d. Chronic diarrhea** with malabsorption is rare and is treated symptomatically. Anorexia, nausea, and vomiting may occur. Medium-chain triglycerides may be of help to decrease stool fat loss and to relieve radiation-induced intestinal lymphangiectasia with protein loss. Steatorrhea may result from bacterial overgrowth; tetracycline, 250 mg q.i.d., may be tried for 10 to 14 days on an empiric basis. Prednisone and sulfasalazine may also be used.

D. Radiation proctitis

1. Acute transient proctitis

- **a. Manifestations.** Tenesmus, diarrhea, and occasionally, minor bleeding develops. Symptoms usually resolve soon after RT is completed.
- **b. Management** is usually not indicated. If symptoms are prolonged or severe, steroid enemas and suppositories, stool softeners, mineral oil, low-residue diet, or paregoric or diphenoxylate-atropine might be helpful.

2. Late radiation proctitis occurs six months to two years after RT.

- **a. Manifestations.** Symptoms include tenesmus, diarrhea, and hematochezia. Proctoscopic examination reveals hemorrhagic, edematous mucosa with decreased pliability and, occasionally, ulcers.
- **b. Management**
    - **(1) For severe inflammation,** treat as described for acute proctitis.
    - **(2) For rectal ulcers** refractory to conservative management (see **1.b**) surgery is advised.
    - **(3) For late rectal narrowing,** treat with dilatations and stool softeners.

VII. Hepatic veno-occlusive disease. Hepatic veno-occlusive disease is a nonthrombotic obliterative process of the central or sublobular hepatic veins characterized by ascites, hepatomegaly, and varied clinical outcome. The diagnosis is established by liver biopsy, which should be done early when hepatic dysfunction is evident because alteration of therapy may improve subsequent clinical outcome.

The hepatotoxic pyrrolizidine alkaloids that occur naturally in plants (other implicated dietary contaminants include aflatoxin and nitrosamines) are the most common cause worldwide. Chemotherapy and irradiation, especially in patients who have had bone marrow or kidney transplants and graft-versus-host disease, are important causes in the Western world.

Azathioprine, 6-mercaptopurine (a metabolite of azathioprine), 6-thioguanine (a compound related to 6-mercaptopurine), and dacarbazine have been implicated as causes of hepatic vascular damage. Other causes include postnecrotic cirrhosis, metastatic or primary hepatic malignancy, myeloproliferative disorders (particularly polycythemia vera), and a variety of other hypercoagulable states.

VIII. Paraneoplastic GI tract syndromes. The etiology of paraneoplastic gastrointestinal tract syndromes is not known.

A. Esophageal achalasia may accompany gastric cancer and is reversible when the cancer is resected. Patients present with dysphagia for all foods and liquids.

- **1. Diagnosis.** The barium esophagogram reveals a large, aperistaltic esophagus. Esophageal manometry shows weak contractions with a "hypertensive" lower esophageal sphincter.
- **2. Therapy.** Patients with achalasia and unresectable cancer must have gas-

trostomy, an esophageal tube (e.g., Celestin tube), or forced pneumatic dilatation.

   B. Intestinal pseudo-obstruction occurs in patients with peritoneal carcinomatosis in the absence of mechanical obstruction. Signs of obstruction are crampy abdominal pain, absence of stools, nausea, vomiting, hyperactive bowel sounds, and nonlocalized air-fluid levels on abdominal plain films.

   1. Diagnosis. Pseudo-obstruction and mechanical obstruction are clinically indistinguishable. Pseudo-obstruction, however, often remits spontaneously. Hypokalemia, hypomagnesemia, fecal impaction, history of vincristine use, and other causes of ileus should be sought.

   2. Therapy is the same as for suspected bowel obstruction (see sec. **II**).

IX. Symptom care for alimentary canal problems are discussed in Chapter 5.

   A. Oral problems including stomatitis, xerostomia, abnormal taste, halitosis, caked material in the mouth, and dysphagia. See Chap. 5, sec. **II**.

   B. Nausea and vomiting. See Chap. 5, sec. **III**.

   C. Colorectal symptoms, including constipation and rectal discharge. See Chap. 5, sec. **IV**.

   D. Anorexia, including hyperalimentation. See Chap. 5, sec. **XII**.

Selected Reading

Edney, J. A., Hill, A., and Armstrong, D. Peritoneovenous shunts palliate malignant ascites. *Am. J. Surg.* 158:598, 1989.

Hohn, D. C., et al. A randomized trial of continuous intravenous versus hepatic intra-arterial floxuridine in patients with colorectal cancer metastatic to the liver: NCOG trial. *J. Clin. Oncol.* 7:1646, 1989.

McDermott, W. V., and Ridker, P. M. The Budd-Chiari syndrome and hepatic veno-occlusive disease. *Arch. Surg.* 125:525, 1990.

Pockros, P. J., et al. Mobilization of malignant ascites with diuretics is dependent on ascitic fluid characteristics. *Gastroenterology* 103:1302, 1992.

Rothchild, J. G., et al. Management of biliary obstruction. A comparison of percutaneous endoscopic and operative technique. *Arch. Surg.* 124:556, 1989.

Runyon, B. A., et al. The serum-ascites albumin gradient is superior to the exudate-transudate concept in the differential diagnosis of ascites. *Ann. Intern. Med.* 177:215, 1992.

Silen, W. Hepatic resection for metastasis from colorectal carcinoma is of dubious value. *Arch. Surg.* 124:1021, 1989.

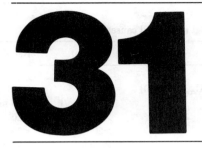

Renal Complications

David W. Knutson and
Dennis A. Casciato

I. Prerenal failure

A. **Pathogenesis.** In all patients with prerenal failure, a decrease in effective circulating volume (ECV) leads to a decrease in renal blood flow with a consequent reversible decrease in glomerular filtration rate (GFR). Decreased ECV provides a baroreceptor-mediated stimulus for the secretion of antidiuretic hormone (ADH). The simultaneous decrease in renal blood flow stimulates the production of renin with consequent increases in circulating levels of angiotensin II (AII) and aldosterone. The combined effects of decreased renal blood flow and increased levels of ADH, AII, and aldosterone result in excretion of urine that is low in volume, highly concentrated, and contains little sodium but relatively large amounts of potassium. (See Table 31-1 for laboratory values that distinguish prerenal failure from renal failure.)

1. **Decreased GFR** leads to a retention of urea and creatinine. Reabsorption of filtered urea is increased in the distal nephron due to slow tubular flow, a high concentration of urea in tubular fluid, and elevated ADH. Thus more urea than creatinine is retained, leading to a characteristic elevated blood urea nitrogen (BUN):serum creatinine ratio.

2. **Creatinine production** is proportional to muscle mass and **urea production** is dependent on protein intake. Thus, these values may be lower than normal in the wasted patient with cancer who often has poor nutritional intake. In such patients, normal or borderline high values of BUN and serum creatinine may suggest significant impairment of renal function.

3. **Chronic renal insufficiency** may predispose to prerenal failure due to obligate fluid losses of kidneys damaged by disease or nephrotoxic therapeutic agents.

B. **Causes of prerenal failure.** Table 31-2 shows general causes of prerenal failure with specific factors that may predispose patients with malignancies to prerenal failure.

C. **Diagnosis and management.** The history often reveals likely causes of increased fluid loss (e.g., diarrhea, vomiting) or sequestration (e.g., congestive heart failure [CHF], edema). Decreased intake may be more difficult to elicit. The physical examination is of paramount importance in assessing volume status and should be used to seek specific evidence of dehydration, hypotension, jugular venous distension, infection, ascites, etc.

1. **Supine systolic blood pressure** of less than 90 mm Hg, **orthostatic decreases** of greater than 10 mm Hg, or orthostatic increases in pulse rate of more than 10 per minute suggest intravascular volume depletion.

2. **Flat neck veins** (in patients whose neck veins can be demonstrated by gentle occlusion) suggest volume depletion.

3. **In patients without findings of volume depletion,** careful palpation and percussion of the bladder, rectal examination of the prostate of males and pelvic examinations in females may divert attention to an obstructive cause.

4. **Insertion of a Foley catheter** should be considered in patients without an overt prerenal cause.

5. **Occult prerenal failure** may be present that escapes detection by any of the above measures. Thus, many clinical scenarios require the careful adminis-

Table 31-1. Distinguishing prerenal from renal causes of azotemia

Characteristic	Prerenal	Renal
Fractional sodium excretion $[FE_{Na} = (U_{Na} \times S_{creat}) \div (S_{Na} \times U_{creat}) \times 100]$	≤ 1	≥ 2
U_{Na}	<15 mEq/l	>30 mEq/l
$U_{creat} : S_{creat}$ ratio	>40	<20
$BUN : S_{creat}$ ratio	>20	<20
Response to fluid or loop diuretics	Positive	Negative

Key: U = concentration in urine; S = concentration in serum; Na = sodium; creat = creatinine.

Table 31-2. Cause of decreased effective circulating volume and prerenal failure in patients with malignancies

General cause	Predisposing factors in patients with malignancies
HYPOVOLEMIA	
Decreased intake	Anorexia from malignancy or chemotherapy, intercurrent illness, obtundation, neglect
Increased loss	
Vomiting	Intestinal obstruction, chemotherapy
Diarrhea	Enteral hyperalimentation, carcinoid, VIPoma, chemotherapy, antibiotic-associated
Renal	
Diabetes insipidus (DI)	Primary pineal tumor, craniopharyngioma, metastasis (breast)
Nephrogenic DI	Chronic renal insufficiency myeloma kidney, lithium, demeclocycline, nephrocalcinosis
Osmotic diuresis	Hypercalcemia, hyperglycemia
Blood loss	Tumor- or chemotherapy-related
Hypoalbuminemia	Poor nutrition, severe liver disease, nephrotic syndrome
INTRAVASCULAR SHIFTS	
Congestive heart failure/ low cardiac output	Malignant pericardial effusion, radiation-induced pericarditis/myocarditis
Sepsis/Shock	Lymphoma/leukemia/myeloma, neutropenia due to chemotherapy
Renal artery obstruction	Tumor (rare)

tration of a fluid challenge. In the absence of clear physical findings of fluid overload, one liter of normal saline can be safely administered to the vast majority of normal-size adults without untoward effect. Often a gratifying increase in urinary output results, and BUN and serum creatinine values subsequently return to normal.

6. **Loop diuretics** given as an IV challenge are often used in acutely oliguric patients. An increased urinary output suggests that obstruction is not present and that the renal tubules are functioning. However, such response does not clarify or correct the underlying abnormality causing the initial decrease in urine production, and, except for overload states such as CHF, the diuretic may make the prerenal failure worse.

7. **Overall management** of prerenal failure is to correct the underlying cause and, when possible, restore ECV to normal. In hypovolemic patients, this

usually requires large volumes of salt-containing solutions. Although albumin solutions specifically increase intravascular volume, they are expensive and the effect is often transient. Obstruction to urinary outflow should be considered in all patients who do not respond to a fluid challenge. In such patients (especially males), insertion of a Foley catheter should be performed. If the problem is still not corrected, all such patients should undergo an imaging procedure to visualize the kidneys and collecting system. Ultrasound is often the safest and most convenient choice.

II. Obstructive uropathy causing renal failure
A. Pathogenesis
1. **Ureteral obstruction.** Uremia may result from bilateral obstruction (or unilateral obstruction in the case of a single functioning kidney) from
   a. **Bladder tumors and tumors of the collecting systems.**
   b. **Uterine tumors,** especially carcinoma of the cervix.
   c. **Retroperitoneal tumors** (rare) including lymphoma, sarcomas, and metastatic tumors.
   d. **Intrinsic renal tumors** (rare).
   e. **Retroperitoneal fibrosis** including that induced by irradiation, drugs (busulfan), carcinoid tumors (especially rectal), Gardener's syndrome (intestinal polyposis), or desmoplastic reactions to metastases.
2. **Outlet obstruction of the urethra.** Causes include primary cancer of the prostate, urethra, cervix, ovary, bladder, or endometrium. Metastatic cancer from the lung, GI tract, breast, and melanoma to the pelvic organs, prostate, or urethra can cause this complication.
B. Diagnosis
1. **Symptoms** are often absent or insidious in onset. Anuria is highly suggestive, but partial high grade obstruction of ureters can occasionally cause renal failure with a normal urine volume. A very variable urine output or overflow incontinence causing dribbling (and the strong smell of urine during physical examination) suggest bladder outlet obstruction.
2. **Physical findings** are those of the underlying disease. Dullness to percussion in the suprapubic region suggests a mass or distended bladder.
3. **Postvoid residual urine** determination is often useful in evaluating for outlet obstruction.
4. **Ultrasonography** may show hydronephrosis. However, acute obstruction or chronic obstruction wherein the collecting system is encased in tumor may show minimal abnormalities. A normal appearing but full collecting system in an oliguric patient suggests obstruction.
5. **Cystoscopy** demonstrates bladder outlet obstruction, shows the extent of bladder tumors, and permits retrograde ureterography.
C. Management
1. **Lymphomas and Hodgkin's disease** are usually successfully managed with chemotherapy, with or without focal RT.
2. **Solid tumors** usually require percutaneous catheter placement under combined ultrasound/fluoroscopic guidance. Stents placed from below are less commonly used. Systemic chemotherapy may be considered for responsive tumors. High-dose pelvic irradiation may be considered as an alternative, as may diverting urethral surgery. However, most patients with pelvic tumors causing obstruction are at an advanced stage of disease; therapy, including percutaneous drainage of the renal pelvis, must be carefully considered in light of the potential for palliation, the extent of disease, and the overall prognosis.
III. Intrinsic renal disease causing renal failure
A. Acute renal failure may have an abrupt onset immediately following renal insult (e.g., radiocontrast administration). Acute renal failure may also arise more insidiously over days to weeks as an indirect consequence of malignancy (e.g., hypercalcemia, myeloma kidney due to deposits of Bence Jones proteins) or therapy (e.g., hyperuricemia following tumor lysis, nephrotoxicity, interstitial nephritis following administration of certain therapeutic agents). Although

acute renal failure is often transient and reversible, certain causes can result in permanent renal failure (e.g., cisplatin toxicity, mitomycin-induced hemolytic uremic syndrome). Oliguria is often present in more dramatic episodes of acute renal failure; in this case, laboratory parameters in Table 31-1 may be useful in distinguishing it from prerenal failure. However, most causes of acute renal failure and many patients with acute renal failure present with normal or near normal urine volumes.

B. **Acute tubular necrosis (ATN)** usually has an abrupt onset and is often oliguric. Urine specific gravity is usually near isosthenuria, and mild proteinuria is typical. ATN can often be suspected by the presence of many "dirty brown" granular casts in the urine. Usually only small numbers of WBCs, RBCs, and tubular epithelial cells are present. Early on, the sediment may be remarkably bland. RBC casts are rare.

1. Several **pathogenetic mechanisms** are recognized, and multiple mechanisms may be responsible in a given patient. Direct tubular toxicity is likely the mechanism for ATN due to aminoglycosides. Intratubular obstruction with cellular debris, protein casts, or (in the case of hyperuricemia) uric acid crystals may play a role. Ischemic injury contributes in ATN due to sepsis or shock.

2. The **major histologic finding** is death and sloughing of tubular epithelial cells with preservation of tubular basement membranes and evidence of epithelial regeneration (mitotic figures). Proteinaceous casts and inflammatory cells may be present. Glomeruli are generally preserved. The lesion may be spotty with some nephrons appearing nearly normal. Disruption of tubular basement membranes (tubulorrhexis) and disrupted glomeruli suggest cortical necrosis, which carries a poor renal prognosis. Management includes avoidance of fluid imbalance and other supportive measures until function returns. Dialysis may be needed in some cases.

3. **Radiocontrast** is a particularly important cause of acute renal failure in patients with malignancies because of the frequency with which these patients undergo radiocontrast studies.

   a. **Predisposing factors** include age over 60 years, diabetes mellitus, volume depletion, other recent radiocontrast studies, high dose of contrast, concomitant nephrotoxic drug therapy, and, possibly, hyperuricemia.

   b. **Prevention** is the best management by hydrating patients and avoiding serial studies in a short period of time. Our routine in high-risk patients is one liter of normal saline IV over 12 hours preceding the study, 12.5–25 gm of mannitol IV "on call" to radiology suite, 40–80 mg furosemide at the end of the procedure, and, importantly, replacement of urinary losses for 8 to 12 hours with half normal saline. We have not encountered a single case of acute renal failure in which either the serum creatinine doubled or the patient required dialysis using this approach in high-risk patients.

C. **Tubulointerstitial nephritis** occurs acutely following the administration of a growing list of drugs but can occur more insidiously following 6 to 12 months of therapy with NSAIDs (see **D**). The acute presentation is that of nonoliguric acute renal failure with variable systemic findings of allergic skin rash, fever, or arthralgias. Leukocytosis with eosinophilia may be seen, but pyuria with eosinophiluria is probably more common. Microscopic hematuria is a remarkably frequent finding.

1. **Histologically,** there is a diffuse inflammatory reaction in the interstitium, sometimes with invasion of tubules by white cells. Eosinophils may dominate or may be only minimally present.

2. The **renal prognosis** is good if the offending agent is discontinued. Anecdotal evidence favors the use of a short course of corticosteroids (40–60 mg/day of prednisone) if renal failure is severe or persists. Dialysis is only rarely required.

D. Drugs that affect the kidneys of cancer patients
   1. Acute tubular necrosis
      a. Antibiotics. Aminoglycosides, amphotericin, pentamidine, cephalosporin (rare), vancomycin (rare, but especially with aminoglycosides)
      b. Chemotherapeutics. Methotrexate, cisplatin (often irreversible damage), streptozocin (and other nitrosoureas), cyclosporine (acute, hydrodynamic changes; chronic, interstitial fibrosis)
   2. Acute interstitial nephritis. Penicillins, cephalosporins, sulfa drugs, thiazide, furosemide, bumetanide (but not ethacrynic acid), antituberculous drugs, NSAIDs (usually after 3 to 6 months of use)
   3. Chronic irreversible renal failure
      a. Acute hemolytic uremic syndrome. Mitomycin, cyclosporine (rare)
      b. Tubular interstitial fibrosis. Cisplatin, cyclosporine
E. Tumor invasion
   1. Primary renal tumors commonly invade renal parenchyma, of course, but renal failure requires extensive bilateral renal involvement and is a rare event. The more common cause of renal failure in patients with primary renal tumors is surgical ablation of renal tissue, the consequence of attempts to extirpate the tumor. Because renal cell carcinomas occur bilaterally in at least 5 percent of patients, preservation of renal tissue by segmental or heminephrectomy is an option to consider; it is a necessity in the patient with only one kidney if dialysis is to be avoided. Such selective ablative surgery may be impossible if tumor has invaded the renal vein (as it tends to do). Patients with renal vein involvement extending into the inferior vena cava often have degrees of renal thrombosis and occasionally consequent renal failure.
   2. Solid tumor metastasis to kidneys occurs frequently late in the course of many tumors but is a rare cause of renal failure or death.
   3. Lymphoid tumors. Renal involvement is common in acute lymphoblastic leukemia (about 50% of cases), Hodgkin's disease, and lymphoma. Renal failure is less common but does occur. Urinary findings include mild proteinuria, hematuria, and often tumor cells which, when present, are highly suggestive of renal invasion. Imaging studies show large poorly functioning kidneys without hydronephrosis. Treatment with local irradiation or chemotherapy is associated with resolution of renal failure and diminution of renal size to or towards normal; both abnormalities may recur.
F. Acute glomerulonephritis causing renal failure is as rare in patients with underlying malignancies as it is in the general population. Certain lymphoproliferative disorders may result in mixed cryoglobulinemia that can cause rapidly progressive (crescentic) glomerulonephritis. Occasionally tumor antigens can cause membranoproliferative glomerulonephritis, a presumably immune complex–mediated process that can result in renal failure (see sec. **IV,** in nephrotic syndrome).
G. Radiation nephritis can occur 6 to 12 months after doses to the kidneys exceeding 2000 cGy as a function of dose and proportion of kidney tissue irradiated. Earlier onset cases may manifest as severe or malignant hypertension, proteinuria of less than 2 gm/day, and an active urinary sediment with microscopic hematuria and granular casts. Later occurring cases mimic chronic interstitial nephritis with a bland urinary sediment, possible salt wasting, or hyporeninemic hypoaldosteronism. Treatment of either presentation is to control blood pressure when elevated.
IV. Immunologic glomerular injury: the nephrotic syndrome. The nephrotic syndrome is an unusual but recognized complication of neoplasms. The syndrome may be caused by glomerular deposits of amyloid, by the deposition of immune complexes, or by less well defined immunologic mechanisms.
A. Incidence. The incidence of nephrotic syndrome as a consequence of malignancies is unknown. From 6 to 10 percent of patients with nephrotic syndrome eventually manifest a malignancy, but the duration before clinical onset of the

malignancy, the large number of patients with a wide variety of malignancies, and the number of isolated (single) case reports make some associations questionable. Accordingly, the clinical maxim that "patients over 50 with nephrotic syndrome should have a diligent search for cancer" probably overstates the case. Our approach in such patients is to perform a careful history and physical examination with attention to the lymphatic system, coupled with a CBC, chest x-ray, and stool for occult blood unless symptoms or findings suggest the need for further workup.

B. Associations exist with Hodgkin's disease (most common); other lymphoproliferative disorders; squamous cell carcinoma; and adenocarcinomas of the lung, kidney, thyroid, cervix, and GI tract (including esophagus, stomach, pancreas and colon). The nephrotic syndrome may occur simultaneously with the clinical manifestation of malignancy. More often, what appear to be true associations of nephrotic syndrome occur months before or after the tumor manifestations, and such associations may occasionally exceed a year. Recurrence of previously treated tumor may be heralded by the return of the nephrotic syndrome by weeks or months.

C. Pathology is correlated with the commonest tumors as follows:

	Minimal Change	Membranous Nephropathy	Membranoproliferative Glomerulonephritis
Carcinoma	4–6%	80%	4–6%
Hodgkin's disease	50–67%	8–12%	—
Non-Hodgkin's lymphoma	33%	33%	33%

D. Pathogenesis. Because of the similarity between the minimal change lesion seen in lipoid nephrosis and the lesion sometimes seen with Hodgkin's disease, a defect in T lymphocyte function causing the generation of an aberrant T cell factor (yet to be defined) has been postulated for both of these lesions. Glomerular deposition of immune complexes containing specific tumor antigens, viral antigens, and normal autoantigens have been described in single case reports regarding a number of tumors.

E. Management. Remission of nephrotic syndrome may occur with partial or complete elimination of the tumor, especially in Hodgkin's disease. Corticosteroid therapy for tumor-associated nephrotic syndrome is usually ineffective if the tumor cannot be controlled.

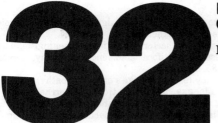

Neuromuscular Complications

Ellen E. Mack

I. Metastases to the brain

A. Pathogenesis

1. **Incidence.** Autopsy series show that 25 percent of patients who die of cancer have brain metastases.
2. **Tumor of origin** (see Table 1-2). The tumor that most commonly metastasizes to the brain is lung cancer, which is responsible for 30 percent of brain metastases. Brain metastases from pulmonary tumors tend to occur early in the course of malignancy, and their diagnosis is synchronous (i.e., before or at the same time as the primary tumor) in approximately one-third of cases. Other types of tumors that commonly metastasize to the brain include renal cancer, breast cancer, and melanoma (each 10 percent of cases), and metastases from tumors of unknown primary sites (15 percent). Carcinomas of the ovary, uterus, and prostate rarely produce intracerebral metastases.
3. **Mechanism.** Tumor dissemination to the CNS usually is by the hematogenous route, and the distribution of lesions parallels the distribution of arterial blood flow. Eighty percent of brain metastases are supratentorial, 15 percent are cerebellar, and 5 percent are in the brainstem. Approximately half of metastases are solitary, especially those from breast, renal, and colon cancers; metastases from melanoma and lung cancer are more likely to be multiple. Metastases can be solid, cystic, or hemorrhagic (especially choriocarcinoma, melanoma, and testicular carcinoma).

B. Natural history.
Left untreated, metastatic brain tumors cause progressive neurologic deterioration leading to coma and death; the median survival is only one month. Approximately 50 percent of patients with brain metastases die of their neurologic disease, and the remainder die of systemic causes. Among treated patients, the median survival is three to eight months; patients with breast cancer and those with limited systemic disease who undergo surgical treatment survive longer.

C. Clinical presentation.
The symptoms of brain metastases usually develop insidiously and progress to disability over a few weeks. However, the onset may be sudden, resembling a stroke, and occasionally symptoms may improve spontaneously (particularly in patients with hemorrhagic metastases). Single metastases usually cause focal cerebral dysfunction at presentation; multiple metastases often cause headache and mental status changes, but focal deficits are less common.

1. **Nonfocal signs and symptoms.** The classic morning headache is seen in only 40 percent of patients. Other nonlocalizing findings include papilledema, nausea and vomiting, mental status changes, and in some instances, diplopia. Calvarial metastases over the sagittal sinus may produce headache and papilledema without other neurologic signs.
2. **Focal signs and symptoms,** including hemiparesis, hemisensory loss, and aphasia, depend on the site of metastasis.
3. **Differential diagnosis.** Conditions that should be considered in the differential diagnosis of brain metastasis include
   a. **Metabolic encephalopathy,** including hyponatremia, hypercalcemia, hypoxemia, uremia, hepatic encephalopathy, and hypothyroidism.

   b. Drug-induced encephalopathy from analgesics, sedatives, steroids, chemotherapeutic agents, and other drugs.
   c. CNS infections, including bacterial and fungal meningitis, herpes encephalitis, progressive multifocal leukoencephalopathy, cerebral abscess. (See Chap. 35, sec. II.B).
   d. Nutritional deficiency (e.g., Wernicke's encephalopathy).
   e. Cerebrovascular disease, including stroke, hemorrhage, and venous obstruction due to thrombotic disorders and DIC.
   f. Paraneoplastic disorders, especially subacute paraneoplastic cerebellar degeneration (see sec. **V.A**).
D. Evaluation. Brain metastases are readily detectable by CT or MRI. The great majority of metastatic tumors enhance after administration of contrast material, but a noncontrast study should also be performed to evaluate for hemorrhage. MRI is more sensitive than CT, especially for lesions of the posterior fossa. CT scans, however, particularly if bone windows are used, are more sensitive in detecting bone metastases, especially at the base of the skull. Lesions detectable by CT or MRI that may resemble brain metastases include cerebral abscesses, parasitic disease, and occasionally stroke. Lumbar puncture is not useful in diagnosing brain metastases and is often contraindicated.
E. Management. The aims of therapy for patients with brain metastases are to relieve neurologic symptoms and to prolong survival. Exact treatment recommendations depend on the histology of the tumor, the degree of systemic dissemination of the tumor, and the patient's clinical condition.
   1. Dexamethasone, usually 16 mg IV followed by 4 mg PO/IV q6h, results in dramatic reversal of neurologic deficits and alleviation of headaches. Unfortunately, the effect is short-lived (weeks), but further improvement is possible with dose escalation and with definitive treatment. Dexamethasone should be tapered whenever possible.
   2. Anticonvulsant therapy is usually reserved for patients with suspected seizures and for patients in whom surgical resection is planned. Preference is also given to patients with metastatic melanoma, which is more likely to cause seizures because of its hemorrhagic nature and its predilection for the gray matter of the brain.
   3. RT is the standard treatment for brain metastases. The field usually encompasses the whole brain, and doses range from 2000 to 4000 cGy, administered by larger fractions in the lower dose regimen.
   4. Surgery provides a significant survival advantage to patients with brain metastases. Median survival for surgically treated patients is 10 to 12 months, and 12 percent of patients live five years or more. Candidates for surgical resection should have solitary brain metastases and limited or controlled systemic disease. Surgical resection is considered in other cases on an individualized basis and may be influenced by the need for a tissue diagnosis. RT is given after surgical resection.
   5. Radiosurgery is a noninvasive method of delivering a single large dose of radiation to a well-defined area with a steep dose falloff so that surrounding brain tissue receives little radiation. It is currently used primarily in patients who are not candidates for surgical resection and is given either as adjuvant therapy after whole-brain RT or is administered to lesions that progress.
   6. Chemotherapy. Cytotoxic agents are generally not used to treat brain metastases, but responses have been documented in patients with metastatic breast cancer, small cell lung cancer and lymphoma.
II. Metastases to the meninges
   A. Pathogenesis
      1. Incidence. Leptomeningeal metastases have been demonstrated at autopsy in 8 percent of patients with systemic malignancy.
      2. Associated tumors. Although any systemic tumor can metastasize to the leptomeninges, those which do so most commonly are lymphoma, leukemia

(especially acute), lung carcinoma (especially small cell), breast carcinoma, and melanoma.

3. **Mechanism.** Metastasis to the leptomeninges occurs by hematogenous spread through arachnoid vessels or the choroid plexus, by infiltration along nerve roots, and by extension from CNS metastases. The sites of heaviest infiltration are usually at the base of the brain, the major brain fissures, and the cauda equina.

B. **Natural history.** Leptomeningeal metastasis causes an inflammatory response that produces signs of meningismus and results in neurologic symptoms by several mechanisms. Direct invasion of cranial and spinal nerve roots as they traverse the subarachnoid space can cause radiculopathies. Invasion by neoplastic cells in the subarachnoid space can cause focal brain and spinal cord dysfunction. Decreased absorption of CSF due to obstruction of the arachnoid villi can cause hydrocephalus.

C. **Clinical presentation.** The hallmarks of leptomeningeal metastases are evidence of noncontiguous neurologic dysfunction and an excess of neurologic findings in relation to symptoms. Although the presentation depends on the level of neuraxis involvement and the mechanism of disease production (see sec. **B** above), there are four basic clinical presentations. These may be seen alone or in combination, and meningismus may also be present.

1. **Spinal.** The most common presentation of leptomeningeal metastases is spinal. Signs and symptoms include back pain, radicular pain, weakness and numbness of extremities, and loss of bowel and bladder control.

2. **Cerebral.** Approximately 50 percent of patients present with cerebral signs and symptoms, including headache, lethargy, change in mental status, gait ataxia, and seizures (partial and generalized).

3. **Cranial nerve.** Signs and symptoms include visual loss, diplopia, facial numbness, facial weakness, dysphagia, and hearing loss.

4. **Hydrocephalic.** Signs and symptoms of increased intracranial pressure, including headache, decreased level of consciousness, gait apraxia, and urinary incontinence.

D. **Evaluation.** Although the diagnosis of leptomeningeal metastases is often strongly suspected on a clinical basis, it can sometimes be difficult to make a definitive diagnosis. The general approach is to demonstrate disease radiographically and to confirm the diagnosis by examination of CSF.

1. **Imaging studies.** Images of the brain and full spine should be obtained because the entire neuraxis is at risk and will require treatment. MRI after administration of contrast material is the preferred modality. If MRI is unavailable, CT scans of the head in conjunction with myelography can be performed instead. Priority should be given to imaging the clinically involved portion of the neuraxis. Hydrocephalus in the absence of an obstructing lesion or contrast enhancement in the distribution of the spinal fluid suggest leptomeningeal involvement. Enhancement is most commonly seen in the basal cisterns, along the Sylvian fissures, and along the nerve roots of the cauda equina, but can also be seen along the sulci of the cerebral hemispheres, around the spinal cord, and rarely within the ventricles.

2. **CSF examination.** To confirm the diagnosis, the CSF is examined for protein and glucose content, cell counts, and cytology. Routine bacterial and fungal cultures should also be performed, because the differential diagnosis often includes infectious meningitis. CSF may be obtained by lumbar puncture or, in cases of suspected spinal block, by cervical puncture with radiographic guidance.

   a. **Routine studies.** Elevated protein and pleocytosis (usually lymphocytic) are nonspecific findings consistent with metastatic disease. A low glucose level occurs in about 25 percent of cases and is thought to indicate more severe disease. The absence of infection should be confirmed.

   b. **Cytologic examination** confirms the diagnosis in approximately 50 percent of cases on the first tap. False-negative cytologic findings are not infrequent. The diagnostic yield increases to approximately 90 percent by the third tap.

   c. Tumor markers can occasionally be helpful when the cytologic findings are nondiagnostic.

   (1) β_2 **microglobulin and** β-**glucuronidase** are elevated in leukemia and lymphoma. β-glucuronidase may also be elevated in solid tumors.

   (2) LDH profile may be altered in lymphoma and leukemia, as there is a preponderance of isoenzymes 4 and 5 in the presence of neoplastic disease.

   (3) CEA is not normally found in CSF. Its presence indicates metastatic solid tumors, especially lung and breast cancer and melanoma.

   (4) HCG and α-**FP**, although useful in diagnosing primary germ cell tumors of the CNS, have limited use in the detection of systemic germ cell tumors metastatic to the meninges.

E. Management. The optimal therapy for neoplastic meningitis has not been established. The basic premise involves irradiation of clinically involved areas and treatment of the rest of the neuraxis with intrathecal chemotherapy. A response can be achieved in approximately 50 percent of patients, but median survival is only about six months. Patients with breast cancer and lymphoma have the best prognosis.

   1. Dexamethasone is of limited benefit in patients with leptomeningeal disease. A trial of low doses (4 to 16 mg/day) is warranted, however.

   2. RT is limited to areas of clinical involvement or bulky disease seen radiographically. This is done to prevent severe marrow depression. The typical dose is 3000 cGy delivered in 10 fractions.

   3. Intrathecal chemotherapy is used to treat the remainder of the neuraxis. The drug can be administered by lumbar puncture or by intraventricular reservoir. The drug is usually given twice weekly until no abnormal cells are found in CSF and is then given at progressively longer intervals. Preservative-free agents should be used.

   a. Methotrexate, 7 mg/m^2 (15 mg maximum) twice weekly followed by leucovorin rescue

   b. Cytarabine, 30 mg/m^2 twice weekly

   c. Thiotepa, 7 mg/m^2 twice weekly

III. Metastases to the spine can result in epidural cord compression, which is a neurooncologic emergency. Any cancer patient with back pain should receive a prompt and thorough evaluation. Patients with neurologic compromise localizing to the spinal cord or cauda equina require emergent evaluation and treatment.

A. Pathogenesis

   1. Incidence. Approximately 5 percent of patients with cancer develop clinical evidence of spinal cord compression (about one-third the incidence of intracerebral metastases).

   2. Distribution. About 10 percent of epidural metastases occur in the cervical spine, 70 percent in the thoracic spine, and 20 percent in the lumbosacral spine. Approximately 10 to 40 percent of cases are multifocal.

   3. Responsible tumors. Any tumor capable of metastasizing can cause spinal cord compression. Lung cancer accounts for 15 percent of cases; breast carcinoma, prostate carcinoma, carcinoma of unknown primary site, lymphoma, and myeloma each account for approximately 10 percent of cases.

   4. Mechanisms. Spinal cord dysfunction arises by several mechanisms. The most common is direct extension of tumor from the vertebral bodies (a common site of metastasis) to the epidural space, resulting in cord compression. Other tumors, such as neuroblastoma and lymphoma, encroach upon the spinal cord through the intravertebral foramina. Secondary vascular compromise can also occur, resulting in cord infarction that may cause the sudden irreversible deterioration seen in some patients. Direct metastasis to the spinal cord parenchyma is a much less common cause of spinal cord dysfunction in cancer patients.

B. Diagnosis

1. **Natural history.** The progression of disease from the spinal column to the epidural space with neural encroachment is manifested clinically as local back pain followed by radicular symptoms and eventually myelopathy.

   a. The initial stage of localized pain can last for several weeks or, in tumors such as breast cancer and lymphoma, for several months.

   b. Radicular symptoms usually herald further progression of the metastatic tumor but are still a relatively early symptom.

   c. Once symptoms related to compression of the spinal cord or cauda equina occur, the progression is usually extremely rapid; a complete myelopathy may develop within hours. Rapid progression is especially common with lung cancer, renal cancer, and multiple myeloma.

2. **Clinical presentation** depends on the level of spinal involvement.

   a. **Midline or paravertebral back pain** is the initial symptom in more than 90 percent of patients with spinal cord compression due to malignancy. The pain is dull and aching and is caused by involvement of bone by the malignancy. Tenderness over the appropriate spinal level is usually readily elicited.

   b. **Radiculopathy** is usually manifested by pain in a dermatomal distribution, but can also include sensory or motor loss in the distribution of the involved roots. Cervical disease and lumbar disease usually cause unilateral radiculopathy, whereas thoracic disease causes bilateral radiculopathy, resulting in a band-like distribution of pain. The pain from thoracic radiculopathies can sometimes be similar to pain from pleurisy, cholecystitis, or pancreatitis. The pain from cervical or lumbar radiculopathies can simulate disk herniation.

   c. **Myelopathy** can rapidly result from further disease progression. Depending on the level of spinal involvement, the signs of myelopathy include bilateral weakness and numbness in the lower extremities and loss of bowel and bladder function. Associated neurologic findings include hyperactive deep-tendon reflexes, Babinski responses, and decreased anal sphincter tone. Disease at the level of the cauda equina usually causes urinary retention and saddle anesthesia. Unusual presentations of spinal cord compression include ataxia without motor, sensory, or autonomic dysfunction. A metastasis to the spinal cord parenchyma can cause a myelopathy without back pain.

3. **Evaluation.** Because the prognosis worsens when myelopathy develops, the diagnosis of epidural metastasis should be established before the onset of spinal cord injury. The extent of workup depends on the clinician's suspicion for metastatic disease and the degree and rate of neurologic progression of the patient.

   a. **Plain x-ray films** correctly predict the presence or absence of epidural metastases in more than 80 percent of cases. Loss of pedicles, destruction of the vertebral body, and vertebral body collapse are the most common abnormalities of cord compression seen on plain films. However, plain films provide no information about the degree and extent of neural impingement and therefore should only be used to evaluate patients without neurologic symptoms or where the index of suspicion is low.

   b. **Bone scans** may be useful in cases in which plain x-rays are normal but there is still a low index of suspicion for epidural cord compression.

   c. **MRI** is usually the procedure of choice for evaluating patients with suspected cord compression. MRI accurately defines the degree of neural impingement and the extent of bone involvement, is noninvasive, and accurately detects other entities in the differential diagnosis of myelopathy (see sec. **d**). Images should be obtained after the administration of a contrast agent. The procedure is usually performed in patients with neurologic dysfunction or where the index of suspicion for cord compression is otherwise high.

   d. **Myelography** may be used when MRI is unavailable, when multilevel disease is suspected and MRI of the entire spine is not feasible, or when CSF sampling is also required. If myelography shows a complete block, contrast material may need to be administered at both the lumbar and high cervical levels to establish the extent of disease. If myelography is performed, CSF should always be sent for routine studies and cytologic examination. Myelography is contraindicated in patients with coagulopathy and may worsen a neurologic deficit below the level of a spinal block.

 e. Lumbar puncture is usually performed in patients with epidural cord compression only if there is a suspicion of concomitant leptomeningeal dissemination of tumor.

 4. Differential diagnosis
  a. Structural lesions. Epidural hematoma (may occur spontaneously or after invasive procedures, especially in patients with a coagulopathy), epidural abscess, benign tumors (e.g., meningioma), herniated disk, osteoporotic vertebral collapse.
  b. Nonstructural lesions. Paraneoplastic syndromes (see sec. **V**), radiation myelopathy (see sec. **VI.B.3**), Guillain-Barré syndrome.
  c. Back pain in the absence of neurologic symptoms or findings in patients with normal imaging studies of the spine may be due to retroperitoneal metastases, which can be diagnosed by CT or ultrasound imaging.

C. Prognosis. The outcome is greatly improved if treatment is initiated before spinal cord symptoms appear. Other prognostic factors include the level of spinal cord involvement and the rate of neurologic progression. Patients with breast cancer and lymphoma tend to do better because their tumors progress less rapidly and respond to multimodal therapy. Patients with carcinomas that progress more rapidly and are less responsive to chemotherapy and RT tend to do less well. True paraplegia (strength zero on a scale of 5) that is not reversible with dexamethasone virtually never improves, even with surgical decompression.

D. Management. If neurologic symptoms have developed or if there is radiographic evidence of epidural encroachment of tumor, rapid therapeutic intervention is essential.

 1. Dexamethasone is very useful for alleviating neurologic symptoms and helps to control pain associated with epidural cord compression. Treatment should begin immediately, even before diagnostic studies are performed. Dosing depends on the degree of neurologic involvement. For radiculopathy only, doses are usually 16 mg IV followed by 4 to 6 mg IV/PO q6h. For rapidly evolving disease, or for evidence of myelopathy, treat with 100 mg IV followed by 24 mg IV q6h. Begin tapering once benefit from definitive therapy has been demonstrated or the neurologic deficits become irreversible.

 2. RT is the primary treatment for spinal cord compression. It not only retards tumor growth but also greatly alleviates pain. RT is especially useful for tumors that are sensitive to radiation (e.g., lymphoma, myeloma), early and slowly progressive lesions, and metastases below the conus medullaris. The usual dose is 3000 to 4000 cGy over two to four weeks.

 3. Surgery is used in the treatment of some patients with tumor metastatic to the spine. If there is spinal cord compression and severe neurologic symptoms of recent, rapid onset, an emergent decompression can be accomplished by a laminectomy (posterior approach). If both systemic and spinal involvement of tumor are limited, and especially if the tumor is relatively resistant to radiation, the tumor and involved vertebral bodies can be resected from an anterior surgical approach, and the spine can be stabilized with prosthetic devices. RT is performed in addition to surgery, preferably after the operation. Other specific indications for surgery include
  a. Unclear pathologic diagnosis on a clinical and radiographic basis.
  b. Progression of neurologic abnormalities during RT.
  c. Spinal cord compression in a previously irradiated area.
  d. Spinal instability.

4. **Chemotherapy** is not usually used for local treatment of malignant spinal cord compression. Some oncologists may advocate its use in highly responsive tumors, such as lymphoma, if neurologic involvement is limited.

IV. Metastases to the peripheral nervous system

A. Brachial plexus

1. **Anatomy.** The brachial plexus involves the C5 through T1 nerve roots. The upper portion of the plexus (C5 and C6) innervates the proximal arm musculature and sensation to the thumb. The lower portion (C8 and T1) innervates the hand musculature and sensation to the fifth digit. In the axillary region, the lower portion of the plexus is in close proximity to the lymphatic system.

2. **Mechanism.** Tumor is most likely to involve the brachial plexus by direct invasion. Indeed, lung and breast cancer are the most commonly involved tumors. Other tumors that involve the brachial plexus usually metastasize to the upper lobe of the corresponding lung and then spread to the plexus via the lymphatic system.

3. **Clinical presentation.** The most common presenting symptom is pain, which tends to radiate from the shoulder to the digits in a radicular fashion and is exacerbated by shoulder movement. Paresthesias and weakness, with loss of deep-tendon reflexes and evidence of muscle atrophy, occur in relation to the extent of involvement of the brachial plexus. Associated findings may include lymphedema of the arm, a palpable axillary or supraclavicular mass, and Horner's syndrome.

4. **Differential diagnosis.** The primary entity to be differentiated from metastatic brachial plexopathy is radiation plexopathy. Other causes of plexopathy include surgical trauma, trauma secondary to poor limb placement during anesthesia, and radiation-induced tumors of the plexus. Metastatic tumors tend to involve the lower trunk of the plexus because of its close proximity to lymphatic vessels, whereas RT plexopathy is more likely to involve the upper trunk.

   a. **Metastatic plexopathy** is suggested by early severe pain, hand weakness, and Horner's syndrome.

   b. **Radiation plexopathy** is suggested by absent or mild pain, weakness of the shoulder girdle, and progressive lymphedema.

5. **Evaluation.** Imaging with CT or MRI may be useful in demonstrating tumor mass in the region of the plexus. Surgical exploration and biopsy may be required to confirm the diagnosis, but false-negative biopsies are not uncommon. Epidural disease due to infiltration along nerve roots is seen in some patients with metastatic plexopathy; therefore, additional imaging of the spine may be required, especially in patients with Horner's syndrome.

6. **Management.** The tumor is treated with RT or chemotherapy as indicated. The primary management problem is usually pain control, as neurologic function usually does not return. Many patients develop chronic pain that is refractory to analgesics. Consultation for ablative procedures is often required.

B. Lumbosacral plexus

1. **Mechanism.** Malignant lumbosacral plexopathy is caused mostly by direct extension of intra-abdominal tumors, but one-fourth of cases are from metastases of extra-abdominal tumors. Nearly one-half of patients with metastatic plexopathy also have spinal epidural disease. Radiation plexopathy can result from pelvic irradiation and can present in a similar fashion.

2. **Clinical presentation.** The most common presenting symptom is pain; usually unilateral, severe, unremitting low back or pelvic pain radiates into the leg. Pain is later followed by paresthesias, weakness, and loss of deep-tendon reflexes. Bladder function is usually preserved.

3. **Evaluation.** CT scans are useful for detecting presacral masses or sacral erosion. Evaluation of the spine, usually by MRI, may also be required.

4. **Management.** RT and chemotherapy are used to treat the malignancy as indicated. The goal of treatment is usually pain control, which is often difficult to achieve.

C. **Peripheral nerves.** Spread of systemic tumors to peripheral nerves is an unusual neurologic complication of malignancy. It occurs primarily in two settings:

1. **Infiltrative polyneuropathy** can result from invasion of the endoneurium by lymphoma and leukemia. This syndrome is underrecognized by autopsy reports. Over weeks to months, it causes a widespread, asymmetric, multifocal neuropathy, which may be fulminant in some cases and lead to death. The diagnosis is made by biopsy of an involved sensory nerve.

2. **Perineural spread of tumors** is seen with cutaneous and primary cancers of the head and neck (i.e., cancers of the larynx, pharynx, and tongue). Tumors invade the perineural space, spread proximally along the nerve, and may even enter the intracranial cavity and extend into the brainstem. The trigeminal and facial nerves are most commonly involved, often together, probably because of their rich coinnervation of the face. Orbital nerves may also be involved. The tumors most likely to disseminate along nerves are spindle-cell variant and atypical squamous cell carcinomas. The diagnosis is based on clinical suspicion and is confirmed by biopsy. CT scans may show thickened, enhancing nerves.

V. **Paraneoplastic syndromes** are rare neuromuscular complications of cancer. They are important to recognize as they may herald early, potentially curable malignant disease. Paraneoplastic syndromes frequently present before the cancer is diagnosed and can be associated with neoplastic disease that is not radiographically detectable. Patients with paraneoplastic syndromes are believed to have a prolonged survival with respect to the underlying malignancy. Several syndromes are now clearly defined and have been demonstrated to have an autoimmune pathogenesis.

A. **Paraneoplastic cerebellar degeneration (PCD)** is a syndrome of pancerebellar dysfunction of subacute onset. Manifestations include truncal and appendicular ataxia, dysarthria, and nystagmus (often downbeating); patients are usually so severely affected that they are bedridden, have unintelligible speech, and are unable to care for themselves. Associated neurologic syndromes such as dementia or neuropathy may be present, but they tend to be much less severe.

1. **Pathogenesis.** This disorder is associated with circulating antibodies that bind to both tumor and cerebellar tissue samples. The tumors in patients with PCD express antigens normally present only in the cerebellum, and the paraneoplastic syndrome is believed to result as a consequence of an immune response against the tumor. About one-half of affected patients have antitumor antibodies. The most common is anti-Yo, which binds to the Purkinje cells of the cerebellum, and is seen in females with breast and gynecologic malignancies. Other antibodies that may be associated with this syndrome include anti-Hu (mostly with small cell lung cancer), and anti-Ri (breast cancer). This disorder is also seen in patients with Hodgkin's disease, especially men, and in conjunction with the Lambert-Eaton myasthenic syndrome in patients with malignancy (mostly small cell carcinoma).

2. **Diagnosis.** The diagnosis should be suspected on clinical grounds because the neurologic presentation is distinct. A definitive diagnosis is possible in patients with anti-Yo, anti-Hu, and anti-Ri antibodies. Other diagnostic features include inflammatory cells in the CSF, normal brain scans, and the absence of other causes of cerebellar dysfunction. If there is no known underlying malignancy, a thorough systemic search for cancer must be undertaken. The diagnosis is sometimes not made until autopsy, when an occult malignancy is discovered, and examination of the brain shows loss of Purkinje cells of the cerebellum.

3. **Therapy** is ineffective. Patients with PCD do not respond to plasmapheresis, immunosuppressive treatment with steroids and cytotoxic agents, or treatment of the underlying malignancy.

B. **Paraneoplastic sensory neuronopathy/encephalomyelitis (PSN/PEM).** PSN, also referred to as dorsal root ganglionitis, is a syndrome of subacute progressive loss of proprioception and vibratory sense. Pain, temperature, and touch modalities of sensation are also affected, but to a lesser degree. Painful dysethesias and paresthesias are usually present. The result is a severe sensory ataxia that leaves patients bedridden. The neuropathy may affect the autonomic system, causing urinary retention, hypotension, pupillary changes, impotence, and hyperhidrosis. Sparing of the motor system is a hallmark of the syndrome, although patients are usually so impaired that they may have mild weakness from disuse atrophy. In patients with more widespread neurologic disease, such as dementia, myelopathy, or cerebellar dysfunction, the disorder is referred to as PEM.

1. **Pathogenesis.** A circulating antibody, called anti-Hu, has been demonstrated in patients with PSN/PEM and malignancy, mostly small cell lung cancer. This antibody reacts with tumor specimens as well as with neurons throughout the nervous system. Often the antibody binds predominantly to the dorsal root ganglia, causing inflammation and loss of neurons. The source of this antibody appears to be present in most small cell carcinomas. The paraneoplastic syndrome is thought to occur as a result of cross reactivity during an immune response directed against the tumor. Despite the widespread presence of the antigen in tumors, only certain patients develop the antibody. Anti-Hu antibody causes other neurologic paraneoplastic syndromes associated with small cell carcinoma (see sec. **A, F, G, H**), and sites of antibody binding in the nervous system correlate roughly with the neurologic presentation of patients with these various disorders.

2. **Diagnosis.** The diagnosis should be expected on clinical grounds, as the neurologic syndrome is often highly specific. Electromyographic (EMG) studies in patients with PSN usually show a total absence of sensory action potentials and normal or nearly normal compound muscle action potentials. A definitive diagnosis can be made by detecting the anti-Hu antibody. CSF studies show increased protein, a mild pleocytosis, and oligoclonal bands. A thorough attempt to diagnose an underlying malignancy must be made in patients who present without known cancer.

3. **Therapy** is ineffective. Plasmapheresis, immunosuppressive therapy, or treatment of the underlying malignancy have not proven to be beneficial.

C. **Opsoclonus-myoclonus.** Opsoclonus is an ocular motility disorder consisting of irregular, involuntary, multidirectional eye movements that persist with eye closure and sleep. It may be associated with myoclonus (brief, jerking contractions of flexor muscles). Opsoclonus-myoclonus is classically associated with neuroblastoma in children, where it heralds a good prognosis. Less commonly, it is associated with ataxia and encephalopathy in adults with breast cancer. In the latter disorder, opsoclonus-myoclonus is associated with the anti-Ri antibody. Unlike PCD and PSN/PEM, opsoclonus-myoclonus can be remitting-relapsing in nature and may resolve spontaneously.

D. **Cancer-associated retinopathy** is a syndrome of visual loss that begins with obscurations and night blindness and proceeds to total blindness. It is most commonly associated with small cell lung carcinoma. A specific circulating antibody has been demonstrated in some cases but has not been characterized. Pathologically, a loss of photoreceptor cells and nuclei from the outer nuclear layer of the retina occurs.

E. **Limbic encephalitis.** Early manifestations of this disorder include personality changes (depression and anxiety), which are followed by a profound loss of short-term memory. Seizures, hallucinations, and hypersomnia may also be present. Limbic encephalitis is most commonly associated with small cell lung cancer and in some cases is attributable to the anti-Hu antibody.

F. **Brainstem encephalitis** causes vertigo, nystagmus, facial numbness, oculomotor disorders, dysphagia, dysarthria, deafness, and long-tract signs. It is most commonly seen in small cell lung carcinoma and may be associated with the anti-Hu antibody.

G. **Motor neuronopathy/motor neuron disease** is a spectrum of disorders involving the motor system for which the association with malignancy is still poorly characterized. Unlike most other paraneoplastic disorders, this syndrome can arise late in the course of the malignancy, even during remission. It is most commonly seen in lymphoma (both non-Hodgkin's lymphoma and Hodgkin's disease), where it is frequently associated with a paraproteinemia. A similar condition can be seen as part of the spectrum of disease associated with the anti-Hu antibody and small cell lung carcinoma.

These disorders are characterized by a progressive loss of motor function with sensory sparing that may resolve spontaneously. Loss of anterior horn cells is seen pathologically. A viral etiology has been speculated. EMG studies can help establish the diagnosis.

H. **Neuropathies associated with plasma cell dyscrasias.** A symmetric, distal sensorimotor polyneuropathy can be associated with plasma cell dyscrasias, including monoclonal gammopathy of undetermined significance (MGUS), multiple myeloma with or without systemic amyloidosis, osteosclerotic myeloma, and Waldenström's macroglobulinemia. The polyneuropathy can be associated with other findings as part of the POEMS syndrome (polyneuropathy, organomegaly, endocrinopathy, monoclonal gammopathy, and skin changes). It is often associated with a monoclonal paraprotein (often IgM-κ), which reacts with a myelin-associated glycoprotein, resulting in a demyelinating neuropathy. The neuropathy is progressive, but usually no pain or autonomic involvement occurs. Treatment with plasmapheresis is beneficial in some patients.

I. **Polymyositis/dermatomyositis.** These disorders cause symmetrical, proximal muscle weakness, characterized by difficulty rising from a chair, combing hair, etc. Only a small minority of cases of polymyositis and dermatomyositis are associated with malignancy. These disorders are discussed further in Chapter 28, sec. II.E.

J. **Myasthenia gravis** causes progressive fatigue with exercise. It occurs in 30 percent of patients with thymomas; 10 percent of patients with myasthenia gravis are found to have thymomas. The syndrome is due to an antibody that binds to the acetylcholine receptor at the postsynaptic membrane of the neuromuscular junction. The diagnosis is made by detecting the antibody in the serum, by the response to edrophonium chloride (the Tensilon test), and by the characteristic EMG response to repetitive stimulation. Treatments include pyridostigmine bromide (Mestinon), steroids, plasmapheresis, resection of an associated thymoma, and sometimes resection of the thymus. Myasthenia gravis is quite difficult to treat, especially during the period of tumor resection. Treatment should be undertaken only by those familiar with the disorder.

K. **Lambert-Eaton myasthenic syndrome** is characterized by proximal muscle weakness, especially of the pelvic girdle. In contrast to myasthenia gravis, the weakness improves with exercise, and therefore the physical examination may fail to substantiate the patient's complaints. Hyporeflexia, muscle tenderness, and autonomic dysfunction (orthostatic hypotension, impotence, dry mouth) may be associated with the condition. Lambert-Eaton myasthenic syndrome results from an autoantibody that reacts with voltage-gated calcium channels of peripheral cholinergic nerve terminals and tumor cell membranes.

  1. **Associated tumors.** Mostly small cell lung cancers are found. One-third of patients have no malignancy.

  2. **Diagnosis.** Characteristic EMG findings include small compound muscle action potentials that increase after brief exercise or repetitive stimulation at high frequencies (20 to 50 Hz).

  3. **Therapy.** Effective therapies include treatment of the underlying malignancy, guanidine hydrochloride (125–500 mg PO t.i.d. or q.i.d.), 3-4-diamino-pyridine, steroids, and plasmapheresis.

VI. **Adverse effects of radiation to the nervous system**

A. **Mechanism.** The nervous system is highly susceptible to damage from radiation. The degree of neural dysfunction depends on the total radiation dose and fraction size, the volume of irradiated tissue, and the time elapsed since RT. Reactions are classified as acute, early delayed, and late delayed. Acute reactions during RT are believed to be due to a transient breakdown in the blood-brain barrier, leading to increased intracranial pressure. The risk of acute reactions increases with larger fraction sizes. Early delayed reactions, occurring weeks to months after irradiation, are usually self-resolving and are thought to be due to demyelination. Late delayed reactions, usually occurring months to years after irradiation, have been demonstrated pathologically as a coagulative necrosis of the involved white matter. Hyalinization of blood vessels is associated with vascular thrombosis and accumulation of fibrinoid material.

B. Radiation syndromes. Specific neurologic syndromes occur in response to RT, depending on the site of irradiation. The skin, hair, subcutaneous tissues, and bone are at risk as well. Hair loss occurs when the dose to the brain exceeds 2000 cGy over two weeks and is rarely permanent when supervoltage equipment is used. Hair regrowth usually occurs within three months, but this may be greatly impeded by chemotherapy.

1. **Radiation encephalopathy.** Acute encephalopathy manifests as headache, nausea, vomiting, somnolence, and worsening of neurologic deficit. Early delayed encephalopathy often mimics tumor recurrence, both clinically and radiographically, and consists of headache, lethargy, fever and worsening of neurologic symptoms. In children undergoing prophylactic whole-brain RT for acute lymphoblastic leukemia, this condition is referred to as the "radiation somnolence syndrome." Chronic radiation encephalopathy is associated with atrophy of the brain and is more likely to occur after whole-brain RT than after focal RT. Clinical findings include memory loss, cognitive dysfunction (learning disabilities in children), gait abnormalities, and urinary incontinence. This chronic disorder sometimes responds to CSF shunting.

2. **Radiation necrosis** is a late delayed reaction to RT that mimics tumor recurrence. It causes worsening focal neurologic deficits and progressive enhancing lesions on imaging studies. PET imaging can be useful in differentiating radiation necrosis from tumor recurrence. Because the necrotic lesion has mass effect, surgical extirpation is often useful.

3. **Radiation myelopathy.** No acute reactions to irradiation of the spine usually occur. However, early delayed reactions usually manifest as electric shock-like sensations in the arms or legs that last for several seconds and are precipitated by flexion of the neck (Lhermitte's sign). The condition is usually self-limited. Late delayed damage to the spinal cord results in a progressive myelopathy that may be asymmetric in onset. This disorder is secondary to necrosis of the white matter and usually occurs with doses greater than 5000 cGy given over five weeks by conventional fractionation.

4. **Radiation plexopathy.** Brachial and lumbosacral plexopathy are a late delayed reaction to RT and are discussed in sections **IV.A.4** and **B.1.** Early delayed reactions cause transient, self-limited paresthesias and weakness.

5. **Loss of special senses.** Loss of vision and hearing are relatively common sequelae of cranial irradiation. Visual loss can result from radiation-induced optic neuropathy, retinopathy, glaucoma, cataract formation, and dry eye syndrome. Hearing loss is due to otitis media (acute or early delayed effect) or to sensorineural damage (late delayed effect).

6. **Hormonal deficiencies** occur as a result of hypothalamic and pituitary dysfunction after irradiation. The most common deficiency involves growth hormone, but thyroid, adrenal, and gonadal dysfunctions also occur.

C. Management. Acute and early delayed reactions are self-limited but often respond to treatment with steroids. Late delayed reactions, which are usually due to neuronal and glial necrosis, do not respond to treatment.

D. Radiation-induced tumors tend to occur decades after irradiation and include meningiomas, nerve sheath tumors, astrocytomas, and sarcomas.

E. Radiation-induced cerebrovascular disease is caused by severe advanced atherosclerosis that occurs years after irradiation. It is thought to be due to occlusion of the vasa vasorum. Patients are at high risk for transient ischemic attacks and strokes.

VII. Neurologic complications of chemotherapy
  A. Drugs associated with central abnormalities
    1. Altered mental state (confusion, depression, drowsiness) is associated with the administration of methotrexate, cytarabine, procarbazine, mitotane, L-asparaginase, ifosfamide, α-IFN, pentostatin, tegafur, levamisole, and, rarely, hexamethylmelamine, fludarabine, and 5-azacytidine.
    2. Cerebellar dysfunction is associated with the use of cytarabine, procarbazine, fluorouracil, and nitrosoureas.
    3. Seizures are rare and are associated with use of vincristine, cisplatin, hydroxyurea, L-asparaginase, ifosfamide and procarbazine.
    4. Myelopathy is seen with use of intrathecal methotrexate.
  B. Drugs associated with peripheral abnormalities
    1. Peripheral neuropathy occurs with vincristine, vindesine, vinblastine, procarbazine, hexamethylmelamine, etoposide, teniposide, taxol, and cisplatin.
    2. Cranial neuropathy is seen with use of vincristine, nitrosoureas (optic neuritis uncommonly), and cisplatin (ototoxicity, loss of taste).
VIII. Other complications of cancer
  A. Cerebrovascular disease (CVD). Strokes and hemorrhages are the second most common cause of CNS lesions in cancer patients. (Metastases are the most common.) Autopsy series show that 15 percent of cancer patients have CVD, of whom half have symptoms during their lifetime. In addition to risk factors that apply to the general population, patients with cancer have additional factors that predispose them to CVD.
    1. Cerebral embolisms can result from
      a. Nonbacterial thrombotic endocarditis, seen especially with adenocarcinoma of the lung and GI tract, is the most common cause of cerebral infarction in patients with carcinoma.
      b. Septic emboli from systemic fungal infections, most commonly *Aspergillus*.
      c. Tumor emboli (uncommon).
    2. Thrombosis can cause strokes as well as occlusion of the superior sagittal sinus. The latter syndrome presents with headache, obtundation, and sometimes bilateral strokes. Thrombotic disorders in cancer are caused by
      a. DIC.
      b. Hyperviscosity syndromes.
      c. Chemotherapy, especially with L-asparaginase.
      d. Vasculitis, usually as a complication of infection.
    3. Hemorrhages are especially common in patients with leukemia, but are associated with many malignancies. Specific etiologies include
      a. Thrombocytopenia.
      b. DIC.
      c. Hyperleukocytosis (acute myelogenous leukemia).
      d. Tumor invasion of blood vessels.
      e. Bleeding diatheses (e.g., in hepatic failure).
    4. Subdural hematomas can result from
      a. Dural metastases.
      b. Lumbar puncture.
  B. CNS infections are discussed in Chap. 35, sec. **II.B.**
  C. Ocular complications in cancer
    1. Metastases to the eye and orbit
      a. Etiology. Ocular and orbital metastases occur most frequently in breast cancer. Hematogenous dissemination to the eye also complicates acute leukemia, melanoma, and sarcomas and carcinomas of the lung, bladder, and prostate. Several head and neck cancers can directly invade the orbit.
      b. Diagnosis
        (1) Signs. Patients develop eye pain, diplopia, loss of vision, and exophthalmos. Fundal hemorrhages, leukemic infiltrates, or masses may be evident on ophthalmoscopy.

(2) **CT scans** of the orbits, brain, and surrounding tissues must be obtained in patients with symptoms of ocular or orbital metastases.

(3) **Biopsy** is performed if the retro-orbital mass is the sole site of disease.

c. **Management.** Prednisone, 40 mg/m^2 PO daily, should be given if vision is threatened. RT to the orbit is the treatment of choice for metastatic disease but may result in blindness. On the other hand, emergency treatment of the eye with small doses of RT may prevent blindness in patients with ocular involvement from acute leukemia.

2. **Thrombosis of the central retinal vein**

a. **Etiology.** Central retinal vein thrombosis occurs in hyperviscosity syndromes associated with Waldenström's macroglobulinemia and occasionally with plasma cell myeloma. Marked erythrocytosis from polycythemia vera may also cause the problem.

b. **Diagnosis.** Patients develop a sudden, often painless loss of vision. "Sausage-link" widening of conjunctival and fundal veins may be present. The fundus may also have hemorrhages, hard and soft exudates, and microaneurysms.

c. **Management.** Plasmapheresis is used for malignant paraproteinemias (see Chap. 22), and phlebotomy for polycythemia vera (see Chap. 24, *Polycythemia Vera*).

3. **Retinal artery occlusion**

a. **Etiology.** Embolic retinal artery occlusion is most commonly due to atherosclerosis but may rarely be seen with atrial myxoma, marantic endocarditis, and cryoglobulinemia.

b. **Diagnosis.** Patients develop sudden, painless loss of vision and a pale fundus with a bright red spot over the fovea.

c. **Management.** Ophthalmologic consultation should be obtained immediately in all cases. Emergent measures include vigorous massage of the eye, administration of tolazoline (Priscoline, 75 mg IV) as a vasodilator, and aspiration of aqueous humor.

4. **Amaurosis fugax** can occur in patients with marked thrombocytosis (usually greater than 800,000/μL) caused by myeloproliferative diseases, especially primary thrombocythemia or polycythemia vera. Treatment consists of antiplatelet drugs (e.g., aspirin, 300–900 mg/day) and chemotherapy. Plateletpheresis may also be used in severe cases.

Selected Reading

Anderson, N. E., Cunningham, J. M., and Posner, J. B. Autoimmune pathogenesis of paraneoplastic neurological syndromes. *Crit. Rev. Neurobiol.* 3:245, 1987.

Byrne, T. N. Spinal cord compression from epidural metastases. *N. Engl. J. Med.* 327:614, 1992.

Graus, F., Rogers, L. R., and Posner, J. B. Cerebrovascular complications in patients with cancer. *Medicine* 64:16, 1985.

Kori, S. H., Foley, K. M., and Posner, J. B. Brachial plexus lesions in patients with cancer: 100 cases. *Neurology* 31:45, 1981.

Patchell, R. R., and Posner, J. B. Neurologic complications of systemic cancer. *Neurol. Clin.* 3:729, 1985.

Portenoy, R. K., Lipton, R. B., and Foley, K. M. Back pain in the cancer patient: An algorithm for evaluation and management. *Neurology* 37:134, 1987.

Sheline, G. E., Wara, W. M., and Smith, V. Therapeutic irradiation and brain injury. *Int. J. Radiat. Oncol. Biol. Phys.* 6:1215, 1980.

Sundaresan, N., and Galicich, J. H. Surgical treatment of brain metastases: Clinical and computerized tomography evaluation of the results of treatment. *Cancer* 55: 1382, 1985.

Wasserstrom, W. R., Glass, J. P., and Posner, J. B. Diagnosis and treatment of leptomeninges metastases from solid tumors: Experience with 90 patients. *Cancer* 49:759, 1982.

Zimm, S., et al. Intracerebral metastases in solid-tumor patients: Natural history and results of treatment. *Cancer* 48:384, 1981.

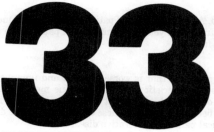

Bone and Joint Complications

Dennis A. Casciato

I. Metastases to cortical bone. Metastases to bone marrow are discussed in Chap. 34, *Cytopenias,* sec. **I.A.**

A. Pathogenesis. Bone metastases commonly develop in the course of many cancers (see Table 2-1). The bones most frequently involved are the femur, pelvis, spine, and ribs. Tumor cells may metastasize to vertebral bodies or the skull without entering the systemic circulation by seeding through Batson's vertebral venous plexus (a valveless system of veins along the entire vertebral column that communicates with other venous systems, from the pelvis to the brain).

   1. Mechanisms. Osteoclasts mediate bone resorption in health and disease. Osteoclast activation is the key step in the establishment and growth of all bone metastases; stimulation of osteoblastic activity also occurs. Malignant cells secrete many factors known to both stimulate the proliferation and activity of osteoclasts and produce osteolysis, possibly indirectly through the osteoblasts. These factors include:

     a. Transforming growth factors

     b. Prostaglandins

     c. Tumor necrosis factors

     d. Parathyroid hormone-related protein

     e. Cytokines, such as interleukins, which activate osteoclasts either directly by tumor cells or indirectly by tumor-stimulated immune cells

   2. Frequency. A relatively small number of malignancies account for the majority of tumors that spread to bone.

     a. Tumors that commonly metastasize to bone. Carcinomas of unknown primary site, the lung, breast, kidney, prostate, and thyroid; plasmacytoma; melanoma; and Ewing's sarcoma

     b. Tumors that rarely metastasize to bone. Ovarian carcinoma and most soft tissue sarcomas

B. Natural history. Bone metastases are usually confined within the bony substance and generally do not cross joint spaces. They lead to pathologic fractures and progressive crippling. A variety of complications can result in death.

   1. Cervical spine metastases with pathologic fracture can damage the spinal cord above the respiratory muscle nerve supply (C1–C4).

   2. Extraosseous extension of bone metastases may compromise neurologic function.

   3. Dense sclerosis of bones (e.g., with prostate cancer) or extensive involvement of bone marrow spaces can result in refractory pancytopenia.

   4. Crippling bone disease can make bedridden patients susceptible to decubitus ulcers, hypercalcemia, and infections.

   5. Pathologic fractures are uncommon in prostate cancer even though the skeleton is the main site of distant metastases, perhaps because of the predominantly osteoblastic response to these lesions.

C. Prognosis. The expected survival of patients with skeletal metastasis varies. Patients with lung cancer survive only a few months. The median survival of patients with breast cancer and only skeletal metastases, however, is two years. The median survival of patients with stage IV renal cancer is 11 months, but 20 to 30 percent of those with a solitary metastasis survive five years after the lesion is surgically resected. About 20 percent of patients with skeletal metastases from prostate cancer survive five years. The majority of patients die within six months of a pathologic fracture.

D. Diagnosis

1. **Symptoms and signs**
   a. Dull, aching, or boring pain that is worse at night and improves with physical activity is characteristic of pain from bone metastases. This pain pattern also occurs with malignant invasion of retroperitoneal structures without bony involvement. These characteristics are directly opposite to the typical pain of degenerative diseases.
   b. Bone pain intensified by activity is often the first symptom of imminent fracture. On the other hand, pathologic fractures can also be painless. Patients often report falling down, but it is often not clear if the fracture was the cause or effect of the fall.

2. **Serum alkaline phosphatase** levels are usually elevated in patients with bone metastases. Elevations appear to reflect an osteoblastic (or healing) response to tumor destruction. In pure osteolytic tumors, such as plasma cell myeloma, the serum alkaline phosphatase level is normal. Non-neoplastic causes of increased *bone* alkaline phosphatase include
   a. Primary hyperparathyroidism, thyrotoxicosis, acromegaly
   b. Renal disease
   c. Paget's disease
   d. Osteomalacia
   e. Healing fractures
   f. Physiologic increases occur in
      (1) Pediatric age group (before bony epiphyseal closure)
      (2) Pregnancy (placental source)

3. **Radionuclide bone scan,** utilizing Tc-99m-methylene biphosphonate, is the most effective screening test for skeletal metastases. The scan often detects metastases several months before radiologic changes are evident.
   a. **Specificity.** Patients with a known cancer and bone pain have positive bone scans in 60 to 70 percent of cases; patients without bone pain have positive scans in 10 to 15 percent of cases.
      (1) Multiple "hot spots" are more specific than one or two. In cancer patients without known metastases, the appearance of new abnormalities on bone scan represents metastasis in only 10 percent of patients with one lesion and in 25 percent of patients with two lesions.
      (2) Retroperitoneal tumors often cause a bony response, characterized by diffuse isotope uptake over the anterior aspect of the spine.
      (3) Patients with bone metastases from breast or prostate cancer may develop new abnormal areas on scans because of bone healing while improving clinically on endocrine therapy.
      (4) Multiple myeloma is the most frequent cause of false-negative bone scans. These patients rarely have positive bone scans except in fractured areas.
      (5) Decreased uptake of radioisotope is seen in irradiated bone that never did contain metastases and thus cannot be interpreted as a sign of absence of metastases or of reduced tumor burden.
   b. **Benign conditions that can cause a positive bone scan**
      (1) Bone healing after fracture
      (2) Radiation osteitis
      (3) Arthritis and spondylitis
      (4) Osteomyelitis
      (5) Osteonecrosis
      (6) Regional osteoporosis
      (7) Paget's disease of bone
      (8) Hyperostosis frontalis interna
      (9) Osteopetrosis (Albers-Schönberg disease)
      (10) Osteogenesis imperfecta

Table 33-1. Radiologic characteristics of bone metastases

Predominantly lytic tumors	Mixed lytic and blastic tumors	Predominantly blastic tumors	Other causes of blastic bone lesions
Non-small cell lung cancer Renal cancer Multiple myeloma Melanoma Thyroid cancer	Breast cancer Squamous cell cancers (most primary sites) Gastrointestinal cancers (most)	Small cell lung cancer Prostate cancer Carcinoids Gastrinoma Gastric cancers (some) Hodgkin's disease Lymphomas Mastocytosis	Tuberculosis Fluorosis Osteoarthritis Osteopetrosis Paget's disease Tuberous sclerosis

4. **Plain x-rays** remain essential for the diagnosis and characterization of bone metastases. Metastatic lesions must involve 30 to 50 percent of bone matrix to be visualized on plain x-ray films. Some tumors typically produce osteolytic or osteoblastic metastases, but most tumors produce mixed lesions (Table 33-1). *Diffuse osteoporosis* may be the only radiologic abnormality in some patients with extensive bony involvement (e.g., multiple myeloma). *Skeletal infections* with many pyogenic bacteria are frequently associated with sclerotic reactions; chronic granulomatous infections, however, may result in purely lytic lesions.
   a. **Indications.** X-ray films should be obtained and compared with previous films of the involved areas in patients with
      (1) Bone pain
      (2) Abnormalities on physical examination suggestive of fracture
      (3) Asymptomatic abnormalities in bone scans
   b. **Routine skeletal surveys** are not indicated except in patients with plasma cell myeloma that may be associated with painless osteolytic lesions in critical bone sites, such as the femora or cervical spine.
   c. **Vertebral involvement** from metastatic cancer is manifested by loss of the pedicles or lateral spinous processes, and vertebral collapse with sparing of the intervertebral space. Infections that involve the intervertebral disc space destroy it. Some chronic infections (e.g., tuberculosis or brucellosis), however, may involve the vertebrae and not the intervertebral spaces, result in vertebral collapse, and thereby mimic malignancy.
   d. **Postirradiation osteitis** produces irregular, diffuse (rather than localized) lytic or mixed lesions confined to the radiation portal.
5. **CT scan** is useful to diagnose early metastases of bone, particularly the spine, when hot spots are detected on the radionuclide scan but corresponding plain x-rays are normal. CT scans elucidate cortical erosion, subtle fractures, and matrix calcification or ossification. In addition, they are useful to evaluate epidural compression, the extent of metastases (e.g., in the femur), and areas difficult to image by conventional x-ray (e.g., costovertebral junction, sternum and sacrum).
6. **MRI scan** is best at delineating the extraosseous extension of a soft tissue mass through the bone cortex (e.g., epidural compression). This technique is also ideal for demonstrating the intraosseous extension of tumor into the cancellous bone.
7. **Biopsy.** If a fracture has already occurred, care must be taken to sample the tumorous area adequately rather than the healing area of fibrous tissue and osteoid formation. Specific expertise in bone histopathology must be available.

   a. Indications. If other sites associated with a lower risk of morbidity are not available, biopsy is done on an accessible site. Bone biopsy for the differential diagnosis of cancer is indicated in patients with
   - **(1)** An isolated bone lesion that the radiologist interprets as being compatible with a primary bone tumor
   - **(2)** An osteolytic bone lesion in a critical area (e.g., cervical spine or femoral neck) and no history of cancer
   - **(3)** A history of a cancer that metastasizes to bone, localized bone pain, normal x-ray films of the area, equivocal bone scan and alkaline phosphatase results, and no evidence of disease elsewhere
   - **(4)** Isolated bone pain in a region that was previously irradiated and x-ray findings that are not typical of postirradiation osteitis
   b. Contraindications. Bone biopsy should not be done in asymptomatic patients with isolated, osteolytic lesions in noncritical areas that are suspected to be benign lesions or metastatic disease. Biopsy in these patients often results in chronic pain at the biopsy site. If a cancer is discovered, it is a metastasis for which treatment could have awaited the development of more widespread symptomatic disease.

E. Management
 1. **Medical management** is necessary in patients with multiple painful metastatic sites.
   a. Chemotherapy and endocrine therapy are useful for treating metastatic tumors known to respond to these modalities. Chemotherapy doses may need to be attenuated because of compromised marrow function from neoplastic invasion or irradiation.
   b. Osteoclast inhibition. Biphosphonates (such as pamidronate or clodronate) are specific inhibitors of osteoclast-mediated bone resorption. Long-term treatment with biphosphonates or stable gallium nitrate to decrease the occurrence of bone pain and pathologic fractures is being investigated in patients with accelerated bone resorption secondary to malignancy. Alternatively, calcitonin or plicamycin could be used for these effects, but are not recommended.
   c. Criteria for response of bone metastases to therapy. The appearance of new osteoblastic lesions on x-ray or bone scans or increasing size of sclerotic lesions does not necessarily indicate progression of metastases. Indeed, these findings may represent clinical improvement. Although the response of bone metastases to treatment is difficult to quantitate, it may be evaluated by assessing
   - **(1)** Pain relief and quality of life
   - **(2)** Serum tumor markers
   - **(3)** Biochemical markers of bone resorption (e.g., hydroxyproline urinary excretion)
   - **(4)** CT scans
   d. Bracing of the vertebral column helps relieve pain and protect neurovascular structures while the lesions are resolved with RT or chemotherapy. Bony strength to resist gravitational forces must be adequate. Bracing of the extremities is seldom helpful.
   e. Analgesic therapy is discussed in Chap. 5, sec. I.
   f. Hypercalcemia is discussed in Chap. 27, sec. I.
 2. **RT** ameliorates pain and may produce bone union and prevent fracture. The optimal dose of RT has not been defined. Smaller doses (e.g., 800 cGy given once) may be as effective as 2500 to 4000 cGy given over two to four weeks.
   a. Pathologic fractures. RT given 10 to 20 days after orthopedic fixation of pathologic fractures is generally considered standard therapy, but the clinical benefit of this additional treatment has *not been demonstrated*.
   b. Isolated sites of bone pain. RT controls local pain from bony metastases in more than 80 percent of patients within two weeks to three months. Irradiating a few severely painful sites may reduce the analgesic dose needed to manage patients with multiple sites of pain.

    c. Asymptomatic osteolytic lesions of the cervical spine and long bones are irradiated to prevent complications.

    d. Hemibody irradiation is used by some centers for control of pain caused by bone metastases. The treatment is effective in about 60 percent of patients, but it is associated with GI upset and hematosuppression, particularly transfusion-dependent anemia.

3. Radiopharmaceuticals, especially ^{89}Sr (Metastron), can decrease pain for several months in about 75 percent of patients with skeletal metastases from breast or prostate cancer. Such agents are useful when endocrine therapy fails to control the disease (see Chap. 2, sec. **IV.B**).

    a. ^{89}Sr is preferentially taken up and retained at sites of increased bone mineral turnover; uptake in bone adjacent to metastases is up to five times greater than for normal bone. This agent appears to provide effective adjuvant therapy to local field RT with decreased new sites of pain, decreased need for further RT, decreased analgesic requirement, and improved quality of life.

    b. Hematologic toxicity is the major precaution, but is usually transient. Other agents (including ^{32}P, ^{153}Sm, and ^{186}Re) generally are associated with more hematologic toxicity or have undergone fewer clinical trials than ^{89}Sr.

    c. Unfortunately, substantial numbers of patients achieve incomplete pain resolution and some patients get no pain relief at all. None of the radiopharmaceuticals affect survival. Relatively few patients exhibit antitumor activity when treated with radiopharmaceuticals.

4. Surgery plays a critical role in managing bony metastases that endanger neurologic function or ambulation. Surgery can usually be avoided when RT or chemotherapy is effective and adequate stability of the bone permits natural repair.

    Orthopedic consultation should be obtained in all patients with metastatic lesions of the femoral neck or shaft or with pathologic limb fracture. When considering operative treatment, the major factors include the patient's general medical condition, functional goals, and comfort and quality of life; the ease of delivering nursing care; and the morbidity of the contemplated procedure.

    a. Methyl methacrylate bone cement greatly enhances the ability to utilize metal implants of either the prosthetic or the fracture-fixation type. It increases binding and torsional stability, promotes hemostasis, and should be used with fixation devices whenever possible.

    b. Methods

        (1) Reinforcement of the involved bone with internal splints (bone plates, hip nails, intramedullary rods)

        (2) Removal of the metastatic tumor from the bone, replacement with methyl methacrylate cement, and insertion of an internal metal splint

        (3) En bloc excision of involved segments of periarticular bone and reconstruction of the joint with a prosthesis bonded to bone with methyl methacrylate cement

        (4) Amputation of painful, dysfunctional extremities riddled with tumor in patients with a reasonable life expectancy

    c. Complications. Surgical treatment for pathologic fractures is associated with an operative mortality of about 8 percent and an infection rate of about 4 percent. Common reasons for failure of internal fixation include poor initial fixation, improper implant selection, and progression of disease within the operative field.

    d. Blood loss during surgical stabilization or biopsy of a metastatic lesion may be life-threatening. Myeloma, breast cancer, and renal cell cancer are notoriously hypervascular. Preoperative angiography and occlusion of feeding vessels, particularly for lesions of the acetabulum, may be indicated.

    e. Rehabilitation. Patients treated surgically for pathologic fractures caused by metastases are good candidates for intensive rehabilitation programs unless they have hypercalcemia or require parenteral narcotics, which are associated with very short survival.

5. Surgical management of specific sites

    a. Upper extremities. Pathologic fracture of the humerus usually occurs at the junction of its proximal and middle thirds; fracture is often treated by stabilizing the extremity in a cast or sling. If the fracture interferes with the functional goals of the patient or if pain is refractory to RT, then excision of tumor, replacement with bone cement, and internal fixation must be considered.

    b. Lower extremities: prophylactic orthopedic surgery. Prophylactic internal fixation is always considered in patients with lytic lesions in the femoral neck or shaft that are at risk for pathologic fracture. Prophylactic surgery should be considered if

      (1) The patient is in good general medical condition, *and*

      (2) The lytic lesion is more than 2.5 cm in diameter (especially if in the femur or tibia), *or*

      (3) The lesion has destroyed at least 50 percent of the cortex of any long bone, *or*

      (4) Spontaneous avulsion of the lesser trochanter has occurred, *or*

      (5) Pain from lytic lesions persists despite RT, regardless of the size of the lesion

    c. Lower extremities: pathologic fractures. Internal fixation is indicated for pathologic fractures of the femur or tibia to decrease pain and to permit early ambulation.

      (1) Femoral head and neck fractures. Internal fixation may be considered but is usually inadequate. Cemented hemiarthroplasty is safe, provides long-lasting relief from pain, permits early ambulation without the need for postoperative RT, and is preferred. Prosthetic replacement is particularly required if bony destruction that would not allow a stable construction even with bone cement augmentation is extensive. A prosthesis with a cemented acetabular cup also should be used if there is a concomitant acetabular lesion. The complication rate is 25 percent.

      (2) Intertrochanteric fractures. Nail-plate devices are used when sufficient residual bone is present to allow stable bony fixation and support body weight, but intramedullary devices (such as the Zickel nail) are frequently required. Prosthetic replacement is considered if there is extensive bony loss, if pathologic fracture has developed slowly, or if there is no possibility of obtaining structural stabililty; the complication rate, however, is substantial.

      (3) Subtrochanteric fractures are more difficult to repair because the fracture often extends into the intertrochanteric area or femoral shaft. Nail-plate devices are associated with a high frequency of implant failure, but intramedullary devices are helpful, especially with the use of methyl methacrylate.

      (4) Femoral shaft fractures require rigid fixation with bone cement and various intramedullary rods, plates, or nails. Nonoperative treatment is generally unsuccessful and causes prolonged periods of pain and difficulty in nursing care.

      (5) Acetabulum. Although lesions of the acetabular roof may respond to chemotherapy, they still leave the patient with an unstable hip if collapse of the roof has already begun. Reconstructive surgery with total hip replacement is often beneficial in patients with reasonable life expectancy (e.g., those with breast cancer).

    d. Cervical spine lesions must be irradiated regardless of symptoms. Patients with cervical spine metastases from any tumor require external immobilization of the head. A soft cervical collar is the least uncomfortable method but should be used only in patients with minimal disease. A rigid two-poster or similar collarlike brace is adequate support if there is some intrinsic stability. If there is gross instability and the integrity of the spinal cord is in jeopardy, it may be necessary to rigidly fix the head with a special brace and the placement of screws into the skull. Since RT rarely produces healing, these prosthetic devices are often permanent.

   e. Thoracolumbar spinal metastases
      (1) Painful lesions should be irradiated. MRI should be done first to search for potential sites of epidural compression and to plan radiation fields. Many patients have evidence of a soft tissue mass extending around the involved vertebrae. These masses compress nerves, contribute to pain, and should be included in the radiation port. Fiberglass braces and corsets may reduce back pain and help stabilize the spine. The patient may be weaned from the supports as the spine stabilizes with therapy.
      (2) Rapidly progressive metastases that are refractory to RT may be manifested by increasing pain, worsening destruction on x-ray films, or the development of neurologic deficits. Open decompression of the spinal cord and internal fixation with rods or plates to permit early mobility (3–4 weeks) should be considered, but the outlook for these patients is poor.

II. Paraneoplastic bone and joint conditions. The mechanism for the development of paraneoplastic rheumatologic conditions is unknown.
   A. Hypertrophic osteoarthropathy is manifested by clubbing of the fingers, pain and effusion in large joints, and periosteitis. The ankles, knees, elbows, and wrists are the most frequently involved joints. The extremely painful periosteal reaction usually involves the extensor surfaces of the legs and forearms. The change in the overlying skin resembles cellulitis with induration, erythema, and peau d'orange.
      1. Associated tumors. Hypertrophic osteoarthropathy develops most frequently with lung adenocarcinomas, less frequently with other lung carcinomas, and occasionally with GI adenocarcinomas and intrathoracic sarcomas.
      2. Benign causes of clubbing
         a. Hereditary clubbing
         b. Lung abscess
         c. Bronchiectasis
         d. Tuberculosis
         e. Endocarditis
         f. Biliary cirrhosis
         g. Crohn's disease
         h. Cyanotic congenital heart disease
      3. Diagnosis. Clubbing should be self-evident; patients should be questioned about the duration of the abnormality. Sponginess, by palpation, of the proximal nail beds may indicate early clubbing. X-ray films of painful joints or long bones will often show periosteal reactions.
      4. Therapy. Control of the associated tumor usually alleviates symptoms of hypertrophic osteoarthropathy. The pain can be relieved by a variety of NSAIDs. Patients with severe pain from periosteitis require narcotic analgesics.
   B. Pachydermoperiostosis associated with lung cancer consists of a dense overgrowth of periosteum resulting in clubbing and leonine facies (see Chap. 28, sec. II.I).
   C. Joint pain, subcutaneous fat necrosis (panniculitis), and eosinophilia occasionally constitute the presenting features of pancreatic cancer.
   D. Rheumatoid arthritis starting after the age of 50 years or suddenly worsening after a long dormant period may be a prodrome of cancer, particularly pancreatic carcinoma. However, an increased incidence of cancer with late onset rheumatoid arthritis has not been demonstrated.

E. Hypercalcemia and hypocalcemia. See Chap. 27, sections **I.A.** and **II.A.**

F. Acute leukemic arthritis is caused by leukemic infiltration of synovium. It is usually symmetric and may resemble rheumatic fever or juvenile rheumatoid arthritis. Effusions may occur. In 25 percent of cases, adjacent bone may develop lytic lesions, osteoporosis, or osteoblastic changes. Brief symptomatic responses can be obtained with ibuprofen or aspirin. Treatment of the underlying leukemia resolves with arthritis.

G. Chronic leukemic arthritis is uncommon; it is usually symmetric but is otherwise similar to the acute type both in roentgenographic patterns and response to therapy.

H. Hairy-cell leukemia arthritis is occasionally associated with vasculitis and rheumatoid arthritis.

I. Myeloma-induced amyloidosis produces carpal tunnel syndrome and, rarely, a rheumatoid arthritis-like syndrome. Synovial tissues may be densely infiltrated with myeloma cells.

J. Serologic abnormalities including antinuclear antibodies, rheumatoid factor, and immune complexes are found in a variety of leukemias, lymphomas, and solid tumors.

III. Adverse effects of radiation to bone

A. Radio-osteonecrosis of the mandible may complicate RT of head and neck cancers. The problem occurs more often in patients with large tumors, bone invasion, history of large alcohol intake and heavy smoking, poor dentition, poor oral hygiene, and poor nutritional status. The mandible becomes brittle and superinfected, resulting in pain, fractures, and draining fistulae.

1. Diagnostic criteria
   a. Localized pain and tenderness.
   b. Mucosal ulceration or necrosis (occasionally, a fistula) with exposure of bone and, occasionally, cutaneous fistulae.
   c. Loose teeth in the suspected area.
   d. X-ray films show a lytic lesion of the mandible, sometimes with a radiodense sequestrum or involucrum.
   e. Manifestations should not be clinically evident for at least four months after completion of treatment.

2. Prevention of radio-osteonecrosis involves proper dental extractions before RT and oral hygiene and fluoride treatment regimen during and after RT. If possible, the patient should not have any dental extractions for two years after RT. Even with these precautions, osteonecrosis develops in 5 to 10 percent of patients when a high-dose RT portal overlies the mandible.

3. Treatment
   a. Conservative management
      (1) Frequent mouthwashes with dilute hydrogen peroxide, or a baking soda and salt solution
      (2) Systemic antibiotics, usually penicillin
      (3) Topical nystatin or bacitracin ointment
      (4) Analgesics
      (5) Gentle debridement
   b. Aggressive management
      (1) Hyperbaric oxygen treatments
      (2) Surgical resection of the nonviable portion of the mandible
      (3) A combination of hyperbaric oxygen and surgical resection

B. Radiation osteitis may mimic bony metastases. Differentiation of these disorders is discussed in sec. **I.D.** Postradiation pathologic fractures of the femoral neck may rarely complicate pelvic irradiation.

C. Radiation-induced bone sarcomas have been reported following high-dose irradiation of both benign and malignant lesions. The incidence is less than 0.1 percent of all five-year survivors; the latent period is more than five years.

D. Premature closure of bone epiphyses and apophyses can result in shortening, kyphosis, and asymmetry of osseous structures in children who have received RT.

IV. Adverse effects of chemotherapy on bone

A. Aseptic necrosis of the hip is a complication of high doses of glucocorticoids. The risk is proportional to the dose of drug and not to the duration of therapy. Increased pressure in the intramedullary space causes the sudden onset of hip pain. Capsular pain is demonstrated by flexing the hip and medially rotating the thigh. Early diagnosis is best established by MRI. Radionuclide bone scan is the diagnostic test of second choice. Orthopedic removal of bone cores decompresses the affected bone and prevents necrosis; this procedure must be done before plain x-ray studies show changes or irreversible bone necrosis that make hip replacement necessary.

B. Postchemotherapy rheumatism is a syndrome of myalgias and arthralgias that develops within one to three months after completing adjuvant chemotherapy for breast cancer utilizing cyclophosphamide and 5-fluorouracil. Mild periarticular swelling occurs in some cases. NSAIDs are not effective. Symptoms are self-limiting and generally resolve over several months. Extensive workups for breast cancer recurrence or for inflammatory rheumatologic disease are not needed in this setting.

C. Raynaud's phenomenon is a common toxicity of treatment with cisplatin, vinblastine, or bleomycin.

Selected Reading

Body, J. J. Metastatic bone disease: Clinical and therapeutic aspects. *Bone* 13:S57, 1992.

Bunting, R. W., et al. Functional outcome of pathologic fractures secondary to malignant disease in a rehabilitation hospital. *Cancer* 69:98, 1992.

Coleman, R. E. and Purohit, O. P. Osteoclast inhibition for the treatment of bone metastases. *Cancer Treat. Rev.* 19:79, 1993.

Kanis, J. A., et al. Rationale for the use of biphosphonates in bone metastases. *Bone* 12(Suppl. 1):S13, 1991.

Loprinzi, C. L., Duffy, J., and Ingle, J. N. Postchemotherapy rheumatism. *J. Clin. Oncol.* 11:768, 1993.

Mertens, W. C. Radionuclide therapy of bone metastases: Prospects for enhancement of therapeutic efficacy. *Semin. Oncol.* 20(Suppl. 2):49, 1993.

Porter, A. T., et al. Results of a randomized phase-III trial to evaluate the efficacy of strontium-89 adjuvant to local field external beam irradiation in the management of endocrine resistant metastatic prostate cancer. *Int. J. Radiat. Oncol. Biol. Phys.* 25:805, 1993.

Wilkins, R. M., Sim, F. H., and Springfield, D. S. Metastatic disease of the femur. *Orthopedics* 15:621, 1992.

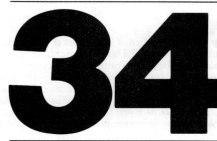

Hematologic Complications

Dennis A. Casciato

Increased Blood Cell Counts

I. **Erythrocytosis (polycythemia).** Erythrocytosis is defined as an elevation of the hematocrit, hemoglobin, and red cell count above the *upper limits of normal.* Normal limits in adults are

	Men	Women
Hematocit	52%	47%
Hemoglobin	17.7 gm/dl	15.7 gm/dl
Red cell count	$5.9 \times 10^6/\mu L$	$5.2 \times 10^6/\mu L$
Red cell mass	36 ml/kg	32 ml/kg

A. **Relative polycythemia** is characterized by normal red cell mass and decreased plasma volume. Causes of relative polycythemia include dehydration, diuretics, burns, capillary leak, decreased oncotic pressure ("third-spacing"), hypertension, and stress ("Gaisböck's syndrome").

B. **Primary polycythemia** (polycythemia vera, PV) develops independently of serum erythropoietin (EP) concentration. Uncontrolled proliferation of marrow elements results in an increased red cell mass. Diagnostic criteria for PV are discussed in Chap. 24, *Polycythemia Vera.*

C. **Secondary polycythemia** is associated with increased red cell mass and increased EP levels.

   1. **Appropriate erythrocytosis**

      a. **Chronic hypoxemia** is a potent stimulus for erythropoietin production. Causes of hypoxemia include pulmonary diseases, right-to-left intracardiac shunts, low atmospheric pressure (high altitudes), and alveolar hypoventilation (brain disease or Pickwickian syndrome). Intermittent arterial desaturation and erythrocytosis may be caused by supine posture, particularly in obese patients with pulmonary disease.

      b. **Heavy smoking.** Excessive and sustained exposure to carbon monoxide from cigarettes or cigars, which produces an increased affinity between the remaining oxygen and the hemoglobin molecule, is a very common cause of erythrocytosis.

      c. **Congenital disorders** include hemoglobinopathies with high oxygen affinity (abnormal oxyhemoglobin dissociation), decreased erythrocyte 2,3-diphosphoglycerate (rare), and overproduction of EP.

      d. **Androgen therapy** stimulates erythropoiesis.

   2. **Inappropriate erythrocytosis** occurs with elevated EP levels in the absence of generalized tissue hypoxia and is seen in a variety of diseases.

      a. **Renal diseases** account for approximately 60 percent of all cases of inappropriate erythrocytosis, and **renal adenocarcinomas** account for half of those cases. Cysts, other tumors, hydronephrosis, and transplantation make up the remaining renal causes of erythrocytosis.

         (1) **Renal cell carcinomas** are associated with erythrocytosis in 1 to 5 percent of cases. The tumor cells are the site of EP synthesis.

         (2) **Renal transplantation** is associated with erythrocytosis in 10 per-

cent of patients. The erythrocytosis has been ascribed to transplanted artery stenosis, graft rejection, hypertension, hydronephrosis, diuretic use, and EP overproduction from residual renal tissue, especially in polycystic disease.

b. **Hepatocellular carcinoma and cerebellar hemangioblastoma** each account for 15 to 20 percent of cases of inappropriate erythrocytosis in the literature.

c. **Other causes** of inappropriate erythrocytosis are rare. Huge uterine leiomyomata and ovarian carcinoma can cause renal hypoxia or ectopic EP production. Pheochromocytomas and aldosteronomas cause erythrocytosis through multiple mechanisms.

D. **Evaluation of patients with polycythemia**

1. **Screening evaluation.** The following studies are obtained in all patients with persistent polycythemia:

a. Perform a **complete history and physical examination** to search for known causes of erythrocytosis. Search for treatments that are associated with erythrocytosis (androgen therapy, renal transplantation). Diligently search for **splenomegaly,** which would suggest PV.

b. Evaluate for **intravascular volume depletion** (e.g., are diuretics being administered?); replete the volume and then reassess.

c. Analyze the **CBC.** The presence of granulocytosis, eosinophilia, basophilia, or thrombocytosis suggests PV.

d. Measure **arterial oxygen** partial pressure and saturation. The red cell mass is roughly proportional to the degree of arterial desaturation. Arterial oxygen saturation less than 90 percent and PaO_2 less than 60 to 65 mm Hg may result in erythrocytosis. Oxygen saturations of greater than 92 percent are required for the diagnosis of PV.

e. If the patient smokes tobacco, measure the **carboxyhemoglobin concentration;** values over 5 percent are associated with erythrocytosis. Note that smoking may also cause granulocytosis.

2. **Special diagnostic studies**

a. **Red cell mass** determination is paramount for distinguishing absolute polycythemia from relative polycythemia. Red cell mass must be measured with ^{51}Cr-labeled erythrocytes to confirm absolute erythrocytosis. Plasma volume is measured concomitantly with ^{125}I-labeled albumin to demonstrate relative erythrocytosis.

b. **Abdominal radiography** (IVP, renal ultrasonography, or abdominal CT scanning) is indicated in all patients with absolute erythrocytosis that is not explained by either PV or appropriate erythrocytosis because the frequency of renal causes is high.

c. **Serum EP concentration** can be measured if the diagnosis is in doubt. If the EP level is high in the presence of erythrocytosis, EP is being produced inappropriately. If the EP level is not high, PV or a genetic disorder of EP production is present.

d. **Oxyhemoglobin dissociation curve** is indicated in patients with a family history of unexplained erythrocytosis. An abnormal P50 indicates the decreased oxygen unloading associated with abnormal hemoglobins.

e. **Other diagnostic studies** for inappropriate erythrocytosis are obtained *only if* the screening evaluation exposes abnormalities that could indicate pathology of a specific organ.

f. **Bone marrow examination** is not diagnostic of any disorder associated with erythrocytosis. Fibrosis is present in some PV cases. Cytogenetic studies are rarely abnormal in PV. In vitro studies of hematopoiesis may be helpful in difficult cases when PV is suspected.

II. **Granulocytosis**

A. **Definitions**

1. **Granulocytosis.** The upper limit of normal for neutrophils is 8000/μL.

2. **Leukemoid reactions.** The term *leukemoid reaction* should be restricted to

granulocytosis with circulating promyelocytes and myeloblasts. Rarely, a WBC exceeding $100,000/\mu L$ with immature forms (including myeloblasts) is seen in response to solid tumor (especially cancer of the breast, lung, or stomach).

3. **Leukoerythroblastic reactions** are characterized by immature granulocytes in association with nucleated erythrocytes and poikilocytes in the peripheral blood. Platelet counts may be normal, increased, or decreased. **Differential diagnosis** includes
   a. Metastatic tumor in the marrow
   b. Marrow fibrosis with extramedullary hematopoiesis
   c. Marrow recovery following severe hematosuppression
   d. Shock, hemorrhage
   e. Brisk hemolysis, hereditary anemias

B. Causes of granulocytosis

1. **Increased proliferation in the marrow** is seen in the MPDs, marrow rebound after suppression by drug or virus, and as a chronic response to infection, inflammation, or tumor. The mechanism of tumor-induced granulocytosis most often involves increased production of granulocyte- and granulocyte-macrophage colony stimulating factors (G-CSF, GM-CSF), IL-1, and IL-3.

2. **Increased marrow proliferation and increased granulocyte survival** is seen in chronic myelogenous leukemia (CML).

3. **Shift from the marrow storage pool into the circulation** is seen in response to stress, endotoxin, corticosteroids, and etiocholanolone.

4. **Demargination** (resulting in granulocytosis involving only mature neutrophils) is seen in stress, including emotional upset, epinephrine administration, exercise, infection, hypoxia, and intoxication.

5. **Decreased egress into the tissues** is seen following chronic treatment with corticosteroids.

C. Differentiation of leukemoid reactions from MPDs and CML involves complete clinical evaluation, especially for the history and presence of splenomegaly. The leukocyte differential count, neutrophil alkaline phosphatase score, and, occasionally, cytogenetics may be helpful (see Table 24-1). Bone marrow biopsies are frequently not diagnostic.

III. Thrombocytosis

A. Thrombocytosis in cancer patients. Persistent thrombocytosis may indicate cancer. Thrombocytosis in neoplastic disease may be idiopathic or the result of bleeding or bone marrow metastases. Generally, thrombocytosis associated with solid tumors is mild, but may exceed $1,000,000/\mu L$.

B. Common causes of transient thrombocytosis

1. Acute hemorrhage or phlebotomy
2. Acute infection
3. Recovery from myelosuppression (viruses, ethanol, cytotoxic agents)
4. After surgery (persists for about 1 week)
5. Response to therapy for folic acid or vitamin B_{12} deficiency
6. Certain drugs (epinephrine, vinca alkaloids, and perhaps miconazole)

C. Causes of chronic thrombocytosis

1. Iron deficiency (the most common cause of thrombocytosis)
2. MPDs
3. Neoplasms (idiopathic or bone marrow metastases)
4. Chronic inflammatory diseases
5. Hyposplenism (postsplenectomy states, hemolytic anemias, regional enteritis, sprue, and splenic atrophy from repeated infarctions)

D. Differentiation of causes of chronic thrombocytosis. After history and physical examination, helpful screening tests for the evaluation of chronic thrombocytosis include

1. **Peripheral blood.** Megathrombocytes and fragments of megakaryocytes are rarely seen in disorders other than the MPDs and CML. A normal mean platelet volume (MPV) suggests reactive thrombocytosis. The granulocyte

differential is helpful for recognizing MPDs and CML. The presence of hypochromia and microcytosis supports iron deficiency.

2. **Serum iron, iron-binding capacity, and serum ferritin.**
3. **Bone marrow** aspirate examination will demonstrate panmyelosis in MPDs and CML. Bone marrow biopsy may detect tumor involvement. Iron staining is unreliable in patients with cancer or chronic inflammatory diseases if the results show low or absent iron stores.

IV. Eosinophilia

A. **Definition.** The upper limit of normal in absolute cell count is 550/μL.

B. **Non-neoplastic causes of eosinophilia**
1. Allergies and drug hypersensitivities
2. Skin diseases (many types)
3. Infection with fungus, protozoan, or metazoan; convalescence following a febrile illness
4. Eosinophilic gastroenteritis, inflammatory bowel disease
5. Eosinophilic pulmonary syndromes (e.g., Löffler's syndrome)
6. Collagen vascular diseases, especially rheumatoid arthritis and polyarteritis nodosa
7. Contaminated tryptophan eosinophilia-myalgia syndrome
8. Chronic active hepatitis, pernicious anemia, immunodeficiency syndromes
9. Hyposplenism (see sec. **III.C.5**)
10. Hypereosinophilic syndromes (see Chap. 23, *Hypereosinophilic Syndrome*)

C. **Eosinophilia associated with neoplasia**
1. Hodgkin's disease (up to 20% of cases)
2. MPDs and CML (common)
3. Immunoblastic lymphadenopathy (more than 30% of cases)
4. Acute lymphocytic leukemia and lymphoma (especially T cell types)
5. Angiolymphoid hyperplasia with eosinophilia (Kimura's disease)
6. Pancreatic acinar cell carcinoma (syndrome of polyarthritis, subcutaneous panniculitis, and peripheral eosinophilia)
7. Tumors undergoing central necrosis or metastasizing to serosal surfaces
8. Malignant histiocytosis
9. Eosinophilia related to treatment: RT to the abdomen, hypersensitivity to cytotoxic agents.

V. Basophilia

A. **Definition.** The upper limit of normal is 50/μL.

B. **Causes of basophilia**
1. Hypersensitivity reactions
2. Myeloproliferative disorders
3. Chronic granulocytic leukemia
4. Mastocytosis
5. Hyposplenism (see sec. **III.C.5**)
6. Infections: tuberculosis, influenza, hookworm
7. Endocrine: diabetes mellitus, myxedema, menses onset
8. Miscellaneous: hemolytic anemia, ulcerative colitis, carcinoma

VI. Monocytosis

A. **Definition.** The upper limit of normal is 500 to 800/μL.

B. **Causes of monocytosis**
1. Hematologic neoplasms, preleukemia, neutropenia, hemolytic anemias, and other hematologic disorders
2. Solid tumors with and without metastases
3. Tuberculosis, subacute bacterial endocarditis, syphilis, and resolution from acute infection
4. Inflammatory bowel disease and sprue
5. Collagen vascular disease
6. Hyposplenism (see sec. **III.C.5**)
7. Factitious monocytosis may occur when blood samples are taken from finger tips affected by peripheral vascular disease

VII. Lymphocytosis (discussed in Chap. 23, *Chronic Lymphocytic Leukemia*, sec. **III.D**).

Table 34-1. Hematopoiesis, cell kinetics, and bone marrow injury

Characteristic	Erythrocytes	Platelets	Neutrophils	Lymphocytes
Bone marrow				
Storage cell	Reticulocyte	Megakaryocyte ($32n$ ploidy); platelets	Metamyelocyte	Lymphocyte
From blast to storage cell	3 days	5 days	5 days	Unknown
Storage time	2 days	<1 day	3–4 days	Unknown
Circulation				
Cells replaced daily	1%	10%	300–400%	25–40%
Half-life	60 days	5 days	7 hours	Days to years
Onset of cytopenia[a]	5 days[b]	3–30 days	5 days	2–3 weeks

[a]The type, severity, and duration of cytopenia depends on the etiology of the injury, its dose and exposure time, and other factors.
[b]Reticulocytopenia; anemia requires prolonged and repeated arrests of erythropoiesis.

Cytopenia

Decreased formed elements in the circulating blood can result from decreased or ineffective production within the bone marrow, increased destruction of cells, or sequestration in the spleen. Patients with cancer often have a combination of these abnormalities, but bone marrow failure is the most common cause of cytopenia. The type and duration of cytopenia depend on several factors (Table 34-1).

I. **Pancytopenia because of bone marrow failure** is treated by administering blood components. Recombinant human erythropoietin or androgen therapy may reduce the red cell transfusion dosage in some patients.

   A. **Metastases to the marrow**

      1. **Occurrence.** Carcinomas of the breast, prostate, and lung are the solid tumors most likely to be associated with extensive marrow metastases. Melanoma, neuroblastoma, and carcinomas of the kidney, adrenal gland, and thyroid also frequently have marrow metastases.

      2. **Findings.** Tumor volume in the marrow does not correlate directly with the degree of hematosuppression. Marrow metastases are often found in patients without any hematologic abnormality. The majority of patients have bone pain, bone tenderness, or x-ray film evidence of cortical bone involvement.

         a. **Bone marrow paraneoplastic alterations** can result in qualitative and quantitative abnormalities in hematopoiesis. In the absence of marrow metastases, changes can develop that are comparable to those seen in the primary myelodysplastic syndromes, including myelodysplasia in all cell lines, marked reactive changes, stromal modifications, and bone marrow remodeling.

         b. **Desmoplastic reactions** to metastases can result in severe myelofibrosis.

         c. **Bone marrow biopsy** is superior to aspiration (with examination of the clot specimen) for detection of metastases; both techniques are complementary. Cytologic preparations of bone marrow aspirates must be inspected at the edges of the smears for clumps of tumor cells.

d. Peripheral blood abnormalities. Nearly all patients with solid tumors and leukoerythroblastosis have demonstrable metastases. Thrombocytopenia (in the absence of RT or chemotherapy) is the next best indicator. Leukocytosis, eosinophilia, monocytosis, and thrombocytosis each are associated with positive bone marrow biopsies in only 20 to 25 percent of cases.

e. Radiographs. Bone scans are positive in 70 percent of patients with bone marrow metastases proved by biopsy, and bone x-ray films are positive in 80 percent of cases.

B. Marrow fibrosis

1. **Occurrence.** Extensive primary marrow fibrosis is characteristic of myelofibrosis with agnogenic myeloid metaplasia and late-stage polycythemia vera. Marrow fibrosis may also be secondary to neoplastic infiltration with leukemia or metastatic carcinoma or as a distant effect of some tumors without demonstrable tumor cells in the marrow. *Secondary fibrosis* in the marrow may also be seen in reaction to

   a. Collagen vascular disorders (particularly systemic lupus erythematosus, in which the fibrosis can reverse following treatment with high dose corticosteroids)

   b. Toxic agents (benzene, radiation, cytotoxic agents)

   c. Infectious agents (especially tuberculosis and syphilis)

   d. Hematologic diseases (myelodysplasia, pernicious anemia, hemolytic anemia)

   e. Miscellaneous disorders (osteopetrosis, mastocytosis, renal osteodystrophy, Gaucher's disease, giant lymph node hyperplasia, angioimmunoblastic lymphadenopathy with dysglobulinemia)

2. **Findings.** Splenomegaly and a leukoerythroblastic blood smear are characteristic of marrow fibrosis of any cause.

C. Marrow necrosis

1. **Occurrence.** When diagnosed antemortem, marrow necrosis nearly always is due to either sickle cell disease or a malignancy, particularly a hematologic neoplasm. Systemic embolization of fat and marrow frequently occurs. The median survival of patients with marrow necrosis from a malignancy is less than 1 month.

2. **Findings.** Patients have severe bone pain (in back, pelvis, or extremities), cytopenias, and a leukoerythroblastic blood smear.

   a. Serum levels of alkaline phosphatase, LDH, uric acid, and bilirubin are usually elevated.

   b. X-ray films are normal.

   c. Bone marrow aspiration demonstrates characteristic findings: Individual hematopoietic cells are not recognizable, and cells with indistinct margins and intensely basophilic nuclei are usually surrounded by amorphous acidophilic material.

D. Bone marrow failure secondary to treatment.
Ionizing radiation and most chemotherapeutic agents cause suppression of bone marrow function. While recovery is usual after chemotherapy, recovery after irradiation is inversely proportional to dose and volume treated and may never be complete. Indeed, after doses in excess of 3000 cGy, the bone marrow may be replaced by fatty and fibrous tissue. The distribution of marrow in the human skeleton is shown in **Fig. 34-1.** The induction of short-term cytopenias by anticancer therapies is discussed in Chap. 4. *Principles.* sec. **VI.B.2.**

The occurrence of **therapy-related myelodysplasia and AML** is even more worrisome for the development of treatment strategies. In order to develop this complication, the patient must have been treated long enough and then live long enough to manifest this long-term toxicity.

1. **Occurrence.** Nearly half of patients have a primary hematologic malignancy. The risk of AML is increased 10- to 50-fold in patients treated for multiple myeloma, Hodgkin's disease, non-Hodgkin's lymphoma, ovarian cancer, germ cell tumors, small cell lung cancer, and childhood ALL. For

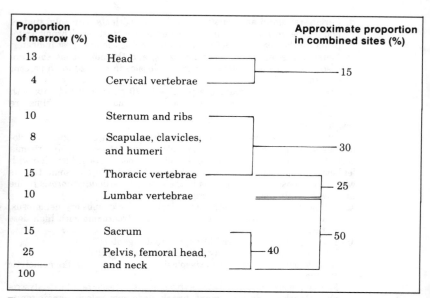

Proportion of marrow (%)	Site	Approximate proportion in combined sites (%)
13	Head	15
4	Cervical vertebrae	
10	Sternum and ribs	30
8	Scapulae, clavicles, and humeri	
15	Thoracic vertebrae	25
10	Lumbar vertebrae	
15	Sacrum	50
25	Pelvis, femoral head, and neck	40
100		

Fig. 34-1. Distribution of bone marrow in healthy 40-year-old human beings. Marrow cellularity is relatively decreased and amounts of fat increased in the elderly. (Data are adapted from R. E. Ellis, The distribution of active bone marrow in the adult. *Phys. Med. Biol.* 5:255, 1961.)

children with ALL who achieve complete remission, the risk for developing therapy-related AML is greater than the risk for developing relapsed ALL. Adjuvant chemotherapy for breast cancer is associated with only a minimally increased risk for the development of AML.

2. **Leukemogenic agents.** The risk of inducing AML is directly related to the total cumulative dose. The risk may also depend on the schedule of administration; for example, the risk in children with ALL is greatest in those undergoing weekly or biweekly therapy with epipodophyllotoxins.

   a. **Alkylating agents** are the drugs with the most clearly demonstrated leukemogenic potential. Melphalan and chlorambucil are the strongest and cyclophosphamide is the weakest leukemogenic agent in this class of drugs.

   b. **Other drugs.** Epipodophyllotoxins (etoposide, teniposide), nitrosoureas, and procarbazine are also proven to be leukemogenic. Cisplatin is not a classical alkylating agent and is possibly leukemogenic; however, it is nearly always given in combination with other drugs, some of which are leukemogenic.

   c. **RT** is associated with a minimally increased risk for AML when given alone, but with a synergistically increased risk when combined with leukemogenic drugs.

3. **Chromosome abnormalities,** particularly involving chromosomes 5q or 7q, are found in 70 percent of therapy-linked AML associated with alkylating agents. These same aberrations are seen in patients developing AML following exposure to leukemogenic solvents and pesticides. In contrast, certain balanced translocations involving 11q23 seem to be characteristic of myelodysplasia and AML occurring after treatment with cytostatic agents acting on DNA-topoisomerase II, such as etoposide.

4. **Natural history.** AML develops three to five years after initiation of therapy

but can arise after 10 or more years; the syndrome rarely develops within one year. Therapy-induced AML is usually preceded by months to years of myelodysplasia (see Chap. 25, sec. I.C). Once AML develops, the course is rapid and usually refractory to treatment. Death usually occurs within two to four months of diagnosis. An important predictive factor for favorable response to intensive antileukemic therapy is the absence of a preceding myelodysplastic phase.

II. Pancytopenia because of hypersplenism
A. Pathogenesis
1. **Hypersplenism.** Splenic enlargement from any cause (including carcinomatous metastases) may result in phagocytosis of the circulating blood cells and the development of cytopenias.
2. **Erythrophagocytosis** that causes anemia is a characteristic finding in the bone marrow and the remainder of the reticuloendothelial system of patients with malignant histiocytosis. Erythrophagocytosis by macrophages surrounding tumor sites has also been demonstrated in lymphomas and Hodgkin's disease.

B. Diagnosis.
The diagnosis of hypersplenism is based on clinical judgment. The only true diagnostic test for hypersplenism is improvement in the cytopenias after splenectomy.

C. Treatment
1. **Indications for splenectomy** are *all* of the following:
   a. The patient has palpable splenomegaly.
   b. The cytopenia is severe (e.g., anemia requiring frequent transfusions; severe neutropenia associated with recurrent, serious bacterial infections; or thrombocytopenia with petechiae, purpura, or other hemorrhagic manifestations).
   c. Other causes of cytopenia have been ruled out (e.g., DIC).
   d. A reasonable survival following splenectomy is expected.
   e. The patient's general medical condition is satisfactory enough to make the operative mortality risk acceptable.
   f. Surgeons experienced in performing splenectomy under adverse conditions are available.
2. **Consequences of splenectomy**
   a. **Postsplenectomy blood picture** is characterized by Howell-Jolly bodies, neutrophilia, eosinophilia, basophilia, lymphocytosis, monocytosis, and thrombocytosis.
   b. **Postsplenectomy sepsis** is a potentially fatal complication, especially in children less than six years of age. The most common infecting organisms are *Streptococcus pneumoniae* and *Haemophilus influenzae*. The incidence of sepsis in patients with Hodgkin's disease who undergo splenectomy has been reported to be 1 to 3 percent. Immunization may be helpful. Febrile episodes must be treated immediately and agressively.
   c. **Accessory spleens** are rarely of concern in patients with malignancy. The presence of Howell-Jolly bodies on the peripheral blood smear means that the patient has functional asplenia.

III. Anemia in patients with cancer
A. Anemia because of blood loss or iron deficiency
1. **Pathogenesis** includes ulcerating tumors, extensive surgery, benign GI tract diseases, gastrectomy (unable to use heme iron but able to use ferrous salts), and hemosiderinuria from chronic intravascular hemolysis.
2. **Diagnosis.** Patients with known GI tract malignancies must not be presumed to be bleeding from an ulcerating tumor (see Chap. 30, sec. I).
   a. **Physical examination** may reveal obvious sites of bleeding. Stools for occult blood should be obtained.
   b. **Blood studies** may demonstrate microcytosis and hypochromia. Important clues that may signify a recent hemorrhage are polychromasia (often prominent five to ten days after acute hemorrhage) or thrombo-

cytosis (as a reaction to bleeding). Hypoferremia and hypertransferrinemia are often masked in cancer patients by the concomitant anemia of chronic disease.

  c. Bone marrow examination demonstrating the absence of stainable iron is unreliable in patients with cancer.

  d. Therapeutic trials. Ferrous sulfate, 325 mg PO t.i.d. for 30 days should elevate the hemoglobin concentration in patients with iron deficiency.

B. Anemia because of nutritional deficiencies results in megaloblastic anemia, macro-ovalocytosis, neutrophil hypersegmentation, and, in severe cases, pancytopenia.

 1. Folic acid deficiency is by far the most common cause of megaloblastic anemia in cancer patients. Decreased intake of folate is common with any advanced cancer or myelofibrosis. Increased requirements for folate develop with the competitive use of folate by rapidly proliferating tumor cells, autoimmune hemolytic anemia, and prolonged IV therapy of septic patients. Folate deficiency may also develop following the use of folate antagonist drugs (e.g., methotrexate).

 2. Vitamin B_{12} deficiency is usually seen in cancer patients who have undergone gastrectomy (the site of intrinsic factor production) or who have malabsorption secondary to lymphoma that involves the ileum (the site of vitamin B_{12} absorption).

C. Anemia of chronic diseases (ACD)

 1. Pathogenesis. ACD is caused by immune activation in reaction to foreign antigens with the production of cytokines that directly inhibit both the action and production of EP. ACD is more severe with widespread metastases but may be observed in patients with localized tumors.

  The increased levels of TNF and IL-1 seen in malignancies and inflammatory conditions result in anemia indirectly. TNF stimulates marrow stromal cells to produce β-IFN and IL-1 acts on T lymphocytes to produce γ-IFN. Both β-IFN and γ-IFN inhibit erythropoiesis directly.

  Neopterin levels, which indicate the activation of macrophages by γ-IFN, are also increased in malignancies. The hemoglobin concentrations are inversely proportional to the blood concentrations of neopterin and γ-IFN. γ-IFN also inhibits granulocytopoiesis, but neutropenia is not a manifestation of ACD. IL-1 also stimulates the release of G-CSF and GM-CSF, which can overcome the inhibitory effects of γ-IFN.

 2. Diagnosis

  a. Hemogram. The erythrocytes in ACD are usually normocytic and normochromic. Some patients have microcytosis and hypochromia. The reticulocyte count is normal or slightly increased.

  b. Serum iron studies. The sine qua non for the diagnosis of ACD is the demonstration of decreased levels of both serum iron and transferrin (total iron binding capacity). Serum ferritin values are normal or increased.

  c. Bone marrow studies demonstrate ineffective erythropoiesis that is manifested by decreased polychromasia of nonnucleated marrow red cells, shortened red cell life spans, and decreased numbers of sideroblasts. Reticuloendothelial iron may be normal, increased or decreased.

 3. Treatment. ACD is rarely severe enough to necessitate red cell transfusions. However, recombinant human erythropoietin can correct ACD in most situations where it is encountered. Subcutaneous administration of 100–150 units/kg three times weekly may decrease the transfusion requirement and increase the quality of life within 8 to 12 weeks of starting treatment.

D. Anemia caused by parvovirus B19. Parvovirus B19 is the etiologic agent of transient acute aplastic crises in persons with underlying hemolytic anemias. This complication is also seen in patients receiving chemotherapy, particularly in treatment for leukemia. An acute infection is manifested by worsening anemia, exanthem, and polyarthralgia.

In immunocompromised hosts who are unable to produce neutralizing antibodies against the virus, an infection can persist and cause chronic bone marrow failure, usually manifested by anemia. The viral target is an erythroid progenitor cell. The bone marrow shows erythroid hypoplasia. Treatment with commercial immunoglobulins may be helpful.

E. Pure red cell aplasia (PRCA)

1. **Pathogenesis.** More than 50 percent of cases of PRCA (isolated severe hypoplasia of erythroid elements in the marrow) have an associated thymoma, which is usually noninvasive (see Chap. 19, sec. **I.B.1**). Lymphoproliferative disorders and various carcinomas have also been associated with PRCA. Rare cases of thymoma have been associated with pure neutropenia.

2. **Diagnosis.** A normocytic, normochromic anemia and reticulocytopenia are present. Bone marrow biopsy demonstrates markedly decreased to absent erythroid precursors and normal megakaryocytes and myeloid elements. Chest film demonstrates a mediastinal mass if associated with thymoma.

3. **Treatment.** Removal of a thymoma results in remission of PRCA in about 50 percent of cases. Many patients with and without thymoma have responded to cyclophosphamide therapy.

F. Warm antibody (IgG) immune hemolysis

1. **Pathogenesis.** Autoimmune hemolysis because of IgG antibodies most commonly occurs in patients with lymphoreticular neoplasms. More than 50 percent of patients in some series have an associated malignancy, but only 2 percent of cases are associated with solid tumors. This complication has also been reported following treatment with various cytostatic drugs. The IgG-coated erythrocytes are removed from the circulation by the reticuloendothelial system, predominantly by the spleen (extravascular hemolysis).

2. **Diagnosis.** Patients with warm antibody autoimmune hemolysis usually have an insidious onset of severe anemia, mild jaundice, and splenomegaly. The blood smear shows polychromasia, a significant degree of spherocytosis, and often, nucleated red cells. Reticulocytes are typically increased but may be normal if any other cause of anemia is also present. The direct antiglobulin test (DAT or Coombs' test) is positive with anti-IgG or anticomplement antisera, usually with specificity for the Rh blood group system.

3. **Treatment.** Prednisone and successful treatment of the tumor are necessary. Patients with solid tumors associated with immune hemolysis respond to prednisone infrequently. Patients who have an unsatisfactory response or need chronic corticosteroid therapy require splenectomy if their general condition permits.

G. Cold antibody (IgM) immune hemolysis

1. **Pathogenesis.** Cold agglutinins are IgM molecules that attach to red cell membranes at cold temperatures and fix complement. At 37°C, the IgM molecules dissociate from the cell, but the complement remains fixed. Cold agglutinins are most frequent in lymphoma and are rare in other malignancies. Overt hemolysis (often intravascular) is unusual except in patients with very high titers (greater than 1:1000) of cold agglutinins.

2. **Diagnosis.** Patients with high titers of cold agglutinins may have acrocyanosis or Raynaud's phenomenon. Red cell agglutination may be observed on blood smears, but spherocytes are not prominent. The DAT is strongly positive when performed at 4°C but is positive only with anticomplement antisera at 37°C.

3. **Treatment.** There is no satisfactory treatment for cold agglutinin hemolytic anemia except for control of the underlying disease.

H. Microangiopathic hemolysis (MAHA) with erythrocyte fragmentation has been described in patients with adenocarcinoma (particularly mucin-producing gastric cancer) and hemangioendothelioma. The pathophysiology of MAHA involves fibrin strands of DIC, pulmonary intraluminal tumor emboli, narrowing of pulmonary arterioles by intimal proliferations, or a side effect of chemotherapy. Most patients with MAHA, however, probably have DIC or chemotherapy-associated thrombotic thrombocytopenia (see sec. **IV.C**).

IV. Thrombocytopenia because of increased platelet destruction. Decreased production is by far the most common cause of thrombocytopenia in patients with cancer (see sec. I). Splenic sequestration may cause thrombocytopenia, almost always in association with anemia (see sec. II). *Increased destruction of platelets* is usually associated with normal megakaryocytes in the bone marrow, and decreased platelet life spans.

A. DIC is the most common cause of increased destruction of platelets in cancer patients (see *Coagulopathy*, section II).

B. ITP complicates lymphoproliferative diseases, especially malignant lymphoma and chronic lymphocytic leukemia, and rarely is associated with carcinoma. Thrombocytopenia is due to reticuloendothelial system destruction of IgG-coated platelets.

   1. Diagnosis of ITP is made presumptively in the absence of evidence for DIC or for drug-induced thrombocytopenia with the finding of a nondiagnostic bone marrow containing normal or increased numbers of megakaryocytes.

   2. Treatment. Control of the underlying disease is essential for satisfactory control of ITP.

      a. Patients are treated with prednisone 60 to 80 mg/day PO. Single alkylating agents or vinca alkaloids successfully achieve remission in some patients. Splenectomy is indicated in patients who fail the above measures and have severe or symptomatic thrombocytopenia.

      b. Many cases of ITP are chronic; platelet counts are 50,000 to 80,000/μl. In the absence of symptoms, it is best to observe these patients without giving long-term immunosuppressive therapy.

C. Chemotherapy-induced thrombotic thrombocytopenic purpura (TTP) or hemolytic-uremic syndrome (HUS). TTP/HUS can develop during the treatment of patients with cancer, particularly when using mitomycin C for adenocarcinoma. Therapy with cisplatin and bleomycin have also been associated with this complication.

Chemotherapy-induced TTP/HUS usually occurs two to nine months after cessation of treatment and even when the cancer is in remission (approximately one-third of patients). Noncardiogenic pulmonary edema develops in 65 percent of patients with this syndrome, which is rapidly lethal if not successfully treated.

More than 90 percent of cases have been associated with mitomycin C. Approximately 10 percent of patients treated with mitomycin C develop TTP/HUS, especially when the cumulative dose is more than 60 mg. Manifestations are often precipitated or exacerbated by transfusion of blood products.

   1. Diagnosis. TTP is characterized by the extensive deposition of hyalinlike material in arterioles and capillaries. Diagnostic features of TTP include microangiopathic hemolysis, severe thrombocytopenia, markedly elevated blood LDH levels, rapidly changing neurologic abnormalities, fever, and often, renal dysfunction. Coagulation abnormalities associated with DIC are absent.

   2. Treatment. Transfusion of plasma or intensive plasmapheresis, with or without antiplatelet drugs, has been successful in achieving remissions in classic TTP, which was formerly considered to be uniformly fatal. Treatment of chemotherapy-induced TTP/HUS with staphylococcal protein A extracorporeal immunoabsorption of circulating IgG immune complexes achieves significant responses in 50 percent of patients. Normalization of platelet counts and LDH values are seen seven to fourteen days after starting treatment.

   3. Recommendations

      a. Monitor hematologic parameters and renal function closely in patients being treated with mitomycin C.

      b. Avoid transfusion of blood products in patients suspected of having TTP/HUS.

      c. Consider treatment with staphylococcal protein A immunopheresis in patients with the definite syndrome. Alternatively, standard therapies used for TTP may also be considered.

V. Granulocytopenia. Granulocytopenia in cancer patients is usually the result of chemotherapy, radiotherapy, other drugs, severe infection, or myelophthisis. An immune or cytokine basis is involved in the granulocytopenia associated with T-γ lymphoproliferative disease (syndrome of large granular T lymphocytes) and rare cases of thymoma. Experimental evidence also supports the existence of paraneoplastic suppression of granulopoiesis. All of these entities are discussed elsewhere in the book.

VI. Blood component therapy
   A. Transfusion of erythrocytes
   1. **Indications** for transfusion of packed red blood cells (PRBC) are to increase blood volume (when acute blood loss threatens the integrity of the cardiovascular system) and to increase oxygen carrying capacity (when anemia causes or threatens tissue hypoxia). Most patients tolerate chronic, moderately severe anemia (hemoglobin > 8 gm/dl) well. No specific hemoglobin value mandates transfusion. PRBC are given to increase the oxygen carrying capacity of blood for actual or incipient CHF or to reverse cardiac or CNS ischemic symptoms. When the hemoglobin level that precipitated symptoms is determined, patients with chronic anemias are transfused prophylactically to exceed that level.
   2. **Transfusion reactions**
      a. **Fever and chills.** Most febrile reactions are caused by antibodies in the recipient directed against granulocytic antigens and specific HLA antigens on leukocytes in the donor blood. Febrile reactions occur in up to 80 percent of patients who receive multiple transfusions. The reaction usually does not start until 30 to 120 minutes into the transfusion.
      b. **Allergic reactions** involving urticaria or anaphylaxis develop in 5 percent of transfused patients. Some of these reactions are due to antibodies in the recipient directed against immunoglobulin components and other proteins in the plasma of the donor. These kinds of reactions or anaphylaxis are particularly likely to occur in patients with congenital IgA deficiency (1 per 800 people).
      c. **Major acute hemolytic transfusion reactions** are most likely to occur following human error during blood preparation or administration. Fever and chills usually develop within the first 30 minutes into the transfusion and are often accompanied by tachycardia, hypotension, tachypnea, oliguria, hemoglobinuria, and DIC.
      d. **Delayed hemolytic transfusion reactions** occur five to ten days after transfusion, particularly in association with alloantibodies to antigens of the Kidd blood group system.
      e. **Posttransfusion purpura** is manifested by severe thrombocytopenia developing five to eight days after transfusion and occurs in the 2 percent of patients who lack the platelet antigen Pl[A1].
      f. **Bacterial contamination** occurs rarely in PRBC units (usually with cryopathic gram-negative bacteria), but is more possible with platelet packs that are stored (at room temperature) for more than five days.
      g. **Viral contamination.** The approximate risks of transmitting viruses through transfusion are

      Cytomegalovirus (CMV): 1:14 (7%)
      Hepatitis B or C virus: 1:100–1:200 (0.5–1%)
      Human immunodeficiency virus (HIV): <1:100,000 (<0.001%); 1:50,000 in Los Angeles (0.002%)
      Human T cell lymphotropic virus (HTLV-1 and HTLV-2): 1:200,000 (0.0005%).

      h. **Graft-versus-host disease (GVHD)** can occur following blood cell transfusion in patients who are undergoing a conditioning regimen for BMT or who have acute lymphoblastic leukemia or congenital immunodeficiency. GVHD can also occur in patients who are not immunocompromised if the blood donor is homozygous for one of the HLA haplotypes of the recipient and particularly if the donor is a first-degree relative.

  i. **Other complications** include those associated with massive transfusion (blood volume overload, hypocalcemia, hyperkalemia, hypothermia), iron overload with chronic transfusions, and alloimmunization.

3. **Uses for erythrocyte preparations**
  a. **Fresh whole blood.** None.
  b. **PRBC.** The mainstay of erythrocyte transfusion therapy.
  c. **Saline-washed PRBC.** Patients who have IgA deficiency (particularly those with high anti-IgA titers), prior urticarial reactions with transfusions, or the need to avoid transfusion of complement.
  d. **Leukocyte-filtered PRBC.** Multiply transfused patients with prior febrile transfusion reactions.
  e. **Frozen red cells.** Source for rare blood types, a backup supply for the common blood types, a substitute for saline-washed or leukocyte-filtered PRBC when those methods fail to prevent febrile or allergic transfusion reactions, and an additional method of autologous donation. The extensive washing required to remove the cryopreservatives in frozen red cells renders the suspension totally free of all leukocytes, platelets, and plasma constituents. The major limitations are the cost and the time required to prepare and store cells.
  f. **Gamma-irradiated PRBC** are given to prevent viable T lymphocytes from causing transfusion-induced GVHD in the recipient. A dose of 1500 cGy is usually administered.
  g. **Directed donor PRBC** do not decrease the risk of transmission of any virus. Furthermore, these units are associated with an increased risk of GVHD when provided by first-degree relatives to immunocompromised patients.

B. **Transfusion of granulocytes.** Granulocytes collected by apheresis are rarely helpful in treating patients with granulocytopenia. The paramount factor in determining the outcome of sepsis is the recovery of marrow function. Transfusion of leukocytes often results in GVHD and transmission of CMV. Prophylactic transfusions are useless. If granulocyte transfusion is utilized, the transfused cells should be irradiated for severely immunocompromised patients, and donors who are seronegative for CMV should be used for seronegative recipients. Granulocyte transfusions may occasionally be helpful only *if all of the following criteria are met:*

  1. Recovery of bone marrow function is a reasonable expectation but is not expected to occur for one week.
  2. The absolute granulocyte count is less than 200/μL.
  3. A serious bacterial or fungal infection is proved by culture.
  4. The infection is not responding to the appropriate antibiotics.

C. **Transfusion of platelets**
  1. **Factors influencing the decision to transfuse platelets**
    a. **Platelet count.** Spontaneous hemorrhage rarely occurs with platelet counts above 20,000/μL. Platelet counts under 10,000/μL are associated with an increased risk of spontaneous hemorrhage, especially when the thrombocytopenia results from decreased production rather than increased platelet destruction. Progressively worsening thrombocytopenia is more likely to be associated with active hemorrhage than stable or increasing platelet counts.
    b. **Platelet age.** Young platelets (i.e., produced after peripheral destruction) are larger and better able to provide hemostasis than old platelets. Usually patients with immune or postinfectious severe thrombocytopenia have no serious hemorrhagic sequelae.
    c. **Active bleeding,** uncontrollable by local measures, or bleeding into vital or inaccessible organs, is an absolute indication for platelet transfusion in patients with thrombocytopenia of nearly any severity.

d. Fever, infection, and corticosteroid therapy increase the risk of serious hemorrhage in patients with very low platelet counts.

e. Immune thrombocytopenia usually makes platelet transfusions useless.

f. Drugs and diseases adversely affecting platelet function may necessitate platelet transfusions in times of hemorrhage or surgery despite adequate platelet counts (see sec. **C.6.a**).

g. Patients who are refractory to platelet transfusion may be alloimmunized, but they also may have DIC, HUS, or ITP.

2. **Problems associated with platelet transfusion**

   a. Alloimmunization. Compatibility between donor and recipient for both ABO and HLA antigens is important for achieving a successful platelet count increment following transfusion. Alloimmunization requires the presence of class I and class II HLA antigens. Platelets alone do not result in the development of antibodies because they carry only class I HLA antigens and platelet-specific antigens; the class II antigens necessary for the development of alloimmunization are provided by transfused monocytes, lymphocytes, and dendritic cells. Rh antigens play only a minor role in alloimmunization following platelet transfusions.

   b. Transfusion reactions. Febrile reactions often occur in ABO-compatible transfusions because of the large number of leukocytes that are contained in platelet packs. Hemolysis of the small numbers of contaminating donor red cells in donor platelet concentrates is of minor consequence. Infectious contamination also occurs because platelets are stored at room temperature.

3. **Selection of which preparation to transfuse** depends on expected future transfusions and the presence of alloimmunization.

   a. Random (ABO-compatible) units are obtained from multiple donors of whole blood. Platelet concentrates (without regard to ABO compatibility) may be used in patients with transient thrombocytopenia that is not expected to recur and when platelets are needed immediately.

   b. Single-donor platelets (plateletpheresis packs) are obtained by density centrifugation. Approximately six to eight units may be obtained from one donor two or three times weekly. Single-donor platelet packs are the preferred blood product in conditions that require recurrent platelet transfusions (e.g., aplastic anemia, acute leukemia) because alloimmunization is delayed. Alloimmunization may be prevented when using this blood product in patients on chemotherapy (e.g., acute leukemia).

   c. HLA-compatible platelets. HLA-matched platelets are required in alloimmunized patients but are not always available. The likelihood of an identical HLA match is 1:4 among siblings and 1:1000 in the general population.

   d. Platelets from family members should be avoided in patients who are possible candidates for BMT. The marrow donor may be used as the source of HLA-identical platelets, however, after the transplantation conditioning program has begun.

4. **Prophylactic transfusions**

   a. Acute leukemia. Complete remission after intensive therapy, if achieved, occurs within 12 weeks. Prophylactic transfusion of these patients with platelets is recommended to maintain the count above 10,000/μL.

   b. In aplastic anemia, prophylactic transfusions are avoided if possible.

   c. Pregnancy. Platelet packs are administered to patients with a platelet count less than 100,000/μL just prior to delivery. After delivery, platelet counts should be maintained above 50,000/μL for one week. The possibility of DIC should be evaluated in patients with continued or massive postpartum bleeding associated with thrombocytopenia. Pregnant patients with thrombocytopenia induced by myelosuppressive therapy or leukemia are given platelet transfusions empirically.

5. **Effectiveness of platelet transfusions** is determined by measuring platelet counts just prior to, one hour after, and 24 hours after transfusions. If the patient does not respond with an increase of about 25,000 in the platelet count after one hour, the transfusion should be considered a failure. The result at 24 hours can be further affected by concurrent hematologic complications. The template bleeding time is normal for platelet counts greater than 100,000/μL; the time increases linearly with decreasing platelet counts less than 100,000/μL.

6. **Other measures**

   a. **Diseases affecting platelet function.** Patients with uremia require dialysis, cryoprecipitate, or desmopressin acetate (DDAVP) to improve platelet function. In patients with platelet dysfunction secondary to paraproteins, it is necessary to control the underlying disease or do plasmapheresis.

   b. **DDAVP** may be useful in patients with drug-induced platelet dysfunction. It can also be given as an empiric trial to improve platelet function in difficult situations at a dose of 0.3 μg/kg given over 20 minutes.

   c. **Alloimmunized patients who are refractory to transfused platelets.** High-dose IV gammaglobulin (400 mg/kg/day for five days) occasionally permits better platelet increments in patients who are refractory to platelet transfusion. Plasma apheresis may be tried empirically in difficult situations.

   d. **Menorrhagia in patients with thrombocytopenia** should be treated with medroxyprogesterone, 20 mg PO daily, to induce amenorrhea. Treatment is continued until the platelet count exceeds 60,000/μL.

D. **Transfusion of plasma proteins**

1. **Preparations**

   a. **Fresh-frozen plasma (FFP)** contains all coagulation factors and is useful in replacement of all acquired clotting factor deficiencies (e.g., DIC, massive transfusion, liver disease). The indications for FFP are

      (1) Replacement of isolated coagulation factor deficiencies

      (2) Reversal of documented coagulation factor deficiencies following massive blood transfusions

      (3) Reversal of warfarin effect in patients requiring immediate surgery or having active bleeding

      (4) Treatment of antithrombin III deficiency and thrombotic thrombocytopenic purpura

   b. **Cryoprecipitate** contains the von Willebrand's disease factor, fibrinogen (factor I), factor VIII, and factor XIII. Cryoprecipitate is useful in treating acquired deficiencies of fibrinogen and factor VIII (e.g., DIC) when volume overload from plasma treatment is to be avoided and in severe von Willebrand's disease.

   c. **Plasma protein fractionation** has resulted in the following commercially available products:

      (1) **Fibrinogen.** This form is never indicated because of the 100 percent risk of hepatitis.

      (2) **Prothrombin complex** (factors II, VII, IX, X, protein C, and protein S) is used in congenital factor deficiencies and in occasional cases of coumarin overdose with life-threatening hemorrhage. The risk of hepatitis with this blood product is 60 percent.

      (3) **Albumin and purified protein fraction** have the same concentration of albumin and the same cost. They are useful for blood volume expansion, but their use in chronic hypoalbuminemia of malabsorption, nephrosis, or cirrhosis, or as a nutritional supplement is futile.

      (4) **Gamma globulin** is useful for congenital immunodeficiencies. Intravenous, high-dose IgG is a very expensive product that is of definite therapeutic importance in only a few clinical circumstances.

     d. Hyperimmune IV gamma globulin must be infused at a rate slower than 1 ml/min to avoid complications. This very expensive product is of definite therapeutic importance in only a few clinical circumstances:

        (1) Congenital humoral immunodeficiency states

        (2) Acquired humoral immunodeficiency states (e.g., chronic lymphocytic leukemia, lymphoma, myeloma) when complicated by recurrent bacterial infections that do not respond to prophylactic antibiotics

        (3) Platelet alloimmunization in conjunction with platelet transfusion

        (4) Idiopathic thrombocytopenic purpura when severe or life-threatening hemorrhage occurs, *or* when severe thrombocytopenia refractory to steroids occurs during pregnancy, *or* when splenectomy is performed and hemostasis is a problem.

2. Hazards

     a. Allergy. All plasma preparations are associated with a small incidence of serum sickness reactions. Fever, urticaria, or erythema may also occur in reaction to residual leukocyte antigens.

     b. Volume overload is an important consideration when administering FFP. Citrate toxicity may occur with very rapid transfusion rates (100 ml/min).

     c. Venous thrombosis and DIC occur with prothrombin-complex transfusions.

     d. Infection with hepatitis B, hepatitis C, delta agent hepatitis, HIV, CMV, and EBV is a potential risk for all plasma products.

        (1) Risks for hepatitis

           (a) Very high risk: fibrinogen, prothrombin complex, repeated use of cryoprecipitate.

           (b) Intermediate risk: single-donor units screened for hepatitis B surface antigen of plasma.

           (c) Very low risk: gamma globulin, albumin, purified protein fraction.

        (2) Risks for HIV transmission: nil for gammaglobulin, albumin, and purified protein fraction.

Coagulopathy

I. Thrombosis ("hypercoagulability"). Multiple or migratory venous thrombosis in cancer patients has been repeatedly documented since Trousseau's description in 1865. An accelerated course of intermittent claudication and of ischemic heart disease has also been described in cancer patients and probably represents additional variants of Trousseau's syndrome.

    Fibrin-platelet vegetations may form on mitral or aortic valves and result in noninfectious endocarditis with paradoxical emboli to peripheral organs. Fewer than one-third of affected afebrile patients have heart murmurs. Most vegetations, which are less than 2 mm, are not detected by echocardiography.

    A. Incidence. The overall incidence of thrombotic episodes in cancer patients is 10 to 15 percent, especially during postoperative periods. Up to one-third of apparently healthy adults eventually prove to have a malignancy when they present with otherwise unexplained deep vein thrombosis or idiopathic pulmonary emboli. Pulmonary emboli have been found at necropsy in about 50 percent of patients with disseminated cancer and have antedated the diagnosis of cancer in 1 to 15 percent of patients.

    B. Malignancies most commonly associated with thrombosis:

      1. Carcinoma of the GI tract, lung, or ovary (only 7% of patients with pancreas cancer develop the classic Trousseau syndrome)

      2. Myeloproliferative disorders

      3. Malignant lymphoproliferative disorders

    C. Mechanisms. Cancer can promote clotting by the following means:

1. Cancer is associated with
   a. Thrombocytosis, *and*
   b. Increased plasma levels of fibrinogen and factors V, VIII, IX, and XI, *and*
   c. Decreased plasma levels of antithrombin-III (AT-III)
2. Localized anatomic changes, such as tumor compression and venous stasis, can precipitate thrombosis. The tumor's disruption of blood vessels exposes collagen and basement membrane, which may trigger clotting. Tumor neovascularization activates both factor XII and platelet reactions.
3. Tumor cells may activate blood clotting by
   a. Directly activating platelets
   b. Stimulating monocytes and macrophages to produce procoagulants (such as tissue thromboplastin or prothrombin activators)
   c. Directly producing procoagulants (such as cysteine protease or trypsin, which activates several coagulation factors)

D. Diagnosis
1. The clinical diagnosis of thrombosis is made by physical examination and venography, venous ultrasonography, or radiofibrinogen scan. The presence of venous thrombosis, a heart murmur, and arterial embolism suggests an underlying mucin-producing carcinoma.
2. An occult malignancy should be sought in patients who present with any of the following:
   a. Idiopathic deep vein thrombosis
   b. Idiopathic pulmonary emboli
   c. Combined venous and arterial thrombosis
   d. Thrombosis at multiple sites
   e. Thrombosis that is resistant to anticoagulation therapy
   f. Associated paraneoplastic syndromes
3. A reasonable screening evaluation for occult cancer in patients with thrombotic disease includes a CBC, LDH, CEA, chest x-ray, and abdominopelvic CT scan.
4. Laboratory tests of coagulation are not helpful for defining the presence of a hyperthrombotic state.

E. Management. Thrombosis in cancer patients is often resistant to therapy.
1. **Removal of the tumor** (if possible) may control thrombotic episodes.
2. **Warfarin or heparin therapy** may be used if there is no contraindication. These agents produce a high incidence of potentially fatal hemorrhage in cancer patients. Long-term warfarin and extended minidose heparin (5000–10,000 IU/day SQ), however, have been associated with only limited success. *Contraindications* to anticoagulant therapy include
   a. Preexisting coagulation or bleeding defect or bleeding source
   b. Inaccessible ulceration (e.g., GI tract)
   c. Recent hemorrhage or surgery in the eye or CNS
   d. Severe hypertension or bacterial endocarditis
   e. Regional or lumbar anesthesia; T tube drainage
   f. Pregnancy (if anticoagulation is mandatory, heparin is used because it crosses the placenta less readily than warfarin)
3. **Antiplatelet drugs.** Aspirin (600 mg b.i.d.) and dipyridamole (50–100 mg PO q.i.d.) can be tried.

II. DIC is a frequent complication of metastatic cancer. Local or diffuse thrombosis or hemorrhage, in all combinations, can occur. The incidence depends on the definition and assays used. Severe DIC is common in only two malignancies: carcinoma of the prostate and acute hypergranular promyelocytic leukemia (type M3).

A. Diagnosis
1. **Clinical features**
   a. **Type of bleeding.** Patients with severe DIC bleed from at least three sites simultaneously. Patients with chronic DIC (the usual DIC in malignancy) may have minimal bleeding.
   b. **End-organ damage.** Hemolysis, hypotension, oliguria, and renal failure are frequent complications of serious DIC.

Table 34-2. Comparison of acute disseminated intravascular coagulation (DIC) and primary fibrinolysis

Feature	Acute DIC	Primary fibrinolysis
Incidence	Common	Very rare
Platelets*	Decreased	Usually normal
Paracoagulation test (fibrin monomers)*	Positive	Negative
Clot lysis or euglobulin lysis time*	Normal or long	Rapid
Fibrinogen	Decreased	Decreased
Fibrin degradation products	Variable	Large amounts

*Discriminatory assays.

2. **Laboratory tests.** No single test is diagnostic for DIC.
   a. **Blood smear.** The numbers of circulating platelets are estimated and fragmented erythrocytes or microspherocytes identified. Schistocytosis is present in about 50 percent of cases.
   b. **Platelet count.** Thrombocytopenia occurs nearly always, but DIC rarely causes platelet counts less than 50,000/μL.
   c. **Clotting tests.** Prothrombin time and activated partial thromboplastin time (PTT) may be slightly shortened, normal, or prolonged. Thrombin time (TT) prolongation occurs with severe hypofibrinogenemia (<50 mg/dl) or clinically significant elevation of fibrin degradation products (FDPs); the TT can also be prolonged with heparin therapy, dysfibrinogenemia, or malignant paraproteinemia.
   d. **Fibrinogen titer** is usually decreased. Fibrinogen concentrations greater than 50 mg/dl (normal range is 200–400 mg/dl) should not result in abnormalities of the TT.
   e. **Paracoagulation tests** for fibrin monomers (protamine sulfate or D-dimers) are positive in more than 95 percent of patients with DIC.
   f. **FDP assay** may be normal in patients with chronic DIC. The FDP titer does not correlate with the clinical course or severity of DIC.
3. **DIC versus primary fibrinolysis.** Although primary fibrinolysis is rare and DIC is common, differentiation between these disorders is important to plan treatment. These disorders are compared in Table 34-2. The platelet count, paracoagulation test, and euglobulin lysis separate the disorders.
4. **Severity of DIC manifestations** depends on the underlying diagnosis, the acuteness of the DIC, the integrity of the reticuloendothelial system, and the intensity of secondary fibrinolysis. Some patients hemorrhage profusely and have marked abnormalities of all of the tests for DIC. On the other hand, DIC may be subclinical and manifested only by a positive paracoagulation test and mild thrombocytopenia.

B. **Management.** Very few patients are helped if the underlying problem is not corrected. Patients should be treated *if* the triggering process is ongoing (e.g., an active, acute infection) *and if* DIC is causing end-organ damage. Treatment is not necessary for laboratory manifestations alone. The following sequence is recommended:
   1. **Treat the underlying disease.** For patients with cancer this is often futile, but the possible advantages of antimicrobial therapy, further surgery, RT, or chemotherapy should be considered.
   2. **The clotting process should be stopped with heparin** unless there are contraindications. An IV bolus of 5000 IU is followed by an infusion of heparin to maintain the PTT at 1.5 to 2.0 times the control value. For cancer patients with chronic DIC, minidose heparin may be given SQ (2500–5000 IU q8–12h).

3. **Administration of blood components.** Platelet packs are given in the presence of thrombocytopenia and serious bleeding. One or two units of FFP or 15 bags of cryoprecipitate usually improve factor deficiencies unless the clotting process is severe. Cryoprecipitate is useful in patients with borderline cardiac reserve who cannot tolerate large volumes of FFP.

4. **Fibrinolysis is inhibited only if necessary,** that is, if the patient has documented primary fibrinolysis or DIC with life-threatening bleeding and evidence of extensive secondary fibrinolysis (i.e., shortened euglobulin lysis time). Fibrinolysis may be inhibited by epsilon-aminocaproic acid (EACA, Amicar); renal failure is a relative contraindication for EACA use. A loading dose of 5 gm is followed by 1 gm/hr IV or 2 gm q2h PO. If the episode of DIC has abated, EACA may be given alone. If the status of DIC is uncertain or ongoing, heparin should be given with EACA. Therapy with EACA is usually discontinued after 8 to 24 hours.

5. **Antiplatelet drugs** (aspirin and dipyridamole) may be useful in patients with chronic DIC who are not bleeding.

6. **Patient surveillance.** The platelet count, paracoagulation test, and clinical evaluation are the most useful factors to follow. The *reptilase time* (performed like the TT) is sensitive to the presence of FDP; unlike the TT, the reptilase test is not affected by heparin.

III. **Primary fibrinolysis.** Primary fibrinolysis occurs essentially only in the following conditions: prostatic carcinoma, advanced cirrhosis of the liver, heat stroke, or amniotic fluid embolism.

A. **Malignancies** may promote fibrinolysis by releasing plasminogen activators, such as urokinase or other proteolytic enzymes. Extensive metastatic liver disease may result in decreased clearance of plasminogen and its activators.

1. **Prostatic carcinoma** and, to a lesser extent, benign prostatic conditions are capable of triggering both thrombosis and fibrinolysis.

2. **Other cancers** that have been reported to activate fibrinolysis are sarcoma and carcinomas of the breast, thyroid, colon, and stomach.

B. **Diagnosis of primary fibrinolysis.** See sec. II.A.3.

C. **Management of primary fibrinolysis.** See sec. II.B.4.

IV. **Other hemostatic defects associated with cancer**

A. **Platelet function abnormalities** are very common in malignancies.

1. **Mechanisms**

a. Coating of platelet surfaces by fibrin degradation products with DIC.

b. Coating of platelets by paraproteins with myeloma.

c. Concomitant azotemia.

d. Inherent platelet dysfunction associated with myelodysplastic or myeloproliferative disorders.

e. Patients may be taking drugs with antiplatelet activity.

2. **Diagnosis**

a. **Signs** of platelet dysfunction include easy bruisability, gingival bleeding with toothbrushing, and other minor mucosal bleeding.

b. **Laboratory studies.** The template bleeding time is the best available clinical tool for demonstrating abnormal platelet function. A variety of in vitro platelet function tests have uncertain clinical validity. Thrombocytopenia, DIC, and azotemia should be ruled out by appropriate tests.

3. **Treatment.** Patients with bleeding and platelet dysfunction require treatment of the underlying disorder and may require platelet transfusions. DDAVP, 0.3 µg/kg, may also be helpful temporarily.

B. **Paraproteinemia.** Hemostatic abnormalities associated with plasma cell myeloma were discussed in Chap. 22, sec. VII.A.1.a.(1).

C. **Liver metastases,** when extensive, can result in inability to synthesize clotting factors. Treatment with vitamin K is ineffective. Bleeding must usually be controlled by the administration of FFP.

D. **Dysfibrinogenemia.** Dysfibrinogens are abnormal fibrinogen molecules, which may be inherited or acquired in association with hepatocellular carcinoma or liver metastases. The PT, PTT, and TT are all markedly abnormal. Fibrinogen concentrations are low when measured by clotting methods but are normal when measured by immunologic or physical precipitation methods. Hemorrhage is not common with dysfibrinogenemia but may occur.

E. Acquired circulating inhibitors of coagulation occur in a wide variety of tumors (e.g., a heparinlike inhibitor has been described in mastocytosis). It is doubtful that these inhibitors are responsible for hemorrhage in the absence of other causes, such as uremia or thrombocytopenia.

F. Specific factor deficiencies

1. **Factor XIII deficiency or dysfunction** is common in patients with cancer but usually does not cause clinical problems. The PT, PTT, and TT are normal, but the assay for factor XIII is abnormal. Hemorrhagic episodes are treated with FFP, 5 ml/kg weekly.

2. **Factor X deficiency** may occasionally be an isolated coagulation abnormality in patients with amyloidosis. Hemorrhagic episodes are treated with FFP, or prothrombin complexes.

3. **Factor XII and Fletcher factor (prekallikrein) deficiencies** have been described in patients with cancer but have little clinical significance.

4. **Acquired von Willebrand's disease** has been reported in cancer patients.

G. Hemostatic abnormalities associated with cytotoxic agents

1. **Hypofibrinogenemia** or dysfibrinogenemia is an almost universal complication of treatment with L-asparaginase.

2. **Vitamin K antagonism** occurs with actinomycin D therapy.

3. **DIC** is a common complication of administration of mithramycin.

4. **Primary fibrinolysis** has been reported to be activated by the anthracyclines.

5. **Platelet dysfunction** (of questionable significance) has been reported with cytarabine, daunorubicin, melphalan, vincristine, mitomycin C, L-asparaginase, and high-dose chemotherapy in preparation for BMT.

Selected Reading

Aderka, D., et al. Idiopathic deep vein thrombosis in an apparently healthy patient as a premonitory sign of occult cancer. *Cancer* 57:1846, 1986.

Castello, A., Coci, A., and Magrini, U. Paraneoplastic marrow alterations in patients with cancer. *Haematologica* 77:392, 1992.

Da Silva, J.-L., et al. Tumor cells are the site of erythropoietin synthesis in human renal cancers associated with polycythemia. *Blood* 75:577, 1990.

Kesteven, P. J. L., et al. Hypersplenism and splenectomy in lymphoproliferative and myeloproliferative disorders. *Clin. Lab. Haematol.* 7:297, 1985.

Monreal, M., et al. Occult cancer in patients with acute pulmonary embolism. A prospective study. *Chest* 103:816, 1993.

Naschitz, J. E., Yeshurun, D., and Abrahamson, J. Arterial occlusive disease in occult cancer. *Am. Heart J.* 124:738, 1992.

Snyder, H. W., et al. Treatment of cancer chemotherapy-associated thrombotic thrombocytopenic purpura/hemolytic-uremic syndrome by protein A immunoadsorption of plasma. *Cancer* 71:1882, 1993.

Spivak, J. L. The application of recombinant erythropoietin in anemic patients with cancer. *Semin. Oncol.* 19(3 Suppl 8):25, 1992.

Trousseau, A. Phlegmasia alba dolens. *Clin. Med. Hotel Dieu Paris.* 3:94, 1865.

I. Granulocytopenia with fever and sepsis

A. Principles. The development of fever in patients with granulocytopenia must always be regarded as a medical emergency caused by infection until proved otherwise. The presenting features of infection are altered by the absence of neutrophilic exudation in infected tissues.

1. **Predisposition**

   a. **Defects in the normal mechanical barriers** to infection provide routes for bacterial and fungal invasion. Examples of such defects are mucositis from tumor erosion, chemotherapy, or RT; indwelling catheters and IV sites; organ obstruction or erosion from tumors or catheters; and disturbed cutaneous integrity from shaving or skin metastases and ulceration.

   b. **Neurologic dysfunction,** such as neurogenic bladder or loss of gag reflex, predisposes patients to pyelonephritis or aspiration pneumonia.

   c. **Impairment of cell-mediated immunity** predisposes patients to infections with obligate intracellulare microbes, such as *Pneumocystis carinii* and *Nocardia,* and is thought to be responsible for severe primary infections with varicella, rubeola, and cytomegalovirus (CMV, which occurs after allogeneic BMT).

   d. **Absence or impairment of splenic function** makes patients susceptible to overwhelming septicemia with encapsulated organisms (e.g., *Streptococcus pneumoniae, Haemophilus influenzae*).

   e. **Hospitalization** predisposes patients to any nosocomial infection.

2. **Risk.** Granulocytopenia carries the risk of bacterial infection, and if prolonged, of fungal infection. The risk of infection increases slightly with granulocyte counts below $1000/\mu L$, rises sharply with counts below $500/\mu L$, and is highest with counts below $100/\mu L$. The more rapid the rate of granulocyte decline, the higher the risk of infection.

3. **Infecting organisms.** Approximately 80 percent of infections in neutropenic patients arise from the patient's endogenous flora. About 75 percent of septicemias are caused by gram-negative organisms. Fungal infections are increasing in incidence and occur after prolonged periods of granulocytopenia or antibiotic therapy.

4. **The outcome of a febrile illness** depends on the duration of leukopenia and restoration of normal granulocytes.

B. Diagnostic methods. Blood cultures and biopsies remain the pivotal investigations for diagnosis in granulocytopenic patients.

1. **History and physical examination.** A careful history should be taken. Despite the lack of physical signs of a normal inflammatory response, physical examination should give special attention to the skin, ocular fundus, sinuses, CNS, pelvis, and rectum.

2. **Surveillance cultures.** Blood cultures have been shown to be the only useful surveillance cultures to be performed during periods of persistent fever in these patients.

3. **Special laboratory procedures.** Gallium[67] scans can help define and localize areas of inflammation but may also give false-positive results in patients

with hematologic malignancies. ^{111}In-IgG scans may contribute to early diagnosis and offer better specificity for localization of infections.

C. Initial therapy. Emergent and empirical treatment with IV antibiotics is mandatory for febrile neutropenic patients. The most effective choices for empiric initial IV antibiotic therapy in granulocytopenic patients with clinical sepsis are:

Ceftazidime (2 gm IV q8h) *plus* piperacillin/clavulanic acid (Timentin) (3.1 gm IV q6h), *or*
Ceftriaxone (2 gm IV q24h) *plus* amikacin (500 mg IV q12h), *or*
Imipenem/cilastin (Primaxin) (500 mg IV q6h alone) *or*
Piperacillin/tazobactam (Zosyn) (3.375 gm IV q8h *alone*)

All four of these regimens cover *Escherichia coli, Klebsiella* spp., *Pseudomonas aeruginosa,* and *Staphylococcus aureus.* These bacteria account for 85 percent of pathogens in this setting.

1. **Colony-stimulating factors** (CSFs) should be initiated immediately in patients with granulocytopenia and clinical sepsis except with acute leukemia. Recombinant granulocyte CSF (G-CSF, filgrastin, 5 µg/kg SQ daily) or granulocyte-macrophage CSF (GM-CSF, sargramostin, 250 µg/m^2 daily) quickly increase the neutrophil count in drug-induced agranulocytosis.

2. **Toxicity of antibiotics** is minimal with all of these regimens, although seizures are associated with high doses of imipenem (1 gm IV every six hours). Diarrhea is more frequent in patients receiving cefoperazone, whereas nausea occurs more often with imipenem. Superinfections caused by beta-lactam-resistant, gram-negative bacilli are uncommon, but occur more frequently with double beta-lactam therapy than with imipenem monotherapy. Superinfections with *Xanthomonas maltophilia* occur only in patients receiving imipenem.

D. Ongoing therapy

1. If patients improve on empiric antibiotic therapy, it should be continued for 9 or 10 days, despite negative cultures.

2. If patients do not improve on empiric therapy after four days, antibiotics should be stopped and cultures repeated. Patients are probably either on the wrong antibiotic(s) or have a condition for which antibiotics are ineffective (e.g., viral or fungal infection, abscesses, or noninfectious causes). Antibiotics should be resumed if patients become worse or the fever persists.

3. If fevers persist after seven days of antibiotic therapy, granulocytopenic patients benefit from empirical antifungal therapy (fluconazole, 200 mg PO or IV every 24 hours). The presence of mucositis or esophagitis should prompt empiric antifungal therapy even earlier. The overall survival rate decreases in adults with acute leukemia if antifungal therapy is not initiated empirically before documentation of filamentous deep fungal infection. Fluconazole has replaced amphotericin B for this purpose because of its ease of administration and low toxicity.

E. Prevention of infection

1. **General measures**

   a. Handwashing by the staff before touching patients is the most important preventive technique.

   b. Skin care may be important in preventing infections with *S. aureus* and other pathogens. Occlusive antiperspirants are avoided. Electric shavers are preferred; not shaving at all may be best.

   c. Avoidance of fresh flowers and foods with high bacterial contents (such as fruits, uncooked foods, and tap water) has no established value.

   d. Teeth should be brushed daily. Procedures involving the use of tubes, tapes, and instruments should be minimized because they may be sources of infection.

2. **Isolation methods**

   a. Reverse isolation (caps, masks, gloves, and gowns) has no established benefit. In fact, it probably deters good patient care by limiting patient contact with the hospital staff and family.

b. High-efficiency particulate air filters and laminar air flow rooms, which are expensive, are of questionable benefit.

3. Prophylactic antibiotics. Using prophylactic antibiotics in granulocytopenic patients hypothetically lowers the endogenous flora (particularly in the GI tract) of potential pathogens.

a. Prophylaxis with quinolones (e.g., ciprofloxacin, 500 mg PO b.i.d.) significantly reduces the occurrence of gram-negative bacteremia and delays the onset of fever during periods of neutropenia (thus reducing the number of days that IV antimicrobial agents are required). This drug does not reduce mortality or the occurrence of fever, however. Subsequent infections are mainly due to resistant gram-positive cocci.

b. Prophylaxis with Bactrim plus colistin. Bactrim (trimethoprim-sulfamethoxazole [80 mg/400 mg], 1 ampule IV or 1 tablet PO q8h) plus colistin (400 mg PO b.i.d.) is associated with fewer infective complications and fewer febrile days compared to treatment with quinolones. Subsequent infections are due to resistant gram-negative rods.

F. Investigational agents attempt to reduce mortality in septic shock syndrome caused by gram-negative bacteria by attacking the mediators of inflammation. Such agents include anti-TNF, E5 (mouse antiendotoxin monoclonal antibody), and HA-1A (human monoclonal IgM antibody that recognizes the lipid A component of lipopolysaccharide). HA-1A acts through immune complex clearance of endotoxin and reduces production of TNF-α, IL-1-β and IL-6.

II. Other infections in the compromised host

A. Pulmonary infections

1. Differential diagnosis

a. Noninfectious causes. About 25 to 30 percent of cases of fever with pulmonary infiltrates in cancer patients are due to noninfectious causes, which include radiation pneumonitis, drug-induced pneumonitis, pulmonary emboli and hemorrhage, lipid emboli following lymphangiography, and leukoagglutinin transfusion reaction.

b. Predicting the infecting agent. Acute, severe symptoms that progress in less than one day suggest a common bacterial pathogen or noninfectious process (pulmonary emboli, pulmonary hemorrhage). A subacute course (over several days) suggests viral, pneumocystis, or occasionally, *Aspergillus* or *Nocardia* infection. A chronic course (over several weeks) is more typical of mycobacterial or fungal infections, radiation fibrosis, or drug-induced pneumonitis. Prediction from chest x-ray film is not valid.

(1) Infection acquired outside the hospital. Despite the susceptibility to opportunistic infections, *S. pneumoniae* and influenza virus are the most likely pulmonary infections in cancer patients.

(2) Infection acquired inside the hospital. *Klebsiella, Serratia, Pseudomonas, E. coli, S. aureus,* and *Acinetobacter* are the most frequently acquired nosocomial pathogens. *Candida, Aspergillus, Legionella pneumophila,* and *P. carinii* are also hospital acquired.

2. Diagnostic approach

a. Sputum examination. If the sputum contains neutrophils or macrophages and fewer than 10 epithelial cells per low-power field, the results are probably valid. Problems with interpretation include

(1) Granulocytopenic patients usually have no neutrophils in the sputum.

(2) Mouth flora may cause aspiration pneumonia.

(3) Many patients show negative sputum examination even when *S. pneumoniae* is the responsible organism.

(4) Many opportunistic organisms that produce pneumonia are infrequently retrieved in sputum (e.g., *Mycobacterium tuberculosis, Nocardia asteroides, Aspergillus, Cryptococcus*).

(5) The various classes of penicillins can inhibit recovery of *N. asteroides* in culture. Aminoglycosides inhibit *M. tuberculosis* and *L. pneumophila.*

  b. **Serology** is useful for identifying infection from *Coccidioides immitis, Cryptococcus neoformans, Aspergillus, L. pneumophila, Mycoplasma pneumoniae, Toxoplasma gondii,* and CMV. No serologic test can help diagnose acute infections.

  c. **Blood cultures** must be obtained in all patients. Cultures are useful as surveillance in patients with pneumonia, granulocytopenia, and persistent fever.

  d. **Thoracentesis** should be performed in patients with pleural effusion.

  e. **Lung biopsy procedures.** Diagnosis is paramount in the immunocompromised host. The highest yield and best control of bleeding is by direct visualization with open lung biopsy. This procedure may be mandatory when the patient is rapidly deteriorating. If the pneumonic process is less rapid, then bronchoscopy with lavage appears to be the best approach. Where a mass or consolidation is present, skinny-needle biopsy is more frequently performed because the chance of complication is less. Invasive techniques are often not justified late in the course of malignancy because they often add morbidity without hope of palliation. Empiric antibiotic therapy is justified in these cases.

 3. **Therapy** for acute pneumonia should be initiated immediately after cultures are obtained. Patients with acid-fast bacilli, *N. asteroides, C. neoformans,* or *A. fumigatus* should not be regarded as colonized and should be treated.

B. **CNS infections.** Infections in the CNS can present either with simple changes of cognition or motor skills or with seizures and coma. Meningismus is a hallmark of disease, but this condition may be absent. An MRI scan is indicated when cerebral edema, abscess, or demyelinating encephalitis is suspected. This scan is particularly useful in defining viral encephalitis and areas where enhanced foci are seen, such as in toxoplasmosis.

Special considerations in cancer patients suspected or proven to have CNS infections are as follows:

 1. **Meningitis.** Cancer patients have an increased incidence of atypical pathogens.

  a. **Granulocytopenic patients** rarely develop gram-negative meningitis despite a high incidence of gram-negative bacteremias. When meningitis does develop, the pathogens usually are the enterobacteriaceae, *P. aeruginosa, Bacillus subtilis,* or *Listeria monocytogenes.* Meningitis caused by aspergillosis or zygomycosis has also been described.

  b. **Patients with defects in cell-mediated immunity.** *L. monocytogenes* and *C. neoformans* are the most likely pathogens. Meningitis and meningoencephalitis from varicella-zoster virus (VZV), herpes simplex virus (HSV), JC virus, HIV, CMV, *T. gondii,* and *Strongyloides stercoralis* also occur.

 2. **Brain abscesses** are most likely caused by mixed aerobic and anaerobic bacteria. In the immunocompromised patient, brain abscesses are often due to pathogens such as *Aspergillus,* Zygomycetes, *Nocardia,* or *Toxoplasma.* Toxoplasmosis can produce meningitis, necrotizing encephalitis, or abscess. In atypical cases, brain biopsy is performed at the time of surgical drainage.

 3. **Lumbar puncture (LP)**

  a. **Papilledema.** An emergency CT scan of the brain must be performed first. Patients with space-occupying lesions on CT scan should have LP or cisternal puncture performed by a qualified neurologist or neuroradiologist.

  b. **Thrombocytopenia.** Spinal subdural hematoma occasionally complicates LP in patients with severe thrombocytopenia. Clinical evidence of CNS infection, however, supersedes consideration of risks. The following guidelines are recommended:

   (1) If the platelet count is below 20,000/μL, transfuse platelet packs just before performing LP. Transfuse additional platelet packs if pain or neurologic signs develop.

(2) The most skilled physician available should perform the LP using a 22-gauge needle. The patient should be observed closely afterward. The role of needle aspiration and surgical intervention in patients who develop spinal subdural hematomas induced by LP has not been determined.

  c. CSF should be evaluated for:

   (1) Glucose and protein concentrations, cell counts, routine bacterial culture and sensitivity, Gram's stain, and cytology.

   (2) Acid-fast culture and stain, fungal cultures, India ink preparation, cryptococcal antigen, and coccidioidiomycosis serology (depending on geography and predominant soil fungus).

   (3) Polymerase chain reaction (PCR) assays (e.g., for HIV, mycobacterium, toxoplasmosis, legionella, listeria, JC virus, or herpesviruses) should be performed only if clinical or laboratory findings suggest the likelihood of the pathogen.

   (4) IgG synthesis assays are useful in suggesting certain viral infections. HIV antigen and index are indicated for high-risk patients.

C. Skin infections

  1. Neoplasms invading the skin (e.g., mycosis fungoides) are associated with infections involving common pathogens such as *S. aureus.*

  2. Cell-mediated immunity deficiencies are typically associated with skin infection by herpes zoster or herpes simplex. Kaposi's sarcoma is highly associated with CMV infections.

  3. Granulocytopenic patients may have skin infections with atypical or few physical findings. *S. aureus* and *S. pyogenes* are common. More serious manifestations represent systemic infections; these include bullae, raised ecchymotic plaques or nodules, black necrotic ulcers, or ecthyma gangrenosum. These manifestations of systemic infection may be produced by *Pseudomonas* spp., *Candida* spp., *Aspergillus* spp., *Aeromonas hydrophila,* and Zygomycetes.

D. Alimentary tract and intra-abdominal infections

  1. Esophagitis may be from *Candida* or HSV.

  2. Colitis with ulceration is commonly produced by CMV. Aspergillosis and zygomycosis may also involve the GI tract.

  3. Intra-abdominal abscesses develop when the bowel or genital tract becomes obstructed, necrotic, or perforated because of tumor. Mixed infections with gram-negative enteric organisms are frequent, particularly with species of *Bacteroides* and *Clostridium. Streptococcus bovis* abscess and sepsis may occur with colon, pancreatic, or mouth carcinoma.

  4. Perirectal abscesses frequently develop in granulocytopenic patients, especially those with acute leukemia; usually they are caused by mixtures of aerobic and anaerobic bacteria.

  5. Liver infections. Hepatitis A, hepatitis B, and hepatitis C viral infections are common. Multiple abscesses secondary to systemic bacterial or fungal infection also occur. Even viruses such as VZV, HSV, or CMV can present as mass or necrotic lesions in the liver of immunocompromised patients. The liver is mildly or moderately involved in many opportunistic infections and may be cultured with biopsy specimens.

E. Urinary tract infections are frequent in cancer patients because of obstructive uropathies, the use of urinary catheters, and prolonged and repeated hospitalizations. These infections are often due to resistant gram-negative bacteria or *Candida.*

F. Bone marrow infections are usually due to systemic disease, particularly with tuberculosis, fungi, salmonellosis, listeriosis, or DNA viruses. **Bone marrow suppression** mimicking aplastic anemia occurs with parvovirus B19, mycobacteria, histoplasmosis, and brucellosis.

G. **Central line infections.** The incidences of central line infections for external (e.g., Hickman) and subcutaneous ports (e.g., Portacath) are equal. The majority of central line infections are caused by coagulase-positive or coagulase-negative *Staphylococcus* spp., and about 80 percent of these infections can be treated with 10 days of antibiotics without removing the line. Vancomycin, 500 mg IV q6h can be used, depending on renal function; if the patient is sensitive, oxacillin, 500 mg IV q6h can be given. The **central line must be removed** in the following circumstances:
   1. Exit site infections with *P. aeruginosa*
   2. All tunnel infections
   3. All line infections caused by fungi or *Candida*
   4. Bacteremia persisting beyond 24 hours of antibiotic therapy or caused by *Bacillus* spp., JK diphtheroids, or most gram-negative organisms

III. **Vaccination of immunosuppressed patients**
   A. **Vaccines contraindicated in immunosuppressed patients** are those that contain living organisms. These include measles (rubeola), varicella (chickenpox), rubella, mumps, oral poliovirus, smallpox, yellow fever, and anthrax.
   B. **Permissible vaccines.** Immunosuppressed patients often do not attain an effective response to active immunization. However, permissible vaccines are those for diphtheria, tetanus, pertussis, typhoid, cholera, plague, influenza, and pneumococcus. The pneumococcal vaccine is strongly indicated for all cancer patients. The overall effectiveness is 75 to 90 percent. Diminished efficacy in the severely immunosuppressed is not well defined.

IV. **Viral infections**
   A. **EBV** is the recognized pathogen for infectious mononucleosis, Burkitt's lymphoma in Africa, and nasopharyngeal carcinoma in Asia. The virus is ubiquitous: about 15 percent of healthy adults, 25 percent of patients with solid tumors, 60 percent of renal transplant recipients, and 80 percent of all patients with leukemia or lymphoma are seropositive for EBV. The virus is transmissible in blood transfusions.
      1. **Diagnosis.** Histologic findings are consistent but not helpful.
         a. **EBV-specific antibodies**
            (1) Antibodies to viral capsid antigen (VCA) develop early and persist for life. In contrast, early IgM components of VCA antibodies persist for only four to eight weeks.
            (2) Early antigen antibodies, including anti-D and anti-R, are associated with severe disease and with the neoplasms linked to EBV infection.
            (3) EBV nuclear antibody (EBNA) types 1, 2, or 3, appear after one month of illness, persist for life, and are useful in diagnosing heterophil-negative cases. Anti-EBNA types 1, 2A, and 6 are simultaneously four to ten times higher in chronic reactivation EBV syndromes than in acute EBV disease. Only anti-EBNA type 1 is elevated in nasopharyngeal carcinoma (NPC). Individual EBNA subtype titers appear to be normal in patients with lymphoma or Hodgkin's disease.
            (4) The plasma level of sCD23 is a sensitive and useful marker of EBV-related polyclonal or B cell monoclonal proliferation in transplanted patients with immunosuppression.
            (5) IgA antibodies to EBV membrane antigen indicate a high risk of developing NPC. This enzyme-linked immunosorbent assay (ELISA) has potential use in the diagnosis of NPC and for large-scale screening of individuals at risk for NPC.
         b. **Nucleic acid hybridization techniques** can detect EBV in human tissues. **Southern blot analysis** distinguishes latent EBV from infectious EBV and determines the clonality of infected tumors with respect to the viral terminal repeat sequence structure. **PCR** is exquisitely sensitive for detecting viral DNA.
      2. **Syndromes associated with EBV**
         a. **Mononucleosis syndrome** is typically manifested by fever, malaise,

pharyngitis, lymphadenopathy, splenomegaly (50% of patients), and a peripheral blood smear showing lymphocytosis with atypical cells. Complications include hepatitis, myopericarditis, meningoencephalitis, Guillain-Barré syndrome, cold agglutinin hemolysis, and thrombocytopenia. Infectious mononucleosis occurring in elderly patients may mimic lymphoma or lymphocytic leukemia. Mononucleosis syndrome may also result from infection with CMV, hepatitis virus, mycoplasma, *Toxoplasma,* brucella, mycobacteria, *Yersinia,* or streptococcus.

b. Chronic infectious mononucleosis syndrome is distinguished by subjective findings of fatigue, malaise, low-grade fever, and mild lymphadenopathy associated with depression of cognitive functions. Occasional patients probably do have this illness, but many more are diagnosed inappropriately because they carry chronic antibodies.

c. Chronic active EBV (CAEBV) is associated with significantly increased numbers of a cytotoxic T lymphocyte (CTL) subset (CD8$^+$, CD11$^-$ lymphocytes).

  (1) Defective EBV-CTL activity and anti-EBNA-antibody responses are frequently observed both in children with CAEBV and in their parents, which may suggest a familial basis for the abnormal immune response to EBV.

  (2) Antibodies to the EBV VCA are associated with regression of outgrowths of virus-transformed B cells and their viral load. Decreases of virus-cell associated growth are also associated with sequential increases in IL-2 and γ-IFN and low levels of IL-6 and GM-CSF. Conversely, little or no decrease in cells infected chronically with EBV is associated with undetectable levels of IL-2, low levels of γ-IFN, high levels of IL-6 and GM-CSF, and an increased frequency of cells bearing the phenotype CD20 and HLA-DR.

d. Virus-associated hemophagocytic syndrome is characterized by high fever, liver dysfunction, coagulation abnormalities, pancytopenia, and a benign histiocytic proliferation with prominent hemophagocytosis in bone marrow, lymph node, spleen, and liver. EBV-associated hemophagocytic syndrome has been fatal, particularly in Japan.

3. Malignancies and lymphoreticular disorders associated with EBV

a. Nasopharyngeal carcinoma in Asia.

b. Epidemic Burkitt's lymphoma, an EBV-associated non-Hodgkin's lymphoma, is endemic in an area of Africa known as the "Lymphoma Belt." This zone is demarcated by climatic requirements of temperature and rainfall. The plant *Euphorbia tirucalli,* which possesses EBV-activating substances, can induce the characteristic 8:14 translocation of Burkitt's lymphoma in EBV-infected lymphoblastic cell lines in vitro. Its distribution conforms closely to the climatic requirements of the lymphoma.

c. Cutaneous T cell lymphoma (CTCL) is associated with both human T cell lymphotropic virus (HTLV-I) and EBV. Three distinct clinicopathologic subgroups are associated with EBV (types II, III, and V). No EBV genome has been thus far detected in type I CTCL (classic mycosis fungoides) or in type IV CTCL (HTLV-I-associated adult T cell lymphoma).

  (1) Type II CTCL (T large-cell lymphoma) is either positive or negative for Ki-1 antigen (CD30). Most of affected patients have Ki-1-negative lymphoma, which is a fulminant disease, whereas the course of the Ki-1-positive cases is benign.

  (2) Type III CTCL (angiocentric T cell lymphoma or "lymphomatoid granulomatosis") presents with chronic ulcers or violaceous papules.

  (3) Type V CTCL is secondary to systemic EBV-associated T cell lymphoma. The common features of these EBV-associated CTCLs are resistance to conventional chemotherapy, poor prognosis, and the terminal manifestation of a hemophagocytic syndrome.

   d. **Adult T cell leukemia-lymphoma (ATLL)** is associated with HTLV-1. It is hypothesized that both EBV and HTLV-1 may infect the same T cells in early life and may have a role in the oncogenesis of ATLL.
   e. **Pyothorax-associated lymphoma** is a rare tumor associated with EBV and long-standing tuberculous pyothorax. Most of these cases are high-grade B cell lymphomas. Over 50 cases have been reported in Japan.
   f. **Gastric carcinoma.** EBV is associated with lymphoepitheliomalike gastric carcinoma with marked lymphocytic stroma. The close relationship between EBV and undifferentiated gastric carcinomas and the variable association with gastric adenocarcinomas suggests fundamentally different roles for the virus in the etiology of these two malignancies.
   g. **Warthin's parotid tumor.** In distinct neoplastic cell types of multiple/ bilateral Warthin's tumor of the parotid gland, the EBV genome is frequently detected by in situ hybridization technique.
4. **Management** is supportive. Corticosteroids are not used except in the presence of severe anemia, airway obstruction, myopericarditis, or neurologic complications. High-dose acyclovir (800 mg PO q.i.d.) may have some benefit early in acute EBV syndromes but does not eliminate persistent EBV infection from the oropharynx. Therefore, this agent does not necessarily prevent lymphoma development. Ganciclovir, foscarvir, or specific cytokine therapy may also have potential benefit for this infection.
B. **Cytomegalovirus (CMV)** often presents as EBV-negative mononucleosis. Fever, interstitial pneumonia, and alimentary canal ulcerative disease are the most common manifestations of CMV in adults with neoplasms. CMV, which is tropic for endothelial cells, also causes retinitis, encephalitis, and peripheral neuropathy.
   CMV can suppress cell-mediated immunity, reticuloendothelial cell function, and granulocyte reserves. Cells infected with CMV stimulate production of IL-1 and TNF. Thus, CMV often coexists or activates other opportunistic infections.
   1. **Infection, latency, and recurrence.** Primary CMV infection can occur perinatally or later in life, and inevitably results in latent infection. Infection is especially likely following transfusions of blood that contains granulocytes.
      Latent CMV burden and risk of recurrence is related to the extent of virus multiplication during primary infection. The risk of CMV recurrence is high in immunocompromised individuals and only after neonatal infection in normal hosts.
   2. **CMV infection of the GI tract** can cause serious inflammatory or ulcerative disease in immunocompromised patients. Manifestations include pain, ulceration, bleeding, diarrhea, and perforation. All levels of the GI tract, particularly the stomach and colon, may be involved. Pathologic examination reveals diffuse ulcerations and necrosis with scattered CMV inclusions.
   3. **Diagnosis**
      a. **Culture.** CMV is slow growing (up to six weeks), and culture is generally not practical. Early antibody detected by application of ELISA in cultures does accelerate identification.
      b. **Histiocytology** shows the characteristic enlarged cells with dense nuclear inclusions and wide peri-inclusion halos. Cytoplasmic inclusions are frequent, but multinucleation is absent.
      c. **Serologic assays**
         (1) Seropositivity for antibodies against CMV is indicative of latent infection but is insufficient as a predictor for the risk of recurrence.
         (2) Complement fixation (CF) antibody showing fourfold titer increases is highly suggestive of acute disease.
         (3) Anticomplementary immunofluorescent assay, ELISA, and indirect fluorescent antibody (FA) assays are sensitive indicators of infection. IgG antibody occurs during the acute phase of the illness and persists for life, whereas IgM antibodies occur early and often disappear after four to eight weeks. Recurrent IgM spikes occur in certain patients, indicating either partial immunity to CMV or exposure to new variants of the virus.

(4) Use of monoclonal antibodies to detect antigens that are amplified through coculturing with lymphocytes is becoming the best means of identifying active CMV disease.

d. PCR assay, both in situ and in DNA extracted from gross specimens, is the most useful new tool to isolate and identify the presence and location of CMV in clinical disease.

4. Management

a. Ganciclovir (9-[1,3-dihydroxy-2-proxymethyl]-guanine, DHPG).

(1) The efficacy of this drug for CMV retinitis and colitis is well documented, but it is less effective with CMV pneumonia or meningoencephalitis. In bone marrow transplant recipients, the prophylactic administration of ganciclovir abrogates CMV pneumonitis and considerably reduces the incidence of CMV infection.

(2) Ganciclovir is given for 14 days at a dose of 5 mg/kg IV q12h. Patients with AIDS often require maintenance treatment (5 mg/kg/day). Dosage is modified according to the predicted creatinine clearance and absolute neutrophil count. An oral form of ganciclovir will soon be available.

b. Foscarnet also has proven efficacy but must be monitored for renal toxicity and electrolyte, calcium, and magnesium imbalance. Ganciclovir and foscarnet are probably synergistic, and combination therapy is useful in patients when ganciclovir alone is ineffective.

Foscarnet therapy is begun with a dose of 60 mg/kg IV q8h in 1 L of normal saline for two weeks. Maintenance therapy (90–120 mg/kg/day) is required in patients with AIDS. Dosing is adjusted for predicted creatinine clearance.

c. Hyperimmune CMV globulin appears to be protective and therapeutic in certain patients.

C. Herpes zoster. VZV is the most common infective agent to complicate lymphoproliferative diseases. Zoster (shingles) is the reactivation of VZV. Vesicles form in clusters on erythematous bases, usually distributed along one to three dermatomes. Several lesions outside a dermatomal distribution does not necessarily indicate dissemination. Disseminated VZV infections may be manifested by encephalopathy, Guillain-Barré syndrome, transverse myelitis, myositis, pneumonia, thrombocytopenia, hepatitis, and arthritis.

1. Diagnosis. It is fruitless to search for an underlying undiagnosed tumor in patients with zoster if the history, physical examination, and routine screening studies are normal.

a. Histocytology (multinucleated cells with intranuclear inclusions) is suggestive.

b. Culture. Inoculate early vesicular fluid.

c. Serology. CF antibody titers are useful, although they may not rise for three to four weeks in immunocompromised patients. Using a PCR method to detect VZV DNA before antibody is produced, contacts of patients with varicella have been shown to carry this infection in their nasopharynx. These patients can be a threat to those who are either immunocompromised or have never been exposed to VZV.

2. Management. VZV is transmissible and patients should be isolated.

a. Acyclovir is the treatment of choice for zoster that occurs in immunocompromised patients and for disseminated VZV in any patient. The dosage is 250 mg/m^2 IV q8h or 800 mg PO four times daily for 7 to 10 days. All immunocompromised patients with zoster should be treated in the first 72 hours of illness.

b. Zoster immune globulin modifies or prevents illness in immunocompromised hosts. Passive immunization can be used instead of acyclovir where a rare toxicity is feared.

c. Ganciclovir has considerable activity for VZV as well as for CMV.

d. VZV live vaccine is available for primary immunization against chickenpox but has no role in the immunocompromised patient.

D. Herpes simplex virus (HSV). Patients with reticuloendothelial neoplasms, T lymphocyte defects, or cytotoxic chemotherapy treatment may develop HSV viremia. The viremia often produces alimentary tract ulceration and hemorrhage, hepatitis (occasionally manifested by abscesslike lesions), and respiratory tract infections.

Patients with Sézary syndrome or atopic dermatitis can develop progressive fulminant mucocutaneous disease (eczema herpeticum), which can recur and disseminate to visceral organs. Human herpesvirus-6 sequences are frequently detected by PCR in lymph nodes from patients with angioimmunoblastic lymphadenopathylike lymphoma, suggesting a possible involvement of this lymphotropic virus in the pathogenesis of at least some cases of the disease.

1. Diagnosis

a. Histocytology demonstrates the characteristic intranuclear mass surrounded by marginated chromatosis and often a peri-inclusion halo. Cytoplasmic inclusions are absent. Electron microscopy analysis of vesicular fluid, which can be performed in less than 30 minutes, strongly suggests the diagnosis. Immunofluorescence for HSV antigen is also rapid and specific.

b. Culture. HSV grows rapidly in tissue cultures (24 to 72 hours) and produces a unique cytopathologic picture.

c. Assays. Hemagglutination and indirect FA titers are useful if fourfold increases are demonstrated. Differentiation of IgG from IgM antibody assists in clarifying recent infection. An HSV IgG-capture ELISA has demonstrated intrathecal synthesis of antibodies to the virus. Furthermore, a PCR assay has demonstrated amplification of HSV DNA in CSF. Both ELISA and PCR are rapid, noninvasive means of diagnosing HSV encephalitis in a very early stage of the disease.

2. Management

a. Topical idoxuridine, especially using dimethyl sulfoxide as a carrier, is effective for HSV keratitis.

b. Acyclovir is now widely accepted as a safe, effective treatment for HSV infections in normal and immunocompromised patients. A dose of 200 mg PO five times daily or 10 to 15 mg/kg IV t.i.d. for 7 to 10 days is effective. As an ointment, acyclovir is useful for primary local infections but does not seem to prevent recurrent disease. The virus specific mechanism of action of acyclovir involves thymidine kinase (TK) and DNA polymerase. Resistance in the most part has proven to be due to an inability of the virus to produce TK.

c. Vidarabine is effective topically for keratitis.

d. Ganciclovir has excellent activity against HSV, although its primary usefulness has been directed at CMV.

e. Vaccines are under development both for viral glycoproteins and for viral-induced mammalian cell antigens.

E. Human parvovirus. The family of Parvoviridae is composed of small, nuclear-replicating viruses that have no envelope and contain an essentially single-stranded, linear DNA genome.

1. Oncosuppressive activity. Certain parvoviruses have the remarkable capacity to prevent the formation of spontaneous and induced tumors in laboratory animals. Epidemiologic studies in humans have correlated serologic evidence of parvoviral infection with a lower incidence of certain cancers. Certain parvoviruses preferentially lyse initiated or stably transformed cells in vitro. Parvoviruses can also have a cytostatic effect, causing the reversion of transformation traits, parallel to the down-modulation of the expression of defined genes, particularly oncogenes.

2. Parvovirus B19. The pathogenic human parvovirus B19 has extreme tropism for human erythroid progenitor cells. B19 is a known cause of erythema infectiosum ("fifth disease") and aplastic crisis in patients with hemolytic anemias (see Chapter 34, *Cytopenia,* sec. III.D).

   F. Human papillomavirus (HPV) is closely associated with anal and cervical dysplasia and carcinoma. See Chapter 36, sec. **V.D.2.**

   G. JC virus of the papovavirus family is associated with the development of progressive multifocal leukoencephalopathy. See Chapter 36, sec. **V.E.1.**

V. Bacteria

  A. Mycobacteria. Active tuberculosis (TB) develops in 0.5 to 1.0 percent of patients with malignancies. Infection is predominantly pulmonary in 70 percent, disseminated in 20 percent, and involves lymph nodes or other nonpulmonary sites in 10 percent of cases. Mortality approaches 100 percent for acute TB pneumonia and 90 percent for disseminated TB when cellular immunity is significantly depressed.

    1. The **incidence** of atypical mycobacterium infection (particularly with *Mycobacterium kansasii* and *M. avium* complex (MAC) is significantly higher in patients with cancer or HIV-AIDS than in the general population. *M. kansasii* infection has been associated with hairy-cell leukemia. *M. malmoense* is an opportunistic pathogen mainly isolated in northern Europe, most often from patients with pulmonary infections. *M. genavense* affects children with severe HIV infection. All of these organisms are commonly resistant to isoniazid or rifampin.

    2. Pathogenesis. Natural resistance to TB depends on the ability of the macrophage to control intracellular growth of the organism. The resistant host develops a chronic infection primarily affecting the lungs, whereas the highly susceptible host develops a rapidly fatal generalized illness. Survivors of the initial infection then develop resistance to reinfection by a mechanism based on sensitized T cells. When this system is only partially successful, the host becomes infectious if mycobacteria are shed into open airways. Cutaneous anergy and treatment with corticosteroids, cytotoxic agents, or irradiation predispose to reactivation of *M. tuberculosis*.

      Mycobacteria infection is associated with an initial copious release of both γ-IFN and IL-10. IL-10 production increases as the infection progresses, and γ-IFN levels diminish. IL-10 may have a negative impact on resistance to mycobacterial infections due to decreased macrophage activity, at least in part.

    3. Resistant TB. Immigration from high-prevalence countries, coinfection with HIV, and outbreaks in congregative facilities are primarily responsible for the increased incidence of TB cases during the past decade. Coincident with the increase in TB, outbreaks of multiple drug resistant (MDR) TB have occurred. MDR TB occurs late in the course of HIV infection and is refractory to treatment. A history of antituberculosis therapy is the strongest predictor of the presence of resistance.

    4. Diagnosis

      a. Chest x-ray evidence of infiltrates in apical or posterior segments of the upper lobe or superior segment of the lower lobe are the most frequent manifestations of postprimary TB.

      b. Smears and cultures. Three sputum cultures are necessary; more samples do not increase the yield. Expectorated sputum is the best culture source. Aerosol-induced sputum is superior to gastric juice aspiration in patients who produce little sputum. Diagnostic yield can be further increased using transbronchial biopsy when other material is not diagnostic. The use of PCR in the blood, spinal fluid, and in tissue is the most sensitive, specific, and rapid assay available.

      c. Effusions. Pleural fluid samples yield about 30 percent positive cultures, and percutaneous needle pleural biopsies (three biopsies in three locations) yield about 75 percent. Culture of pericardial fluid yields 50 percent positive results, and pericardial biopsy yields 80 percent positive results on either histology or culture. Analysis of ascitic fluid findings are not helpful unless the fluid is concentrated; peritoneal biopsy is preferred.

d. TB meningitis. Spinal fluid analysis is variable, although mononuclear cell pleocytosis and low glucose concentrations are common. Concentrated spinal fluid reveals TB bacillus on smear in 30 to 50 percent of cases and on culture in about 50 percent. PCR is becoming the best assay to diagnose mycobacterial meningitis.

5. Management

a. TB prophylaxis in cancer patients. Any patient who is to receive immunosuppressive therapy must be skin tested for TB and anergy. Prophylaxis with isoniazid (INH), 300 mg/day for one year, should be given to any cancer patient who has a positive tuberculin skin test.

b. Active TB. INH, 300 mg/day PO, plus rifampin, 600 mg/day PO, is the most effective therapy for active, nonresistant TB. Treatment should continue for a minimum of nine months and for at least six months after culture conversion. The addition of streptomycin or amikacin, 1 gm/day IM for three months, may shorten the duration of therapy. Ethambutol, 15 mg/kg/day PO, can be substituted for the offending drug if INH hepatitis or rifampin toxicity occurs.

c. Resistant TB. MDR TB is readily transmitted among hospitalized patients with AIDS. MDR TB requires treatment with four to six drugs (pyrazinamide, ethionamide, ciprofloxacin, amikacin, ethambutol, clofazimine, and possibly clarithromycin) depending on defined sensitivities.

d. MAC. Treatment for dissemination should include either azithromycin or clarithromycin and ethambutol (used as a second drug when tolerated). When resistance to a two-drug regimen or multisystem disease develops, one or two additional drugs should be selected from the following: clofazimine, rifabutin, ciprofloxacin, or in some instances, amikacin.

B. *Nocardia asteroides* **(nocardiosis).** Several types of cell-mediated immune defects have been described in association with nocardiosis. About 20 percent of cases occur in patients receiving corticosteroids.

In immunocompromised subjects, 75 percent of *Nocardia* infections occur in the lung. Nocardiosis can be asymptomatic, heal spontaneously, or produce a lower lobe bronchopneumonia with cavities, abscesses, or empyema. Disseminated nocardiosis typically involves subcutaneous tissue, muscle, and CNS tissues. Apparently localized soft tissue abscesses or osteomyelitis frequently disseminate.

1. Diagnosis. Gram's stain of sputum reveals gram-positive, beaded, branching filaments. Sputum should also be examined with modified Ziehl-Neelsen stain. Some organisms are acid-fast. Sabouraud dextrose and beef heart infusion culture media is incubated aerobically.

2. Management

a. Sulfadiazine, 6 to 10 gm/day PO in divided doses, is used for six weeks to three months. Most authorities suggest one year of therapy for severe infection.

b. Chloramphenicol (4 gm/day PO), chlortetracycline (2 gm/day PO), or Bactrim-DS (2 tablets q8h PO) can be used in addition to sulfadiazine for severe disease.

c. Cycloserine (15 mg/kg PO in four divided doses), alone or as an adjunct to sulfadiazine, shows promising results.

C. *Listeria monocytogenes* may be confused with gram-positive cocci, *H. influenzae*, or diphtheroids on Gram's stain of specimens. Infections are more common in patients with defects in cell-mediated immunity. *L. monocytogenes* is the most common cause of bacterial meningitis in patients with carcinoma and in patients receiving corticosteroids or other immunosuppressive therapy, especially for lymphoma.

CNS infection with cerebritis or brain abscess accounts for 80 percent of cases. The mortality for CNS infections is 15 to 45 percent. Bacteremia or sepsis accounts for 20 percent of cases in adults. Pulmonary involvement is always in the form of an empyema.

1. **Diagnosis**
   a. **Culture.** Once *L. monocytogenes* is isolated, the organisms have a unique tumbling motion when viewed in a hanging drop.
   b. **Spinal fluid.** Either lymphocytes or polymorphonuclear neutrophils are predominant. Spinal fluid protein concentration ranges from normal to 1 gm/dl. Glucose levels are low in only 50 percent of cases.
2. **Management**
   a. **Sepsis.** Ampicillin, 200 mg/kg/day IV, or penicillin, 300,000 units/kg/day IV, are given in six divided doses. Erythromycin and tetracycline are alternative drugs.
   b. **Meningoencephalitis** is treated in the same manner as sepsis. Intrathecal gentamicin, 3 to 5 mg every 24 hours, may be synergistic with intravenous antibiotics.

D. *Legionella pneumophila.* "Legionnaires' disease" can affect normal and immunosuppressed hosts, especially patients receiving glucocorticoids. The disease typically produces lobar pulmonic consolidation evolving from patchy infiltrates. Features that suggest legionnaires' disease include nonproductive cough, nodular pulmonary consolidation, diarrhea, hyponatremia, and confusion.
   1. **Diagnosis**
      a. **Cultures** on supplemented Mueller-Hinton agar should be obtained.
      b. **Tissue examination.** Dieterle staining can be used to detect bacteria in tissue. Positive direct FA examination of tissue strongly suggests legionnaires' disease. PCR assay is available as a research tool.
      c. **Serology.** Antibody titers do not help early in the disease course.
   2. **Management**
      a. **Erythromycin**, 1 gm IV q6h, should be given for three weeks. Newer macrolides, such as clarithromycin and azithromycin, and several quinolones have efficacy.
      b. **Rifampin**, 300 to 600 mg/day PO, is effective as an alternative and can be added if the patient does not respond to erythromycin.

E. **Salmonella.** Malnutrition, malignancy, gastrectomy, necrotic or ischemic tumor masses, and corticosteroid therapy predispose patients to infection with *Salmonella* species. Salmonella enterocolitis, bacteremia, enteric fever, and localized infection are the predominant infections in patients with neoplastic disease.
   1. **Diagnosis.** Culture is done on selective media. Serology is of minimal value.
   2. **Management.** Ampicillin, 100 mg/kg/day PO, or chloramphenicol, 50 mg/kg/day PO in four divided doses for two weeks is most often used. Osteomyelitis, endocarditis, or deep-seated abscesses may take four to six weeks of therapy. Trimethoprim-sulfamethoxazole (Bactrim) should be used for resistant strains. Abscess formation necessitates surgical drainage.

VI. **Fungi**
A. **Cryptococcosis.** Patients receiving corticosteroids and those with sarcoidosis or Hodgkin's disease have the highest incidence of infection with *Cryptococcus neoformans*. About one-third of these patients show anergy to cryptococcal skin antigens.
   1. **Clinical presentation.** Pulmonary infection can be asymptomatic. Chest film reveals local bronchopneumonia, lobar involvement, or discrete nodules that may cavitate. CNS infection usually presents as insidious meningoencephalitis. The onset can be rapid in immunosuppressed patients.
   2. **Diagnosis**
      a. **Culture.** *C. neoformans* is an encapsulated, yeastlike fungus that replicates by budding; pseudomycelia are not produced. Sputum culture on Sabouraud's agar that reveals cryptococci in an immunocompromised host must be regarded with alarm. The normal population can harbor this organism without symptoms, however.
      b. **CSF** reveals an elevated opening pressure and lymphocytic pleocytosis in cryptococcal meningoencephalitis. A low glucose concentration is found in 50 percent of cases. India ink preparation is positive in only

one-third of patients. Centrifugation of spinal fluid may reveal the organisms. PCR assays for cryptococcal disease appear promising.

c. Serology. The presence of cryptococcal polysaccharide antigen in spinal fluid or blood is key to the diagnosis (detection in 90% of cases of meningitis). Antibody assays are less useful because cryptococcal antibodies are prevalent in the uninfected population. Skin tests are not useful. Low serum cholinesterase and elevated serum BUN are useful surrogate markers that predict high mortality occurring within two weeks after fungaemia.

3. Management

a. Pulmonary disease. Uncomplicated pulmonary disease usually does not need to be treated. Patients with pulmonary infections who are immunocompromised must be treated with agents such as fluconazole or itraconazole (see **F.1**). If these fail, amphotericin B with flucytosine should be tried (see **F.2**). Salvage therapy with a combination of imipenem, cotrimoxazole, and a prolonged course of itraconazole has also proven acceptable.

b. Meningitis or disseminated disease is treated with fluconazole at a dose of 400 mg per day either PO or IV as long as creatinine clearance is normal. The combination of a reduced dose of amphotericin B plus flucytosine for about six weeks is a second-line regimen (see **F.2**). Intrathecal amphotericin B (see **F.3.c**) is indicated only as a salvage therapy when fluconazole has failed. Failures of any regimen are associated with depressed spinal fluid glucose, extremely abundant cryptococci in the spinal fluid, CNS obstruction, or poor renal function.

B. Candidiasis. The major risk factors for systemic candidiasis include immunosuppressives, antibiotics, glucocorticoids, or hyperalimentation therapy. Indwelling catheters, intravenous drug abuse, and underlying diseases that produce defects in polymorphonuclear neutrophil function or cell-mediated immunity (e.g., leukemia, lymphoma, diabetes mellitus) also are associated with this infection.

1. Clinical presentation. Localized candidiasis can involve the skin, mouth, esophagus, rectum, or vagina. Disseminated candidiasis can present with fever alone, sepsis, endophthalmitis, skin nodules, renal disease, arthritis, or myositis. *Candida albicans* and *C. tropicalis* show discrete, yellow-white retinal lesions.

2. Diagnosis

a. Cultures. Finding hyphae in the urine is more suggestive of infection than finding blastospores or positive culture, but positive blood culture is far more important. Although *Candida* grow well in routine, biphasic, and Sabouraud's agar, they may not produce turbidity in liquid media because they sink to the bottom (the laboratory should be informed when this pathogen is suspected).

b. Serology. Agglutinins are usually not helpful. Precipitins, which do not appear until 10 to 14 days after infection, suggest candidal infection when titers exceed 1:8.

c. Esophagogram shows a typical shaggy, moth-eaten appearance in cases of esophageal candidiasis.

3. Management. Infected foreign bodies, such as prosthetic valves or indwelling catheters, must be promptly removed.

a. Local therapy. Nystatin is used either as an ointment or in liquid suspension (100,000 U/ml). Oral candidiasis is treated with 500,000 to 2,000,000 units every four to six hours. If this fails, clotrimazole (Mycelex troches), five times daily, or ketoconazole, 200 to 400 mg once daily, should be used.

b. Prophylaxis. Fluconazole, 200 mg PO once daily or 200 mg IV every 24 hours, can be used for prophylaxis in patients in whom chemotherapy is initiated and neutropenia is anticipated. Prophylactic fluconazole prevents colonization and superficial infections by *Candida* species other than *C. krusei*. This agent is used until recovery of the neutrophil count, development of proven or suspected invasive fungal infection, or the occurrence of a drug-related toxicity.

   c. Systemic therapy (see also sec. **F**)

     (1) Fluconazole also remains the first-line therapy in invasive candidiasis for most species other than *C. krusei*.

     (2) Amphotericin B (20 mg/day IV for two weeks) is recommended only as a second-line therapy for most adult patients with single organ involvement or candidemia. In severe disease, doses up to 50 mg/day IV should be given for six to ten weeks or until a total dose of 1.5 to 2.0 gm is reached.

     (3) Flucytosine, effective in 80 percent of patients, can be used in conjunction with amphotericin when the disease is severe, particularly with CNS infection (see sec. **F.3** for dose). This regimen is a salvage attempt.

C. Aspergillosis. The typical presentation for aspergillosis in immunosuppressed patients is fever and pulmonary infiltrates, often with infarction, hemoptysis, and gangrene from vascular invasion. Nearly one-third of patients have no radiologic abnormalities early in the disease. Dissemination complicates pulmonary disease in 25 to 50 percent of cases. Various skin lesions, multiple abscesses, brain infarction, or GI ulceration with hemorrhage can result.

Aspergillosis is the second most frequent fungal infection that affects the face and mouth of patients receiving chemotherapy. In these patients bone marrow recovery or the use of CSFs may lead to the liquefaction of pulmonary foci. Potentially lethal erosion bleeding may then occur because of the vasotropic nature of the infection.

   1. Diagnosis. Sputum examination showing septate, acutely branching organisms is highly suggestive of aspergillosis. This finding represents a serious problem in immunosuppressed patients. Methenamine silver stains of lung tissue are usually diagnostic. The value of serologic tests is unproved.

   2. Management

     a. Antifungal treatment should include the combination of amphotericin B and flucytosine during periods of granulocytopenia, followed by itraconazole after bone marrow recovery (see **F** for dosages). Itraconazole appears to contribute significantly to therapy, but the drug is not effective during granulocytopenic episodes. Liposomal amphotericin B is a promising drug for this disease.

     b. Fluconazole may obscure the onset of aspergillosis. When aspergillosis is seriously suspected, fluconazole should be given neither prophylactically nor for fever of unknown origin.

     c. Surgical resection of localized invasive pulmonary aspergillosis with a cavitating lesion may prevent hemoptysis and recurrence in selected patients. In leukemic patients the achievement of complete remission combined with aggressive antifungal therapy leads to markedly increased cure of aspergillosis. The combination of a fibrinolytic agent and an antifungal drug may be considered for intractable aspergillus infections, because these organisms are angioinvasive.

D. Zygomycosis. Zygomycetes infection has been recognized with increasing frequency in patients who have leukemia or lymphoma (but not solid tumors). Infections caused by *Cunninghamella bertholetiae* (a fungus of the Zygomycetes class, Mucorales order) are being identified with increasing frequency in immunocompromised patients, including patients undergoing chemotherapy. Other predisposing factors include acidosis, uremia, immunoincompetence, glucocorticoid therapy, diabetes mellitus, malnutrition, and burns.

   1. Manifestations. The genera *Rhizopus, Absidia,* and *Mucor* produce similar pathologic and clinical manifestations because of neutrophil exudation, tissue necrosis, and vascular invasion (resulting in thrombosis and infarction).

     a. Pneumonia can be associated with a dry cough or hemoptysis. X-ray films may show interstitial infiltrates, lobar consolidation, or cavitation.

b. Cerebral disease is usually secondary to pulmonary involvement. Coma and focal neurologic signs represent brain infarcts or abscesses. Spinal fluid studies are not usually helpful. **Rhinocerebral disease** occurs most frequently in uncontrolled diabetes mellitus. Manifestations include bloody nasal discharge, orbital infection, periorbital and perinasal swelling, ptosis, proptosis, loss of vision, trigeminal anesthesia with ophthalmoplegia, facial pain, and facial nerve palsy.

c. Disseminated disease can result in gastroenteritis, bowel perforation or hemorrhage, peritonitis, or abscess in any organ.

2. Diagnosis. Zygomycetes organisms have broad, nonseptate hyphae in tissue specimens and, in culture media, mycelia with hyphae and sporangia. Diagnosis is made by demonstrating the organism by culture or hematoxylin-eosin, periodic acid–Schiff, or methenamine silver stains of preparations.

3. Management. Early diagnosis is paramount. Amphotericin B or its liposomal form is the drug of choice (see sec. **F**). Mortality remains high.

E. Diagnosis of other systemic mycoses

1. *Histoplasma capsulatum, Coccidioides immitis,* and *Blastomyces dermatitidis* have diagnostic culture results and histopathologies. These common human pathogens can also present as opportunistic infections in patients who are immunocompromised. Dissemination is often associated with cutaneous anergy.

2. *Trichosporon beigelii* causes white piedra and an emerging opportunistic mycosis that is frequently difficult to diagnose. This mycosis is associated with a high attributable mortality. Systemic infection has been most frequently described in neutropenic patients receiving chemotherapy.

a. Cutaneous involvement occurs in approximately 30 percent of patients and frequently presents as purpuric papules and nodules with central necrosis or ulceration. Biopsy specimens of these lesions reveal dermal invasion by fungal elements. Culture is positive in greater than 90 percent of the cases. Antigen detection in the blood is an early manifestation of disseminated *Trichosporon* infection.

b. The antifungal triazoles, fluconazole and SCH 39304, are most active. Amphotericin B and liposomal amphotericin B appear to be ineffective.

3. *Hansenula anomala* is rarely pathogenic, but this infection has occurred in patients with small cell lung cancer. Fluconazole treatment appears to be effective.

4. *Pseudoallescheria boydii,* an uncommon cause of infection, may cause CNS disease and positive blood cultures in patients with leukemia. Although infections are usually resistant to amphotericin B, they may respond to itraconazole.

5. Fusariosis. Members of the genus *Fusarium* are ubiquitous fungi uncommonly associated with infection. Disseminated fusariosis typically occurs in neutropenic patients, carries a high mortality rate, and presents with fever and diffuse cutaneous maculopapular necrotizing nodules. *F. verticilloides* can be isolated from culturing the biopsy of skin lesions (hyphae are often observed on direct microscopy) or bronchial aspirates of lung lesions. Liposomal amphotericin B (see **F.3.b**) for three to six weeks may eradicate this infection, although amphotericin B by itself seems ineffective.

6. Alternariosis, another uncommon fungal infection resembling aspergillosis, has been described in both immunocompromised and immunocompetent hosts. Cutaneous alternariosis can occur during neutropenia in bone marrow transplant patients who are receiving antifungal prophylaxis with fluconazole. Therapy requires surgical excision and amphotericin B.

7. Fungemic shock. As the use of empiric antibiotics or prophylaxis for bacteria has increased, organisms such as *C. albicans, Aspergillus niger, F. so-*

lani, and *Acremonium strictum* have been implicated in septic shock occurring in immunocompromised patients.

8. **Radiation port dermatophytosis** is an uncommon condition in which patients receiving RT concurrently have tinea corporis confined primarily to the irradiated skin. Because the cutaneous manifestations may be misinterpreted clinically as acute radiation-induced dermatitis, this condition may be more prevalent than reports suggest.

F. **Therapy of systemic fungal infections**

1. **Fluconazole and itraconazole** have become the primary antifungal agents used in systemic infections. These agents are far safer than amphotericin B and have excellent efficacy.

   a. **Administration.** Because of their safety, these azole agents can be used with little monitoring. Creatinine clearance and liver function dictate significant changes in dosage. Fluconazole can be given up to 400 mg PO or IV b.i.d. Itraconazole can be given at a dose of 100 to 600 mg PO daily depending on the infection.

   b. **Toxicity.** Fluconazole can be associated with GI disturbances and headache. Severe but unusual sequelae are exfoliative skin disorders, thrombocytopenia, and hepatotoxicity. Itraconazole also is mildly toxic, but unlike fluconazole it has no effect on concomitantly administered warfarin, cyclosporin A, or insulin.

2. **Flucytosine** is useful only in combination with amphotericin B for treating *Cryptococcus, Candida,* and other fungi. The drug penetrates the spinal fluid well (thereby having an advantage in CNS infections) and is excreted primarily by the kidneys.

   a. **Dosage** is 150 mg/kg/day PO in four divided doses, adjusted to maintain a serum level of 50 to 75 μg/ml. When the two drugs are given in combination, the dose of amphotericin B is reduced to 0.3 to 0.5 mg/kg/day, and the dose of flucytosine is decreased to 100 mg/day.

   b. **Toxicity.** Granulocytopenia, thrombocytopenia, and elevation of serum levels of hepatic enzymes and creatinine are common side effects. CNS and GI disturbances occur less frequently.

   c. **Dosage modification.** Dosages must be reduced with leukopenia, thrombocytopenia, or deterioration of renal function. (Note: Amphotericin B frequently results in decreased renal function; therefore, toxic levels of flucytosine occur when amphotericin B and flucytosine are used simultaneously.)

3. **Amphotericin B** (and its promising congener liposomal amphotericin B) remains the choice for specific deep-seated or systemic fungal infections or for fluconazole or itraconazole failures. Initially, a test dose of 1 to 5 mg is given. Diphenhydramine (Benadryl), 50 mg PO, is given before the infusion. Hydrocortisone sodium succinate, 25 to 50 mg, and aqueous heparin, 100 units, are added to the amphotericin infusion bottle.

   a. **Dosage.** A dose of 20 mg in 250 ml of 5% dextrose in water is infused over 30 minutes the day after the test dose is given. The dose is slowly raised in 5-mg increments until a maximum of 1.0 mg/kg/day is reached. Usually no more than 50 to 60 mg/day is given. Most deep-seated fungal infections necessitate 2.0 to 3.0 gm of amphotericin when used alone or 1.5 to 2.0 gm when used with flucytosine.

   b. **Liposomal amphotericin B** (AmBisome) is given at a dose of 3 mg/kg/day.

   c. **Intrathecal amphotericin** doses for CNS fungal infections begin at 0.025 mg; the daily dose does not exceed 0.50 mg. The drug is administered every two to seven days either into a reservoir (e.g., Ommaya valve), cisterna, or ventricle, or by LP using a hypertonic technique.

   d. **Toxicity.** Side effects include fever, chills, hypotension, nausea, vomiting, and azotemia. Permanent reduction of glomerular filtration, renal tubular acidosis, phlebitis, anemia, and headache are frequent complications. Serum creatinine and potassium levels are measured daily.

VII. Parasites

A. Toxoplasmosis. The incidence of asymptomatic disease is based on serology ranges from 10 to 40 percent in the United States to 96 percent in western Europe. Of those patients with AIDS who are seropositive for *Toxoplasma gondii,* approximately 25 to 50 percent develop toxoplasmic encephalitis.

Individuals with symptomatic disease present with a low-grade febrile illness characterized by localized or generalized lymphadenopathy, hepatosplenomegaly, malaise, and fatigue. Any organ may become involved. Infection in patients with abnormal cellular immunity may mimic brain tumor or lymphoproliferative disorder.

1. Diagnosis

    a. Histology. Identification of trophozoites rather than cysts is important because cysts can persist for decades. Lymph node pathology is very characteristic of toxoplasmosis.

    b. Culture is rarely used.

    c. Serology usually establishes the diagnosis. IgM and CF antibodies are useful for the diagnosis of early infection. Titers of both assays decrease after six to twelve months. Indirect FA titers are also useful. Sensitive ELISA antibody sandwiches and the use of PCR for *Toxoplasma* DNA have helped differentiate inactive old disease from acute infection.

2. Management. Pyrimethamine (a folic acid antagonist) plus a sulfa derivative are given in divided doses for one month. The development of hematologic toxicity often interrupts treatment.

    a. Pyrimethamine is given with a loading dose of 100 to 200 mg PO followed by maintenance of 50 mg/day. Folinic acid, 5 mg/day, is required when 100 mg/day or more is given.

    b. Sulfadiazine is given with a loading dose of 50 to 75 mg/kg followed by maintenance of 75 to 100 mg/kg/day (1 gm PO q.i.d.).

    c. Other combination therapies for acute disease

        (1) Pyrimethamine (100 mg/day PO) plus clindamycin (1.2 gm/daily IV in divided doses)

        (2) 5-Fluorouracil (1.5 mg/kg/day) and clindamycin, (1.8 to 2.4 gm daily) for treatment of cerebral toxoplasmosis, which may provide a less toxic option

B. Pneumocystis. *Pneumocystis carinii* causes pneumonia in immunodeficient patients, including those with AIDS. Children (in remission) with acute lymphocytic leukemia and patients in whom corticosteroid therapy is being tapered are particularly susceptible to infection.

Manifestations include dyspnea, fever, nonproductive cough, pulmonary rales, hypoxemia, and hypocapnia. Chest x-ray early in the disease may appear benign, while blood gases often demonstrate major hypoxia and gallium scans light up the entire lung. Chest films more typically show diffuse symmetric, bilateral, perihilar infiltrates that spread rapidly. Nodules or cavities develop infrequently.

1. Diagnosis. Methenamine silver and Gram-Weigert's methods stain cyst walls. Giemsa stains sporozoites within the cyst wall but not the wall. Sputum specimens are diagnostic in 10 to 15 percent of cases, bronchoscopic brushings in 65 to 75 percent, and open lung biopsy in 90 percent. Monoclonal antibody assays for *P. carinii* may speed diagnosis and improve follow-up of this infection. In patients who are critically ill or severely thrombocytopenic, lung biopsy should be deferred. Less invasive procedures or possibly empiric trial of therapy should be done, because the biopsy procedure has high morbidity and mortality.

2. Management. In patients with any respiratory difficulties associated with their pneumonia, any therapy for active disease should be used in conjunction with a short, rapidly tapering course of corticosteroids. Treatment is given for 14 to 21 days, and options include:

    a. Bactrim, two double-strength tablets PO or two ampules IV every six to eight hours

   b. Pentamidine, 4 mg/kg IM daily
   c. Mepron may be useful in patients who are intolerant of trimethoprim-sulfamethoxazole (Bactrim).
   d. Trimetrexate in combination with leucovorin appears to be extremely effective even when other regimens have failed.
C. Strongyloidiasis. Humans are infected by both filariform larvae and adult forms, resulting in self-perpetuating autoinfection. Defective cell-mediated immunity, high-dose corticosteroid therapy, and decreased bowel motility enhance the chance of massive GI tract, pulmonary, or CNS infection.
   1. Diagnosis. Larvae can be recovered from the stool in 25 to 60 percent of patients and from duodenal aspirates in 40 to 90 percent. Peripheral eosinophilia is typical but may be absent in the hyperinfected state.
   2. Management. Thiabendazole, 1.5 gm PO b.i.d. for two to four days.
D. Other parasites
   1. _Giardia lamblia_ infection is associated with hypogammaglobulinemia, small bowel lymphoma, and pancreatic carcinoma. Manifestations include diarrhea, nausea, flatulence, and cramps.
   2. Malaria and babesiosis may hyperinfect immunosuppressed hosts, especially after splenectomy. Infection results in high fever and hemolysis.
   3. Cestodes can disseminate in patients with Hodgkin's disease. Invasion of blood vessels and deep organs produces severe symptoms.
      a. Cysticercosis is the systemic infection with eggs of _Taenia solium_. It most frequently presents with brain masses (often with calcified rims on radiographic studies). Craniotomy is necessary for both definitive diagnosis and therapy.
      b. Echinococcosis can present as a space-occupying lesion in several visceral organs. Diagnosis is established by serologic tests and evidence of the organism by histopathology.

Selected Reading

Cohen, P. R., et al. Tinea corporis confined to irradiated skin. Radiation port dermatophytosis. _Cancer_ 70:1634, 1992.

Dreizen, S., et al. Orofacial fungal infections. Nine pathogens that may invade during chemotherapy. _Postgrad. Med._ 91:349, 1992.

Katsikis, P., et al. Antilipid a monoclonal antibody HA-1A: immune complex clearance of endotoxin reduces TNF-alpha, IL-1 beta and IL-6 production. _Cytokine_ 5: 348, 1993.

Martino, P., et al. Fungemia in patients with leukemia. _Am. J. Med. Sci._ 306:225, 1993.

Moreau, P., et al. Localized invasive pulmonary aspergillosis in patients with neutropenia. Effectiveness of surgical resection. _Cancer_ 72:3223, 1993.

Pizzo, P. A. Approach to the patient with prolonged granulocytopenia. Recent results. _Cancer Res._ 132:57, 1993.

Silber, J. L., et al. Fluconazole prophylaxis of fungal infections in patients with acute leukemia. Results of a randomized placebo-controlled, double-blind, multicenter trial. _Ann. Intern. Med._ 118:495, 1993.

Van der Auwera, P., et al. Use of the quinolones in the prophylaxis and treatment of granulocytopenic immunocompromised cancer patients. _Drugs_ 45 (Suppl. 3):81, 1993.

Waage, A., et al. Cytokine mediators of septic infections in the normal and granulocytopenic host. _Eur. J. Haematol._ 50:243, 1993.

Walsh, T. J., et al. Recent progress and current problems in management of invasive fungal infections in patients with neoplastic diseases. _Curr. Opin. Oncol._ 4:647, 1992.

36 Acquired Immunodeficiency Syndrome (AIDS)

Jeffrey E. Galpin and
Dennis A. Casciato

I. Epidemiology and etiology

A. Epidemiology. AIDS is caused by the human immunodeficiency virus (HIV), which is transmitted sexually or by blood components. More than 300,000 cases of AIDS were reported to the Centers for Disease Control and Prevention (CDC) in the United States by 1994. This reported incidence probably represents only 10 to 15 percent of all HIV-1 infected individuals. Worldwide, AIDS may affect 30,000,000 people by the year 2000.

The disease is a pandemic affecting mainly heterosexually active individuals and their offspring, but also attacking intravenous drug users, homosexual men, and recipients of blood products. Homosexual men still account for the majority of AIDS cases in many industrialized countries, but heterosexual acquisition in these countries is steadily growing.

B. Transmission

1. **Sexual transmission.** Unprotected receptive anal intercourse is still thought to be the most efficient mode of sexual transmission for HIV. Heterosexual intercourse probably has a 1 percent chance of transmission per single act. A history of other sexually transmitted diseases triples the odds. The presence of genital ulcers in either sexual partner increases the relative risk of acquiring HIV nearly fivefold.

2. **Blood transfusion.** Nearly all recipients of blood contaminated by HIV become infected. For the general population, the risk of contracting AIDS through transfusion of blood is approximately 1:100,000 per unit of blood. Previously, transfusion of hemophilic factors VIII and IX almost guaranteed transmission of HIV. Current methods of factor preparation, however, have rendered these blood products noninfective for HIV. Albumin, plasminate, and gamma globulin preparations have not been shown to transmit HIV.

3. **Contaminated injection equipment** is the major cause of spreading the epidemic in intravenous drug users worldwide. The risk of acquiring disease through a single contaminated needle stick is approximately 33 percent for HBV compared with less than 1 percent for HIV.

4. **Pregnancy.** Estimates of the transmission frequency from HIV-infected mothers to their children range from 10 to 40 percent. When women have severe immunosuppressive disease, a higher incidence of stillbirth and prematurity is observed. The use of zidovudine dramatically reduces this frequency.

5. **Exposed groups.** No cases of AIDS have occurred in family members of patients with AIDS unless the members had other recognized risk-related behavior (e.g., sharing needles, sexual contact). Few well-defined cases of the development of AIDS in health care workers is the same as in the general population and far less than the risk of death from viral hepatitis caused by needle sticks.

6. **Other methods of transmission.** Low concentrations of HIV have been found in tears and saliva in less than 2 percent of patients with severe AIDS. Viral inhibitors are present in saliva. Tears and aerosols from the lungs do not appear to transmit AIDS.

C. Virology. HIV is a double-stranded RNA virus.

    1. Lentiviruses. AIDS is caused by HIV-1 or HIV-2 lentiviruses, which are retroviruses, because they contain a reverse transcriptase. This transcriptase enables transcription of RNA to DNA.

        a. The remarkable complexity of their viral genomes distinguishes the lentiviruses from other retroviruses. Most retroviruses that are capable of replication contain only three genes: *gag, pol,* and *env.* The *gag* and *env* genes encode the core nucleocapsid polypeptides and surface-coat proteins of the virus, respectively, whereas the *pol* gene gives rise to the viral reverse transcriptase and other enzymatic activities.

        b. HIV-1, however, contains in its nine-kilobase RNA genome not only these three essential genes, but also at least six additional genes: *tat, rev, nef, vif, vpu,* and *vpr.* HIV-2, which is more closely related to simian immunodeficiency viruses than to HIV-1, contains a unique regulatory gene, *vpx.*

    2. HIV is lymphotropic in humans and binds to cells with the CD4 or CD26 antigen on their surfaces. This antigen is found primarily on T lymphocyte-helper cells, but is also present on certain monocytes and macrophages in the GI tract and CNS. HIV is found in high concentration in the follicular dendritic cells of lymph nodes, a critical reservoir for this virus.

        a. In order for the host to recognize HIV and kill infected cells, specific cytotoxic CD8 killer lymphocytes must be activated through close association with antigen-presenting cells such as monocytes and macrophages. This interaction requires CD20, CD28, and CD80 receptors.

        b. A superantigen (SAg), also termed "Vβ-selective element," appears to be associated with HIV-1. Such a SAg could activate targeted T cells for optimal viral replication and viral reservoir establishment during the early stages of infection. Alternatively, SAg could participate in the induction of selective cell death (apoptosis) in the T cell subpopulation targeted by the SAg.

    3. Regulating proteins. HIV produces an early transactivating regulating protein (Tat) as well as an RNA-splicing regulating protein (Rev). Tat increases the level of transcripts derived from the long-terminal repeat (LTR) of HIV-1. Rev interacts with RRE (Rev-responsive element). The Rev-RRE interaction allows unspliced messages to create long RNA transcripts needed for structural proteins. Membrane proteins include gp41 and gp120, and Gag proteins include p17 and p24. Late regulatory proteins include Nef, Vif, Vpu, and an accessory protein, Vpr.

    4. Virus replication

        a. Although HIV may be clinically inapparent for many years after its acquisition, the virus is always replicating. The clinical course of HIV has no real latent periods but rather clinical plateaus with continued viral activity. Using PCRs on either viral RNA or DNA, continuous viral activity has been confirmed.

        b. Early in the asymptomatic period of disease the virus is less infective and less virulent. Late in the clinically symptomatic period, HIV becomes highly infective and replicative. These two phases seem to correlate with the virus either not inducing syncytia (early), or inducing syncytia (late).

    5. Virus evolution. HIV appears to evolve as the disease progresses not only from host to host, but also within the single host. The viral phenotypic evolution is closely related to changes in the V3 loop of the envelope protein gp120.

II. Diagnosis

  A. Clinical presentation

    1. HIV-1 can present acutely as a primary lymphocytic pneumonia or a mononucleosislike syndrome. The infection may also be initially asymptomatic; only many years later do the effects of immune dysfunction emerge. These later clinical scenarios can include night sweats, recurrent sinusitis, pro-

Table 36-1. The 1993 classification system for HIV disease

CD4⁺ T lymphocyte counts	Categories		
	A	B	C
1: > 500 cells/μL	A1	B1	C1
2: 200–500 cells/μL	A2	B2	C2
3: < 200 cells/μL	A3	B3	C3

Category A consists of one or more of the following conditions:
Asymptomatic HIV infection
Acute retroviral syndrome
Persistent generalized lymphadenopathy

Category B consists of conditions formerly classified as AIDS-related complex (ARC):
Bacillary angiomatosis
Candidiasis, oropharyngeal or recurrent vulvovaginal
Cervical dysplasia
Constitutional symptoms for longer than 1 month (e.g., fever or diarrhea)
Hairy leukoplakia, oral
Herpes zoster involving more than one dermatome
Idiopathic thrombocytopenia purpura
Listeriosis
Pelvic inflammatory disease
Peripheral neuropathy

Category C consists of AIDS-defining conditions:
CD4 count less than 200/μL
Candidiasis, esophageal or pulmonary
Cervical cancer
Coccidioidomycosis
Cryptococcosis, extrapulmonary
Cryptosporidiosis
Cytomegalovirus disease, active
Encephalopathy
Herpes simplex: chronic ulcer(s) (>1 month's duration); or, bronchitis, pneumonitis, or esophagitis
Histoplasmosis
Isosporiasis, chronic intestinal
Kaposi's sarcoma
Lymphoma: Burkitt's, immunoblastic, or primary brain (or equivalent)
Mycobacterium avium complex, *M. kansasii,* or other *Mycobacterium* species: disseminated or extrapulmonary
Mycobacterium tuberculosis, any site
Pneumocystis carinii pneumonia
Pneumonia, recurrent
Progressive multifocal leukoencephalopathy
Salmonella septicemia, recurrent
Toxoplasmosis of brain
Wasting syndrome due to HIV

gressive skin lesions (such as psoriasis, folliculitis, bacillary angiomatosis, or seborrheic dermatitis), or entities listed in Table 36-1. Often HIV becomes evident only when an AIDS-defining event occurs (see Category C in Table 36-1).

   2. HIV-2 Clinically, HIV-2 appears to progress more slowly and produce milder immune dysfunction than HIV-1. HIV-2 is particularly associated with CNS disease, such as spastic paraparesis, as well as with chronic diarrhea, thrush, and tuberculosis.

B. Diagnostic tests. Patients with any significant risk of exposure to HIV should be evaluated for its presence. Screening must remain confidential and be used only for evaluation for therapy and control of further transmission.

1. **HIV antibody assays.** The most commercially available method of screening for HIV is the enzyme immunoassay systems. The antibody becomes positive from one to three months after exposure to HIV. Very rarely, the serum can be antibody-negative while it is antigen-positive—as long as 12 to 18 months after the virus is acquired. The false-negative rate is approximately 3 percent when only antibody assays are used. The false-positive rate is only 0.2 percent in high-risk groups but much higher in low-risk groups.

2. **Western blot** is the confirmatory test for HIV antibodies. HIV proteins are separated electrophoretically and stained on film, which is then reacted against the test serum.

3. **HIV antigen assay** (such as p24 antigen) can be used to define the presence and activity of infection and to follow the course of therapy.

4. **Cellular assays.** Determination of the percentage and absolute number of CD4 lymphocytes remains the standard for measuring the immunologic progression of HIV infection. However, assays of CD8 killer cells or cytotoxic T cells may better indicate the viability of the host's immune system.

5. **Other supportive assays**

   a. Polyclonal B lymphocyte proliferation and decreased B lymphocyte response to mitogens are common with HIV infection. Increased levels of gamma globulin, β2-microglobulin, and neopterin are frequently observed.

   b. The so-called TH1-type and TH2-type responses contribute to the immune dysregulation associated with HIV infection. Many seronegative, HIV-exposed individuals generate strong TH1-type responses to HIV antigens. Resistance to HIV infection or progression to AIDS may depend on maintaining dominance by TH1-type responses.

      (1) Asymptomatic patients and those with early disease have increased levels of IL-2 and γ-IFN with low expression of IL-4 and IL-10 (Th1-type response).

      (2) Progression to AIDS is characterized by loss of production of IL-2 and γ-IFN concomitant with increases in levels of IL-4 and IL-10 (TH2-type response).

III. **Classification.** The 1993 revised CDC classification system for syndromes associated with HIV infection (categories A, B, and C) emphasizes the clinical importance of the CD4$^+$ T lymphocyte count (categories 1, 2, and 3). This classification system is shown in Table 36-1. Categories that define the presence of AIDS are A3, B3, C1, C2, and C3. Primarily used for public health practice, this system attempts to reflect the current standards of medical care for HIV-infected persons.

IV. **Treatment of HIV**

A. **Overview.** Early treatment of HIV infection with safe therapeutics while monitoring for progression of disease is mandated today. Prophylaxis against opportunistic infections as immunity reaches critical levels of decay should be provided. The current goal is making HIV infection a long-term, chronic disease that permits quality life for decades. The best way to target HIV involves the combined use of two agents: (1) antiretroviral agents, which attack the virus at different assembly sites, and (2) immune modulators, which specifically stimulate host immunity to kill HIV in its cellular home.

B. **Reverse transcriptase inhibitors** (RTIs) often become ineffective because of mutational emergence within 6 to 18 months. A second agent is often added after 4 to 6 months of therapy. The use of multiple drugs results in additive toxicity, however.

1. **Zidovudine** (AZT, azidothymidine, Retrovir) is a thymidine analogue that inhibits HIV replication by competing with HIV reverse transcriptase and causing premature termination of DNA. Although AZT does not eliminate HIV or cure AIDS, treated patients appear to have longer, better quality survival. AZT therapy is associated with increased weight, decreased neuropsychologic effects of the disease, decreased viral load by PCR, decreased maternal transmission of the virus to fetuses, and, in many cases, reduced p24 antigenemia.

   a. **Dosage** (100-mg capsules) is usually 300 to 500 mg/day PO in divided doses. Intravenous and pediatric liquid forms are available. AZT should be started whenever the CD4 count falls below $500/\mu L$. AZT should be continued as long as CD4 counts and other laboratory and clinical markers of disease progression remain stable, which could be as short as four months or as long as three years.

  b. Toxicity includes headaches, vertigo, insomnia, myalgias, nausea, peripheral neuropathy, bone marrow suppression (agranulocytosis and megaloblastic anemia), and decreased vitamin B_{12} concentration. Toxicity is often more severe when AZT is used in later stages of AIDS.

2. Dideoxycytidine (ddC) is a nucleoside analogue AZT. Dosage is usually 0.375 mg PO t.i.d. Toxicity involves reversible peripheral neuropathy and aphthous stomatitis.

3. Didanosine (ddI, dideoxyinosine) is a purine dideoxynucleoside which is derived from an inactive pro-drug (dideoxyadenosine, ddA) by a ubiquitous enzyme, adenosine deaminase. Dosage is 400 to 600 mg/day in the form of a buffered chewable tablet or powder packet. Toxicity is primarily acute pancreatitis. Diarrhea can occur.

4. Other RTIs. D4T and 3TC, which are both nucleoside RTIs, appear to have efficacy against HIV. D4T is approved at a dose of 40 mg PO b.i.d. Nonnucleoside RTIs (NNRTIs), such as U-90 or DMEA, appear promising.

5. Convergent combination therapy directs several drugs against the viral reverse transcriptase enzyme. The initial approach combined two nucleoside RTIs with a NNRTI. Mutational resistance and additive toxicities continue to be problems. The combination of 3TC plus AZT has demonstrated synergy.

6. Hydroxyurea, an antitumor antimetabolite, may decrease HIV viral load by reducing viral substrate.

C. Investigational therapies

1. Protease inhibitors. Structural proteins (i.e., *gag* and *pol* products) are derived from unspliced mRNA. The synthesized precursor Gag-Pol fusion polyprotein is cleaved by HIV protease to yield mature gene products. The Gag precursor is cleaved into viral capsid proteins [p17 (matrix), p24 (capsid), p7 (nucleocapsid), and p6]. The Pol precursor is cleaved into the individual replication enzymes [protease, RT, and integrase]. Protease inhibitors inhibit cleavage into final proteins and prevent such mature gene products from being assembled.

2. Tat and Rev protein inhibitors. Regulatory proteins, such as the Tat and Rev proteins, are derived from multiply spliced mRNA, which permits formation of necessarily longer transcripts. Long-terminal repeating gene (LTR), which facilitates transcription of viral elements, exists at either end of HIV-1 RNA strands.

  The Tat protein is essential for efficient expression by the LTR of HIV, and the Rev protein is necessary for efficient expression of full-length and singly spliced transcripts. Tat mediates its effect by interacting with a segment of the R region in the 5J LTR, which is termed the "TAR" element (for "trans-activating response"). Rev mediates its effect by interacting with a segment of RNA, or the RRE (for "Rev-responsive element"). Clinical trials have begun with both Tat and Rev inhibitors, which should prevent the transcription of the virus.

3. Gene product therapy. A murine retroviral vector has been used to introduce the HIV envelope and *rev* genes into fibroblasts, attempting to stimulate a more effective cellular immune response against HIV. This treatment theoretically could result in the killing of HIV-infected cells that express the viral envelope glycoprotein and *rev* products. It is being tested in clinical trials.

4. Autologous CD8-positive cytotoxic T lymphocytes that are expanded in vitro, stimulated with IL-2, and reinfused in the HIV-positive individual are being studied in an attempt to increase cytotoxic T cell response to HIV infection.

5. Passive immunotherapy and HIV immune globulin from humans or pigs may prevent maternal-fetal transmission of HIV or be used as primary therapy to stabilize HIV disease. Nonspecific intravenous gamma globulin seems to control certain opportunistic infections, chronic sinusitis, and the specific peripheral neuropathy of HIV disease.

6. **Antisense oligonucleotide therapy** targets the regulatory genes of HIV by providing abnormal oligomers for the virus. Antisense RNA ("complementary RNA") refers to an RNA strand that has the opposite polarity from mRNA and can therefore hybridize to the corresponding mRNA. The longer antisense RNA molecules inhibit mRNA processing or translation and do not affect transcription. Inhibition of virus replication can be achieved without affecting the expression of host genes. A considerable disadvantage of these modified nucleotides is that sequence specificity may be lost. PolyTAR antisense oligodeoxyribonucleotide to HIV for the inhibition of viral replication is being investigated in clinical trials.

7. **Ribozyme therapy.** Ribozymes are catalytic RNA molecules that have recently been cloned into retroviral vectors. These compounds inhibit expression of diverse strains of HIV-1 by transient transfection. Ribozymes theoretically have the potential to cleave messenger RNA molecules continuously. They could cleave HIV either on entering the cell, while being assembled within the cell, or outside the cell. Limiting factors are the abilities to transduce enough cells and to target infected cells.

8. **Cytokine therapy.** Individuals with early HIV disease demonstrate inherent, inducible killer cell cytotoxicity. Late in the disease, inherent cytotoxicity is lost. Reinduction of cytotoxicity may be induced, however, with gene transfer therapy or appropriate cytokines, such as IL-2 or IL-12. Pentoxifylline and dexamethasone suppress the release of TNF, IL-1, and IL-6 and make them interesting research therapies for prevention of HIV-related wasting. IL-12 (or NK cell stimulatory factor) has multiple effects on T and NK cell functions.

9. **BMT** for AIDS is becoming more feasible as better therapies for sterilizing HIV are being developed.

D. **HIV wasting syndrome** affects fat more severely in women and muscle initially in men. High serum levels of triglycerides with low levels of cholesterol are a hallmark of the syndrome.

1. **Pathogenesis.** The underlying causes behind weight loss and negative nitrogen balance in HIV are incompletely understood. Cachectin (endotoxin-stimulated macrophage supernatant) induces severe weight loss in animal models. High levels of IL-1, α-IFN, γ-IFN, and transforming growth factor can cause anorexia and weight loss. Cytokines such as TNF can decrease gastric motility and affect liver metabolism, resulting in high levels of triglycerides. Synergy between cytokines is probably required for significant wasting, which is also magnified by GI disease and malabsorption. Secondary infection appears to trigger the initiation of wasting.

2. **Treatment** involves controlling HIV progression and secondary infection. Megestrol acetate (Megace) and oral marijuana (Marinol) increase appetite, decrease nausea, and can temporize weight loss, if not true wasting. Total parenteral nutrition for more than six weeks probably does not alter the course of wasting. Combination cytokine inhibitors theoretically may block wasting.

V. **Management of opportunistic infections**

A. **Parasites**

1. *Pneumocystis carinii* pneumonia (PCP). The clinical presentation of PCP may be subtle, with gradually increasing dyspnea and nonproductive cough. Patients may present with either a low-grade fever or severe night sweats and high fever. The mortality rate for PCP is 10 to 30 percent for persons who do not require ventilators and as much as 85 percent for persons who do. See sec. **V.F.** for prophylaxis recommendations in patients with HIV. See Chap. 35, sec. **VII.B** for diagnosis and treatment of PCP.

2. **Microsporidiosis and cryptosporidiosis** may produce high mortality in HIV patients with severe immune deficiency who present with severe diar-

rhea, electrolyte imbalances, and wasting. *Enterocytozoon bieneusi* (microsporidia), one of the commonest causes of chronic diarrhea in HIV disease, often occurs with CMV. Affected patients can present with cholangitis, cholecystitis, or kidney dysfunction. Diagnosis of microsporidia requires either electron microscopy or Warthin-Starry stain of punch biopsies of the middle duodenum obtained at endoscopy. Treatment is usually ineffective.

3. **Toxoplasmosis.** Cerebral toxoplasmosis possibly represents the most common CNS opportunistic infection associated with AIDS. Neither the highly variable clinical presentation nor the neuroradiologic imaging (see sec. **E.3**) is pathognomonic.

   a. In patients with AIDS, toxoplasmic encephalitis is almost always a reactivation of a preexisting latent infection, most often occurring when the total CD4 count falls below 100 cells/μL. Toxoplasmosis causes pneumonia, lymphadenopathy, and chorioretinitis outside of the CNS.

   b. Because of its prevalence in the HIV population, many clinicians believe prophylaxis for toxoplasmosis is appropriate. See **V.F** for dosage recommendations for prophylaxis. See Chap. 35, sec. **VII.A.** for diagnosis and treatment of systemic and CNS disease.

B. Bacteria

1. **Mycobacteria.** MAC causes disseminated disease in 15 to 40 percent of patients with HIV infection in the United States. Disseminated MAC typically occurs in patients with advanced disease and peripheral blood $CD4^+$ T lymphocyte counts below 100/μL. Acute disseminated disease is often associated with profound weight loss, anemia, diarrhea, abdominal pain, night sweats, rising serum levels of alkaline phosphatase, intra-abdominal lymphadenopathy, and hepatosplenomegaly. Compared to MAC, patients infected with *Mycobacterium tuberculosis* present with more lung involvement and less blood and lymph node dissemination. See **V.F** for prophylaxis recommendations for MAC. See Chap. 35, sec. **V.A** for diagnosis and treatment of mycobacterial infections.

2. **Pyomyositis** (solitary or multiple pyogenic muscle abscesses) is common in the tropics but rare in temperate climates, where it is associated with recent travel to tropical areas, trauma, diabetes mellitus, neutropenia, and drug use. Nontropical pyomyositis, usually caused by *Staphylococcus aureus,* has been described repeatedly in patients infected with HIV.

   a. Clinically, pyomyositis is characterized by fever and painful muscle swelling, most commonly affecting the quadriceps, gluteal, paraspinal, psoas, pectoral and deltoid muscles. Elevation of skeletal muscle enzyme levels is uncommon.

   b. Early diagnosis of pyomyositis may be difficult because the inflamed muscle is usually deep, and classic signs of inflammation may be absent. Ultrasound and CT scanning are useful in diagnosis, and needle aspiration may yield pus for microbiological investigations.

   c. Failure to institute appropriate treatment for pyomyositis promptly may result in septicemia with metastatic abscesses.

3. **Bacillary angiomatosis** presents as a folliculitis or pustular skin disease. *Rochalimaea henselae* is a causative agent of bacillary angiomatosis, peliosis hepatis, and cat-scratch disease. Erythromycin or tetracycline are the drugs of choice. Zithromycin and clarithromycin also appear to be active.

4. **Bacterial infections.** Pneumonias and focal abscesses with gram-positive and gram-negative bacteria are markedly increased in HIV patients. Therapy is the same as for immunocompromised patients without AIDS.

C. Fungi

1. **Candidiasis** is the most common fungal infection seen in association with HIV infection.

   a. The severity of oropharyngeal candidiasis and the frequency of relapses increase with worsening immunodeficiency. Women with mildly reduced CD4 counts tend to have vaginal candidiasis, often as their first HIV-related illness. Oral candidiasis develops with more severe immunodeficiency (CD4 counts below 300/µL), progressing to candida esophagitis at counts below 100/µL.

b. Although treatment with azole systemic antifungals is usually successful at first, relapses are so frequent that maintenance therapy is nearly always needed (sec. **V.F**). See Chap. 35, **VI.B** for diagnosis and treatment of candidiasis.

2. Cryptococcosis. *Cryptococcus neoformans* is the most common systemic fungal infection associated with HIV infection. Extrapulmonary infection has been reported in up to 13 percent of patients with AIDS.

a. Cryptococcal meningitis can be insidious or acute. Affected patients can present with a mild headache and prolonged fever or with sudden changes in mentation and neurologic function.

b. Up to 35 percent of patients with cryptococcal meningitis die during induction therapy and only 20 to 30 percent survive for longer than 12 months. See Chap. 35, **VI.A** for diagnosis and treatment.

D. Viruses

1. CMV is the most common viral opportunistic infection in patients with AIDS. More than 90 percent of gay men have serologic evidence of CMV exposure, and up to 90 percent of patients with HIV-1 show signs of CMV infection at autopsy.

a. Retinitis, the most common disease manifestation of CMV, affects approximately 20 percent of patients with AIDS. CMV is also estimated to be responsible for about 30 percent of GI disease in AIDS patients, manifesting as colitis, cholecystitis, pancreatitis, and esophagitis. CMV also can present as severe pneumonia and central or peripheral nervous system disease.

b. See Chap. 35, sec. **IV.B** for diagnosis and treatment of CMV.

2. HPV is closely associated with dysplasia and carcinoma of the anus and uterine cervix in both HIV-infected patients and normal hosts. The severity of these lesions, however, often parallels increasing immune deficiency.

a. Among HIV-infected men, immunosuppression has been correlated with the development of anal squamous intraepithelial lesions (ASILs), the detection of specific anal HPV types, and the detection of high levels of anal HPV DNA. Nevertheless, HIV-seropositive men with CD4 counts above 500/µL had a higher prevalence of both anal HPV and ASIL than men without HIV infection.

b. HPV DNA has also been found in cervicovaginal fluids from HIV-1-seropositive female prostitutes with cervical intraepithelial neoplasia. HPV types 16, 18, 31, 33, and 56 and ME180-HPV have been associated with development of neoplasm.

3. Oral hairy leukoplakia (OHL), a benign lesion caused by EBV, is characterized by an asymptomatic thready white pattern seen along the tongue and buccal mucosa of HIV patients. OHL is highly predictive for the development of AIDS.

a. The diagnosis of OHL may be confirmed by ultrastructural examination or in situ hybridization of exfoliative cytologic specimens.

b. Anecdotal experience suggests that high-dose acyclovir improves OHL.

4. Lichen planus causes mucocutaneous lesions that often appear oral and thrushlike. These lesions may respond to ganciclovir.

5. Herpes viruses. Diagnosis and therapy are described in Chap. 35, sec. **IV.D**.

E. CNS demyelinating syndromes

1. Progressive multifocal leukoencephalopathy (PML) is a rare demyelinating disease of the CNS seen in immunocompromised adults. PML is caused by the JC virus (JCV), which belongs to the papovavirus family.

a. Most cases of PML are due to reactivation of latent JCV infection. PML does not appear to be contagious. An estimated 4 percent of AIDS patients develop PML; in 25 percent of these cases it is the AIDS-defining diagnosis. JCV and HIV may possibly act synergistically, which explains

both the increased incidence and the more aggressive course of PML in AIDS patients compared with other immunocompromised populations.
   b. **Symptoms and signs** are diverse and include limb weakness, altered mental status, speech difficulties, and gait disturbance. Monoparesis or hemiparesis, personality changes, dysarthria, dysphasia, visual loss or blindness, tremor, headache, cranial nerve palsies, nystagmus, and visual-field defects can also develop.
   c. **Clinical evolution** is typically rapidly fatal. Patients usually die three to four months after presenting with their first neurologic symptom. Rare cases of remission and prolonged survival have been reported. No treatment is available.

2. **AIDS dementia complex** (ADC), manifested by encephalitis with neuropsychiatric symptoms, can follow HIV-1 replication within the CNS. Although HIV-1 may have a direct role in demyelination, the pathogenesis of ADC is complex.
   a. HIV-1 may promote demyelination indirectly in patients with ADC. The HIV-1 Tat protein secreted by infected microglial cells can penetrate neighboring oligodendrocytes that are latently infected by JCV. The Tat protein can then reactivate the latent JCV and result in PML.
   b. CMV coinfection in the same brain cells can increase HIV-1 viral load in the CNS by transactivating HIV-1 LTR-driven gene expression.
   c. Cytokines and HIV-1-specific cytotoxic T lymphocytes are also involved. Both α-TNF and IL-6 are increased in the CSF of HIV-infected individuals, and both activate HIV-1 expression in cells of monocyte origin, including glial cells. Transforming growth factor β, which is derived mainly from infected brain macrophages in AIDS patients, recruit infected monocytic cells to the CNS. This results in an increased viral load and progression.

3. **Diagnosis of HIV-related CNS disease**
   a. **MRI and CT radiographic findings**
      (1) **Toxoplasmosis.** Multiple ring-enhancing lesions with discrete margins, mass effect, and edema are commonly seen. Most patients have bilateral lesions with basal ganglia involvement. Gray and white matter may be involved.
      (2) **CNS lymphoma.** Lesions are often single and hyperdense, although multiple lesions have been seen in up to 50 percent of cases. Mass effect and edema are frequent. Ring-enhancement is variable. A solitary lesion on MRI is most likely to be lymphoma.
      (3) **HIV encephalopathy and PML** may be indistinguishable. Atrophy may be apparent on CT or MRI. MRI often shows subcortical white-matter abnormalities with increased T2 signal multifocally. These lesions tend to be large, bilateral, patchy-to-confluent areas with ill-defined and irregular margins.
   b. **Brain biopsy** is the gold standard for diagnosis of PML. Two-thirds of brain biopsies lead to treatable diagnoses. Both the patient and clinician benefit from having a definitive diagnosis.

4. **Treatment.** AZT penetrates most efficiently into the CSF and can effectively antagonize HIV-1 replication in macrophages. This drug can improve neurologic dysfunction in AIDS patients. ddI, which is less efficient than AZT in CSF penetration, may cause or exacerbate a painful peripheral neuropathy. Combination therapy with AZT and foscarnet or acyclovir may be beneficial.

F. **Recommendations for antimicrobial prophylaxis**
   1. **Candidiasis.** Fluconazole, 50 mg PO every other day to 200 mg/day, depending on the number of episodes, response to therapy, and severity of immunosuppression, is effective.
   2. **Recurrent herpes simplex.** Acyclovir, 200 mg to 800 mg PO daily. The lowest dosage that inhibits recurrent outbreaks is used.
   3. **Toxoplasmosis.** Trimethoprim-sulfamethoxazole (Bactrim-DS) one tablet

PO daily or b.i.d. for two days per week. Dapsone plus pyrimethamine also has merit for prophylaxis.

4. **PCP.** Trimethoprim-sulfamethoxazole (Bactrim-DS) (one tablet every other day) is the drug of first choice. Dapsone (25 mg PO daily) is a reasonable alternative. Pentamidine, either IV or as an aerosol via nebulizer, is expensive and associated with higher failure rates and toxicity than oral prophylaxis. Prophylaxis for PCP is given to patients who have recovered from the illness or who have less than 200 CD4 cells/µL.

5. **MAC.** Rifabutin, 300 mg/day PO, or biaxin, 500 mg PO b.i.d., is given. Prophylactic treatment to prevent the onset of MAC is indicated in patients who have less than 200 CD4 cells/µL.

VI. Hematologic problems in AIDS

A. **AIDS-associated hematosuppression.** Pancytopenia inevitably occurs during the course of AIDS. Contributing factors to the significant depression of bone marrow function include HIV infection of macrophages, lymphocytes, and stromal cells; autoimmune destruction of mature or immature hematopoietic cells; marrow involvement with lymphoma or granulomatous infection; and anemia of chronic inflammation.

B. **Treatment of anemia and neutropenia**

1. **Erythropoietin** (EPO). Spontaneous anemia in AIDS is successfully treated with 100 to 200 IU/kg EPO IV or SQ three times weekly. Worsening anemia in association with AZT therapy can also be abrogated with decreased transfusion requirement using the same dose of EPO if the endogenous EPO level is less than 500 mU/ml, particularly if the MCV is high.

2. **Hematinics.** Iron and folic acid should be administered to those patients in whom stores of these nutrients may be marginal.

3. **G-CSF** (filgastrim), 2 to 5 µg/kg SQ daily, can improve the neutrophil count in patients who developed neutropenia spontaneously or received hematosuppressive agents, such as AZT.

4. **GM-CSF** can also improve neutropenia associated with AIDS or AZT but may stimulate HIV replication.

C. **HIV-associated thrombocytopenia**

1. **Epidemiology.** Thrombocytopenia is the most common hematologic manifestation of early HIV infection. Only 1 to 2 percent of patients suffer moderate or severe thrombocytopenia (< 50,000/µL). Isolated thrombocytopenia does not appear to be a harbinger of the accelerated development of AIDS.

2. **Pathophysiology.** Impaired thrombocytopoiesis is found almost universally in patients with HIV-associated thrombocytopenia, in contrast to patients with ITP. Qualitative and quantitative abnormalities of megakaryocyte colony growth have been demonstrated. Anti-HIV antibodies found on the platelet surface appear to cross-react with platelet membrane glycoprotein IIb-IIIa.

3. **Clinical features.** Patients with hemophilia and HIV-associated thrombocytopenia may develop spontaneous bleeding when the platelet count is less than 50,000/µL. Other patients with HIV rarely are symptomatic until the platelet count is less than 20,000/µL.

4. **Treatment**

a. **Spontaneous resolution** of thrombocytopenia occurs in 50 percent of patients, particularly in those with platelet counts below 50,000/µL.

b. **AZT** in doses as low as 600 mg/day is the treatment of choice. At least in part, the drug stimulates platelet production, independent of its antiviral effect. Responses are seen in 50 percent of patients within 2 to 4 weeks, are sustained for 18 to 24 months, and cease when the drug is stopped. Continuous therapy is required.

c. **Prednisone** is effective in 50 to 75 percent of patients, but almost all patients relapse when the dose is tapered.

d. **Splenectomy** can be safely performed and should be considered in patients with persistent severe thrombocytopenia. It is helpful in 90 percent of patients. Sustained satisfactory platelet counts (> 50,000/µL) are achieved in the majority of patients.

D. Opportunistic malignancies (see Chapter 37).

Selected Reading

Ballem, P. J., et al. Kinetic studies of the mechanism of thrombocytopenia in patients with human immunodeficiency virus infection. *N. Engl. J. Med.* 327:1779, 1992.

Boyd, M. T., Antisense RNA to treat HIV infections *AIDS* 5:225, 1991.

Dieterich D. T., et al. Concurrent use of ganciclovir and foscarnet to treat cytomegalovirus infection in AIDS patients. *J. Infect. Dis.* 167:1184, 1993.

Fischl, M., et al. Recombinant human erythropoietin for patients with AIDS treated with zidovudine. *N. Engl. J. Med.* 322:1488, 1990.

Geleziunas, R, et al. Pathogenesis and therapy of HIV-1 infection of the central nervous system. *AIDS* 6:1411, 1992.

Hirsch, M. S., et al. Therapy for human immunodeficiency virus infection. *N. Engl. J. Med.* 328:1686, 1993.

Masur, H. Special Report: Recommendations on prophylaxis and therapy for disseminated *mycobacterium avium* complex disease in patients infected with the human immunodeficiency virus. *N. Engl. J. Med.* 329:898, 1993.

Sarver, N., et al. Ribozymes as potential anti-HIV-1 therapeutic agents. *Science* 247:1222, 1990.

Small, P., M., et al. Exogenous reinfection With multidrug-resistant *Mycobacterium tuberculosis* in patients with advanced HIV infection. *N. Engl. J. Med.* 328:1137, 1993.

Taub, D. D., et al. Superantigens and microbial pathogenesis. *Ann. Intern. Med.* 119:89, 1993.

I. Introduction. Over 40 percent of all patients with HIV infection develop malignant disease at some time during the course of infection. Further, as survival in HIV disease is increased, greater numbers of patients with neoplastic disease will be diagnosed.

The cancers that occur in AIDS are similar to the tumors that are known to develop in organ transplant patients who receive immunosuppressive drugs to prevent graft rejection. The most frequent cancers in this setting are Kaposi's sarcoma, lymphoma, and vulvar and cervical carcinomas. Other disorders of immune dysregulation are also associated with an increased risk of lymphoma, as documented in various autoimmune and congenital immune deficiency diseases.

II. AIDS-related lymphoma

  A. Incidence

    1. Lymphoma accounts for approximately 3 percent of all new cases of AIDS. All age groups and all risk groups for acquisition of HIV infection are equally likely to develop lymphoma.

    2. A recent prospective study of 1295 HIV-infected patients with hemophilia has demonstrated a 5.5 percent incidence of lymphoma, at a median interval of 59 months from initial HIV infection. The relative risk of lymphoma was 36 times higher than that seen in HIV-negative hemophiliacs. The mean CD4 cell count at diagnosis of lymphoma was $64/\mu L$.

  B. Pathology. The vast majority of AIDS-related lymphomas are B cell tumors of high-grade pathologic type. Approximately 80 to 90 percent of patients are diagnosed with immunoblastic lymphoma or small noncleaved lymphoma; the latter may be Burkitt or non-Burkitt subtypes. In contrast, only 10 to 15 percent of patients with *de novo* lymphoma are diagnosed with one of these rather unusual forms of lymphoma. Intermediate grade, diffuse large cell lymphomas have also been reported with some regularity in the setting of underlying HIV infection.

  C. Clinical features

    1. Eighty to 90 percent of patients with newly diagnosed AIDS-lymphoma present with systemic B symptoms, consisting of fever, drenching night sweats, or weight loss.

    2. Sixty to 90 percent of patients have far-advanced disease presenting in extranodal sites. This occurrence is in sharp distinction to patients with *de novo* lymphoma, in whom approximately only 40 percent of patients present with extranodal disease.

      a. The more common sites of initial extranodal disease include the CNS (approximately 30% prevalence at diagnosis), GI tract (25%), bone marrow (20–33%), and liver (10%).

      b. Any anatomic site may be involved, with lymphoma reported in the myocardium, ear lobe, gall bladder, rectum, gingiva, and elsewhere.

  D. Diagnosis and staging evaluation

    1. Biopsy. Immunophenotypic or genotypic studies are often helpful to confirm the monoclonality (and thus the malignant nature) of the process.

    2. CT scans. Staging evaluation should begin with a CT scan of the chest, abdomen, and pelvis. Nearly two-thirds of patients with AIDS-lymphoma have evidence of intra-abdominal lymphomatous disease, which most commonly involves the lymph nodes, GI tract, liver, kidney, and adrenal gland. Isolated hepatic or splenic enlargement is not usually seen in the absence of other intra-abdominal findings.

3. **^{67}Gallium scanning** is an important staging tool that may be particularly useful in evaluating residual stable masses after the completion of systemic chemotherapy (see Chap. 2, sec. II.B.).

4. **Bone marrow** aspiration and biopsy should be performed, usually from two sites.

5. **LP.** While not required in most patients with *de novo* lymphoma, LP should be performed routinely as part of the staging evaluation of a patient with AIDS-related lymphoma. Approximately 20 percent of HIV-infected patients are found to have leptomeningeal involvement even when completely asymptomatic with regard to the CNS. Since prophylactic intrathecal chemotherapy has become an integral part of initial therapy, it is now common practice to inject the first dose of methotrexate or cytosine arabinoside at the time of this initial staging LP in an attempt to prevent isolated CNS relapse.

E. Prognostic factors. At the present time, there is no strong evidence to suggest that patients with intermediate grade large cell lymphoma fare any differently from those with high-grade disease.

1. **Decreased survival** in AIDS-related lymphoma is associated with:
   a. A history of AIDS prior to the lymphoma
   b. Karnofsky performance status less than 70 percent
   c. Involvement of bone marrow
   d. Low CD4 cells ($<200/\mu L$)
   e. Stage IV disease
   f. Treatment with dose-intensive regimens.

2. **Lymphoma primary to the central nervous system** (P-CNS). Patients with P-CNS disease fare significantly worse than patients with AIDS-related systemic lymphoma. The median survival is only two to three months despite therapy, probably because of the far-advanced degree of HIV disease (see **G.1**).

3. **Leptomeningeal involvement** in patients with AIDS-related systemic lymphoma is *not* a poor prognostic indicator. Long-term survival is possible in these individuals provided that specific therapy is given.

F. Management

1. **High-dose regimens.** Several dose-intensive regimens were found to be ineffective and associated with high rates (60–80%) of complicating opportunistic infections, often leading to early patient demise. Patients with good prognostic indicators (such as excellent performance status and no history of AIDS prior to the lymphoma), however, may be able to tolerate the dose-intensive regimens that appear overly toxic in patients with poor prognostic features.

2. **Low-dose regimens.** The AIDS Clinical Trials Group (ACTG), sponsored by the National Institutes of Allergy and Infectious Disease (NIAID), studied a low-dose modification of the m-BACOD regimen in patients with AIDS-related lymphoma, in an attempt to evaluate the hypothesis that "less might be better." Intrathecal cytosine arabinoside was administered weekly four times during the first cycle of therapy, in an attempt to prevent isolated CNS relapse. In addition, prophylactic therapy for PCP was mandated. After two cycles, a restaging evaluation was performed. With complete remission, the patient received two additional cycles, at which time all chemotherapy was discontinued, and AZT was begun.

   a. **The low dose m-BACOD regimen** is given at 28-day intervals for four to six cycles as follows:

Bleomycin	4 mg/m^2 IV, day 1
Doxorubicin	25 mg/m^2 IV, day 1
Cyclophosphamide	300 mg/m^2 IV, day 1
Vincristine sulfate	1.4 mg/m^2 IV (not to exceed 2 mg), day 1
Dexamethasone	3 mg/m^2 PO, days 1 to 5
Methotrexate (MTX)	200 mg/m^2 IV day 15, with folinic acid rescue, 25 PO every 6 hours for 4 days, beginning six hours after completion of MTX
Cytosine arabinoside	50 mg intrathecally, days 1, 8, 21, and 28 of first cycle
Helmet-field RT	2400 cGy with marrow involvement; 4000 cGy with known CNS involvement
Zidovudine (AZT)	100 mg q4h for one year, starting after chemotherapy is completed

    b. Results. With 35 evaluable patients, a complete remission rate of approximately 50 percent was achieved, with long-term, lymphoma-free survival in 75 percent of complete responders. The median survival of complete responders was 15 months, whereas that of all evaluable patients was 6.5 months. Complete remissions were seen equally in all pathologic types.

      (1) No patient experienced isolated CNS relapse.

      (2) Patients with history of prior AIDS had a lower CR rate (25%), but this was not the case in patients who had other poor prognostic features, such as low CD4 cells or stage IV disease.

    c. Complications. Despite the low-dose chemotherapy and use of prophylaxis for PCP, approximately 60 percent of patients experienced nadir granulocyte counts less than 1000/μL, 20 percent had nadirs of 500/μL or less, and PCP occurred in 20 percent of patients, representing the only complicating opportunistic infection.

  3. Addition of hematopoietic growth factors

    a. GM-CSF was added to the m-BACOD regimen, with subsequent escalation of m-BACOD to full doses (see Table 21-7). This regimen was found tolerable, with no documented up-regulation of HIV. The efficacy of this approach, when compared to the low-dose m-BACOD regimen, is currently being tested prospectively by the ACTG.

    b. The CHOP regimen, either with or without the addition of GM-CSF, has been used. Patients who received GM-CSF had fewer chemotherapy cycles complicated by neutropenia and fever and fewer days hospitalized for fever, when compared to patients receiving CHOP alone. Serum HIV p24 antigen levels increased during the third week of chemotherapy with GM-CSF, although the clinical significance was not determined.

  4. Addition of antiretroviral agents has also been employed in an attempt to ameliorate the potential for opportunistic infections during chemotherapy.

    a. AZT itself produces significant bone marrow suppression. Regimens consisting of AZT with concomitant chemotherapy (even low dosages) have been associated with significant cytopenias and short survival.

    b. ddC and ddI are not associated with significant bone marrow suppression. With the low-dose m-BACOD regimen with concomitant ddC, a complete remission rate of 56% was found, with complicating opportunistic infections in only 11 percent of cases. Significant bone marrow compromise was not seen, and response rates were equivalent in patients with good or poor prognostic indicators.

G. Primary CNS lymphoma (see also Chap. 21, sec. **VI.B**)

  1. Clinical features. Patients with P-CNS lymphoma present with far-advanced HIV disease, with median CD4 cells less than 50/μL and history of AIDS prior to the lymphoma in approximately 75 percent of cases. Initial symptoms and signs are variable and include seizures, headache, or focal neurologic dysfunction. Isolated subtle changes in personality or behavior may also be seen.

2. **Diagnosis.** Radiographic scanning reveals mass lesions in the brain, occurring at any site. These masses are likely to be relatively large (2–4 cms) and relatively few in number (1–3). Ring enhancement may be seen. No specific radiographic findings are characteristic of P-CNS lymphoma. Definitive diagnosis requires tissue biopsy.

3. **Management.** RT is associated with complete remission in 20 to 50 percent of cases, but the median survival has been only two to three months, with death often due to opportunistic infection. Although RT may not improve the duration of survival, the quality of life does improve, often quite dramatically, in approximately 75 percent of patients. Combined use of chemotherapy and radiation improves survival in P-CNS lymphoma unrelated to AIDS, but such information is lacking in AIDS-related disease.

III. Hodgkin's disease (HD)

A. **Incidence.** HD is not considered an AIDS-defining condition; its incidence has not increased with the AIDS epidemic. HD is seen more frequently in HIV-infected patients with a history of injection drug use compared to other groups at risk for HIV.

B. **Biology.** An association of HD with EBV has been suggested for years based on epidemiologic data. Recently, approximately 50 percent of patients with HD have been shown to contain clonally integrated EBV within the diagnostic Reed-Sternberg cells. No data indicate that EBV is actively replicating within HD tissues. Thus, the use of acyclovir or other agents would not be expected to be efficacious.

C. **Clinical features.** Patients with underlying HIV infection have different clinical and pathologic manifestations of HD than expected in patients without HIV disease.

1. **Sites of disease.** The majority of HIV-infected patients with HD have widespread extranodal disease at diagnosis, with approximately 80 to 90 percent presenting with stage III or IV disease. Systemic B symptoms (e.g., fever, drenching night sweats, weight loss) are seen in approximately 80 to 90 percent of patients.

   Unusual extranodal sites of disease may be seen, including the anus and rectum, and CNS. Bone marrow is commonly involved and may be the only site of disease in patients with B symptoms, either with or without various peripheral cytopenia(s).

2. **Pathology.** Mixed cellularity and lymphocyte depletion subtypes are prominent. Nodular sclerosis and lymphocyte predominant subtypes are relatively decreased in incidence in the setting of HIV infection.

D. **Prognostic factors.** The median survival after definitive therapy is approximately one to two years as opposed to uninfected patients with HD. Eighty to 90 percent of the latter patients may be cured.

E. **Management.** The ABVD regimen is used most frequently, along with hematopoietic growth factors.

IV. Kaposi's sarcoma (KS)

A. **Incidence.** KS has been diagnosed in approximately 20 percent of homosexual or bisexual men with HIV infection, 1 percent of hemophiliacs, and 3 percent of injection drug users or transfusion recipients. Development of KS has been correlated with history of oral-fecal contact during intercourse. KS is extremely unusual in women.

B. **Biology**

1. **Genetic predisposition.** Development of KS has been correlated with HLA-DQ1 in HIV-positive homosexual men. Other HLA associations have also been described.

2. **Factors associated with development of KS.** Immunosuppression is an apparent requisite for KS, due in this case to underlying infection by HIV. HIV-infected CD4 cells produce a protein termed "oncostatin M," which serves as a potent growth factor for KS. Oncostatin M production may be

upregulated by corticosteroids, which are thus contraindicated in patients with KS, or even in HIV-infected homosexual/bisexual men. In addition, the KS cell itself can produce a whole series of cytokines (IL-6, TGF-b, FGF-b, and others), which serve as autocrine growth factors, upregulating the growth of the KS. These cytokines are also responsible for a local "capillary leak syndrome," leading to the lymphedema that may be seen in association with KS.

C. **Clinical features**
1. **Natural history of disease.** Some patients experience a very slowly progressive disease over many years, whereas others have fulminant rapidly advancing KS that rapidly leads to death.
2. **Sites of involvement.** The patient with KS usually presents with disease on the skin that may consist of nodular, hyperpigmented lesions or irregular lesions. The lesions are often remarkably symmetric. Lymphedema may be profound, occasionally in the absence of visible skin lesions. Lymphadenopathy, sometimes in the absence of KS lesions on the skin, is often seen. Another common site of involvement is the oral cavity, which is associated with KS lower in the GI tract approximately 50 percent of the time. Literally any visceral organ may be involved. KS in the lung is associated with a poor prognosis and mandates immediate chemotherapy.

D. **Diagnosis and staging evaluation.** An initial biopsy with pathologic confirmation should be obtained. Routine staging is *not* necessary in the patient with KS. Assessment of visible disease on the skin and oral cavity, a baseline chest x-ray, and determination of the number of CD4 cells in blood should be performed. If the patient has symptoms suggestive of GI involvement (e.g., abdominal pain, weight loss, or diarrhea), endoscopy should be performed. With unexplained abnormalities on chest x-ray, bronchoscopy should be performed; the diagnosis of KS is usually made by visualization and not by biopsy, which may be associated with hemorrhage.

E. **Prognostic factors.** Factors associated with poor prognosis include (1) history or presence of opportunistic infection, (2) presence of systemic B symptoms, consisting of fever, drenching night sweats, or weight loss in excess of 10 percent of the normal body weight; and (3) CD4 cells less than $300/\mu L$. In the absence of all such factors, the median survival is approximately three years. A history of opportunistic infection is the most significant poor prognostic factor, with median survival of only seven months.

F. **Management**
1. **Initial observation.** Because KS is multifocal at initial diagnosis, is not currently curable, and may have an extremely variable pace of disease, the patient can simply be observed without specific therapy until such treatment is deemed necessary.
2. **Treatment of local disease.** Hyper- or hypopigmented scars may remain after successful local treatment of KS lesions.
   a. Specific local lesions may be treated efficaciously with **local injections** of vincristine (0.2 mg), vinblastine (0.1–0.3 mg), or α-IFN (1–2 million units). Liquid nitrogen, sclerotherapy, or surgical excision may also be used.
   b. **Local RT** may also be quite useful, although care must be exercised in radiating the oral cavity, because significant mucositis can occur after relatively small doses.
3. **α-IFN** may be used in patients with more extensive disease than can be managed by local treatment alone.
   a. When used as a single agent, α-IFN is given at a dose of 36 million units/day over a 12-week induction period, followed by 18 million units given three times per week. The response rate is 40 percent (usually partial responses). Patients with poor prognostic factors are not expected to respond.
   b. The combination of α-IFN (10 million units/day) with AZT (500 mg/day) has resulted in both antiretroviral synergy and higher response rates

(30% response in patients with poor prognostic factors; and 50–60% response in those with good prognosis disease).

4. **Chemotherapy** is indicated for (1) rapidly progressive disease, (2) pulmonary KS, (3) symptomatic visceral disease, and (4) lymphedema.

   a. Several agents are effective in KS, including vincristine, vinblastine, etoposide, and Adriamycin. Combination therapy is more effective than single agents, and the regimen of choice is currently the ABV regimen: Adriamycin (20 mg/m^2), bleomycin (10 mg/m^2), and vincristine (2 mg), all given IV every two weeks. Prophylactic therapy for PCP should be given along with chemotherapy.

   b. The response rate to ABV is 88 percent, with complicating opportunistic infections in approximately 20 percent of patients. Unfortunately, with discontinuation of therapy, the KS eventually relapses.

5. **Experimental therapies** currently in trial for KS include (1) liposomal Adriamycin or daunomycin; (2) IL-4, which downregulates the potent growth factor, IL-6; and (3) other antiangiogenesis compounds, such as fumagillan derivatives and SP-PG.

V. **Cervical cancer**

   A. **Incidence.** Cervical cancer is now an AIDS-defining diagnosis. Women currently constitute the fastest rising group of new AIDS cases in the United States. The primary risk factor for HIV infection in these individuals is heterosexual transmission, usually from a partner who was not known to be infected by the woman in question. The precise incidence of cerivcal carcinoma or in situ carcinoma (cervical intraepithelial neoplasia, CIN) is unknown but is expected to increase significantly over the next several years.

   B. **Biologic factors.** Cervical cancer is associated with prior infection by HPV, usually involving serotypes 16, 18, 31, 33, or 35. Immunosuppression may allow more rapid development of in situ or invasive disease in the setting of such HPV infection. Preliminary data indicates that infection by more than one serotype may increase the risk of cervical cancer or CIN.

   C. **Clinical features** of cervical cancer in the HIV-infected woman are not different from those in uninfected individuals (see Chap. 11). However, preliminary evidence suggests that HIV-infected women are more likely to have advanced stage disease, high-grade pathologic type, and relapse after definitive therapy.

   D. **Management.** Because of the aggressive nature of cervical carcinoma in HIV-infected women, it becomes extremely important to diagnose such patients early, at the time of "in situ" abnormalities on the Pap smear. It is recommended that HIV-infected patients undergo routine Pap testing every 6 to 12 months with evaluation of HPV status, although this is not yet well established. Colposcopy and biopsy should be performed in the presence of positive HPV status or any questionable Pap smear results. Invasive cervical cancer is currently treated in the "usual" manner.

VI. **Anal carcinoma.** Although not currently considered part of the AIDS epidemic, the incidence of HPV-related anal carcinoma is known to be increased in homosexual men. Large cohort studies are currently being conducted to determine the natural history of anal cancer in HIV-infected persons and its response to therapy.

Selected Reading

Levine, A. M. Acquired immunodeficiency syndrome-related lymphoma. *Blood* 80:8, 1992.

Levine, A. M. AIDS-related malignancies: The emerging epidemic. *J. Natl. Cancer Inst.* 85:1382, 1993.

Appendixes

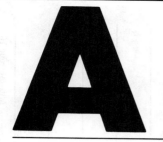

**Combination
Chemotherapy
Regimens**

A-1. Combination chemotherapy regimens for solid tumors[a]

Use	Regimen (cycle)	Cyclo-phosphamide	Adria-mycin	5-FU	Metho-trexate	Etoposide	Cisplatin	Ifos-famide[b]	Other
Breast	CMF (28 d)	100 PO (d 1–14)		600 (d 1,8)	40 (d 1,8)				
Breast	CMF (21 d)	600 (d 1)		600 (d 1)	40 (d 1)				
Breast	CA (21 d)	600 (d 1)	60 (d 1)						
Breast	FAC (21–28 d)	400–500 (d 1)	40–50 (d 1)	400–500 (d 1,8)					
Breast	FNC (21 d)	500 (d 1)		500 (d 1)					Mitoxantrone 10 (d 1)

Disease	Regimen				
GI tract	F-L (28 d)	370 (d 1–5)			Leuc 200 (d 1–5) Give before 5-FU
GI tract	F-L (28 d)	425 (d 1–5)			Leuc 20 (d 1–5) Give before 5-FU
GI tract	F-L (7 d)	425 weekly			Leuc 20 weekly Give before 5-FU
GI tract	ELF (21 d)	500 (d 1,2,3)		120 (d 1,2,3)	Leuc 150 (d 1,2,3) Give before 5-FU
Gestational trophoblastic neoplasia	MAC III (21 d)	3 mg/kg (d 1–5)	1 mg/kg IM or IV (d 1,3,5,7)		Dactin 12 µg/kg (d 1–5); Leuc 0.1 mg/kg PO (d 2,4,6,8)
Gestational trophoblastic neoplasia	EMA-CO (14 d)	600 (d 8)	100 then 200 CVI over 12 hr (d 1)	100 (d 1,2)	Dactin 0.5[d] (d 1,2); and Leuc 15[d] q12h for 4 doses; Vcr 1.0 (d 8)

A-1. (continued)

Use	Regimen (cycle)	Cyclo-phosphamide	Adria-mycin	5-FU	Metho-trexate	Etoposide	Cisplatin	Ifos-famide[b]	Other
GYN: Germ cell (See testicular)	VAC (28 d)	150 (d 1–5)							Dactin 0.3–0.4 (d 1–5); Vcr 1.2[d] wkly × 12
GYN: ovary	PC (28 d)	1000 (d 1)					50 (d 1)		
GYN: ovary	CHAP (28 d)	350 (d 1,8)	20 (d 1,8)				60 (d 1,8)		Hexamethylmela-mine 150 PO (d 1–14)
GYN: ovary	PAC (21–28 d)	500 (d 1)	40–50 (d 1)				50 (d 1)		Or Carb 300 for cis-platin (d 1)
GYN: ovary	PT (21–28 d)	500 (d 1)					75 (d 1)		Taxol 135 (d 1, before cis-platin)
Head and neck	PF-CIV (28 d)			1000 CIV (d 1–5)			100 (d 1)		
Head and neck	MBC (21 d)				40 (d 1,15)		50 (d 4)		Bleo 10 (weekly)

Islet cell	F-St (28–42 d); alternate with ADcz				400 (d 1–5)	St 500 (d 1–5)
Islet cell	ADcz (28–35 d); alternate with F-St			60 (d 1)		Dcz 250 (d 1–5)
Lung; small cell and NSCLC	CE (28 d)		100–200 (d 1–3)			Carb 50–125 (d 1–3)
Lung; small cell and NSCLC	PE (21–28 d)	25–50 (d 1–3)	100 (d 1–3)			
Lung; small cell and NSCLC	ICE (28 d)	25 (d 1–5)	100 (d 1–3)	4000[b] (d 1 CIV)		Or Carb 400 for cisplatin (d 1 only)
Lung; small cell	CAV (21–28 d)				40–50 (d 1)	1000 (d 1) ; Vcr 1.4[c] (d 1)
Lung; small cell	CAE (21–28 d)		50 (d 1–5)		45 (d 1)	1000 (d 1)
Melanoma	DD (28 d)					Dcz 750 (d 1); Dactin 1 (d 1)
Melanoma	VDP (21–28 d)	75 (d 5)				Dcz 150 (d 1–5); Vbl 5 (d 1,2)

A-1. (continued)

Use	Regimen (cycle)	Cyclo-phosphamide	Adria-mycin	5-FU	Metho-trexate	Etoposide	Cisplatin	Ifos-famide[b]	Other
Neurologic	PCV (42 d)								Procarbazine 60 PO (d 8–21) CCNU [Lomustine] 110 PO (d 1) Vcr 1.4[c] (d 8, 29)
Prostate	None	Alone	Alone	Alone					Use sequential single agents
Sarcoma	CyVADic (21 d)	500 (d 1)	50 (d 1)						Vcr 1.4[c] (d 1,5); Dcz 250 (d 1–5)
Sarcoma	A-Dac (21 d)		45–60 (d 1)						Dcz 250 (d 1–5)
Sarcoma	IE (28 d)					100 (d 1–5)		1800[b] (d 1–5)	
Sarcoma	IMAP (28 d)		15 CIV (d 2–5)				120 (d 7)	1200[b] CIV (d 1–5)	

	Regimen				
Testicular	BEP (21 d)		100 (d 1–5)	20 (d 1–5)	Bleo 30 (d 2,9,16)
Testicular	PVB (21 d)			20 (d 1–5)	Vbl 0.15 mg/kg (d 1,2); Bleo 30 (d 2,9,16)
Testicular	EIP (21 d)		75 (d 1–5) over 6 hr	20 (d 1–5)	1200[b] (d 1–5)
Transitional cell	VBP (21–28 d)			20 (d 1–5)	Vbl 6 (d 1,2); Bleo 30 u[d] weekly
Transitional cell	CISCA (21–28 d)	500–650 (d 1)	40–50 (d 1)	60–100 (d 2)	
Transitional cell	MVAC (28 d)	30 (d 2)	30 (d 1,15,22)	70 (d 2)	Vbl 3 (d 2,15,22)

[a] Dosages are expressed in mg/m^2 and given IV by short infusion unless otherwise specified; d = days; PO = by mouth; IM = intramuscular; CIV = continuous IV infusion.
[b] Given with MESNA for uroprotection (e.g., 20% of ifosfamide dose immediately before and at 4 and 8 hours after infusion).
[c] Maximum 2.0-mg dose.
[d] **Total dose; not mg/m^2.**
Key: Bleo = bleomycin; Carb = carboplatin; Dcz = dacarbazine; Dactin = dactinomycin; 5-FU = 5-fluorouracil; Leuc = leucovorin; NSCLC = non-small cell lung cancer; St = streptozocin; Vcr = vincristine; Vbl = vinblastine.

A-2. Combination chemotherapy regimens for lymphoreticular neoplasms[a]

Use	Regimen (cycle)	Cyclo-phosphamide	Vin-cristine	Vin-blastine	Prednisone	Adria-mycin	Bleomycin	Procarbazine	Other
ML	C & P (14 d)				40 (d 1→5)				Chlorambucil 16–30 PO (d 1)
ML	CVP (21 d)	750 (d 1)	1.4[b] (d 1)		100 (d 1→5)				
ML	CHOP (21 d)	750 (d 1)	1.4[b] (d 1)		100[c] (d 1→5)	50 (d 1)			
ML, HD	COPP (28 d)	650 (d 1,8)	1.4[b] (d 1,8)		40 (d 1→14)			100 (d 1→14)	
ML, HD	CVPP (28 d)	300 (d 1,8)		10[c] (d 1,8,15)	40 (d 1→15)			100 (d 1→15)	
ML, HD	BCVPP (28 d)	600 (d 1)		5 (d 1)	60 (d 1→10)			100 (d 1→10)	BCNU 100 (d 1)
HD	MOPP (28 d)		1.4 (d 1,8)		40 (d 1→14)			100 (d 1→14)	Mechlorethamine 6 (d 1,8)
HD	ABVD (28 d)			6 (d 1,15)		25 (d 1,15)	10 (d 1,15)		Dacarbazine 375 (d 1,15)
HD	MOPP/ABV (28 d)		1.4[b] (d 1)	6 (d 8)	40 (d 1→14)	35 (d 8)	10 (d 8)	100 (d 1→7)	Mechlorethamine 6 (d 1)
ML, HD	Salvage and other regimens								See Table 21-3 and Table 21-7

[a]Dosages are expressed in mg/m² and are given IV by short infusion unless otherwise specified; d = days; PO = by mouth; CIV = continuous IV 24-hour infusion. [b]Maximum 2.0-mg dose. [c]Total dose, not mg/m². Key: HD = Hodgkin's disease; ML = malignant lymphoma.

B

Toxicity of Chemotherapy

B-1. Toxicities and dose modifications for antineoplastic agents

Drug	Vesicant[b]	↓ WBC	↓ Plts	N & V	Alopecia	Other[c]	Dose modification for dysfunction[d]
Alkylating agents							
Amsacrine	+ + +	+ +	+	+	+ + +	M, H	(L)
Busulfan	PO	+ + +	+ + +	+	+	P	(R)
BCNU (carmustine)	+ +	+ + +	+ + +	+ + +	+	P, R	(R)
CCNU (lomustine)	PO	+ + +	+ + +	+ +	+	P, R	(R)
Carboplatin	0	+ +	+ + +	+	0		R*
Chlorambucil	PO	+ +	+ +	0	0	Leuk	
Cisplatin: 20/m²/d for 5 d	+	+	+	+ +	+	R, N	(N)
Cisplatin: 40–100/m² for 1 d	+	+ +	+ +	+ + +	+	R, N	N*
Cyclophosphamide	0	+ + +	+	+ +	+ + +	U	(L)
Dacarbazine (DTIC)	+	+ +	+ + +	+ + +	+	Flu syndrome	L*, R*
Hexamethylmelamine	PO	+	+	+ + +	0	N	(L)
Ifosfamide	0	+ +	+ +	+	+ + +	N, U	R*

Drug						Leuk	Drug interactions
Mustargen	+++	++	++	+++	+		(R)
Melphalan	PO	++	++	+	0	Leuk	L*, R*
Procarbazine	PO	++	++	+	0		R*
Streptozotocin	++	+	+	+++	0	R, L, hypoglycemia	
Antimetabolites							
Azacytidine	0	+++	+++	+++	+++	N, M	L* (N)
Cladribine	0	++	++	+	0		
Cytarabine, 100/m²	0	+++	+++	++	+	M, Chol	(L), (R)
Cytarabine, 2000/m²	0	+++	+++	+++	+	M, N, Chol, Oc	(L), (R)
Fludarabine	0	++	++	++	+	N	R*
Fluorouracil, IV bolus	+	++	++	+	0	N, M, Oc	(L)
Fluorouracil, with leucovorin	+	+++	+++	+	+	D	(L)
Fluorouracil, continuous infusion	+	+	+	++	+	M, D	(L)
Hydroxyurea	PO	+++	+++	+	0	Skin	R*, (L)
Mercaptopurine	PO	++	++	+	0	Chol	L*

B-1. (continued)

Drug	Vesicant[b]	↓ WBC	↓ Plts	N & V	Alopecia	Other[c]	Dose modification for dysfunction[d]
Methotrexate	0	+ +	+ +	+	0	M. N	R*
Mitoguazone	+ +	+ +	+	+	0	M, N	
Pentostatin	0	+	+	+	0	R	R*
Thioguanine	PO	+ +	+ +	+	0	Chol	L*
Thiotepa	0	+ +	+ +	+	0		
Antibiotics							
Actinomycin D	+ + +	+ + +	+ + +	+ +	+ +	M, Skin	L*, R*
Bleomycin	0	0	0	+	+ +	P, Skin, allergy	
Daunorubicin	+ + +	+ + +	+ + +	+ +	+ + +	H	R*
Doxorubicin	+ + +	+ + +	+ + +	+ +	+ + +	H	
Idarubicin	+ + +	+ + +	+ + +	+ +	+ + +	H	
Mithramycin	+ + +	+	+ +	+	0	Hypocalcemia	
Mitomycin C	+ + +	+ + +	+ + +	+	+	R, P, TTP	
Mitoxantrone	0	+ +	+ +	+	+	Chol	

Toxicities[a]

Alkaloids						
Etoposide (VP-16)	+	+	+	+	N	R*
Paclitaxel (Taxol)	++	+++	+++	+	N	(N)
Teniposide (VM-26)	+	++	++	+	N	(N)
Vinblastine	+	+++	+++	+	Cramps	L*, (N)
Vincristine	+	+	+	++	N	L*, N*
Vindesine	+	++	++	++	N	L*
Other agents						
Aminoglutethamide	PO	0	0	+	AI, rash, fever	(R)
Asparaginase	0	0	0	++	N, allergy	
Estramustine	PO	0	0	++	Thromboemboli	
Levamisole	PO	0	0	+	N	
Mitotane	PO	0	0	++	AI	L*
Suramin	PO	+	+++	+	N	

aScale: 0 = rare, + = mild, ++ = moderate, +++ = marked or severe; ↓ WBC = leukopenia; ↓ Plts = thrombocytopenia; N & V = nausea and vomiting.

bUse extravasation precautions for all moderate to marked vesicants.

cAI = adrenal insufficiency; Chol = cholestasis; H = heart; L = liver function tests; Leuk = acute myelogenous leukemia; M = mucositis; D = diarrhea; N = neural; Oc = ocular (conjunctivitis); P = pulmonary; R = renal; TTP = thrombotic thrombocytopenia-like syndrome; U = urothelial.

dL*, N*, R* = Reduce dose for liver, neurologic, or renal dysfunction, respectively. (L), (N), (R) = Use with caution for liver, neurologic, or renal dysfunction, respectively.

B-2. Common toxicity criteria

Toxicity	Grade 1	Grade 2	Grade 3	Grade 4
Hematologic				
Hemoglobin	10.0–N	8.0–10.0	6.5–7.9	<6.5 g/dl
Platelets	75,000–150,000	50,000–<75,000	25,000–<50,000	<25,000/μL
White blood cells	3000–4000	2000–3000	1000–2000	<1000/μL
Neutrophils	1500–2000	1000–1500	500–1000	<500/μL
Lymphocytes	1500–2000	1000–1500	500–1000	<500/μL
Prothrombin time	$1.01–1.25 \times N$	$1.26–1.50 \times N$	$1.51–2.00 \times N$	$>2.00 \times N$
Partial thromboplastin time	$1.01–1.66 \times N$	$1.67–2.33 \times N$	$2.34–3.00 \times N$	$>3.00 \times N$
Fibrinogen	$0.99–0.75 \times N$	$0.74–0.50 \times N$	$0.49–0.25 \times N$	$\leq0.24 \times N$
Clinical hemorrhage	Mild, no transfusion	Gross, 1–2 units transfusion per episode	Gross, 3–4 units transfusion per episode	Massive, >4 units transfusion per episode
Systemic				
Weight gain/loss	5.0–9.9%	10.0–19.9%	>20%	—
Fatigue*	Decrease by one level of performance status score (ECOG), but not to PS 4	Decrease by two levels of performance status score (ECOG), but not to PS 4	Decrease by three levels of performance status score (ECOG), but not to PS 4	Decrease of performance status score (ECOG) to PS 4

Allergy	Transient rash or drug fever ≥38°C (100.4°F)	Urticaria, drug fever ≥38°C (100.4°F), mild bronchospasm	Serum sickness or bronchospasm; requires parenteral medication	Anaphylaxis
Fever without infection	37.1–38.0°C (98.7–100.4°F)	38.1–40.0°C (100.5–104.0°F)	>40.0°C (>104.0°F) for <24 hr	>40.0°C (>104.0°F) for >24 hr or fever with hypotension
Chills	Chilly sensation, no rigors	Mild rigors, no medication required	Severe rigors, requires medication	—
Infection	Mild	Moderate	Severe	Life-threatening
Dermatologic				
Local injection	Pain	Pain and swelling with inflammation or phlebitis	Ulceration	Plastic surgery indicated
Skin	Asymptomatic scattered macular or papular eruption or erythema	Scattered macular or papular eruption or erythema with pruritus or other associated symptoms	Generalized symptomatic macular, papular, or vesicular eruption	Exfoliative or ulcerating dermatitis
Alopecia	Mild hair loss	Pronounced or total hair loss	—	—
Hand-foot syndrome	Mild paresthesias +/or numbness of fingers +/or toes	Moderate paresthesias +/or numbness with or without local dermatitis	Painful swelling of distal phalanges with or without local dermatitis	—

B-2. (continued)

Toxicity	Grade 1	Grade 2	Grade 3	Grade 4
Alimentary				
Stomatitis	Painless ulcers, erythema, or mild soreness	Painful ulcers, erythema, or edema, but still can eat	Painful ulcers, erythema, or edema, and cannot eat	Requires enteral or parenteral support
Nausea	Reduced but reasonable intake	Intake significantly decreased but still can eat	No significant intake	—
Vomiting	One episode in 24 hr	Two to five episodes in 24 hr	Six to ten episodes in 24 hr	>10 episodes in 24 hr, or requires parenteral support
Diarrhea	Increase of 2–3 stools/day over baseline	Increase of 4–6 stools/day, or nocturnal stools, or moderate cramping	Increase of 7–9 stools/day, or incontinence, or severe cramping	Increase of ≥10 stools/day, grossly bloody diarrhea, or requires parenteral support
Liver (clinical)	—	—	Precoma	Hepatic coma
Amylase	<1.5 × N	1.5–2.0 × N	2.1–5.0 × N	>5.1 × N
Bilirubin	—	<1.5 × N	1.5–3.0 × N	>3.0 × N
SGOT, SGPT	≤2.5 × N	2.6–5.0 × N	5.1–20.0 × N	>20.0 × N
Alkaline phosphatase or 5′-nucleotidase	≤2.5 × N	2.6–5.0 × N	5.1–20.0 × N	>20.0 × N

Urinary/Metabolic

Creatinine	$<1.5 \times N$	1.5–$3.0 \times N$	3.1–$6.0 \times N$	$>6.0 \times N$
Proteinuria	1+ or <3 g/L	2 or 3+ or 3–10 g/l	4+ or >10 g/l	Nephrotic syndrome
Hematuria	Microscopic only	Gross, no clots	Gross with clots	Requires transfusion
Hypercalcemia	10.6–11.5	11.6–12.5	12.6–13.5	≥13.5 mg/dl
Hypocalcemia	8.4–7.8	7.7–7.0	6.9–6.1	≤6.0 mg/dl
Hypomagnesemia	1.4–1.2	1.1–0.9	0.8–0.6	≤0.5 mg/dl
Hyperglycemia	116–160	161–250	251–500	>500 mg/dl or ketoacidosis

Pulmonary and vascular

Lungs	Asymptomatic with pulmonary function test abnormalities	Dyspnea on significant exertion	Dyspnea at normal level of activity	Dyspnea at rest
Hypertension	No treatment required; asymptomatic transient diastolic increase by >20 mm Hg or to >150/100 if previously WNL	No treatment required; asymptomatic recurrent or persistent diastolic increase by >20 mm Hg or to >150/100 if previously WNL	Requires therapy	Hypertensive crisis
Hypotension	Changes requiring no therapy (including transient orthostatic hypotension)	Requires fluid replacement or other therapy but not hospitalization	Requires therapy and hospitalization; resolves within 48 hours of stopping the agent	Requires therapy and hospitalization for >48 hours after stopping the agent

B-2. (continued)

Toxicity	Grade 1	Grade 2	Grade 3	Grade 4
Cardiac				
Arrhythmias	Asymptomatic and transient; no therapy required	Recurrent or persistent; no therapy required	Requires treatment	Requires monitoring; or ventricular tachycardia or fibrillation
Cardiac ischemia	Nonspecific T-wave flattening	Asymptomatic ST/T-wave changes ischemia	Angina without evidence for infarction	Acute myocardial infarction
Cardiac function	Asymptomatic decline of resting ejection fraction by <20% of baseline value	Asymptomatic decline of resting ejection fraction by >20% of baseline value	Mild CHF responsive to therapy	Severe or refractory CHF
Pericardium	Asymptomatic effusion, drainage not required	Pericarditis (rub, chest pain, ECG changes)	Symptomatic effusion; drainage required	Tamponade; drainage urgently required
Neurologic				
Myalgias	Mild muscular aching; no medication required	Moderate myalgia requiring medication; no enzyme (CPK) elevation	Severe myalgias requiring medication; enzyme (CPK) elevated	—
Motor	Subjective weakness; no objective findings	Mild objective weakness without significant impairment of function	Objective weakness with impairment of function	Paralysis
Sensory	Mild paresthesias; loss of deep tendon reflexes	Moderate paresthesias; mild or moderate objective sensory loss	Severe objective sensory loss or paresthesias that interferes with function	—

	Mild	Moderate	Severe	Life-threatening
Cortical	Mild somnolence or agitation	Moderate somnolence or agitation	Severe somnolence, agitation, confusion, disorientation, hallucinations	Coma, seizure, toxic psychosis
Seizures	—	Simple partial seizures; consciousness preserved; self-limited or controlled	Complex partial or generalized seizures with altered consciousness; self-limited or controlled	Seizures of any type that are prolonged, repetitive, or difficult to control (status epilepticus)
Cerebellar	Slight incoordination, dysdiadokinesis	Intention tremor, dysmetria, slurred speech, nystagmus	Locomotor ataxia	Cerebellar necrosis
Mood	Mild anxiety or depression	Moderate anxiety or depression	Severe anxiety or depression	Suicidal ideation
Headache	Mild	Moderate to severe but controllable	Unrelenting and severe	—
Vision	—	Blurred vision or diplopia	Symptomatic subtotal loss of vision	Blindness
Hearing	Asymptomatic hearing loss on audiometry	Tinnitus	Symptomatic hearing loss, correctable with hearing aid	Deafness, not correctable
Constipation	Mild	Moderate	Severe	Ileus >96 hours

*See inside back cover for Performance Status Scales (including ECOG).
Key: N = normal; WNL = within normal limits; CHF = congestive heart failure.
Source: Adapted from the National Cancer Institute.

C

Tumor Identifiers

C-1. Microscopic clues of tumor origin

Potentially helpful findings	Probable primary site of tumor type
HISTOPATHOLOGY	
Signet ring cells	Gastrointestinal tract, ovary, breast (lobular carcinoma)
Psammona bodies	Ovary, thyroid, breast
Papillary	Thyroid, ovary, mesothelioma
Nonacinar cell nests	Carcinoid, melanoma, paraganglioma
Rosettes and areas of ganglion cell-like differentiation	Neuroblastoma
Very poorly differentiated small cell neoplasms	See Chap. 20, sec. II.C.3.
HISTOCHEMISTRY	
Mucin stains (e.g., mucicarmine)	Adenocarcinoma (absent in renal cell carcinoma)
Glycogen stains (PAS-positive removed by diastase)	Abundant in renal cell carcinoma, germ cell tumors, and some adrenocortical carcinomas (small quantities not helpful)
Silver impregnation (e.g., Fontana-Masson, Grimelius, Sevier-Munger)	Tumors of polypeptide-forming endocrine cells, enterochromaffin cells, melanoma
HORMONE RECEPTORS	
Estrogen receptor	Breast, endometrium, thyroid, meningioma
Progesterone receptor	Breast
ELECTRON MICROSCOPY	
Lamellar surfactant bodies	Alveolar carcinoma (lung)
Cells united by well-developed cell junctions (desmosomes), intercellular bridges, tonofilaments	Squamous cell carcinoma
Premelanosomes, melanosomes, tubular arrays	Melanoma
Abundant polyribosomes, absence of intercellular junctions	Lymphoma, leukemia
Myofibrils, extracellular osteoid, dilated rough endoplasmic reticulum	Sarcoma
Long surface microvilli	Mesotheliomas (some)
Cytoplasmic "neuroendocrine" secretory granules	Neuroendocrine tumors, including carcinoid
Apical terminal webs	Gut epithelial cells
Acinar spaces, junctional complex, tight junctions, microvilli, desmosomes	Adenocarcinomas
Microvilli, glycocaliceal bodies, terminal webs, apical mucus granules	Adenocarcinoma of colon
Intracellular neolumens, prominent tonofilaments	Adenocarcinoma of breast
Staghorn microvilli	Adenocarcinoma of ovary
Tubulofilamentous structures of cytoplasm	Adenocarcinoma of kidney

C-2. Selected immunohistologic tumor markers*

Detectable antigen	Tumor type
Alpha-fetoprotein (AFP)	Germ cell and trophoblastic tumors, hepatocellular carcinoma
β_1-antitrypsin	Hepatocellular carcinoma
Carcinoembryonic antigen (CEA)	Gut, pancreas, cervix uteri, lung, ovary, breast, urinary tract
Chromogranin	NET
Collagen, type IV; laminin	Sarcomas (neurogenic, smooth muscle)
Cytokeratin	Nonspecific; broad range of carcinomas and sarcomas
Desmin	Sarcomas (smooth or skeletal muscle, glomus tumors); corpus uteri (connective tissue part)
Factor VIII; CD31, CD34	Sarcomas (vascular)
Gross cystic disease fluid protein (GCDFP-15)	Breast
Hormones, specific	Endocrine gland, gut or pancreatic tumors
Human chorionic gonadotropin (HCG)	Trophoblastic, breast and other tumors
Human placental lactogen	Trophoblastic tumors
Immunoglobulin molecules	Lymphomas/leukemias
Involucrin	Squamous epithelia

C-2. (continued)

Detectable antigen	Tumor type
Leucocyte common antigen (LCA)	Lymphomas/leukemias, histiocytic tumors
Lymphoid cell epitopes and activation markers	Lymphomas/leukemias
Milk fat globules	Breast (nonspecific)
Muramidase (lysozyme); CD68	Histiocytic tumors, myelogenous leukemia
Myelin base protein	Sarcomas (neurogenic)
Myoglobin	Sarcomas (neurogenic, skeletal muscle), corpus uteri
Muscle-specific actin	Sarcomas (leiomyosarcoma, MFH)
Neurofilaments	NET: lung (small cell carcinoma)
Neuron-specific enolase	NET: lung (small cell carcinoma); breast carcinoma (some); melanoma
NKI/C3 or MB-5	Melanoma
Pancreatic carcinoma antigen	Pancreas, gut
Prostate-specific acid phosphatase, prostate antigen (PAP, PSA)	Prostate
S100 protein	Melanoma; sarcomas (neurogenic, cartilage); histiocytic tumors
Thyroglobulin	Thyroid
Vimentin	Sarcomas (muscle, cartilage, vessels, bone, synovial, epithelioid, MFH; renal cell carcinoma; lymphomas/leukemias; melanoma

Key: MFH = malignant fibrous histiocytoma; NET = neuroendocrine tumors (neuroblastic, Merkel cell, and carcinoid tumors; paragangliomas; pheochromocytoma).

C-3. Glossary of cytogenetic nomenclature

Symbol	Definition	Example*
p	Short arm of a chromosome [arm above the centromere]; a prefix number gives the number of the chromosome and a suffix number refers to a particular band on the chromosome	22p5 is the 5th band from the centromere on the short arm of chromosome 22
q	Long arm of a chromosome [arm below the centromere]; numbering is the same as for p	22q5 is the 5th band from the centromere on the long arm of chromosome 22
t	Translocation of part of one chromosome to another. The first set of parentheses indicates the chromosomes involved and the second set indicates the bands affected by the break points on the respective chromosomes	t(3;21)(q26;q22) is the translocation of material between the long arms of chromosomes 3 and 21 with break points at band q26 for chromosome 3 and band q22 for chromosome 21
ins	Insertion of extra material [e.g., portions of a chromosome] within a chromosome	ins(3;3)(q26; q21q26) is the insertion of band 26 to a position between bands 21 and 26 in the long arms of chromosome 3 [for different chromosomes being involved, the conventions for t are followed]
inv	Inversion [or turn in the opposite direction] of a portion of the chromosome	inv(3)(q21q26) is inversion of bands of 21 through 26 on the long arm of chromosome 3
+ or −	Before a chromosome: Addition [+] or loss [−] of a whole chromosome	+8 or −7 is an extra chromosome 8 or a missing chromosome 7 [see del]
+ or −	After an arm: Additional material [+] or loss of material [−] in the designated arm of the specified chromosome	7q− is missing material in the long arm of chromosome 7 [see del]
del	Deletion of all or part of a chromosome	del (7q) or del (7)(q22) is deletion of the long arm or of band 22 in the long arm of chromosome 7, respectively [see "+ or −"]
der	Derivative chromosome: an abnormal chromosome resulting from structural rearrangement, generally of a balanced nature, involving 2 or more chromosomes	der(1;7)(q10;p10) [see t, ins, inv]
i	Isochromosome: a symmetric chromosome composed of duplicated long or short arm with associated centromere	i(17q) is chromosome 17 with duplicated long arms
idic	Isocentric: symmetrical abnormal chromosome composed of the duplication of a total arm and its centromere with part of the adjacent other arm	idic(X)(q13)
dic	Dicentric: a chromosome with 2 centromeres	

*All examples presented have been observed in myelodysplastic syndromes.

C-4. Leukocyte differentiation antigens

CD[a]	Cellular distribution[b]	Related functions or proteins [Name]
CD1	Thy, LC, DCI, B sub	MHC-I-like protein; associated with β2-microglobulin
CD2	T, T•, NK	Leuc function antigen receptor
CD3	T prec (cytoplasmic), T (surface)	T-complement receptor
CD4	T sub, Mo	HIV-receptor; MHC-II receptor
CD5	T, B sub	
CD6	T sub, B sub	
CD7	T prec, T sub, NK	Fcµ receptor
CD8	T sub, NK	MHC-I receptor
CD9	B prec, B sub, Mo, Plt	
CD10	B prec, B sub, PMN	CALLA
CD11	Leuc, PMN, Mo, NK, HCL	Leuc function antigen; complement receptor
CDw12	PMN, Mo, Plt	
CD13	PMN, Mo	
CD14	Mo, (PMN), LC	
CD15	PMN, (Mo), Reed-Sternberg cells	[Sialyl Lewis^x]
CD16	NK, PMN, Mp	Fcγ receptor [FcRIII]
CDw17	PMN, Mo, Plt	
CD18	Leuc	CD11
CD19	B, B prec	
CD20	B, B prec sub	[B1]
CD21	DCF, B sub	Complement receptor; EBV receptor
CD22	B, B prec	Myelin-associated protein
CD23	B•, Mo•, Eos	Fcε receptor
CD24	B, PMN	
CD25	T•, B•, Mo•	IL2 receptor
CD26	T•	

C-4. (continued)

CD[a]	Cellular distribution[b]	Related functions or proteins [Name]
CD27	T *sub*	
CD28	T *sub*, B•, PC	Cdw49
CD29	Leuc	
CD30	T•, B•, Reed-Sternberg cells	Ki-1 or Ber-H2 antigen
CD31	Plt, Mo, PMN, B, (T)	Plt glycoprotein-IIa
CD32	Mo, PMN, B, Eos, Bas, Plt	Fcγ receptor [FcRII]
CD33	My *prec*	
CD34	HC progenitors	
CD35	PMN, Mo, B, NK *sub*, RBC	Complement receptor
CD36	Plt, Mo, (B)	Plt glycoprotein-IV and IIIb
CD37	B, (T), (Mo)	
CD38	NK, T•, PC, Lymphoid progenitors	
CD39	B *sub*, (Mo)	
CD40	B, (Mo), carcinomas	
CD41	Plt	Plt glycoprotein-IIb/IIIa complex; glycoprotein-IIb
CD42	Plt	Plt glycoprotein complexes, plt adhesion [GP . . .]
CD43	PMN, Mo, T, NK, brain	Leukosialin
CD44	Leuc, RBC, Plt	Lymphocyte homing receptor [H-CAM, Pgp-1]
CD45	T *sub*, B, PMN, Mo	Leucocyte common antigen
CD46	Leuc	Membrane cofactor protein
CD47	Leuc	
CD48	Leuc	
CDw49	Plt, T•, T	Plt glycoprotein, collagen receptor [α-integrin chain, VLA]
CDw50	Leuc	[ICAM-3]

C-4. (continued)

CD[a]	Cellular distribution[b]	Related functions or proteins [Name]
CD51	Plt	Vitronectin receptor
CD52	Leuc	[Campath-1]
CD53	Leuc	
CD54	Broad; Endo	Leuc function antigen ligand
CD55	All HC	Decay accelerating factor
CD56	NK, T•	[NCAM]
CD57	NK sub, T sub, brain, carcinomas	
CD58	Most cells	Leuc function antigen; CD2 ligand
CD59	Most cells	
CDw60	Plt, T sub	
CD61	Plt	Plt glycoprotein-IIIa; CD41, CD51
CD62	Plt•	[Selectin]
CD63	Plt•, Mo, (PMN,T,B)	Plt activation antigen
CD64	Mo, PMN•	Fcγ receptor
CDw65	PMN, Mo sub	
CD66	PMN	Carcinoembryonic antigen (CEA)
CD67	PMN	
CD68	Mp	
CH69	B•, T•, Mo•, NK•	Activation inducer molecule
CD70	B•, T•, Reed-Sternberg cells	[CD27-ligand]
CD71	B•, T•, M, RBC prec	Transferrin receptor
CD72	B	
CD73	B sub, T sub	
CD74	B, Mo	MHC-II invariant chain
CD75	B sub, (T sub)	
CD76	B sub, T sub	Neuramidase sensitive epitope
CD77	B•, follicular center B	

C-4. (continued)

CD[a]	Cellular distribution[b]	Related functions or proteins [Name]
CDw78	B, (Mo)	
CD79	B, (PC); ZM	Igα-receptor/Igβ-receptor complex [MBI, B29]
CD80	B sub, T sub; Mp sub, DC, HD	CD28; upregulated by EBV; on HTLV-1 transfused T [B7]
CD81	B, PC, T, Mo sub, Endo, Epi	B cell adhesion [TAPA-1]
CD82	Broad (neg on RBC), Endo, Epi	Signal transduction [R2, 4F9, IA4]
CD83	DCC, DCI (neg on DCF); LC, ZG	Marker for DCC [HB15]
CDw84	B, T sub, Mo, Plt	Expressed from pre-B to pre-PC (neg on PC) [2G7]
CD85	PC, B, Mo	Marker for PC, expressed on HCL [VMP55]
CD86	B•, blasts, Mo, ZG	Activation marker for B [FUN-1]
CD87	PMN, Mo, Eos, Endo tumor cells	Binds urokinase plasminogen activator [UPA-R]
CD88	PMN, Mo, Mp, Eos, mast cells, smooth muscle	Receptor for C5a; cell activation, chemotaxis [C5aR]
CD89	PMN, Mp, T/B sub, Eos	IgA receptor, PMN respiratory burst [FcαR]
CDw90	Stromal cells; 5–25% CD34+ cells	Thy-1/CD34+ progenitors [Thy-1]
CD91	Mo, Mp, ExHC	Differentiation of Mo, Mp [α2M-R]
CDw92	PMN, Mo, Plt, Endo	[VIM15]
CD93	My, PMN, Mo, Endo	[VIMD2]
CD94	NK; sub of γ/δ γ/β T cells	Regulates cytolytic activity and adhesion [Kp43]
CD95	My/T lymphoblastoid cell lines	Apoptosis [APO-1, FAS]
CD96	> 60% of T-ALL (neg on most T-lymphomas)	T activation? <10% of resting hematolymphoid cells [TACTILE]
CD97	T sub, NK sub, Eos	[BL-KDD/F12]
CD98	T•, NK•, Thy; heart, skin (neg on B, PMN)	Regulation of calcium fluxes in heart and skeletal muscles [4F2, 2F3]
CD99	T and B dependent areas of lymph nodes, ZG	Adhesion [E2, MIC2]
CD100	Broad; T (neg on B, CD34+, Endo, My)	Amplifies CD-2 induced PBL proliferation [BD16, BB18]

C-4. (continued)

CD[a]	Cellular distribution[b]	Related functions or proteins [Name]
CDw101	PMN, Mo, CD4 *sub*, CD8 *sub*	CD28 [BA27, BB27]
CD102	Leuc, Plt, Endo	Ligand for CD11a/CD18 [ICAM-2]
CD103	T memory *sub*; 2–6% of PBL	T adhesion and interaction with Epi; HCL marker [HML-1]
CD104	Epi; Endo keratinocytes; Thy, B	Cytoskeleton anchorage [β4-integrin chain]
CD105	Endo Mo•, RBC *prec*, CD34+ *sub*	Transforming growth factor receptor, adhesion [Endoglin]
CD106	Endo Mo, bone marrow stromal cells, DCF	[VCAM-1, INCAM-110]
CD107	Plt	Lysosomal associated membrane protein [LAMP]
CDw108	T•, spleen•, some stromal cells, HD	Cell activation [MEM]
CDw109	T•, Plt•, Endo	Activation, proliferation, signaling [7D-1, 8A3]
CD115	Mo, Mp; committed bone marrow progenitors	c-fms gene product growth, signaling, adhesions [CSF-1R]
CDw116	My, PMN, Eos, Mo, Mp; ExHC, marrow progenitors; AML	Stimulation of PMN, Eos, MP; stem cell growth [GM-CSF-R]
CD117	Mast cells; melanocytes, LC; CD34+ *sub;* Endo ExHC; AML	c-kit gene product; binds Stem Cell Factor [SCF-R c-kit]
CDw119	Broad; T, B, Mo, ZM, Epi, Endo	Mo•, B differentiation; MHC I & II expression [γ-IFN-R]
CD120	Broad; ZG ExHC	[TNF-R]
CDw121	Broad; T, B, Mo, fibroblasts; Endo HC, ExHC	IL-1 receptor on fibroblasts, T activation [IL-1R]
CD122	T, B, NK; AML, ALL, HD	CD25; activation of B, T, Mo [IL-2R]
CDw124	HC, ExHC, fibroblasts, Epi	Growth factor receptor on T, B, Mo• [IL-4R]
CD126	T, Epi, myeloma, bacteria	Growth factor receptor for HC and myeloma cells; associated with gp130 [IL-6R]
CDw127	My, Lymphoid cells	Proliferation of Pro-B, pre-B, T [IL-7R]
CDw128	PMN, Eos, B, Mo, melanoma, keratinocytes	Activation and chemotaxis of PMN and Eos [IL-8R]

C-4. (continued)

CD[a]	Cellular distribution[b]	Related functions or proteins *[Name]*
CD130	Broad, HC, ExHC	Signal transducer; associated with receptors for IL6, IL11, leukemia inhibitory factor, and oncostatin-M *[gp130]*

[a]The antibody *clusters of differentiation (CD)* are designated at international workshops. Many CD designations also have subtypes (e.g., a, b, . . .). More than 1400 antibodies have been analyzed by the workshops. The related functions and proteins represented are highly selected and very incomplete.
[b]● = activated form of cell, *neg* = negative, *prec* = precursor, *sub* = subset.
Key: ALL = actute lymphoblastic leukemia; AML = acute myelogenous leukemia; B = B cells; Bas = basophils; DC = dendritic cells; DCC = circulating DC; DCF = follicular DC; DCI = interdigitating DC; EBV = Epstein-Barr virus; Endo = endothelial cells; Eos = eosinophils; Epi = epithelial cells; ExHC = extra HC; HC = hemopoietic cells; HCL = hairy cell leukemia; HD = Hodgkin's disease; HIV = human immunodeficiency; IL = interleukin; Leuc = leucocytes; LC = Langerhans cells; MHC = major histocompatibility complex class; Mo = monocytes; Mp = macrophages; My = myeloid cells; NK = natural killer cells; PBL = peripheral blood lymphocytes; PC = plasma cells; Plt = platelets; PMN = neutrophils; RBC = erythrocytes; T = T cells; Thy = thymocytes; ZM = mantle zone of lymph node; ZG = germinal center of lymph node.
Source: Adapted from Pinto, A., et al. New molecules burst at the leukocyte surface. A comprehensive review based on the 5th International Workshop on Leukocyte Differentiation Antigens (Boston, USA, 3–7 November 1993) *Leukemia* 8:347–358, 1994.

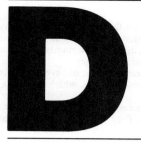

Carcinogenic Viruses and Oncogenes: A Primer

I. A glossary of basic jargon

Jargon is the use of pseudo-words (like the word "pseudo-words") plucked from a "word-salad" and used either to make the simple appear arcane, to disguise one's ignorance of a subject, or to have secret codes which can be used to gain entry into a boys club.

— B.B.L.

A. Molecular biology terminology

Amplification—the production of many copies of a gene. This process can occur normally in certain phases of development, but is also seen when a gene, such as *c-myc*, loses its transcriptional controls.

Antisense nucleotides—a DNA or RNA sequence that is complementary to the protein coding sequence of a gene or mRNA. Antisense nucleotides can adhere to a specific coding sequence of DNA or RNA and potentially block transcription or translation. Antisense sequences are also used as molecular probes.

Apoptosis—"programmed cell death," such as is seen in normal tissue reabsorption during development (e.g., tadpole tails). Apoptotic cells show clumps of intracellular organelles in the absence of associated inflammation or necrosis and are phagocytosed. Apoptosis may be the mechanism by which tumor cell populations are decreased by hormones, cytotoxic chemotherapy, and radiation therapy. Apoptosis is genetically regulated. For example, the p53 tumor suppressor oncogene stimulates apoptosis, but the *BCL*-2 oncogene inhibits apoptosis, decreases normal cell death, and increases cell populations.

Breakpoint cluster regions (BCRs)—regions in the genome where chromosome translocations are likely to occur, which are often situated close to a protooncogene. In chronic myelogenous leukemia (CML), a part of a BCR on chromosome 22 near the *sis* oncogene is exchanged with a portion of chromosome 9, which contains the *abl* gene, to form the Philadelphia chromosome. The normal *c-abl* protein is a membrane tyrosine kinase. Infection with retroviruses containing the new *abl-bcr* fusion gene from chromosome 22 can cause CML in mice.

CDs—"cluster of differentiation" antigens, which appear on leukocyte surface membranes and change as various leukocyte lines differentiate. The type of leukocyte and the stage of differentiation can be determined using monoclonal antibody assays of these CDs. CDs on malignant leukocytes are useful for diagnosis and prognosis of leukocyte malignancies. See Appendix **C-4.**

Codon—an ordered set of three nucleotides that code for an amino acid or termination code during RNA translation.

Complementary RNA and DNA—RNA or DNA sequences whose codon sequences are mirror images of each other. Complementary sequences adhere to each other. A known RNA or DNA can be used as a molecular probe to look for its complement. The degree of adherence is a measure of how closely the complementary nucleotides mirror each other.

Chromosome rearrangements (see Appendix C-3 for nomenclature)—various inversions, translocations, and additions that can alter the environment of growth-controlling genes and lead to malignancy. A number of these rearrangements are specific for a given type of malignancy.

Cyclins—proteins that trigger the entry of cells into the cell cycle by activating the transcription of *c-myc* and *c-mos* oncogene proteins, which stimulate DNA synthesis.

Double minutes (DMs)—small extrachromosomal globs of DNA without a centromere that are seen under the microscope. They often indicate abnormal gene amplification in transformed cells.

DNA—deoxyribonucleic acid.

DNA polymerases—a group of enzymes that joins deoxynucleotides aligned along a complementary DNA sequence. Some of these polymerases are used for DNA replication and others for repair.

Exons—Sequences in a gene that code for polypeptides.

Gene—a DNA sequence that codes for a single type of polypeptide. Normal cell genes contain subsequences ("introns") scattered through the main sequence that are not used for making polypeptides.

Heterogeneous nuclear RNA sequences—a mixture of nuclear RNA sequences of different sizes. Most of this RNA consists of primary RNA transcripts in the process of rapidly losing their introns to form mRNA.

Homologous sequences—segments of different RNA or DNA nucleotides with the same or complementary nucleotide sequences.

Hybridoma—a hybrid cell that makes a specific monoclonal antibody. The hybrid cells are made from normal mouse lymphocytes that produce antibodies and immortalized mouse plasmacytoma cells that do not make antibodies. The lymphocytes are taken from the spleens of mice exposed to foreign antigens such as human leukocytes. Each splenic lymphocyte makes an antibody to one foreign antigen. These lymphocytes do not replicate, but can survive in a toxic medium (HAT medium). In contrast, the plasmacytoma cells can reproduce but cannot survive in HAT medium. The hybrid cells produce specific antibodies, can reproduce, and can survive in HAT medium, which destroys unhybridized plasmacytoma cells. After the hybrid cells are separated, they are allowed to reproduce several times. This procedure allows the isolation and expansion of clones of cells that produce antibodies to a specific antigen.

Insertional mutagenesis—transformation of a cell by a sequence of viral or cellular DNA, which is inserted into the normal host genome. Inserted sequences that cause transformation may be promoters that deregulate normal genes, or may be cellular proto-oncogenes or viral pro-oncogenes that produce growth control substances. The inserted DNA can also disrupt or combine with normal gene sequences, which then produce abnormal polypeptides. LTRs (see retrovirus terminology) are powerful promoters and can cause abnormal activation of nearby control genes that control normal growth.

Introns—noncoding gene sequences. After a gene is transcribed into RNA, the corresponding RNA intron folds back on itself to form loops, or "lariats," that are removed, degraded, and not used for translation of mRNA into protein. Introns appear to regulate transcription and shuffle nucleotide sequences around to produce new proteins and genetic diversity. Introns are present in normal cells but are absent in oncogenic retroviruses.

Kinases—enzymes that regulate a variety of proteins and nucleotides by phosphorylation.

Messenger RNA (mRNA)—RNA with all introns removed and ready to be translated into protein.

Mis-sense sequences—DNA sequences with sections of abnormal codons, whose protein products function abnormally or not at all.

Monoclonal antibody—an antibody made by hybridoma cell cultures that is highly specific for a specific cell surface antigen.

Nucleosides—a purine or pyrimidine base combined with a sugar (i.e., ribose or deoxyribose for RNA or DNA).

Nucleotides—a nucleoside joined with a phosphate group.

Oncogene—a gene that can cause cells to manifest a malignant phenotype.

Polymerase chain reaction (PCR)—a technique for expanding the amount of very small sequences of DNA.

Promoter—a sequence of DNA near a particular gene that initiates the transcription of that gene.

Proto-oncogenes—normal cell genes that are homologous to viral oncogenes (*v-onc*) or cellular oncogenes (*c-onc*) and which typically code for proteins that are essential for control of proliferation and differentiation. Their names are written in italics and begin with a c-plus a three letter symbol for the particular gene (e.g., *c-mos*).

RNA—ribonucleic acid.

Signal transduction—the mechanism by which extracellular molecules affect intracellular chemistry and biology. Signal transduction is essential for growth and differentiation in multicellular organisms.

Transcription—the production of a complementary (mirror image) RNA sequence from a DNA template.

Transcription factors—specific proteins that bind to control elements of genes. Families of transcription factors include helix-loop-helix proteins, helix-turn-helix proteins and leucine zipper proteins.

Transfection—The introduction of DNA sequences from one cell into the genome of another. Several cellular oncogenes (*c-onc*) were discovered by transfecting normal cells with DNA taken from cancer cells. After several generations of transformed daughter cells, all of the transfected DNA is lost except the *c-onc*.

Translation—the production of proteins by ribosomes from mRNA in the cell cytoplasm.

B. Retrovirus terminology

Capsid—proteins that form the protein core of the virus and are coded by the viral *gag* gene.

Envelope—the outer lipid and protein bilayer of the virus that is formed from the cell membrane of the previously infected cell plus the proteins coded by the viral *env* gene. For a specific type of cell to be infected, it must have a specific membrane receptor that "recognizes" the envelope of a particular retrovirus. For example, CD4 ("helper T4") cells have specific receptor sites for HIV capsid antigens.

Long-terminal repeats (LTRs)—DNA transcripts of the ends of a provirus that help the virus to become incorporated into cell chromosome DNA. LTRs signal the start and stop points for transcription of proviral RNA.

Provirus—the double-stranded DNA copy of a retroviral RNA.

Replication competent retroviruses—retroviruses with the full complement of sequences necessary for reproduction.

Replication deficient viruses—retroviruses that have lost some of the normal coding for proteins necessary for viral replication. These retroviruses typically have a *v-onc* and rapidly transform cells in animal tissues and in culture into malignant phenotypes.

Reverse transcriptase—a DNA polymerase that is part of the retroviral core and uses the viral RNA template to make a double strand of complementary DNA. This enzyme is coded by the viral *pol* gene.

Short-terminal repeats—located at both ends of the entire viral RNA sequence. These are reverse transcribed after viral infection into DNA LTR.

Viral oncogenes (v-onc)—transforming genes with close homology to normal cell genes.

Viral RNA—two identical strands are present in each virus and consist of several coding sequences. The special sequences *pol, gag,* and *env* are unique to certain retroviruses that regulate viral gene expression and reproduction. Examples of unique genes include the TAX gene of HTLV I and the TAT gene of HIV. See **II.A.3.a.** and **II.A.3.c.** of this appendix.

II. Carcinogenic viruses

Several different types of virus cause cancer to develop in animals and transform cells in tissue culture. Viral infection contributes to the development of a few human tumors, but cell gene mutations, host immune deficiency or stimulation, and other viral infections are required before cells actually become malignant.

A. RNA retroviruses cause cancers in animals and cause malignant transformation of human and animal cells in culture. As a rule, retroviruses do not kill the host cell but allow it to survive. Studies of these viruses have been essential in understanding growth control in normal and malignant human cells.

1. **Molecular biology of retroviral infections**
   a. After infecting the cell, all retroviruses are reverse-transcribed into provirus DNA, which is incorporated randomly into the host genome (DNA).
   b. Replication competent provirus DNA is transcribed into RNA, which is subsequently translated into viral proteins. The RNA and some viral proteins form new retroviruses that leave the cell, take some of the membrane along as their envelope, and then infect other cells.
   c. Some retroviruses, such as human T cell lymphotropic virus type 1 (HTLV-1), transform cells by being inserted next to normal cellular oncogenes. These *c-onc* become abnormally activated. Such retroviruses do not have oncogenes themselves, and malignant transformation is a slow process.
   d. Viral DNA can also combine with DNA of a normal cell gene and make new retroviruses that contain RNA copies of a normal host gene. If the normal host gene is a cellular oncogene (proto-oncogene or *c-onc*), the new virus can insert the oncogene into ectopic locations in the cell genome of newly infected cells and cause malignant transformation. Some of these viruses lose their own genes when they combine with host DNA and become replication deficient.

2. **Nomenclature of retroviral oncogenes** is usually based on the name of the animal tumor from which the retrovirus is extracted. Examples include *src*—Rous sarcoma virus of chickens (the first oncovirus discovered); *sis*—simian sarcoma virus; *erb*—erythroblastosis virus of chickens; *H-ras*—Harvey rat sarcoma virus; *K-ras*—Kirsten rat sarcoma virus; *myc*—myelocytoma; *ras*—rat sarcoma.

3. **Retroviruses and human cancer**
   a. **Human T cell lymphotropic virus type 1 (HTLV-1)** causes lymphoblastic leukemia in southern Japan and other countries. It is the only virus to date that has been clearly shown to cause a human cancer. HTLV-1 is a replication competent virus that does not possess an oncogene. Part of its transforming activity occurs by insertional mutagenesis. It also codes for the TAX protein, which induces infected lymphocytes to produce interleukin-2 receptor proteins. Interleukin-2 attaches to these receptors and stimulates infected cells to proliferate. Other unclear events are necessary, however, for leukemia to develop, and only a very small percentage of infected persons develop leukemia.
   b. **HTLV-2** may be causal for a small percentage of hairy cell leukemias and a variety of T cell lymphoproliferative disorders.
   c. **HTLV-3** (human immunodeficiency virus [HIV]) is associated with aggressive B lymphocyte malignancies in patients with AIDS. It also produces the TAT protein, which stimulates proliferation of Kaposi's sarcoma cells. These cells are not infected by the virus.

B. DNA viruses may become incorporated into the cell genome, but this step is not always necessary. Oncogenic DNA viral genes code for proteins that affect growth regulating substances in the cell.

1. **Mechanisms of DNA oncogenesis** include:
   a. Interference with cellular inhibitors of growth, resulting in uncontrolled cell replication (e.g., the retinoblastoma gene product).
   b. Activation of cellular DNA and RNA synthesis by viral protein products.
   c. Insertional mutagenesis; viral DNA is inserted into the host genome and disrupts normal growth control.

   d. Gene translocation and rearrangement.
2. **DNA viruses shown to have an oncogenic role in human malignancies** include:
   a. **Human papilloma virus (HPV)** DNA sequences are found in over 80 percent of human uterine cervical cancer cells. HPV appears to be necessary but not sufficient for the development of most cervical cancers. See Chap. 36, sec. **V.D.2** and Chap. 11, *Cancer of the Uterine Cervix*, sec. **I.C.**
   b. **Epstein-Barr virus (EBV)** infects more than 90 percent of individuals in the first two decades of life, but generally causes no illness. EBV infects B lymphocytes and nasopharyngeal epithelium, both of which have a specific surface receptor for the virus. When EBV-infected cells are exposed to other proliferative stimuli, such as malaria, malignancy can result. EBV is a cofactor for the development of nasopharyngeal carcinoma in Asia, epidemic Burkitt's lymphoma, B-cell lymphomas in immunocompromised patients, cutaneous T-cell lymphoma (with HTLV-1), and gastric carcinoma. See Chap. 35, sec. **IV.A.3.**
   c. **Hepatitis B** viral DNA sequences are found in the genomes of essentially all hepatocellular carcinomas. These sequences are translated into proteins that stimulate transcription. They also may cause cell transformation by insertional mutagenesis, which disrupts growth regulating genes.
   d. **Adenoviruses and polyoma viruses** cause transformation of cells in cell culture but have not yet been shown to cause or contribute to human malignancy.
   e. **Human parvovirus oncosuppressive activity** is discussed in Chap. 35, sec. **IV.E.1.**
III. Oncogenes. Oncogenes are genes that cause malignant transformation of normal cells. They are consistently associated with malignancy and may be of either cellular or retroviral origin. In general, more than one oncogene is abnormally active in cancer. The multiple interactions among oncogenes that are necessary for cell division typically result in activation of many otherwise normal oncogenes. A one-to-one correspondence between most cancers and a single oncogene abnormality generally cannot be determined.
   A. Definitions and description
   1. **Retroviral oncogenes *(v-onc)*** were first discovered in rapidly transforming retroviruses extracted from animal tumors. Approximately 20 oncogenes of this type have been described.
   2. **Cellular oncogenes** were discovered by extracting DNA from cancer cells and inserting it into normal cells, which then become malignant (DNA transfection). More than 20 oncogenes of this type have been described.
   3. **Inhibitory genes** produce proteins that inhibit cell proliferation. Abnormalities in these genes can lead to abnormal proliferation of cells. About 12 such genes have been described.
   4. **Proto-oncogenes** (*c-onc* or normal cell genes) control proliferation and differentiation in normal cells and appear to be the source of all oncogenes. RNA from transforming retroviruses is homologous with various proto-oncogenes, which is evidence for this conclusion.
      a. **Proto-oncogenes are highly conserved through evolution.** Many of the same oncogenes are found in life forms as diverse as humans and yeast. They appear to be essential to life.
      b. **Each proto-oncogene makes protein products that are differentially expressed** during the cell cycle or at specific stages of development of a particular tissue.
   5. **Differences between *c-onc* and proviral *v-onc***
      a. Cellular oncogenes have both introns and exons, and viral oncogenes have only exons.
      b. Proviral DNA possesses LTRs, which are powerful promoter genes not found in *c-onc*. When LTRs are inserted near a *c-onc*, they can deregulate it and transform the cell into a malignant phenotype.

B. Steps of signal transduction: A model for understanding oncogene biology

Step 1: Growth factors of both proto-oncogene and non–proto-oncogene origin combine with specific growth factor receptors (GFRs) on target cells, activating tyrosine kinase activity on the GFR (see step 2). The growth factor-GFR complex itself is taken up by the cell and deactivated. Some growth factors and their associated proto-oncogenes are fibroblast growth factors (*Int-2* and others) and platelet-derived growth factors (*sis*).

Example: *sis* oncogene

    a. Normal function. The *sis* oncogene codes for one of the chains of platelet-derived growth factor (PDGF). PDGF is manufactured in megakaryocytes and packaged in platelets. When platelets become activated, they release PDGF, which stimulates its surface receptor to produce tyrosine kinase activity and stimulates the proliferation of fibroblasts.

    b. Abnormalities in cancer cells involve unregulated production due to ectopic location of gene, possible amplification, and truncated protein.

    c. Associated human cancers include some squamous cancers, glioblastomas, acute myelogenous leukemia (AML), and osteosarcomas. The *sis* oncogene is possibly activated by HTLV-1.

    d. Effect of abnormalities on prognosis. None are known.

Step 2. Growth factor receptors (GFRs) and some hormone receptors are proto-oncogene proteins that traverse the cell membrane. The cell surface part of the protein has sites for specific extracellular growth factors. When GFRs are activated by their growth factors, their cytoplasmic sites become active tyrosine kinases. Some GFRs and their proto-oncogenes are colony-stimulating factor receptor-1 (*fms*) and epidermal growth factor receptor (*erb*-B).

The activated tyrosine kinases transduce the extracellular signal to cytoplasmic proteins and to the nucleus by a variety of mechanisms. For example, they activate cytoplasmic proto-oncogene proteins. They also increase the levels of diacylglycerol, which then activate protein kinase C (PKC); PKC activates a number of proteins that stimulate DNA synthesis. They also phosphorylate guanosine 5'-diphosphate (GDP) to make the triphosphate (GTP), which activates p21 (a *c-ras* protein); the GTP-p21 complex stimulates DNA transcription in the nucleus.

Example: *erb*-B oncogene (Others: *fms, ros, sea*)

    a. Normal function. The proto-oncogene counterpart of *erb*-B produces cell surface receptors for EGF and has tyrosine kinase activity when activated by EGF.

    b. Abnormalities in cancer cells. The *erb*-B gene product produces a truncated product with unregulated protein kinase activity. It delivers a constant proliferative signal to the cell.

    c. Associated human cancers are squamous cancers and glioblastomas.

    d. Effect of abnormalities on prognosis. Survival is poor with increased expression of *erb*-B for patients with breast cancer, upper respiratory tumors, and uterine cervix cancer.

Step 3. Cytoplasmic kinases that modulate the activity of key cellular enzymes are activated by membrane receptor kinases. These proteins typically have serine or threonine kinase phosphorylating activity and some have GTPase activity. These kinases have an extensive variety of effects in activating nuclear proteins and in direct activation of DNA promoter regions. For example, the cell division cycle kinase (*cdc*) is found in all eukaryotic cells and is essential to the transition of cells from the G_2 phase to the M phase. Its activity is regulated by cyclin proteins and phosphorylation and it appears to act by destabilizing the cytoskeleton in preparation for mitosis.

Example: *ras* oncogene (Others: *raf, mos, src, yes, fps, abl, crk, cdc*)

    a. Normal function. Proto-oncogene precursors of *c-ras* proteins transduce signals from the cell surface to the nucleus. The proteins combine with GDP and GTP. The protein-GTP complex (e.g., p21-GTP) is the chemically active form, which then activates a variety of nuclear promoter proteins. The protein has GTP-ase activity that is enhanced by a cytoplasmic protein called GAP. The GTP-ase converts its own bound GTP to GDP, inactivating the complex; this phenomenon is thought to be a self-regulatory activity of the protein. The *ras* protein also increases levels of diacetylglycerol, which activates PKC, an important initiator of DNA transcription (see step 4).

   b. Abnormality in cancer cells. The *ras* oncogenes are a group of five related oncogenes with most of the activities of their normal proto-oncogene counterparts. Several defects, including defective GTPase, have been found. This abnormality leads to a constant presence of the GTP form of the molecule, which continuously activates nuclear proteins and DNA transcription.

   c. Associated human cancers. These include AML, some melanomas, neuroblastomas, breast cancers, bladder cancers, and lung cancers.

   d. Effect of abnormalities on prognosis. The prognosis is poor for AML.

Step 4. Proteins directly controlling gene expression ("transcription factors") are involved in the final step of signal transduction. Some of these factors are short-lived and never leave the nucleus. For example, *c-jun* and *c-fos* proteins are among the first proteins transcribed at the G_0-S interface and appear to initiate the cell cycle. Cyclins appear to trigger the cell's entry into the cell cycle and into mitosis by activating the transcription of *c-myc* and *c-mos*. Proteins from *c-myc* and *c-mos* also reside in the nucleus and form complexes that stimulate DNA synthesis. Other factors enter from the cytoplasm (e.g., *ras*, *myc*); these are transcribed and activated by cytoplasmic kinases (see step 3). Several normal products of proto-oncogene kinases in the cytoplasm also activate gene transcription, particularly PKC, which acts directly as a DNA promoter and stimulates the production of *c-jun* and *c-fos* proteins; this *jun/fos* complex binds to specific promoter regions of DNA and stimulates DNA transcription.

Example: *c-myc* oncogene (Others: *jun, fos, erb-A, rel, ski, myb*)

   a. Normal function. The *c-myc* are a family of proteins with direct nuclear regulatory activity. The presence of active *myc* appears necessary for cell division. Dimethylsulfoxide inhibits *myc* transcription, stops cell division, and can cause differentiation of leukemic blast cells in culture. High levels of *c-myc* are found in immature blood cells and gastrointestinal cells. Both *c-myc* and the *c-jun/c-fos* protein products form dimers connected at a leucine-rich region called the "leucine zipper" near the site of attachment to promoter genes.

   b. Abnormalities in cancer cells. Amplification of the *myc* gene can be so prolific that the multiple copies sometimes cannot remain on a chromosome. Extrachromosomal "double minutes" often microscopically give visible evidence of such amplification, with high quantities of active gene product being formed.

   c. Associated human cancers include Burkitt's lymphoma, B-cell lymphomas, promyelocytic leukemia, neuroblastoma, small cell lung cancer, and colon cancer.

   d. Effect of abnormalities on prognosis. In neuroblastoma the prognosis is poorer in direct proportion to levels of N-*myc* (N = neuroblastoma) for this member of the *myc* gene family.

Step 5. Growth inhibitor genes produce substances, typically phosphatases, which normally inactivate growth-promoting oncogene products and inhibit cell proliferation. Mutations that make these genes nonfunctional lead to uncontrolled cell proliferation and malignancy. Examples of these mutations and their associated tumors include RB1 (retinoblastoma and some osteosarcomas), WT1 (Wilms' tumor), NF1 (neurofibromatosis), MEN1 (multiple endocrine neoplasia), and FAP1 (familial adenomatous polyposis of the colon).

Index